AN ADVANCED LIFESPAN ODYSSEY *for* COUNSELING PROFESSIONALS

1e

Bradley T. Erford

Loyola University Maryland

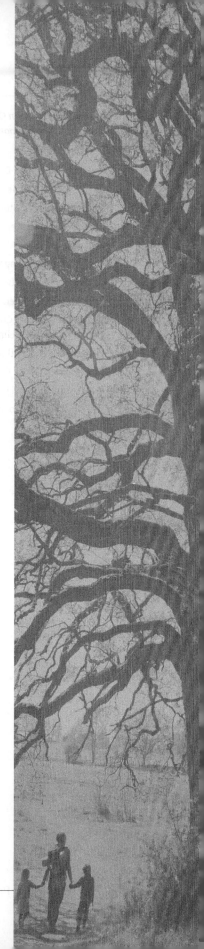

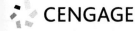 **CENGAGE**

Australia • Brazil • Canada • Mexico • Singapore • United Kingdom • United States

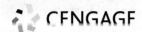

An Advanced Lifespan Odyssey for Counseling Professionals
Bradley T. Erford

Product Director: Jon-David Hague

Product Manager: Julie Martinez

Content Developer: Stefanie Chase

Product Assistant: Stephen Lagos

Marketing Manager: Margaux Cameron

Content Project Manager: Rita Jaramillo

Art Director: Vernon Boes

Manufacturing Planner: Judy Inouye

Production Service & Compositor: Jitendra Kumar, MPS Limited

Text Researcher: Kavitha Balasundaram

Text Designer: Cheryl Carrington

Cover Designer: Caryl Gorska

Cover Image: Getty/Johner Images

For product information and technology assistance, contact us at **Cengage Customer & Sales Support, 1-800-354-9706.**

For permission to use material from this text or product, submit all requests online at **www.cengage.com/permissions**. Further permissions questions can be e-mailed to **permissionrequest@cengage.com**.

Library of Congress Control Number: 2015932615

Student Edition:

ISBN: 978-1-285-08358-2

Loose-leaf Edition:

ISBN: 978-1-305-85756-8

Cengage
200 Pier 4 Boulevard
Boston, MA 02210
USA

Cengage is a leading provider of customized learning solutions with employees residing in nearly 40 different countries and sales in more than 125 countries around the world. Find your local representative at **www.cengage.com**.

To learn more about Cengage platforms and services, register or access your online learning solution, or purchase materials for your course, visit **www.cengage.com**.

Printed in Mexico
Print Number: 03   Print Year: 2021

This effort is dedicated to The One:

the Giver of energy, passion, and understanding;

Who makes life worth living and endeavors

worth pursuing and accomplishing;

the Teacher of love and forgiveness.

Brief Contents

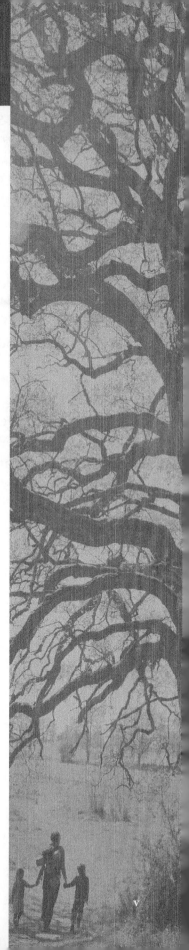

Contents

CHAPTER 16

Middle Adulthood: Social/Emotional, Family,
Career, and Spiritual Development   367
By Robin Lee, Jennifer Jordan, Michelle Stevens, and Andrew Jones

CHAPTER 17

Later Adulthood and Old Age: Physical
and Cognitive Development   389
*By Cecile Yancu, Debbie Newsome, Joseph Wilkerson,
and Shannon Mathews*

Preface

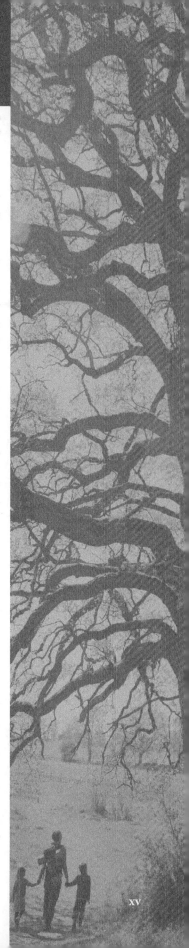

Welcome to the lifespan odyssey! This text was designed to align with CACREP standards for counselor training programs. The background education and experiences of counselors in training are quite diverse: many have undergraduate degrees in psychology, education, or human services, while others have undergraduate degrees in business, the humanities, or some other discipline. Thus, some start with a basic understanding of human development and perhaps an undergraduate course on the topic, while others have no previous exposure to the content domain. The alignment with CACREP standards helps all counselors-in-training to master the core knowledge of lifespan development, but more importantly to apply this knowledge to helping people resolve difficulties they may encounter on their lifespan odysseys. These issues might include the implications of substance abuse for development, behavioral or emotional issues associated with trauma or an unstable environment, interventions that have been shown to be effective when working with clients along the spectrum of developmental problems, and the normal and abnormal human developmental processes that counselors must master and apply during clinical experiences—and when they take their rightful place as counseling professionals!

This text covers human development from womb to tomb across all developmental areas (e.g., physical, cognitive, language, social, emotional, career), and reflects the trend toward empirically supported practice in the application of lifespan theories. Each life stage from infancy/toddlerhood (Chapters 5–6) to later adulthood (Chapters 17–18) is subdivided into the following sections: physical development (A), cognitive development (B), social/emotional development (C), and social/career development (D), as applicable. With an engaging writing style, a multitude of real-life examples make the content concrete, understandable, and applicable to counselor training. Each chapter includes case studies, reflections, and discussions of current issues, all while focusing on cross-cultural variations. Descriptions of more than 30 major developmental theories and perspectives are provided, and abnormal psychological development and mental and emotional disorders are integrated into all chapters, from infancy through later adulthood, as appropriate. Reflections from counselors and parents that give counselors-in-training ideas for how the theoretical and content pieces can be integrated into real-life practice applications. Lifespan instructors will also be pleased to know that a comprehensive instructor's manual is available from Cengage, with chapter outlines, summaries, and a test bank of multiple-choice, true/false, and extended response questions.

Chapter 1, "Important Fundamental Principles in Lifespan Development," by Katie Sandberg and Bradley T. Erford, introduces some fundamental topics and principles of lifespan development, how current knowledge about human development was derived, and methods used to pursue emerging knowledge and understanding. A brief overview of the "stages of development" is followed by aging processes, the nature of development, important principles and issues in human development, and how developmental theories are categorized. Finally, we turn our attention to how, as humans, we generate knowledge and understanding of complex human phenomena through human development research.

Chapter 2, "Theories of Human Development: Psychosocial, Sociocultural, Multicultural, Biological, and Learning Theories," by Caroline O'Hara, Lindy K. Parker, and Catherine Y. Chang, explores how human development is influenced by multiple factors (e.g., biology, society, culture, environment) and how various theorists over the years have attempted to explain how humans grow and develop. In this and in Chapter 3, brief overviews of the major theories of human development are provided. In Chapter 2, human development is explored from historical, psychosocial, sociocultural, and multicultural perspectives. Biological and learning theories are also examined. While Chapter 2 serves as an introduction and overview of the myriad theories attempting to explain human development, many of these theories will be discussed in later chapters, embedded in the context of the appropriate life stage.

Chapter 3, "Theories of Human Development: Cognitions, Morality and Faith, and the Human Experience," was also written by Lindy K. Parker, Caroline O'Hara, and Catherine Y. Chang. Chapter 3 examines theories of cognitive and intellectual development, moral development, humanism, and faith development. The chapter ends with a brief introduction to adult development theories, with a special focus on developmental theories of womanhood.

Chapter 4, "Genetics, Heredity, Environment, and Prenatal Development," by Taryn Richards and Bradley T. Erford, proposes that human beings are complex creatures whose similarities and differences are determined in large part by genetics and heritability. From conception, a person's physical and cognitive development unfolds in a predictable manner according to information encoded in DNA. As the embryo or fetus develops, environmental influences become more important, and trauma in the prenatal environment can have significant long-term effects—and can even result in death. Chapter 4 reviews the importance of genetics and heritability to the developing human being, and normal and abnormal developmental processes throughout the trimesters of the prenatal period, which begins at conception and culminates in the birth of new living, breathing human being just waiting to embark on a lifespan odyssey!

Chapter 5, "Physical and Cognitive Development in the Infancy and Toddlerhood Years," was written by Nadine E. Garner and Julia M. Dunn. The years from infancy through toddlerhood, spanning approximately birth through age 3, serve as a bridge between life in the womb and the more independent functioning of preschoolers. This chapter explores the tremendous changes that occur in the physical and cognitive domains of the infant and toddler. The rapid brain and body growth during this developmental period are highly context-dependent, shaped by nutrition, sleep, parenting, the broader culture, and the child's own temperament. The child's unique pattern of development lays the groundwork for the continuing adventure across the lifespan.

Chapter 6, "Emotional and Social Development in the Infancy and Toddlerhood Years," was also written by Nadine E. Garner and Julia M. Dunn. It explores the tremendous changes that occur in the emotional and social domains of the infant and toddler. The rapid changes during this developmental period are highly context-dependent, shaped by the broader culture and the child's own temperament. The child's unique pattern of emotional and social development lays the groundwork for the continuing adventure throughout the lifespan.

Chapter 7, "The Preschool Years: Early Childhood Physical and Cognitive Development," was written by Charlotte Daughhetee and Stephen Parker. In the odyssey of human development, the preschool years are a time of many momentous challenges and changes. This chapter provides an overview of both physical and cognitive development during the preschool or early childhood years (approximately ages 2 or 3 through 6 years of age), a time when children make substantial developmental advances in their lifespan journey. Issues related to growth and health, as well as the progression of cognitive processes, are explored. The preschool years are a time of tremendous growth for children, and healthy physical and cognitive growth and development are essential for well-being.

Chapter 8, "The Preschool Years: Early Childhood Emotional and Social Development," was also written by Stephen Parker and Charlotte Daughhetee. They propose that life is not a solitary journey, that we traverse our lifespan in relationships with others. The formation of a sense of self and the extent of one's ability to form bonds and connections with others is a crucial aspect of development during the preschool years. Through multifaceted familial and societal influences, individuals form a basis of emotional and social competence that will guide their personal odyssey across the lifespan.

In Chapter 9, "Middle Childhood: Physical and Cognitive Development," by Stephanie Puleo, the lifespan odyssey proceeds through middle childhood, beginning around age 6 with the adventure of entering elementary school, and continues until about age 11. In Chapter 9, changes in physical and cognitive functioning that occur during middle childhood are discussed. As attention is focused on these domains, it is important to keep in mind that each develops in conjunction with emotional and social development and is influenced by environmental factors. The development of each child is unique, contingent on the interaction of a variety of factors, so a range of phenomena that occur during middle childhood is presented.

Chapter 10, "Middle Childhood: Emotional and Social Development," was also written by Stephanie Puleo. While family influences remain important, the school environment plays an increasingly greater role in the child's cognitive, emotional, and social development during middle childhood. Before they can learn to read, write, and compute, children must be able to function in the absence of their primary caretakers for extended periods of time. As their attention shifts from home to school and from fantasy to reality, children in middle childhood acquire skills and concepts necessary for daily living. Their attention spans increase, their motor abilities grow more complex, they gain better understanding of right and wrong, they begin to think logically, they become integrated into social networks, and their developing self-awareness permits them to compare themselves to others and refine their self-concepts.

Chapter 11, "The Adolescent Years: Physical and Cognitive Development," by Ann Vernon, revisits adolescence, a unique and important stage of development that marks the passage from childhood to adulthood, by looking at what occurs with regard to physical and cognitive development. It is important to note that there are some significant dynamics of early adolescence (about ages 11–14) that are different from middle adolescence (about ages 15–18). Parents, teachers, and adolescents welcome this change, although, depending on the rate at which they reach formal operational thinking, some older adolescents still appear much like young adolescents.

Chapter 12, "The Adolescent Years: Emotional, Identity, and Social Development," also by Ann Vernon, explores the emotional, identity, and social development that occurs during adolescence. Early adolescence is generally considered to be a more emotionally volatile time, while mid-adolescence is a more emotionally stable period, where the "yo-yo" nature of early adolescence is replaced by greater stability, less dependence on peers, greater self-reliance, and more flexible and rational thought patterns. In addition to the challenges associated with "mood management," adolescents also are faced with the very major task of developing an independent identity and navigating more complex social relationships. Parents, teachers, and adolescents welcome these changes, although, depending on the rate at which they reach formal operational thinking, some older adolescents may still appear much like young adolescents.

Chapter 13, "Young Adulthood: Physical and Cognitive Development," by Stephanie Crockett, proposes that in Western cultures, the journey to adulthood is marked more by the achievement of certain developmental tasks rather than a specific chronological age, although young adulthood is normative from the age range of 18 years through the 30s. Young adulthood is frequently associated with achieving the following tasks: accepting responsibility for oneself, making independent decisions, and becoming financially independent. Chapter 13 provides an overview of the characteristics and developmental tasks that define young adulthood. The physical and cognitive changes that young adults experience are explored in detail.

Then in Chapter 14, "Young Adulthood: Social, Emotional, and Career Development," also written by Stephanie Crockett, young adulthood marks a transitional period full of social-emotional and career developmental changes as well. Most young adults have sufficiently resolved the identity issues associated with adolescence and can begin to focus on establishing intimate relationships and starting a career. Social development in young adulthood is characterized by the development and maintenance of close relationships with intimate partners, friends, and family. In addition to establishing relationships, young adults focus on becoming productive workers and achieving the tasks associated with finding and maintaining a career. This chapter examines the ways in which young adults go about establishing and maintaining intimate relationships, and the vast variety in lifestyle choices made. Personality development and mental health in young adulthood are also discussed. The second half of the chapter focuses on career selection, vocational preparation, transitioning to the workforce, and balancing work-life roles.

Chapter 15, "Middle Adulthood: Physical and Cognitive Development," was authored by Robin Lee, Jennifer Jordan, Michelle Stevens, and Andrew Jones. In the past decade, middle adulthood has been redefined by society. No longer is middle adulthood considered to be the beginning of the aging process; rather, it is recognized that this group of people may be entering an exciting chapter in their lives. Middle adulthood can be an incredibly rich stage of life, with a variety of life experiences. Many in middle adulthood are raising young children; others are enjoying grandchildren. Some are rediscovering their partners or significant others after years of focusing on children or careers. With the momentous developments in medical technologies, many in middle adulthood are finding ways not only to delay aging, but also to prevent it in some ways. While some in middle adulthood can face negative changes to their physical health, they can also experience significant positive changes in all areas of development including physical, cognitive, and social/emotional. People in middle adulthood have experienced a wide variety of social events that have defined them, from the civil rights movement to the women's movement, as well as the development of technologies we all use today. All these significant experiences have created a rich developmental stage of life we call middle adulthood.

Chapter 16, "Middle Adulthood: Social/Emotional, Family, Career, and Spiritual Development," was also authored by Robin Lee, Jennifer Jordan, Michelle Stevens, and Andrew Jones. Middle adulthood brings about myriad social and emotional developmental changes; it is a transition between being the younger generation beginning their adult lives and being the older generation and slowing down. This stage within the lifespan introduces new situations: establishing a career, raising children, caring for the older generation, and preparing for retirement. Middle adulthood describes a developmental stage that often gets "stuck" and overlooked but given greater responsibility. Is this the cause of the "midlife crisis"? Does the "midlife crisis" really exist? Middle adulthood also presents different challenges and opportunities, such as maintaining marital relationships, ending them, or beginning new relationships. But relationships change because the self-concept of a middle adult is often one of confidence and insecurity.

And, finally, the odyssey transitions through older adulthood and ultimate demise. Chapter 17, "Later Adulthood and Old Age: Physical and Cognitive Development," by Cecile Yancu, Debbie Newsome, Joseph Wilkerson, and Shannon Mathews, starts with the notable supposition that, globally, the population is aging. Those aged 60 and older have increased from 8% of the total population in 1950 to 11% in 2011 and are expected to reach 22% by 2050. Among the elderly, the 80 years and over group is also growing exponentially. In the United States, the leading edge of the "Baby Boomer" generation, a large cohort of people born between 1946 and 1964, has reached the age of Medicare and Social Security. Although population aging raises important challenges for every society, the good news is that while people are living longer, they are also living healthier for more years of life. With the help of modern medicine, a healthier lifestyle, and a cleaner environment, older people are often able to delay debilitating illness until shortly before death. As a result, our ideas about growing older have evolved from being a time of social withdrawal and frailty to a period of vitality, community engagement, and tackling challenges head on. Older people are now seen by many as a valuable social and economic resource capable of contributing to the economy in myriad ways, from volunteerism to skills experience to consumer power.

Chapter 18, "Relationships and Psychosocial Aspects of Later Adulthood," was also written by Debbie Newsome, Cecile Yancu, Joseph Wilkerson, and Shannon Mathews. This final chapter discusses the ways social relationships evolve and change in older adults, as well as two important societal concerns: ageism and elder abuse. Next, socioemotional theories related to aging are introduced, as well as theories related to personality stability and change in older adulthood. A special focus involves ways in which older adults deal with adversity and what makes some older adults more resilient than others as they age. Issues of spirituality and religion in later life are also addressed. Enjoy the odyssey!

About the Editor

Bradley T. Erford, Ph.D., LCPC, NCC, LPC, LP, LSP, was the 2012–2013 President of the American Counseling Association (ACA) and a professor in the school counseling program of the Education Specialties Department in the School of Education at Loyola University Maryland. He is the recipient of the American Counseling Association (ACA) Research Award, ACA Extended Research Award, ACA Arthur A. Hitchcock Distinguished Professional Service Award, ACA Professional Development Award, and ACA Carl D. Perkins Government Relations Award. He was also inducted as an ACA Fellow. In addition, he has received the Association for Assessment in Counseling and Education (AACE) AACE/MECD Research Award, AACE Exemplary Practices Award, AACE President's Merit Award, the Association for Counselor Education and Supervision's (ACES) Robert O. Stripling Award for Excellence in Standards, Maryland Association for Counseling and Development (MACD) Maryland Counselor of the Year, MACD Counselor Advocacy Award, MACD Professional Development Award, and MACD Counselor Visibility Award. He is the editor/co-editor of numerous texts including: *Orientation to the Counseling Profession* (1st and 2nd editions, Pearson Merrill, 2010, 2014), *Group Work in the Schools* (Pearson Merrill, 2010), *Transforming the School Counseling Profession* (1st, 2nd, 3rd, and 4th editions; Pearson Merrill, 2003, 2007, 2011, 2015), *Group Work: Processes and Applications* (Pearson Merrill, 2010), *Developing Multicultural Counseling Competence* (1st and 2nd editions, Pearson Merrill, 2010, 2014), *Crisis Intervention and Prevention* (1st and 2nd editions, Pearson Merrill, 2010, 2014), *Professional School Counseling: A Handbook of Principles, Programs and Practices* (1st and 2nd editions, pro-ed, 2004, 2010), *Assessment for Counselors* (1st and 2nd editions, Cengage, 2007, 2013), *Research and Evaluation in Counseling* (1st and 2nd editions, Cengage, 2008, 2014), and *The Counselor's Guide to Clinical, Personality and Behavioral Assessment* (Cengage, 2006); and co-author of three more books: *35 Techniques Every Counselor Should Know* (Merrill/Prentice-Hall, 2010), *Educational Applications of the WISC-IV* (Western Psychological Services, 2006), and *Group Activities: Firing Up for Performance* (Pearson/Merrill/Prentice-Hall, 2007). He is also the General Editor of *The American Counseling Association Encyclopedia of Counseling* (ACA, 2009). His research specialization falls primarily in development and technical analysis of psychoeducational tests and has resulted in the publication of dozens of refereed journal articles and book chapters, and eight published tests. He was a member of the ACA Governing Council and the ACA 20/20 Visioning Committee. He is Past President of AACE, Past Chair and Parliamentarian of the American Counseling Association—Southern (US) Region; Past Chair of ACA's Task Force on High Stakes Testing; Past Chair of ACA's Standards for Test Users Task Force; Past Chair of ACA's Interprofessional Committee; Past Chair of the ACA Public Awareness and Support Committee (Co-Chair of the National Awards Subcommittee); Chair of the Convention and Past Chair of the Screening Assessment Instruments Committees for AACE; Past President of the Maryland Association for Counseling and Development (MACD); Past President of the Maryland Association for Measurement and Evaluation (MAME); Past President of the Maryland Association for Counselor Education and Supervision (MACES); and Past President of the Maryland Association for Mental Health Counselors (MAMHC). He is also a past action editor and board member of the *Journal of Counseling and Development*. Dr. Erford has been a faculty member at Loyola since 1993 and is a Licensed Clinical Professional Counselor, Licensed Professional Counselor, Nationally Certified Counselor, Licensed

Psychologist, and Licensed School Psychologist. Prior to arriving at Loyola, Dr. Erford was a school psychologist/counselor in the Chesterfield County (VA) Public Schools. He maintains a private practice specializing in assessment and treatment of children and adolescents. A graduate of the University of Virginia (Ph.D.), Bucknell University (M.A.), and Grove City College (B.S.), he has taught courses in Testing and Measurement, Psycho-Educational Assessment, Lifespan Development, Research and Evaluation in Counseling, School Counseling, Counseling Techniques, and Stress Management, as well as practicum and internship student supervision.

About the Authors

Catherine Y. Chang, Ph.D., is an associate professor and program coordinator of the counselor education and practice doctoral program in the Department of Counseling and Psychological Services at Georgia State University. She received her doctorate in counselor education from the University of North Carolina at Greensboro. Her areas of research interest include multicultural counseling and supervision, professional and social advocacy in counseling, Asian and Korean concerns, and multicultural issues in assessment.

Stephanie A. Crockett, Ph.D., is an assistant professor and director of the Adult Career Counseling Center in the Department of Counseling at Oakland University. She received her doctorate in counselor education from Old Dominion University. Her areas of research interest include career development and counseling, research methods and assessment, and clinical supervision.

Charlotte Daughhetee, Ph.D., LPC, LMFT, NCC is a professor of counseling at the University of Montevallo. She has a B.S. in early childhood education from Indiana University, and an M.Ed. in counseling and Ph.D. in counselor education, both from the University of South Carolina. She has worked as a teacher and counselor in K–12 and in higher education settings, and her current teaching interests include school counseling, marriage and family counseling, and professional issues in counseling. In her clinical experience, she has worked with children, families, and individuals in a variety of school, agency, and private practice settings. She has published in counseling journals and textbooks on school counseling, continuing competency, and crisis management. Her three adult children have given permission for her to use the amusing family anecdotes in Chapter 5.

Julia M. Dunn, B.S., is a graduate student in the School Counseling program at Millersville University of Pennsylvania and the graduate assistant for the School Counseling program.

Nadine E. Garner, Ed.D., LPC, is an associate professor in the Psychology Department and graduate program coordinator of the school counseling program at Millersville University of Pennsylvania. She is co-author of *A School with Solutions: Implementing a Solution-Focused/Adlerian-Based Comprehensive School Counseling Program*. She provides training in solution-focused counseling to counselors and educators both nationally and abroad. She also consults with school districts that seek to implement a solution-focused approach to their comprehensive developmental school counseling curriculum. As a former K–12 professional school counselor at Scotland School for Veterans' Children, she developed a comprehensive conflict resolution/peer mediation program.

Andrew Jones is a master's degree candidate in the professional counseling program at Middle Tennessee State University, where he will shortly complete his degree in mental health counseling. He plans to pursue a Ph.D. in counselor education in the future. His interests include working with college students and individuals with bipolar disorder.

Jennifer Jordan, Ph.D., LPCS, NCC, is an associate professor in the counseling and development program at Winthrop University. She is past president of the Southern Association of Counselor Education and Supervision (2011–2012). She specializes in group counseling and working with children and adolescents.

Robin Wilbourn Lee, Ph.D., LPC, NCC, is an associate professor in the professional counseling program at Middle Tennessee State University. She also serves as the director of the MTSU Center for Counseling and Psychological Services. She received her doctorate in counselor education and supervision from Mississippi State University. Her areas of research interest include legal and ethical issues in counseling, counselor training program issues, sexual assault, and domestic violence.

Shannon Mathews, Ph.D., is an assistant professor and program coordinator for the gerontology program in the Department of Behavioral Sciences and Social Work at Winston-Salem State University. She received her doctorate in gerontology from the University of Kentucky, where she also received a master's degree in medical anthropology. Her research interests include disadvantage in later life, caregiving, aging in place, and issues related to poverty across the life course.

Debbie W. Newsome, Ph.D., LPC, is an associate professor and program director of the clinical mental health counseling program in the Department of Counseling at Wake Forest University. She received her doctorate in counseling and counselor education from the University of North Carolina at Greensboro. Her areas of research interest include clinical mental health counseling, outcome assessment, and holistic approaches to counseling.

Caroline O'Hara is a doctoral student in the counselor education and practice program at Georgia State University (GSU). She received her M.S. and Ed.S. degrees in professional counseling from GSU. Her research interests include identity development, social justice counseling, multicultural counseling competence, sexual and gender diversity, supervision, and advocacy (both client and professional).

Lindy K. Parker, Ed.S., LPC, NCC, is a doctoral student in the counselor education and practice program at Georgia State University. She has clinical experience working in an alternative school setting, and in an adolescent inpatient and outpatient psychiatric and substance abuse hospital.

Stephen Parker is an associate professor of sociology at the University of Montevallo. He received his B.A. and M.A. from Baylor University. He completed his Ph.D. at Indiana University. He is co-author (with Donna Eder and Cathy Evans) of *School Talk: Gender and Adolescent Culture* (1995). He has published in the *American Journal of Sociology*, *Sociology of Education*, and the *Journal of Contemporary Ethnography*. His research on child development and adolescent culture in no way prepared him for parenting his two wonderful children. His teaching interests include sociology of culture, gender, sociological theory, and popular music.

Stephanie Puleo, Ph.D., LMFT, LPC, NCC, is a professor in the Department of Counseling, Leadership, and Foundations at the University of Montevallo in Montevallo, Alabama. She is certified by the American Red Cross in disaster mental health. Dr. Puleo earned her Ph.D. in counselor education at the University of Alabama. She also has earned master's degrees in community counseling and school psychology. In addition to coordinating the marriage and family counseling program track at the University of Montevallo, she provides counseling and psychometric services to individuals, couples, and families in the Birmingham and central Alabama area.

Taryn E. Richards, M.Ed., is a nationally certified counselor and a professional secondary school counselor in Maryland. She has authored textbook chapters, supplemental instructional materials, journal articles, and a book in the areas of lifespan development, mental health treatment, and assessment.

Katie M. Sandberg, M.A., is a mobile mental health counselor, nationally certified counselor, and a member of both Psi Chi, the International Honor Society in Psychology, and Chi Sigma Iota, the International Honor Society in Counseling. She has authored numerous textbook chapters and supplemental instructional materials in the fields of lifespan and human development and assessment.

Michelle Stevens, Ph.D., is an assistant professor and practicum coordinator of the professional counseling program in the Educational Leadership Department at Middle Tennessee State University. She received her doctorate in counselor education from Kent State University. Her areas of research interests include multicultural counseling and awareness, supervision, effective practicum and counselor training, and minority graduate student concerns.

Ann Vernon, Ph.D., NCC, LMHC, is professor emeritus and former coordinator of counseling at the University of Northern Iowa, and is a counselor in private practice, where she works extensively with children, adolescents, and their parents. Dr. Vernon is the former Director of the Midwest Center for REBT and Vice-President of the Albert Ellis Board of Trustees. She is the author of numerous books, chapters, and articles, including *Thinking, Feeling, Behaving* and *What Works When with Children and Adolescents*

Joe Wilkerson, M.A., LPCA, is a graduate of the clinical mental health counseling program at Wake Forest University. He works in community mental health in the mountains of western North Carolina.

Cecile Y. Yancu, Ph.D., is an associate professor of sociology in the Department of Behavioral Sciences and Social Work at Winston-Salem State University. She received her doctorate in socio-medical sciences from Columbia University of the City of New York. Her research focuses on disparities in health-related quality of life. Specific areas include the impact of chronic daily stress on obesity-related health disparities, underuse of hospice and palliative care by African-Americans, and high-risk sexual behavior among young African-American adults.

Ancillaries

MindTap

MindTap™ Counseling for *Erford's A Lifespan Odyssey for Counseling Professionals*, 1st Edition is a digital learning solution that helps instructors engage and transform today's students into critical thinkers. Through paths of dynamic assignments and applications that you can personalize, real-time course analytics, and an accessible reader, MindTap helps you turn cookie cutter into cutting edge, apathy into engagement, and memorizers into higher-level thinkers.

Online Instructor's Manual

This manual provides an overview of the text and a summary of the chapter to assist instructors in teaching the course.

Online Test Bank

Organize your course and capture your students' attention with the resources found in the Test Bank, including multiple-choice, true/false, and essay questions—most with answers.

Online PowerPoints

Helping you make your lectures more engaging while effectively reaching your visually oriented students, these handy Microsoft PowerPoint® slides outline the chapters of the main text in a classroom-ready presentation.

Acknowledgments

A heartfelt thank you to Julie A. Martinez, Stefanie Chase, Rita Jaramillo, and Jitendra Kumar. In addition, I would like to thank the following people, who provided thoughtful feedback throughout the writing process.

Jen Alexander, Harding University Leah Alviar
Anne Andrews, Thomas Nelson Community College
Naveeda Athar, Concordia University Chicago
Victoria Bacon, Bridgewater State University
Alan Basham, Eastern Washington University
Thomas Blume, Oakland University
Judith Bomar, University of Connecticut
Steve Bradshaw, Bryan College
Leilani Brown
Lori Bruch, University of Scranton
Michelle Bruno, Indiana University of Pennsylvania
Nona Cabral, California Baptist University
Tamara Calhoun, Schenectady County Community College
Amy Carrigan, University of Saint Francis
Walter Chung, Eastern University
Arthur Clark, St. Lawrence University
Bonnie Colon, Purdue University Calumet
Jeffrey Cornelius-White, Missouri State University
Walter Crockett, Jackson State University
Judy Daniels, University of Hawaii
Trent Davis, Jefferson College of Health Sciences
Kim Desmond, IUP
John Dewell, Loyola University
Carol Erbes, ODU
John Farrar, Central Michigan University
Gerard Geoffroy
Jackie Goldstein, Samford University
Eric Green, UNT Dallas
Lucy Jones
Patrick Kariuki, Milligan College
Kim Kjaersgaard, Alaska Pacific University
Rich Lanthier
George Leone, New Mexico Highlands University
Susan Lester, University of Saint Joseph, Connecticut
Linda Lopez Chaparro, Oxnard College
Christopher Maglio, Truman State University
Jeana Magyar-Moe, University of Wisconsin–Stevens Point
Bill McHenry, Texas A&M University–Texarkana
Michael Milco
Christopher Moore, Oregon State University
Barbara Nicoll, University of La Verne

Heidi Nightengale, Empire State College
Sue Norton, Edinboro University
James O'Neil, University of Connecticut
Margaret Parker, California State University Dominguez Hills
Cathleen Paterno, Saint Xavier University
John Pellitteri, Queens College–City University of New York
Kristi Perryman, Missouri State University
Sherry Pickover, University of Detroit Mercy
Karen Polite, Harrisburg Area Community College
Michael Poulakis, University of Indianapolis
Carolyn Rollins, Albany State University
Fay Roseman, Barry University
Chadwick Royal, North Carolina Central University
Paul Schwartz, Mt. St. Mary College
Stephanie Scott, Walden University
Misty Silver, Mayland Community College
Tod Sloan, Lewis and Clark
LeAnn Solmonson, Stephen F. Austin State University
Debbie Stout, California State University–Fullerton
Janet Trotter, University of La Verne
Heather Whaley, Carson Newman University
Susan Wycoff, California State University Sacramento
Riva Zeff, Seattle University
Ken Zelinski, Monmouth University

Important Fundamental Principles in Lifespan Development

By Katie Sandberg and Bradley T. Erford

T his initial chapter introduces some fundamental topics and principles of lifespan development, how current knowledge about human development was derived, and methods used to pursue emerging knowledge and understanding. A brief overview of the "stages of development" is followed by aging processes, the nature of development, important principles and issues in human development, and how developmental theories are categorized. Finally, we turn our attention to how, as humans, we generate knowledge and understanding of complex human phenomena through human development research.

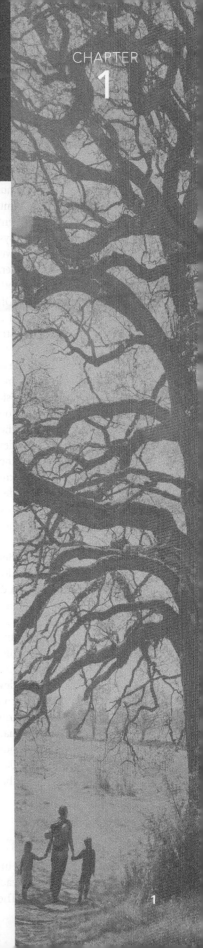

Important Fundamental Principles in Lifespan Development

Welcome to the exciting journey of human development, an odyssey that lasts a lifetime! This book was designed to help counselors in training to understand and apply their knowledge and principles to aid all their clients, regardless of the clients' current age or developmental challenges. As such, the entire lifespan from conception to death is covered. Understanding human development is a complex undertaking, and counselors are well served to learn as much as possible about all its stages and facets in order to maximize their helpfulness to clients. It is essential to understand that an individual client is embedded in rich and complex systems of social and cultural contexts which the client has constructed and given meaning; while it is important for counselors to understand the client's developmental issues and challenges, it is equally essential to consider the developmental issues and challenges of those other individuals and groups that comprise that individual's social and cultural contexts. Often, it is not just the "client's presenting problem" that brings that client to counseling, but a complex interplay of overlapping systems and relationships that are creating challenges, stresses, and sometimes even turmoil expressed as "symptoms" by the client.

This initial chapter is a whirlwind tour through some fundamental topics and principles essential to understanding lifespan development, how current knowledge was derived, and methods used to pursue emerging knowledge and understanding. A brief overview of the "stages of development" is presented first, representing a socially constructed sequence used to structure Chapters 4–18 of this book. Next, processes of aging are reviewed, followed by the nature of development, important principles and issues in human development, and how developmental theories are categorized. This will be followed by a wealth of developmental, theoretical, and practical knowledge in Chapters 2 and 3. Finally, the focus shifts to how knowledge and understanding of complex human phenomena are generated through human development research, including: data collection procedures, specialized developmental research designs, the ethics of research involving humans, and the importance and consequences of framing human developmental issues in counseling as both normal and abnormal.

This last issue is particularly critical in one's development as a professional counselor. Because diagnosis and treatment are usually within the scope of practice of most professional counselors, and because third-party payers (e.g., insurance companies) often require a diagnosis for reimbursement of services, a working knowledge of abnormal developmental features is necessary. But professional counselors also believe in client wellness, resiliency, and the use of positive psychological principles to help clients and students attain and maintain a healthy lifestyle. This is a particularly important distinction to consider in a lifespan development course: Most individuals attain normal development functioning and maintain that functioning for long periods of time; but sometimes events and issues create developmental challenges and "abnormal" manifestations. These manifestations are socially constructed, culturally dependent, and change over time with the expansion of knowledge, innovations in treatment, and even the revision of diagnostic protocols. This is why potential clients seek the services of professional counselors. The more a counselor knows about human development, the better able the counselor will be able to understand and help students and clients—and the deeper the possibilities for one's own self-understanding. So, let the odyssey commence!

Stages of Life

The Prenatal Period through Old Age

Human development is often discussed and analyzed in terms of stages. Individuals within each stage are presumed to have similar cognitive, physical, and socioemotional abilities. They also typically encounter similar experiences and psychological processes related to developmental progression. Although developmental scientists used to focus almost exclusively on the great deal of change apparent from birth to adolescence, many now acknowledge the substantial changes that occur throughout the entire lifespan.

Because these stages are social constructions, meaning that they are created within and by individuals from particular societies, not all cultures will agree on exactly when a child becomes an adult. The Chippewa Native Americans, for example, divide childhood into only two stages, the boundary between them being the ability to walk. Then, once a child hits puberty, he becomes an adult; adolescence does not exist in their society (Broude, 1995). However, although not all cultures, or even all subcultural groups, agree on the specific stages and age boundaries within each stage, there is general agreement on the eight periods or stages typically accepted within Western industrialized societies. The eight periods most professionals use to characterize development include the prenatal period, infancy/toddlerhood, early childhood, middle childhood, adolescence, young adulthood, middle adulthood, and later adulthood/old age. Consequently, two chapters in this textbook are dedicated to each of these stages, except the prenatal stage.

Because each developmental stage will be elaborated upon in much greater detail in later chapters, only a brief description of each stage will be provided here. The **prenatal period** lasts from conception until birth, when a tremendous amount of rapid growth and organ development takes place. **Infancy** is the period from birth to about 2 years; it encompasses great gains in sensorimotor and cognitive development. The period from about 2 to 3 years ordinarily is termed **toddlerhood**. Children in this period further develop their language skills and begin mastering such tasks as potty training and feeding and dressing themselves.

Children aged about 3 to 6 years usually are in **early childhood**. Children in early childhood further refine their gross and fine motor skills and make gains in independence, self-control, language, and memory. Individuals in **middle childhood**, the period from about six to 12 years, begin to think more logically and concretely in the structured educational environment they now inhabit. They experience incredible gains in language and learning. Peer relationships increase in importance until they become paramount in **adolescence**, the period from about 12 to 19 years. Adolescents experience substantial changes, including puberty, the capacity to think abstractly, and the search for identity. Mental disorders often begin in adolescence. Some researchers have expanded the stage of adolescence into early adolescence (about 12 to 14 years), middle adolescence (about 15–18 years), and later adolescence (about 19 to 22 years) because of the prominence of the university experience. Thus, in some Westernized cultures, late adolescence overlaps with the early years of what has traditionally been called young adulthood. Again, because the stages of human development are socially constructed, our understanding and categorization of human developmental occurrences continue to emerge.

In **young adulthood**, the period from about 19 to 30 years, individuals face the challenges of establishing a career and seeking out intimate relationships. Often the end of young adulthood is marked by marriage and starting a family. In **middle adulthood**, the longest lifespan period, lasting from about 30 to 60 years of age, many adults either experience career success or reevaluate and change their careers. Family obligations are extremely important for those who choose to have children, and the responsibility of caring for both children and aging parents may be stressful. **Late adulthood** characterizes the period of life from about 60 to 75 years, when most individuals are nearing the end of their career and are launching children, if they have not already done so. These substantial life changes may cause individuals in late adulthood to reflect on their lives and the impact they have made. The extension of this developmental stage is **old age**, which includes individuals over the age of about 75. People in old age face challenges such as retirement and loss of a spouse.

Most of the reflections and personal reflections in this book involve authors' or contributors' recollections and anecdotes. But for this first reflection, think about your own development up to this point in your life. Has your development been "normal"? Have you attained developmental milestones on time? Ahead of time? Late? Which developmental stage are you currently in? How has your developmental trajectory influenced the opportunities you have experienced in your family, peer group, community, and culture? Consider who you were "as a person" (e.g., physically, cognitively, socially, emotionally) at 4 years of age; at 8 years of age; at 14 years of age; at 21 years of age. How have YOU grown and developed?

As physical health and cognitive abilities gradually decline, the support of close relationships and the search for life's meaning become quite important.

Of course, while individuals within each stage generally have similar capabilities and experiences, there is also a great deal of variability among individuals in each stage due to their unique genetic makeups and environmental influences. Because age is not an exact indicator of developmental status, some individuals may reach developmental milestones in each designated stage substantially before or after same-aged peers. Consider, for example, the young boy who begins reading at the age of 4 or 5, much earlier than the average child. Although this child, according to chronological age, is technically transitioning between toddlerhood and early childhood, the child is displaying cognitive capabilities that do not usually emerge until the beginning of middle childhood. So, while periods of life are a useful way to talk about most individuals in each stage, it is important to realize that individual variability within stages can be immense.

Aging Processes

Humans all grow and develop in ways both similar and different throughout their lives. Likewise, all individuals have varying perceptions of their age across the lifespan. These varying perceptions and domains of development can be explained via a discussion of biological, psychological, and social aging processes, which are inextricably intertwined.

Biological Aging

Biological aging processes refer to changes in how the human body functions across the lifespan. Understanding the reciprocal metabolic processes of anabolism and catabolism can help to better comprehend the typical progression of biological aging. **Anabolism** involves one's body building up to peak biological performance. Individuals may reach their full biological potential at varying times throughout their lifespan, depending on socioeconomic status, self-care strategies, and environmental impacts. For example, a single mother living in poverty with inadequate access to appropriate nutrition and opportunities to exercise will likely reach her biological peak potential much sooner than an upper-class male who follows a strict diet and exercise regimen. This anabolic period from birth until peak is highly valued in Western societies, and many people seek to sustain anabolic growth as long as possible.

Following the attainment of peak potential, the human body inevitably begins to slowly deteriorate, a process termed **catabolism**. Although the onset for catabolism varies, once begun, it continues until death. The slow deterioration of many physical abilities and cognitive capacities as chronological age progresses can be the cause of much stress and anxiety as people begin to lose skills and functioning they once possessed. Fortunately, there are strategies available for aging individuals to maintain their physical and cognitive abilities. It is well documented that aging people can enhance their health prospects by maximizing positive social exchanges and social support and by minimizing negative social interactions (Rohr & Lang, 2009). Increasing positive social interaction and support can also help

You have heard of anabolic steroids, the drugs some athletes use (illegally) to build muscle strength and endurance in order to achieve higher levels of performance in competition. These drugs are used because high performance is valued in our society, especially in athletics, and can reap large economic and social rewards. Question: Have you ever heard anybody say, "Hey, buddy. You wanna buy some catabolic steroids?" In Western cultures, high performance—and attractiveness—are valued; decline is to be delayed (sometimes at any cost).

aging individuals boost their cognitive functioning (Seeman, Lusignolo, Albert, & Berkman, 2001). Therefore, engaging in positive social interaction and support are important ways to sustain both physical and cognitive functioning as the body ages. Thus, although catabolism cannot be reversed, it can be slowed with appropriate strategies and lifestyle choices.

Psychological Aging

Psychological aging processes refer to an individual's perception of his or her age. In other words, psychological age encompasses how old an individual "feels." For example, an adolescent girl who becomes pregnant may have to grow up fast to face the challenges associated with motherhood at such a young age. Thus, she might feel old. In contrast, a healthy 65-year-old man may engage in vigorous exercise daily and continue to pursue various fulfilling occupational, social, and leisure activities. He might view himself as still quite young—"I feel much younger than 65!"

Social Aging

The social process of aging can be described as the way individuals view aging within their own culture or society. **Social aging** perceptions are mediated by culture, vocation, and socioeconomic status. Professionals (e.g., doctors, lawyers, professors) tend to gain prestige as they age, because additional years in their fields are associated with experience and knowledge. Thus, a 70-year-old doctor is likely to be afforded much greater social respect than a retired factory worker of the same age.

Interestingly, the perception of when people become "old" varies not just within cultures, but cross-culturally as well. In New Zealand, as in many other cultures, becoming a grandmother is a significant marker of being considered "old" for a woman (Armstrong, 2003). People in Turkey saw themselves as "old" at a younger age than Americans did (McConatha, Hayta, Rieser-Danner, McConatha, & Polat, 2004). McConatha et al. suggested that this perception may be due to the smaller numbers of people over the age of 65 years in Turkey, the limited amount of available information about the elderly, or the fact that Turkey is a less technologically advanced society. McConatha and associates also found that young adults from both Turkey and America perceived entrance into old age at a younger age than middle-aged adults. They suggested that older individuals tend to acquire a more realistic perception of aging.

Perceptions of aging are also linked to beliefs and stereotypes about old age. Many people worry about losing physical and cognitive capacities as they age. Women especially fear the physical changes associated with age, likely because Western media so pervasively promotes the beauty ideal of a youthful appearance (McConatha et al., 2004). Slevec and Tiggemann (2010) have even shown that aging anxiety and media exposure can predict motivation for and consideration of cosmetic surgery, showing just how important it is for many women to look young. Men, on the other hand, can still attain attractiveness and power as they grow older, even without a youthful appearance.

This fear of aging is likely related to perceptions of the elderly in our society. Elderly people are often stigmatized and attributed more negative than positive characteristics (Widrick & Raskin, 2010). As people look older and older, the likelihood that they will be perceived as fitting negative stereotypes about old age increases (Hummert, Garstka, & Shaner, 1997). This finding illustrates the connection between physical aging and social aging. The abundance of negative stereotypes, coupled with the cultural stigma ascribed to aging, can intensify feelings of fear and anxiety around growing older (McConatha et al., 2004).

Think About It   1.2

When describing how old someone is, we often immediately think of chronological age. But we have all heard the expression "you are as young as you feel!" Thus, a person can be 29 years old socially and chronologically, have the physical and biological body of a 39-year-old due to bodily deterioration and physical difficulties, but "feel" like a 19-year-old teenager, psychologically speaking. Likewise, that same 29-year-old may look very young and attractive and be in great physical condition, having "the body of a 19-year-old," but have been run through the emotional wringer for most of the past three decades because of physical, sexual, or emotional abuse, and thus "feel" (psychologically) weary, burnt out, and far older than a 29-year-old.

Fortunately, Pinquart (2002) found that when confronted with negative stereotypes about competence in old age, most elderly people use these stereotypes as a basis for downward comparison rather than internalization into self-perceptions. In other words, exposure to negative stereotypes about older people resulted in negative peer appraisals rather than negative self-appraisals. In contrast, Garstka, Schmitt, Branscombe, and Hummert (2004) found that the psychological well-being of older individuals in their study suffered when they believed themselves to be the target of age discrimination.

It is important to remember that not all cultures view aging processes similarly. Although the perception of markers for old age in New Zealand seemed similar to what we might expect in America, differences in old age perception were apparent between Turkish and American citizens. Many Americans view and respond to aging in greater detail, but these results are not necessarily applicable across cultures. For instance, in more traditional East Asian cultures, adults are often afforded greater respect with increasing age (Sung, 2001). When working with clients from various cultures, therefore, it is important to assess how their worldviews may differ regarding the aging process.

As a future helping professional, it is important both to consider the many challenges associated with aging, and to familiarize oneself with the multitude of protective factors that can serve to enhance client functioning as one ages. Additionally, you should become aware of your own age stereotypes so you can guard against using patronizing communication such as a markedly slower pace or obviously amplified articulation of speech. Given that the population of older adults will continue to expand as people live longer and longer lives, Laidlaw and Pachana (2009) called attention to the need for increased supervised training opportunities with older adults.

The Nature of Development

There are many guiding principles that can help you understand the overall nature of human development. Development is cumulative, variable, cyclical, and repetitive, and it is characterized by cultural differences, individual differences, and both stability and change. Each of these characteristics of development will be elaborated upon below.

Human Development Is Cumulative

Throughout the entire human lifespan, development occurs continuously and builds upon itself. The possibility for change always exists. Although many believe that the early years of development lay the groundwork for an individual's future, there is no one period of development that is more important than others, according to the lifespan perspective (Baltes, 1987). However, looking back to earlier periods of development can provide information to help understand an individual in the present. For example, the quality of responsive parenting and subsequent attachment behaviors in infancy shape how the individual learns to perceive the world and establish relationships with friends and lovers later in life. Thus, to reach an optimal understanding of current development, individuals must be viewed in the context of their entire lifespan.

Human Development Is Variable

There is no set developmental trajectory that will make development exactly the same for any two individuals. Although development prior to conception follows very similar pathways for all individuals, once born, individuals follow increasingly diverse pathways as they become older. Each individual will respond to various life events in unique ways, which will then shape his or her future experiences. While some abilities increase with time, others decrease or remain the same. Rates of change also differ for the various capacities that change over time. For example, while perceptual speed, memory, and fluency decline with age, knowledge of vocabulary usually remains stable until the age of 90, when it begins to slowly decline (Singer, Verhaeghen, Ghisletta, Lindenberger, & Baltes, 2003). In addition, the priorities placed on different aspects of social, emotional, cognitive, and physical development are subject to change throughout the lifespan.

Human Development Is Cyclical and Repetitive

Development throughout the lifespan follows a **cyclical** and **repetitive** pattern. Throughout each phase of the lifespan, individuals experience changes, gains, and losses. Baltes (1987) believed that loss and gain were inextricably linked, with loss always bringing some sort of gain and gain always bringing some sort of loss. For example, as school-aged children begin to gain the capacity for logical thought, their imaginative ability for thought also changes as they learn new social norms around the expression of creative, rare, and even bizarre thoughts. Individuals are constantly learning, growing, and adapting their prior knowledge to incorporate new knowledge. Thus, the cycle of development continues throughout life.

Human Development Is Influenced by Cultural Differences

Various cultures can include, but are not limited to, groups of people from different countries, races, ethnicities, sexual orientations, religions, gender identities, socioeconomic status, and disability status. **Cultural differences** vary in their ability to influence different dimensions of development. For example, infant babbling is a universal phenomenon, regardless of the culture into which the baby is born. Remarkably, though the onset is delayed, even babies born with deafness across the world learn to babble (Oller, 2000). This suggests that babbling is an innate, maturational trait that exists cross-culturally. However, there are many aspects of development that are highly influenced by the culture in which one is raised.

Culture can have a profound effect on the development of countless skills and abilities, as well as the reactions of individuals to various experiences throughout their lifespan. For example, many people might be surprised to learn that the seemingly individual phenomenon of memory is actually affected by culture. Maternal reminiscing style varies cross-culturally and greatly affects the child's capacity for autobiographical memory. European-American mothers are more evaluative and elaborative when reminiscing, and their children focus more on personal attributes when recalling memories (Wang, 2006a). This is likely due to the individualistic focus of mainstream American culture, and as a result, children learn to tell personal narratives as a way of forming their identities. However, in China, collectivism and interdependence have a higher cultural value, so mothers use a low-elaborative, directive, and sometimes mother-centered conversational style to connect the child and mother in a relational hierarchy. This structuring of relationships is more important than teaching children to use memory to tell elaborate personal narratives. As a result of maternal reminiscing style and the child's self-concept, among a host of other factors, European-American children can recall earlier memories than their Chinese counterparts. The ability to focus on specific episodes that is cultivated in European-American children transfers into their ability to recall specific facts about other people as well. The cultural roots of these abilities is important to keep in mind in order to avoid taking the view that Chinese children are less intelligent or less able to recall memories. Chinese children are simply not socialized to focus on detailed individual events the way European-American children are.

This comparison of Chinese and European-American children demonstrates how cultural practices can affect the development of autobiographical memories. An example of how reactions of individuals to various experiences can be culture-dependent as well is provided by Lansford, Deater-Deckard, Dodge, Bates, and Pettit's (2004) research on child discipline. They found that physical discipline, such as corporal punishment (e.g., spanking), in childhood led to higher levels of behavior problems for European-American adolescents but lower levels of externalizing disorders for African-American adolescents. They attributed this finding to the fact that in White culture, children perceive spanking to be scary, but in African-American culture, children view spanking as a legitimate parenting practice which their parents do for their own good. Here, culture affects the meaning of the parenting behavior, and thus children from different cultures have different developmental reactions to the same parental behavior. The finding that the relationship between corporal punishment and adverse child outcomes is weakened when corporal punishment is perceived as a culturally normative disciplinary practice has been extended cross-culturally in China, India, Italy, Kenya, the Philippines, and Thailand as well (Lansford et al., 2005).

As helping professionals, we should strive to take an **emic**, or culture-specific, approach to truly understand the cultural meaning behind different practices and behaviors. Taking an **etic**, or universal, approach can limit one's ability to understand the insider's perspective and bias the counselor toward assuming certain psychological constructs are valid everywhere regardless of culture. It is best to always examine the cultural implications behind various developmental phenomena.

Think About It   1.3

How does culture influence a person's self-perceptions related to achievement? Beauty? Intelligence? Kindness? Friendship? Moral behavior?

Human Development Involves Vast Individual Differences

While development is almost always influenced by cultural context, **individual differences** also play a role in the unique paths each person's development takes. The experiences that individuals seek out, coupled with their genetic predispositions, interact to produce unique developmental trajectories.

Maguire et al. (2003) found interesting evidence for the plasticity of the human brain in response to environmental stimuli. They found that London taxi drivers, who must rely on extensive knowledge of spatial relations to navigate through the city daily, have increased gray matter in the posterior hippocampus, which plays a large role in spatial navigation. Maguire and colleagues ruled out the possibility that those with greater hippocampal volume sought out jobs requiring navigational expertise by showing that other participants with navigational expertise, but who were not taxi drivers, showed no marked increase in hippocampal volume. Thus, it seems that the incredible amount of spatial navigation required of London taxi drivers has enabled their hippocampi to actually expand. Clearly, individual differences in experience can play a large role in development.

Human Development Involves Both Stability and Change

Development is characterized by both stability and change. While these two concepts may seem contradictory, they are often complementary in development. While some aspects of development, such as intelligence, remain relatively stable throughout the lifespan, others, such as memory, are quite amenable to change given the right environmental influences, such as training and practice.

Both positive and negative experiences have the power to change the developmental trajectory of an individual. For example, children who grow up in violent, abusive homes learn violent behavior; their chronic exposure to violence may actually change the shape of the brain, creating a predisposition toward violent behavior (Perry, 1997). For these children, early exposure to violence can have a lifelong impact on how they handle their own aggression and frustration. Although research regarding resiliency factors in children exposed to intimate partner violence is in its infancy, competent parenting, social competence, easy temperament, and intellectual resources have been identified as protective factors for such children (Gewirtz & Edleson, 2007). Thus, children exposed to violence at home are not as likely to suffer long-lasting effects on their well-being if some of these resiliency factors are in place.

In conclusion, change can occur at any time throughout the lifespan, but we have yet to pinpoint exactly which abilities have limited modifiability at various ages. The search for plasticity and its constraints is an important topic for developmental research (Baltes, 1987). Evidence does exist that an enriched environment and new learning can promote neuroplasticity in late adulthood (Goh & Park, 2009). Goh and Park further asserted that determining how to preserve cognitive functioning in late adulthood is a critical topic for future developmental research.

Important Human Development Principles and Issues

There are multiple principles and issues that underlie human developmental science. These themes are often posed as dichotomies. Through exploration of the themes of discontinuous versus continuous development, qualitative versus quantitative changes, nature versus nurture, predictable and historical changes, critical periods versus flexibility and plasticity, and active versus passive, it becomes evident that most of these dichotomous variables may be better viewed as ends of a continuum because some measure of both variables is often important. Think about where you lie on the continuum as you read about each theme. Do you agree completely with proponents of one perspective or the other, or do you fall somewhere in between? Determining your personal views about these themes will help you to conceptualize how you view lifespan development.

Discontinuous versus Continuous Development

Developmental scientists debate whether human development occurs in a discontinuous or continuous fashion. Those who promote the **discontinuous**, or stage, view believe that children go through relatively stable periods of development that culminate in abrupt transformations as they transition to the next stage of functioning. Each stage is characterized by new behaviors, cognitions, and emotions that are seen as fundamentally different from the behaviors, cognitions, and emotions that characterized the previous stage of development. Regardless of the speed at which people move through these stages, all people are believed to progress through them in a fixed order. You can understand the discontinuous perception of development by imagining a child progressing up a staircase (see Figure 1.1). Each step represents a stage in the child's development. There are long plateaus in growth followed by dramatic spurts where the child learns and grows a great deal in a short period of time, leaping to the next level of more advanced functioning.

In contrast, theorists who view development as **continuous** believe that developmental change is continually occurring at a gradual, steady pace. An example of quantitative, incremental growth would be a child adding a new word to his vocabulary. Learning the meanings of new words does not require large-scale changes in development; rather, it enables the child to build on existing knowledge. Rather than moving

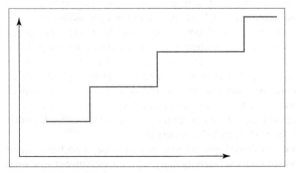

Figure 1.1 Discontinuous development.

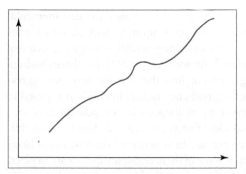

Figure 1.2 Continuous development.

abruptly up a staircase, continuous development looks more like the smooth upward progression seen in Figure 1.2.

The majority of developmental psychologists now believe that development is characterized by both continuity and discontinuity. Indeed, continuous change may ultimately lead to more stage-like developments. One may also hear this manifestation of the continuity–discontinuity issue referred to as the quantitative–qualitative issue.

The continuity–discontinuity issue is also related to perceptions of whether or not the personality traits of a young child and the effects of early experiences will persist across time. Do you believe that a defiant, oppositional child will inevitably develop into a defiant, oppositional adult? Or do you believe that the environment the child grows up in will determine whether these traits persist or change over time? It is likely that some inherent personality traits are resistant to change. However, it is also possible that parenting practices and cultural norms can encourage or discourage the expression of various traits. For example, making excuses for the child's inappropriate behavior might facilitate the continuity of his recalcitrance, while firm rules and direct approaches to conflict resolution might help him become less oppositional. Thus, a multitude of factors interact to determine whether a child's traits will prove continuous or discontinuous over time.

The effects of early childhood experiences may or may not have long-term implications, depending on the personal characteristics of the child and the type of experience. Early childhood experiences can range from stressful, abnormal events like abuse or loss, to normal events like potty training during the toddler years. The issue is whether these early childhood experiences have long-term implications. You will recall from the previous section about stability and change that exposure to violence in the home in early childhood can have long-lasting deleterious effects. It is less likely that minor, sporadic conflicts with siblings in early childhood would have similar long-lasting implications. It is important to be aware of whether you view development as discontinuous or continuous, because this will have implications for how you view clients and their problems. Consider for a moment Joey in Case Example 1.1.

➤ CASE EXAMPLE **1.1** JOEY.

Joey is a 17-year-old 12th grader who comes to see you because he is struggling to determine what he wants to do with his life after graduation. You learn that Joey's parents have been pressuring him to pursue a career in the medical field like his father. They expect him to spend the majority of his time at home studying and do not permit him to date or engage in extracurricular activities. Joey tells you that he feels isolated from his peers and is unsure of himself in social settings. He feels uncomfortable interacting with peers outside of school. He struggles with math and science and is not sure that he is suited for, or interested in, a career in the medical field. However, he does not want to upset his parents by telling them this, and he is unsure of what other career options might be good for him. Think about how you view Joey's situation and what you would do.

If you subscribe to a discontinuous view of development, you may think that Joey's problems are a result of his struggle in resolving Erikson's identity versus role confusion stage. (This stage will be explained in greater detail in Chapter 7.) He is definitely dealing with confusion as he attempts to establish his social and occupational identities, and he is at the right age to be dealing with the identity versus role confusion crisis. However, a rigid view of when people should enter and resolve each stage could prevent you from considering that Joey is struggling to resolve guilt about choosing goals that conflict with parental expectations, or that he has not sufficiently mastered the necessary social and academic skills to feel competent.

If you subscribe to a continuous view of development, you may view Joey's problems quite differently. You may notice that his unresolved social identity mirrors his unresolved occupational identity. Perhaps Joey has not been given sufficient opportunities to learn appropriate social skills or advance his academic skills. It is also possible that his avoidance and complacency have been reinforced by his parents or teachers, and now these behaviors are no longer working for him. This continuous view would be helpful in understanding the contextual influences on Joey's behavior, but it would obscure any potential stage issues that might be influencing Joey's problem.

Therefore, it is important for counselors to be aware of their predispositions toward discontinuous or continuous views of development so that they can be cognizant of areas they may be overlooking. Knowing one's own personal biases is an important step in self-awareness for all counselors. Furthermore, taking a multidimensional view of Joey's situation to examine all the potential factors and avenues for intervention would be advantageous in finding an effective way to help Joey. The potential roles of his social and academic abilities, developmental stage, family, peers, school, and culture would all be important areas to assess. This assessment would provide a comprehensive view of Joey's situation and the most effective interventions to apply.

Predictable and Historical Changes

Developing children will encounter both predictable and historical changes as they grow and learn. Baltes (2003) maintained that just as humans change and develop, so do the contexts they live in. As a result, an individual's context exerts three types of influence that can affect development. These influences are normative age-graded influences, normative history-graded influences, and nonnormative or highly individualized life events.

Normative age-graded influences are the predictable changes that every individual will encounter throughout his or her lifespan. Every developing individual will experience certain similar biological and social processes at about the same chronological age. For example, all children will begin puberty within the same range of time and all adult women will experience menopause at around the same age. These processes are universal. Social processes, such as beginning formal education, will occur at about the same age for most children but may vary slightly across cultures.

Normative history-graded influences are the historical circumstances that affect people of common generations similarly. Depending on an individual's age at the time of a significant historical event, it will likely affect him differently than a much older or much younger individual. For example, events such as the Great Depression of the 1930s, World War II, the civil rights movement, the technological age, and the terrorist attacks of September 11, 2001, all affected members of diverse generations differently. Growing up in the age of global terrorism will provide the current generation with a different outlook on life than the perspectives of those who grew up during the prosperity of the 1950s. As a result, the children growing up in the age of global terrorism will respond in certain ways that will carve out new or distinct values, beliefs, and social roles.

Nonnormative or highly individualized life events are those unusual occurrences that greatly affect an individual's life. Nonnormative influences are considered unusual either because they occur at an atypical time of life or because they are rare and uncommon events. These unusual events do not happen to all people or affect all people in similar ways. Because they are not connected with age or history, they can occur at any time in an individual's lifespan. Examples include experiencing the death of a parent or sibling at a young age, giving birth as a teenager, experiencing a natural disaster, winning the lottery, making a career change in midlife, or taking up a risky new hobby later in life.

In conclusion, all of these normative and nonnormative influences combine in unique ways to affect the development of every individual. While some contextual influences are predictable, others are highly variable and their effects are dependent on the developing person's age and reaction to the various events throughout their lives.

Think About It   1.4

What normative age-graded influences, normative history-graded influences, and nonnormative or highly individualized life events influenced your development—and perhaps even your decision to become a professional counselor? How were these influences different from those of your parents, siblings, and friends?

Critical Periods versus Flexibility/Plasticity

There is ongoing debate regarding whether humans must develop certain skills at critical periods or whether they have the ability to develop skills equally well at any point in their lives. Proponents of **critical periods** believe that a certain limited period of time exists when humans have the maximum opportunity for optimal development given appropriate environmental inputs. For example, a pregnant woman with certain diseases or who takes certain drugs at various points throughout pregnancy increases the risk of harming the baby's development. During the first eight weeks of pregnancy, the baby's organs and structures are beginning to develop, making this a critical period for healthy development. Mothers who contract rubella (German measles) during their first trimester place their babies at increased risk for eye, ear, and heart defects, since these organs are forming at this time. After the first trimester, having rubella is still dangerous to the developing baby, but the risk of serious damage decreases, since these organs have already been formed.

Evidence for the importance of critical periods has also been found in the **imprinting** behaviors of new ducklings, which will bond with the first moving object they see, even if it is a human instead of another duck. Imprinting illustrates how animals have a predisposition toward learning certain information at a certain point in their lifespan (Papalia, Olds, & Feldman, 2009).

Along with research regarding the effects of teratogens (DNA-altering substances) on prenatal development, many researchers have used the acquisition of language as evidence for the existence of critical periods in human development. Because children learn language from approximately ages 1 through 5 years, this age span has been termed a critical period for language development. However, because it seems that the window of opportunity may never completely close (Bruer, 2001), many scientists now believe that the term "sensitive period" more accurately describes child development in various domains. A **sensitive period** refers to a timeframe when responses to development in certain areas will be optimal. The boundaries of a sensitive period are more flexible than those of a critical period. Proponents of sensitive periods believe that development in certain areas is still possible outside of the normally occurring period, but it is more difficult (Bjorkland & Pelligrini, 2002). So, while it is possible to learn a new language later in life, it will not be learned as well or as easily as it would have been during the first few years of life (Pinker, 1994).

Researchers continue to search for the reasons critical or sensitive periods exist. Is it because the brain is especially suited to learn certain types of information at certain times? Is it because humans are more susceptible to environmental inputs regarding certain types of learning at specific times? Both of these explanations may play a role in explaining the sensitive period for language acquisition. Young children lack the cognitive sophistication to analyze large amounts of knowledge at once, so they learn language bit by bit, making it easier to understand. However, once new language learners become older, their inability to "turn off" their interpretation and analysis of new vocabulary and grammar makes it harder for them to comprehend a new language (Papalia et al., 2009). So the cognitive development of young children makes them more suited for language acquisition. Their environmental inputs may also make them especially responsive to language acquisition. Young children can learn language by becoming totally immersed in it rather than through formal schooling because they have no other language system through which to filter communication (Broderick & Blewitt, 2014).

While language provides an excellent example of the existence of critical or sensitive periods for one aspect of development, not all facets of human development are confined to critical or sensitive periods. These various aspects of development that can be modified throughout the lifespan show plasticity. In other words, aspects of behavior that are amenable to influence and change throughout the entire lifespan are plastic. For example, older adults can work to improve their memories with training and practice. Physical exercise can even stimulate the formation of new neurons in the hippocampus, the area of the brain responsible for memory (Pereira et al., 2007). Thus, memory is an aspect of development that can be influenced at any time in life by environmental inputs. **Plasticity**, or flexibility, is an important characteristic of much of human development.

Active versus Passive Development

Developmental theorists also debate whether child development is an active or a passive process. Proponents of the **active development** viewpoint believe that children actively construct their own worlds and initiate their own growth. The active theme extends even to unconscious choices made by individuals that affect their development. In other words, developmentalists consider a child to be active in development whenever some characteristic of that child influences the environment he is experiencing (Shaffer & Kipp, 2010). For example, a child who lags behind his peers in physical development did not choose to appear this way. However, the child's small stature will likely affect the way he experiences both his environment and his treatment by others. Counselors who embrace the active viewpoint will likely use more humanistic approaches to facilitate personal expression and meaning making.

Those who espouse the **passive development** perspective maintain that children are passively shaped by their environments. These people believe that humans have little control over the external forces that shape their development. Thus, proponents of this viewpoint believe that the environment and parents of developing children have enormous effects on a child's ultimate developmental outcomes. This perspective is indicative of behavioral counseling theories, which hold humans to be highly malleable and receptive to environmental influence.

Clearly, like many of the seemingly dichotomous themes discussed in this section, it would be inaccurate to only believe humans to be either active or passive in their development. As you will see in the discussion about nature and nurture, both the developing person and the environment can mutually influence each other. Thus, while the developing person takes in information from the environment, the person also influences the environment experienced through subsequent reactions. Furthermore, understanding of the information one continues to take in from the environment is influenced by prior experiences and knowledge. This constructivist process can be embraced in therapy to help clients reevaluate the way they make meaning in their personal narratives.

Nature versus Nurture

Which do you think plays a more important role in influencing child development, nature or nurture? If you are having trouble deciding, you are in the company of the many philosophers, psychologists, and developmental scientists who have argued over this issue for years. **Nature** refers to the biological characteristics and predispositions that an individual inherits, while **nurture** refers to environmental influences and experiences. As you think about the importance of both nature and nurture on child development, keep in mind that there are various forces and processes that can fall under these two categories. For example, "nature" encompasses heredity, universal maturational processes, biological predispositions, and hormones (Papalia et al., 2009). "Nurture" ranges from the interactions between a child's family members, peers, school, neighborhood, government, and culture, to the internal environment of their genes and cells.

Developmental scientists have been in contention for centuries regarding whether nature or nurture is more influential in child development. Prior to 1690, most people assumed that human nature was predetermined (Steinberg, Bornstein, Vandell, & Rook, 2011). In contrast, John Locke, an English philosopher, contended that an infant's mind was a *tabula rasa*, or blank slate, so that everything in a child's development was the result of experience and environment. In the late 19th century, Sir Francis Galton, who invented the term "nature versus nurture," presented the opposite viewpoint by proposing that biological characteristics were the main determinants of human nature (Sameroff, 2010). In the 1920s, John Watson and other behaviorists contended that learning and experience accounted for differences in individual development. For the remainder of the 20th century, various movements and key people swayed the debate in terms of nature or nurture. For example, the cognitivist revolution of Piaget in the 1960s positioned the mind of a child, rather than experience, as the essential location of individual differences. However, Bronfenbrenner's ecological model, developed in the 1970s, explained child development as influenced by the various influences of family, school, work, and culture, and the interactions between these systems. The continual oscillation between showing nature or nurture to be more important has obscured the importance of integrating the two influences on child development.

Recently, however, more and more scientists are beginning to appreciate and integrate the importance of both nature and nurture on human development (Dacey, Travers, & Fiore, 2009; Papalia et al., 2009). Sameroff (2010) is one of the biggest proponents of an integrated theory of human development, stressing not just nature and nurture, but nature and nurture interacting together. He insists that nature and nurture must be viewed as unified and continually influencing one another. Their interdependence can be understood by comprehending that nature and nurture modify each other, so depending on their unique combinations, they will produce unique outcomes. For example, individuals with the same genes, like twins, will develop differently if raised in different environments. Also, individuals in similar environments, like siblings or peers, will experience the same environment differently as a result of their different genetic makeups. Overall, it is essential to keep in mind the mutually important influences of both nature and nurture, since many complex human attributes such as intelligence, temperament, and personality are the result of the complicated interaction of biological and environmental forces (Shaffer & Kipp, 2010).

The Interaction of Genetics and Environment

Genetics and environment interact to influence development, but exactly how genes and the environment interact to produce various developmental outcomes varies according to the different attributes in question. For some traits, humans are restricted to a small number of outcomes simply as a function of their genes. This is referred to as **canalization** (Waddington, 1966). Traits that are mostly genetically predetermined, with little opportunity for environmental influence, are thus said to be canalized (Shaffer & Kipp, 2010). Close to conception, prenatal development is highly canalized; as individuals become older, their environments become increasingly influential. One example of a highly canalized trait is children's language acquisition (Lightfoot, Cole, & Cole, 2008). All children will develop language capacities unless they are exposed to severe environmental deprivation or extreme genetic disorders.

Environments are also capable of canalizing child development, meaning that some environmental conditions can be so potent that they affect child development regardless of genetic characteristics. For example, children who grow up in economically disadvantaged environments are at risk for permanently impaired cognitive, academic, and socioemotional development (Votruba-Drzal, 2006). Thus, even children with a genetic disposition to be smart may struggle in school as a result of their deprived home environments.

However, most attributes are not determined by rigid canalization (Shaffer & Kipp, 2010). While genes often set the boundaries for trait expression, other genes and environmental input determine exactly where a trait's expression will fall within that genetically predisposed range (Gottesman & Hanson, 2005). Thus, genes set the upper and lower limits on trait expression, and the environment determines the final outcome. So, while genes determine what we are capable of doing, the environment determines what we actually do. This principle is evident in recent research indicating that genes determine the stability of cognitive ability in adulthood, while environmental inputs determine the change in cognitive ability (Lyons et al., 2009).

Not only do genes determine our range of outcomes, they can actually influence the environments that we experience (Scarr & McCartney, 1983). This is because our environments are affected by both our genes and the genes of our parents. Scarr and McCartney proposed three types of bidirectional genotype-environment interactions, including passive genotype-environment correlations, evocative genotype-environment correlations, and active genotype-environment correlations.

In **passive genotype-environment correlations**, the child is reared in an environment influenced by the genotypes of the parents (Scarr & McCartney, 1983). The child's own genotype is also provided by the biological parents; thus, the parents provide both genes and environment, which influence the child's development. An example of this would be if a child has parents who enjoy and have talent in artistic endeavors such as painting and drawing. These parents are likely to provide their child with art materials and instruction and practice creating art. Thus, the child is likely to become a skilled artist who enjoys expressing himself creatively, due to both his genotype and the environment provided by his parents.

In **evocative genotype–environment correlations**, the features of the child, which are influenced by his genes, evoke reactions from others toward him (Scarr & McCartney, 1983). These responses then further shape the child's development. For example, a child who has long, thin fingers might be encouraged to play the piano by his parents. His parents might then purchase a piano or send him to piano lessons. Thus, the child's genotype influences the environment that is provided for him.

In **active genotype–environment correlations**, the child seeks out environments consistent with his genetic makeup and thereby creates his own environment, which then strengthens his inherent qualities (Scarr & McCartney, 1983). So, by selecting activities and environments that match his genetic predisposition, a child perpetuates and strengthens his inherent qualities. For example, a child who is genetically predisposed to be open to new experiences will actively seek out new activities to pursue and new people to meet. The more the child seeks out new experiences and enjoys them, the more likely he will be to continue to seek out additional new experiences. Thus, the initial experiences driven by a child's genotype lead to further experiences. The active genotype–environment correlation gets stronger with age, because children are increasingly able to select their own environmental niches. Thus, genes and environments can interact to restrict the range of attribute expression, or they can combine when the genes of children and their parents elicit various environments. It is important to remember that genes *influence*, rather than *determine*, environments.

Genetic Contributions

An understanding of human development would not be complete without knowledge of the specific contributions of genetics to growth and development. **Epigenesis** is the idea that environments shape our genetic expressions, which in turn further shape our environments. Thus, epigenesis goes one step further back than Scarr and McCartney's (1983) model by positing the importance of the environment and experience on initial gene expression. For example, hormone levels are affected by experiences in our environment such as the length of sunlight on a given day, nutrition, toxins, and stress. These hormone levels then affect protein production, and can thus turn on certain genes to allow for their phenotypic expression or keep them shut off.

The concept of the environment acting to "turn on" certain genes is well illustrated by Kim-Cohen and Gold's (2009) research on the link between early childhood abuse and resilience. Among the children who experienced early childhood abuse, a certain genetic subset showed resilience and effectively avoided maladaptive development. Children who had certain genetic structures (i.e., high-activity MAOA or long 5-HTT alleles) were resilient in the face of child abuse. So those with resilient alleles had less chance of psychopathology compared to those without the resilient alleles, even in situations of high environmental risk. In situations of low environmental risk, however, the two groups of children had similar outcomes because the allele was not "turned on" by experience. This provides evidence that children may experience similar things differently due to their different genotypes.

Many developmental scientists have attempted to determine the **heritability** of a trait, or the extent to which the outward expression of a trait is genetically determined. Heritability is usually represented as a heritability quotient, or the percentage of variation in trait expression that can be attributed to genetic factors. For example, researchers have demonstrated that children's activity level has high heritability (Wood, Rijsdijk, Saudino, Asherson, & Kuntsi, 2008). This means that genetics plays a large role in the hyperactivity and impulsivity that characterize children with attention-deficit/hyperactivity disorder (ADHD).

Twin studies have provided valuable information regarding genetic contributions to development. Because identical twins are genotypically identical, any differences between them must be due to their environments. Fraternal twins, on the other hand, are no more genetically similar than ordinary siblings. Thus, if the expression of a trait is mainly genetically determined, identical twins should look much more similar than fraternal twins. For example, twin studies have shown intelligence to have high heritability (Brant et al., 2009).

It is important to keep in mind that while heritability and genes are influential, the environment is always influential to some extent. Simply knowing the heritability of a trait does not guarantee that you know exactly how it will be expressed in various individuals. Unfortunately, knowing the heritability of a trait does not give us any information regarding the ease or difficulty of attempting to alter that trait (Mullen, 2006). This is important information to be aware of for counselors trying to help clients achieve change and parents trying to nurture their children. In brief, regardless of whether a characteristic is attributed mainly to genetics or experience, the possibility of affecting change does exist. This is essential for professional counselors to understand and to convey to clients and students who may believe they have little control over the expression of their genes—or thoughts, feelings, or behaviors.

The contribution of genetics to mental disorders has been widely studied. Most recent evidence has suggested that the most common and most severe mental disorders have moderate to high heritability (Keller, 2008). This means that individual genetic variance is largely responsible for the development of most mental disorders. Autism spectrum disorder is one of the mental disorders with the highest heritability, at 90%. Schizophrenia also has a high heritability (80%), while bipolar disorder has a more moderate heritability estimate, at 60%. The heritability of depression varies according to gender, with women having 40–42% heritability and men having 29–31% heritability (Verhagen et al., 2008).

Just like all other human characteristics, mental disorders are not due solely to genetic factors even if they are highly heritable. Wermter and colleagues (2010) posited the importance of using gene–environment interactions in understanding the factors that lead to the development of mental disorders, since these interaction effects have been noted in ADHD, anxiety, schizophrenia, and substance use disorder. For example, in a classic study, Caspi et al. (2003) found that differences in the promoter region of the serotonin transporter gene resulted in differential responses to stressful life events. Carriers of two long alleles were less likely than carriers of one or two short alleles of this gene to exhibit depression and suicidality after experiencing stressful life events. Thus, while having one or two short alleles did not necessary predict depression, the experience of stressful life events could make such a person more prone to depression than a more resilient carrier of two long alleles.

In summary, it is important to consider both genetic contributions, like heritability, and gene–environment interactions to fully understand the causes of most major mental disorders and other human characteristics. It seems impossible to disentangle nature from nurture.

Environmental Contributions

While you have just seen how genetics is often extremely influential, the environment in which a child grows up has the potential to be just as influential. We will first discuss the various potential influences of family, socioeconomic status, poverty, neighborhood, school, and culture. We will then place these factors in a broader ecological model to facilitate your understanding of the contributions of the environment to child development.

The family is an incredibly important and influential context of development for children. Because the family is the main developmental context for children until they enter school, it is hugely important in influencing early development and creating enduring patterns. While the nuclear family used to be considered the norm, various other family structures are becoming increasingly common, including single-parent families, blended families, multigenerational families, and families headed by same-sex parents. Only 60% of U.S. children in 2009 lived in nuclear families, a notable decline from 84% of children in 1970 (Kreider, 2007; U.S. Census Bureau, 2010b). Of children, 23% now live in single-mother families, and this pattern is even more pronounced for minority and low-income children (Brown, 2010).

There is much debate regarding which types of family structures are optimal for child development. While children in families headed by two married, biological parents experience better educational, social, cognitive, and behavioral outcomes (Brown, 2010), divorce can actually be beneficial for children when their parents' marriage is characterized by high levels of conflict and abuse (Amato, 2004). Children living in a family with intimate partner violence (IPV) are at risk for a host of negative outcomes, including, but not limited to, pervasive fear, mood disorders, academic difficulties, and aggression (Bedi & Goddard, 2007). So divorce would likely be beneficial for these children. Keep in mind that while children are influenced by their parents' marital satisfaction, their behavior also influences their parents' marital functioning (Schermerhorn, Chow, & Cummings, 2010). Furthermore, the negative effects of not being in a nuclear family are more pronounced for Whites than for ethnic minorities (Brown, 2010). Lack of economic resources, inconsistent and unresponsive parenting patterns, and family turbulence are all cited as potential reasons for the more negative outcomes experienced by children not living in two-parent, married families.

Although marital status and biological parentage are both important for children's well-being, children raised by lesbian couples fare just as well as children of married, heterosexual, biological parents (Biblarz & Stacey, 2010). The data regarding the outcomes of children raised by gay men is sparse, but it is promising and favorable thus far. Biblarz and Stacey suggest that the presumption that men and women parent in different but equally necessary ways holds true in parent–child relationships but does not affect children's ultimate well-being and success. It is important to keep in mind that lesbian and gay parents are highly motivated to become parents and self-select into parenthood, unlike the range of motivations among heterosexual parents. This bias may affect the positive outcomes of the children raised in lesbian and gay families (Tasker, 2010).

Children living in single-parent families may find themselves in these family situations for a host of reasons, including parental separation, death, incarceration, and military deployment. Parental military deployment places the child at risk for various problems, including neglect, lower test scores, and both internalizing (e.g., anxiety, depression) and externalizing (e.g., oppositional, aggression) emotional and behavioral problems (Sheppard, Malatras, & Israel, 2010). However, military families often have strong support systems and active coping strategies, so many are quite resilient. Overall, children living in single-parent families are more likely to experience greater economic hardship and suffer negative effects on their well-being. Like European-Americans and African-Americans, Mexican-American children living in single-parent families report greater school misconduct and depressive symptoms, but their strong sense of family can serve as a protective factor (Zeiders, Roosa, & Tein, 2011). For Latina/o children, living with a single parent is also associated with less parental monitoring, which is associated with greater adolescent substance use (Wagner et al., 2010). Thus, living in single-parent homes may influence children based on the context of the home as well as the parenting behaviors influenced by the single-parent structure.

Socioeconomic status (SES) also has a substantial influence on child development. SES is based on parental income levels as well as such markers of "cultural capital" as educational attainment. Children from affluent homes usually fare better than children from poorer homes. For example, family income is strongly inversely related to aggression, so children from wealthy families are the least likely to behave aggressively (Vanfossen, Brown, Kellam, Sokoloff, & Doering, 2010). However, children from economically privileged families may suffer from the pressure to achieve and literal and emotional isolation from busy parents, which can result in anxiety, depression, and substance abuse (Luthar & Latendresse, 2005).

Overall, children living in poverty have an increased risk for health, behavioral, and social problems. For instance, children living in low-income families have an increased likelihood of lead exposure, which is linked with lower IQ scores and lower behavior regulation (Dilworth-Bart & Moore, 2006). Homeless children become sick more often (Markos & Lima, 2003) and are more likely than their housed peers to have problems with anxiety, depression, poor social skills, delays in speech and language development, aggression, and withdrawal (Walsh & Buckley, 1994). The various effects of poverty will be discussed later in this section in regard to Bronfenbrenner's model.

Neighborhood is often closely linked with SES, since parental income determines where the family can afford to reside. Across various outcomes, the economic status of the neighborhood seems to matter even more than other dimensions of the neighborhood, such as ethnic heterogeneity or stability (Vanfossen et al., 2010). Children who grow up in poor, dangerous communities are likely to have poor social skills and adjustment outcomes (Criss, Shaw, Moilanen, Hitchings, & Ingoldsby, 2009). Children residing in impoverished neighborhoods are also likely to be exposed to higher levels of both community and home violence (Fitzgerald, McKelvey, Schiffman, & Montanez, 2006). Exposure to neighborhood violence is associated with increased aggression in boys, while for girls neighborhood family structures seem to have the most impact on their aggression levels. For girls, increases in single male- and female-headed households are linked with an increase in aggression (Vanfossen et al., 2010). Clearly, residing in unsafe neighborhoods places children at risk for a host of problematic outcomes. Research on resiliency factors has identified social support from the family, peers, and community as critical elements of positive developmental outcomes for youth in such indigent conditions (Chapin & Yang, 2009).

Given the sizable amount of time children spend in school, the school has great potential to affect child development. Teachers, peers, and the school climate all interact to influence how the child feels about school and learning. The people and climate of the school can potentially serve as either protective or risk factors. For example, in regard to depression, school climates, teacher and peer relations, and academic achievement that provided opportunities for support, independence, and nurturing relationships were protective factors for children. School contexts that placed students at risk for depression were marked by criticism, rejection, and neglect (Herman, Reinke, Parkin,

Traylor, & Agarwal, 2009). Herman and colleagues have also suggested that schools can protect students by increasing perceptions of cohesion, cooperation, and satisfaction with classes, and decreasing competition and conflict. Thus, it is evident that the influence of the school climate can extend beyond academic engagement and perceptions of safety to mental health and well-being.

Finally, the influence of culture plays a critical role in child development. **Culture** encompasses the worldview of a group of people, including their beliefs, values, attitudes, language, and knowledge. Because culture influences the way people think about the world, people from different cultural backgrounds may perceive the world in diverse ways. Although there is great diversity among Americans, the majority of Americans espouse **individualistic values** and strive to teach their children to be independent. Thus, Americans engage in practices designed to help children learn to value independence and individualism. This individualistic viewpoint stands in stark contrast to the **collectivistic worldview** held by many in other cultures such as the Japanese and Mayans.

We can see how worldviews can have a profound influence on the way people perceive child-rearing practices in the example of co-sleeping, the practice of parents and children sharing the same bed or bedroom area. Based on their opposing worldviews of individualism and collectivism, Americans and Mayans had extremely different reactions to the practice of co-sleeping. Americans thought co-sleeping was strange and dangerous, while Mayans viewed making the child sleep alone as equivalent to child neglect (Morelli, Rogoff, Oppenheim, & Goldsmith, 1992). Thus, cultural values prescribed how parents should raise their children. The impact of culture on child-rearing practices then extends to how the child develops as a result of those practices. The importance of culture will be discussed again in regard to Bronfenbrenner's ecological model and the developmental niche model.

The **ecological model of child development** can be used as a broad theoretical framework to understand environmental contributions. Bronfenbrenner (1994) created the ecological model of human development in the 1970s, and it has become incredibly influential and widely accepted since then. Bronfenbrenner believed that the developing child is continually influenced by the systems within which the child is embedded. The reciprocal, enduring interactions between the developing child and his environment are termed **proximal processes**. Examples of proximal processes would include parent–child activities or play with a group of peers. Furthermore, not only does the child interact with these various systems, but the systems also interact with each other to influence the child's development.

Bronfenbrenner (1994) has likened the developmental context to a series of nested Russian dolls that fit within each other. You can also imagine Bronfenbrenner's model as an individual child in the center surrounded by concentric circles which increase in size, as depicted in Figure 1.3. Each of these concentric circles represents the four nested systems of the ecological model, which are the microsystem, mesosystem, exosystem, and macrosystem. As the systems

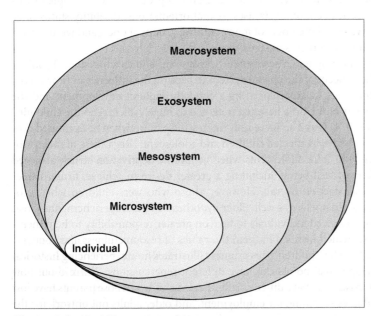

Figure 1.3 Bronfenbrenner's model.

increase in distance from the center of the circle, so they also increase in distance from the individual child to broader, cultural concepts. We will discuss each of these systems in detail.

Bronfenbrenner (1994) defines the **microsystem** as a pattern of "activities, social roles, and interpersonal relations experienced by the developing person in a given face-to-face setting with particular physical, social, and symbolic features that invite, permit, or inhibit engagement in sustained, progressively more complex interaction with, and activity in, the immediate environment" (p. 39).

It is within these immediate, face-to-face settings that proximal processes operate to drive individual development. The settings of the microsystem vary depending on a person's age. For example, an infant will likely primarily experience the family microsystem. As the child develops, he will come into contact with various other microsystems, such as extended family, day care, the neighborhood, school, and peer groups. Remember that the influences in the microsystem, as in all of Bronfenbrenner's systems, are reciprocal. So not only is the child influenced by his family, community, school, and peers, but he influences them as well. The various factors of family, neighborhood, and school discussed above would be considered microsystems.

The **mesosystem** is defined as the connections and relationships between two or more microsystems. Examples of mesosystems include the linkages between home and school or neighborhood and school. Problems in one microsystem can spill over into other microsystems, affecting them as well.

The **exosystem** is defined as the connections and relationships between two or more settings, at least one of which the developing child does not experience directly. Even though the child does not experience these settings directly, the exosystems still indirectly influence the development of the child by shaping the behavior of people who interact with the child or by defining a larger context that affects the child's life (Steinberg et al., 2011). Examples of exosystems include the relationships between the home and a parent's workplace or between the school and the community.

The outermost system in Bronfenbrenner's (1994) model is the **macrosystem**, which is the overarching cultural context in which the other systems are embedded. The macrosystem includes the various beliefs, values, customs, lifestyles, and political and social institutions and events that characterize a culture. Cultural groups include people of different ethnic heritages, socioeconomic statuses, sexual orientations, disability statuses, or religious worldviews. We are all members of many cultural groups at once, and we are influenced by all of these cultural contexts in some way.

In addition to the microsystem, mesosystem, exosystem, and macrosystem, Bronfenbrenner introduced the concept of the **chronosystem** to capture the influence of time on the developing person. The changes experienced by a child throughout development and the historical and social events of the time have the potential to hugely affect who the child ultimately becomes. Elder (1974) found an incredibly interesting pattern when he examined how the Great Depression of the 1930s affected children and adolescents. Regardless of their prior economic status, those who were adolescents when economic deprivation struck achieved various positive markers of well-being, including a greater desire to achieve, firmer career goals, and greater life satisfaction overall. However, those who were children when economic deprivation struck did not fare as well. Elder hypothesized that experiencing the Great Depression as a teenager enabled individuals to take on greater responsibility to help themselves and their families, which instilled in them the values of resourcefulness and cooperation to a higher degree than for children. This example illustrates how experiencing historical events at various developmental points can have different repercussions. Think about how more recent economic crises may have differentially affected children whose parents have lost their jobs, college graduates searching for employment, and older adults out of work for the first time in their lives. Bronfenbrenner's framework is demonstrated in Case Example 1.2.

➤ CASE EXAMPLE **1.2**   AN APPLICATION OF BRONFENBRENNER'S THEORY.

The achievement gap is a serious problem in America today. Children of low socioeconomic status are consistently outperformed by their higher socioeconomic status peers. One explanation is that children of poverty generally do not receive as much cognitive stimulation in a warm, supportive environment as their more economically advantaged peers (Votruba-Drzal, 2006). Here we see how a lack of stimulation and warmth at home can result in problems with emotional regulation and academic achievement at school (mesosystem).

Expectancies and values in various microsystems can also either support or conflict with each other. Conflicts between expectancies and values at home and in school can prove especially problematic. Using the conflict of microsystems as a basis for explanation, another reason for the achievement gap is that expected modes of interaction at home and in school conflict for low-SES children and match for middle- and high-SES children (Payne, 2008). Thus, the relationship between the microsystems of home and school for children of lower economic means results in a problematic mismatch that harms their academic potential.

Children growing up in poverty also experience less cognitive stimulation at home and learn modes of interaction with their parents that do not match the way they are expected to behave in school. Living in impoverished circumstances can result in chronic economic stress, which can cause parents to experience more mental health problems, less marital satisfaction, and lower self-esteem (Votruba-Drzal, 2006). The emotional distress thus experienced by many parents living in poverty is linked to less nurturing and less responsive parenting practices, which can be harmful for children's well-being and academic achievement. So one can see how the reciprocal relationship between the parent and neighborhood (exosystem) can influence a child's development.

At the macrosystem level, values and lifestyles of children growing up in poverty may look somewhat different from "typical" American values and lifestyles espoused by the middle class. Economically disadvantaged children are likely to place a strong value on family relationships and view obtaining daily necessities for survival as paramount (Daniels, 1995). This contrasts with the middle-class values of negotiation, competition, individualism, and future orientation. It is easy to see how the pervasive influence of social and historical contexts affects child development, especially when one considers the overlay of the chronosystem—such as during an economic downturn that might reduce the earning ability of a family already in a dire economic state.

Another useful framework for understanding how the environment affects the development of a child is Super and Harkness's (1994) **developmental niche model**. The developmental niche model is very similar to Bronfenbrenner's ecological model, but it places increased emphasis on the overarching effects of culture on all of the systems influencing child development. The central point of the Super and Harkness model is that physical and social settings, customs of child rearing, and caretaker psychology all exist under the umbrella of overarching cultural values. These three components interact to shape how a child in a particular culture is raised, and they influence each other bi-directionally as well. Case Example 1.3 provides an illustration of the developmental niche model.

➤ CASE EXAMPLE **1.3**   THE DEVELOPMENTAL NICHE MODEL.

It is perhaps easiest to understand the concept of the developmental niche by looking outside U.S. culture, although it certainly operates in the various facets of American culture as well. The Yoruban practice of sending their children on community errands as toddlers (Zeitlin, 1996) is illustrative of the developmental niche model. The Yoruban cultural values and ideologies, or macrosystem, include the belief that childhood is a time to develop the skills to become self-reliant in order to help the family. Thus, their caregiver psychology is that social development and self-reliance should be promoted in children to ensure that they become autonomous and able to care for themselves by the age of 7. Errands are a custom that enables the Yoruban child to learn and practice self-reliance. As the child is entrusted with responsibility and engages in social interaction with others, he or she is being socialized into becoming a valuable member of society.

So errands are much like education. Also, the Yoruban people live in a rural African community where they can trust their neighbors, so their physical setting allows them to promote their child's social development without having to worry about the child's personal safety. Their social setting of large families and friendly neighbors also supports this practice. Thus, the Yoruban practice of errands is influenced by their macrosystem, caregiver psychology, and physical and social settings, culminating in the developmental outcome of early self-reliance, responsibility, and social skills. In summary, avoiding using false dichotomies and maintaining an awareness of the interacting and equally important contributions of genetics and the environment will help you to become a more effective professional counselor.

Types of Theory Structures Common in Human Development

There are three types of theories commonly used in understanding the vast majority of developmental research. These include stage theories, incremental theories, and multidimensional theories. Each will be discussed in turn.

Stage Theories

Stage theories propose that human development across the lifespan changes abruptly via rapid transformations that propel individuals from one stage of functioning to the next, where they remain quite stable for long periods of time. Each stage of functioning is seen as qualitatively different from the previous stage because individuals have achieved markedly new ways of thinking and behaving. Although some children move through these designated stages faster or slower than others, all children are believed to progress through these stages in the same order. Recall from the previous section regarding discontinuous versus continuous development that stage theorists view child development as akin to a staircase, where long periods of stability are interspersed with dramatic surges forward, in which the child attains advanced physical and cognitive functioning. Thus, stage theories are viewed as the opposite of incremental theories, which describe development in terms of more gradual, continuous growth. However, there is of course continuous growth within stages.

Stage theories are thus characterized by discontinuous development and periods of relative stability upset by dramatic transformations in functioning in which physical and cognitive abilities are propelled to a qualitatively different level than before. Another characteristic of stage theories is that specific stages are defined as much by what is included within them as by what is not included within them. In other words, explicit contrasts between functioning at various stages are very important.

Piaget's (1970) famous theory of cognitive development provides an excellent illustration of a stage theory. While Piaget's theory will be explained in greater detail in later chapters, in short, Piaget proposed four distinct stages of cognitive functioning from birth to adolescence. The first stage, the sensorimotor stage, encompasses the time from birth until 2 years. Infants in this stage hone their sensory and motor capabilities as they attempt to learn about the world through their actions on it. In the second stage, preoperational thought, children aged 2 to 7 gain the capacity to generate mental images of objects not present in their environment. This symbolic functioning is the precursor to language development. Children in the preoperational stage are also characterized by egocentrism, the tendency to think everyone else shares their perspective. This hampers reasoning skills and communication. Children in the preoperational stage are also limited by centering on only one aspect of a problem at a time and by their inability to reverse mental operations. By the time most children reach age 7, they are catapulted into the concrete operational stage, which is marked by their ability to think logically and understand the perspectives of others. They can focus on more than one aspect of a problem at a time, to integrate knowledge and reach rational conclusions. Not all individuals reach the fourth and final stage, formal operations. If individuals do reach the formal operations stage, it is typically attained between ages 11 and 15, when they demonstrate abstract thinking, along with advanced logic and reasoning skills.

Piaget's cognitive developmental theory is characteristic of a discontinuous stage theory for many reasons. First, there are four distinct stages that are seen as qualitatively different from each other. Children in each stage perform similarly across cognitive domains within their stage but are quite different from children in other stages. Second, individuals remain in these periods for extended periods of time until changes in the way they are able to think propel them to the next level of functioning. You can see how the development of symbolic functioning is a necessary achievement of the sensorimotor developmental period in order for children in the preoperational stage to achieve gains in language. Third, each stage is defined both by what is included and by what is excluded. For example, children in the preoperational stage are defined as much by their ability to engage in symbolic functioning (which was not present in the previous stage) as by their inability to focus on more than one aspect of a problem (which they are able to do in the next stage). Finally, the stages are invariant in sequence. Children could not possibly enter the formal operations stage without first progressing through the concrete operations stage because the cognitive accomplishments of the concrete operations stage are necessary for progression into the formal operations stage.

Incremental Theories

Incremental theories are essentially the opposite of stage theories. Rather than viewing development as long periods of stability interrupted by drastic, qualitative changes in functioning, incremental theorists believe development progresses along a gradual, continuous path, constantly building upon itself little by little. Recall from the previous section regarding discontinuous versus continuous development that incremental theorists conceptualize development as following the smooth path of an escalator. In summary, incremental theorists see change as gradual, steady, and specific to particular abilities rather than encompassing broad reorganizations.

B. F. Skinner's theory of operant conditioning (see Chapter 2) is perhaps one of the best examples of an incremental theory. Based on his research with animals, Skinner proposed that random behaviors produce either favorable or unfavorable outcomes (Skinner, 1953). Whether a behavior is met with a favorable or unfavorable outcome affects the likelihood that that behavior will be repeated in the future. Favorable outcomes, or reinforcers, increase the likelihood that a behavior will be repeated, thus strengthening the behavior. Reinforcers can be either positive, such as providing a desired reward, or negative, such as removing an aversive stimulus. Unfavorable outcomes, or punishments, decrease the likelihood that a behavior will be repeated, thus weakening or suppressing the behavior. Punishments can also be positive or negative. A positive punishment is one in which a negative stimulus is added, while a negative punishment is one in which a desired reward is removed.

This gradual shaping of behaviors by various outcomes over time leads to steady and continuous change. Skinner's theory of operant conditioning calls attention to the importance of many responses to a behavior, ultimately shaping that behavior. This slow, steady change is not marked by rapid, qualitatively different changes in functioning like the change of stage theories. Furthermore, the incremental change illustrated by operant conditioning is specific to one ability or skill at a time. The infant whose mother becomes excited and supportive when he babbles is likely to repeat this random occurrence because he gained a pleasant outcome, his mother's support and excitement. However, this shaping of babbling, a precursor to language, is not related to the infant's overall cognitive development in other domains.

Multidimensional Theories

Multidimensional, or systems theorists, suggest that development is characterized by both continuity and discontinuity. In effect, **multidimensional theories** integrate stage and incremental theories, acknowledging the importance of both. Multidimensional theories therefore describe both large and small qualitative and incremental changes. Broderick and Blewitt's (2014) suggestion that continuous change may ultimately lead to more stage-like developments fits well with a multidimensional outlook. Another important aspect of multidimensional theories is the fact that these theories acknowledge the complexity of reciprocal influences in development. Individuals are not simply influenced by their environment and heredity; rather, they exert influences on their environment and the expression of their genes as well.

Bronfenbrenner's ecological theory, described above in the nature versus nurture section, is an excellent example of a multidimensional theory. In brief, Bronfenbrenner's model describes the multitudinous mutual influences of various cultural systems and societal values on the developing individual. The developing child is influenced by, and influences, his relationships with family, school, the community, and peers, as well as the relationships among these systems and the overarching values and norms of his culture. Thus, Bronfenbrenner's ecological theory represents the epitome of the importance of interrelated causal processes in development.

Additionally, changes in Bronfenbrenner's model can be qualitative or incremental. For instance, a child moving toward more logical thought is likely doing so as a result of cognitive maturation and the influences of school and possibly family, community, and peers as well. As the child tests out new ideas and explanations for phenomena, he is likely to be reinforced for positive progress. Once the child develops a more logical understanding of the world around him, he can both act on the world in different ways and gain new experiences based on his newfound knowledge. His attainment of logical thought is likely to be an incremental process. However, once he pieces many new bits of knowledge together, the child is likely to experience a qualitative shift in which he will use his newfound logical way of thinking in various domains.

Counseling Perspectives: Normal versus Abnormal Development

Framing Situations from a Normal Developmental Perspective

As helping professionals, it is critical to understand the implications of approaching client situations from both normal and abnormal developmental perspectives. Counselors must always be aware that culture determines what is considered good versus bad, healthy versus unhealthy, and normal versus abnormal. Recall from above that while most Americans viewed co-sleeping as strange and dangerous, Mayans thought that making a child sleep alone constituted child neglect (Morelli et al., 1992). Differences between cultures do not necessarily imply that one culture or the other is deficient. Rather, what is considered normal and healthy must be viewed with cultural relativity, since the definitions of normality and abnormality are completely context dependent.

With this caution in mind, there are aspects of development that can be viewed from a normative perspective for children of most cultures. For instance, the developmental milestone of maturation, and the task approach of Arnold Gesell (1929; Gesell, Ilg, & Ames, 1974) provide physical, cognitive, language, and personal-social developmental markers that should be achieved by certain ages. If a child is not meeting developmental milestones within the expected timeframe, this should alert parents to the possibility of underlying problems. Additionally, if a child meets developmental milestones but then regresses, this could be a cause for concern. For instance, most infants experience separation anxiety by about 12 months of age. This distress, exhibited when the primary caregiver leaves the child's presence, is normal and developmentally appropriate. Separation anxiety may reappear during significant transitional times, such as when a child begins preschool or kindergarten. Children who cannot get past this latter bout of separation anxiety, or who exhibit it for longer periods of time later in childhood, are not displaying developmentally appropriate behavior. Because this behavior is no longer considered normative in middle childhood, an 8-year-old child exhibiting such behaviors may be diagnosed with separation anxiety disorder.

In summary, knowledge of appropriate physical, cognitive, social, and emotional capabilities throughout the lifespan provides counselors with an understanding of which client behaviors and cognitions are developmentally appropriate and which may necessitate intervention.

Nosological Systems of Problem Identification and Intervention Selection

Within the traditional medical model, practitioners are concerned with the classification of physical and mental illnesses. Some helping professionals focus on identifying mental illnesses. **Abnormality** is defined as behavior that is deviant from the norm, distressing, dysfunctional, or potentially dangerous to the individual or others.

Because norms for conduct differ cross-culturally, and even across subgroups within cultures, the definition of abnormality may vary across cultures. However, any thoughts, behaviors, or emotions that break the norms of psychological functioning in a given society are considered abnormal. Determination of abnormality also depends on the specific circumstances surrounding the seemingly deviant thoughts, emotions, or behavior. Natural disasters, war, loss of a loved one, and terminal illness can all result in long periods of sadness that might resemble depression. However, with knowledge of the special circumstances preceding a client's seemingly abnormal functioning, counselors can gain greater understanding of the reasons behind the client's seemingly abnormal behavior. Sadness would surely be a normative response for a victim of a natural disaster who lost relatives and belongings and had to start over in a new location and job.

Another critical part of the definition of abnormality is that it must be **dysfunctional**. This means that the individual experiencing abnormal thoughts, behaviors, or emotions is so distracted by them that he can no longer go about his everyday activities appropriately or productively.

The above definition of abnormality is somewhat vague and can leave clinicians wondering if a client's behavior is in fact abnormal or simply unusual. The best way to determine abnormality is to use a **nosological classification system** like the *Diagnostic and Statistical Manual of Mental Disorders* (DSM). The current edition of this manual is the DSM-5 (American Psychiatric Association, 2013). The DSM-5 provides descriptions of symptoms and guidelines for determining if an individual meets the clinical diagnosis for any of about 400 mental disorders. Likewise, the World Health Organization (WHO, 2011) produces the *International Classification of Diseases—10th Edition—Clinical Modification* (ICD-10-CM). The ICD-10-CM provides descriptions and symptoms for more than 1000 medical and psychological disorders.

When clinicians decide that a client's pattern of abnormality matches the description of symptoms within a particular disorder, they are able to make a diagnosis. Clinical diagnosis is helpful because it allows clinicians to understand more about the disorder in general and then apply that knowledge to select appropriate interventions to effectively help their clients.

Understanding of the DSM-5 would not be complete without knowledge of the basic criticisms of this widely used classification system. To begin with, some researchers question whether mental disorders should be classified according to a categorical or a dimensional system (Widiger & Samuel, 2005). Widiger and Samuel assert that categorical classification presupposes that the conditions in the DSM are qualitatively different from normal functioning and discrete from one another. The fact that many disorders occur together but are still considered discrete is a major problem with the current DSM. Additionally, the DSM is plagued by problematic boundary disputes. Thus, many clinicians may have a difficult time deciding where to draw the line between two very similar disorders. Widiger and Samuel suggested that boundary disputes may be challenging because the DSM forces clinicians to decide where clients lie on artificial categories imposed on continuums of functioning. Thus, they argue for an approach that focuses not just on discrete categories but on degrees of functioning.

Others criticize the dominance of the DSM in making judgments about abnormal behavior. Overreliance on the DSM clouds the clinician's ability to consider alternative explanations for seemingly abnormal behavior (Duffy, Gillig, Tureen, & Ybarra, 2002; Saleebey, 2001). Additionally, because the DSM is guided by the views of the dominant majority, it may discount the perspectives of marginalized subcultures (Duffy et al., 2002).

Marginalized populations, as well as the dominant populations, are also disadvantaged by the DSM due to its assumption that the problem at hand lies within the individual rather than in the environment (Ivey & Ivey, 1998). For example, women diagnosed with premenstrual dysphoric disorder are more likely to be in stressful life situations, yet by labeling these women with a mental disorder, their problems are determined to be internally caused rather than the result of systemic barriers and external circumstances (Duffy et al., 2002).

As a result of the problems inherent in use of the DSM for classification and description of mental disorders, some have suggested that using a medical model may be inappropriate (Duffy et al., 2002). Society attaches a stigma to mental illness, and diagnostic labels may exacerbate the stigma by enhancing the public's view of those with mental illness as different from themselves (Corrigan, 2007). Given the repercussions of being a member of a stigmatized group and the potential harmful effects of labeling, it seems that a strengths-based approach focused more on wellness than on deficits may be beneficial. Because the current DSM disregards the potential strengths of individuals, which may be the most important potential resources in recovery, Saleebey (2001) has suggested that positive traits, talents, knowledge, capacities, and personal and environmental resources should be assessed as another axis of the DSM.

Emphasis on a wellness model has grown in recent years. The positive psychology movement that appeared at the turn of the century promotes meaning, virtue, resilience, and well-being as the four pillars of the good life (Wong, 2011). The wellness and positive psychology movements acknowledge that all of these pillars are shaped by culture, so positive outcomes may be defined as beneficial for the individual or for the group. Proponents of positive psychology maintain that it is essential to understand what makes life meaningful, how life can be improved for all people, and how to maximize the positives in one's life to eliminate the negatives.

Building up positive resources as a preventive measure is the cornerstone of a wellness-based model. Davis and Asliturk (2011) maintain that those who are resilient in stressful situations are those who have engaged in proactive coping and preventive problem-solving measures. They assert that learning to anticipate and plan for potentially necessary alternative options in life is a skill that can be taught.

The focus of wellness and positive psychology on resilience and positive rather than negative aspects of a person's life and functioning is echoed in the driving principles behind solution-focused brief counseling (SFBC) as well. SFBC is characterized by a focus on what is working rather than what is not working for a client. Research has shown that a solution-focused orientation increases client self-confidence and positivity (Wehr, 2010).

The second wave of the positive psychology movement addresses concerns raised by some that ignoring a problem results in an unbalanced approach. The new wave of positive psychology endorses the importance of both enhancing the positive aspects of an individual's life and functioning and effectively managing negative aspects (Wong, 2011). This balanced approach has the potential to both increase positive well-being and decrease negative mental health aspects. Wellness and positive psychology further advocate for a systemic viewpoint. Wong identifies the development of a more civil society as a positive context for living as key to a future agenda. This work has been expanded by Magyar-Moe (2009) and Seligman, Rashid, and Park (2006).

Clinicians will have to weigh the costs and benefits of strict adherence to a nosological classification system such as the DSM-5 against taking a wellness-based approach. It is recommended that helping professionals gain understanding of, and competence in, using the DSM-5 as well as knowledge of its limitations. Incorporation of a wellness-based approach commensurate with the positive psychology or wellness movements or SFBC can be a proactive, preventive, and effective approach.

Studying Human Development

Human development is studied to better understand human beings and to better predict normal and abnormal processes. The better our understanding of normal and abnormal processes, the more efficient and effective our counseling interventions can become. In order to study human development, researchers must determine what type of design to use in their study and how to go about collecting data. The focus of this section will be on data collection methods and research designs. There are various advantages and disadvantages to each data collection method and research design, so researchers must carefully choose which method best meets their needs.

Researchers seek to have both internal and external validity in their studies. **Internal validity** refers to the soundness of the study. When a study is internally valid, the researcher can confidently determine that the change in the dependent variable (outcome) is due to the conditions the researcher introduced in the independent variable, and not due to other potentially confounding variables. Thus, all sources of potentially confounding variables must be controlled or removed. This ensures that the study has high internal validity. But as experimental control increases, applicability and generalizability to the real world, or **external validity**, sometimes decreases. In other words, if a study is externally valid it has high generalizability to other samples and to the real world. As experimental environments become increasingly controlled for internal validity, some of the real-world generalizability may be lost. Thus, researchers should seek to maximize both internal validity and external validity in their data collection and research study designs.

Data Collection Methods

Researchers use various data collection methods to gather data for their studies. Here we will discuss standardized testing, naturalistic observation, case study, and self-report methods. Although this list does not include all of the potential avenues for data collection, those outlined in this section are the most commonly used by researchers studying human development.

Standardized Testing

Researchers can use **standardized testing** to obtain measures of behavior and personality attributes such as intelligence, memory, and self-esteem. Standardized tests are given and scored using uniform procedures for all test takers. Because standardized tests are normed on large populations, researchers can compare the performances and individual differences among participants. An example of a standardized test is the Scholastic Assessment Test

(SAT-I). Your score on the SAT tells you how you compare with the millions of other students who have taken the test.

Standardized tests can be quite expensive for researchers to purchase, and their administration, scoring, and interpretation can be time consuming. However, if a standardized test is available for the construct the researcher is interested in studying, many consider its use a good idea. This is because scores on standardized tests often have high levels of documented score reliability and validity. This means that the results of standardized tests are generally consistent over time and the test accurately measures what it is designed to measure.

Standardized tests have some inherent weaknesses, as the uniform administration procedures do not allow administrators to vary from them or to collect additional information about a potential problem area until after the testing has concluded. Also, because the tests are "objective," the questions and answers tend to be written to capture presupposed answers that can be easily categorized and scored for accuracy. Thus, participants often must answer briefly (e.g., coloring in a bubble on a multiple choice test), rather that provide a rich description of the reasoning process they used to arrive at an answer. Standardized tests also tend to be expensive to administer and score, although many publishers offer discounted pricing for use of instruments in research studies.

Naturalistic and Structured Observations

Naturalistic observation is used when researchers want to unobtrusively observe people going about their usual business in everyday settings. These settings can include school, home, the workplace, parks, or any place where people carry out the activities of their everyday lives. The researcher does not seek to manipulate the environment or the behavior of the participants in any way. It is important for researchers to define exactly which behaviors they plan to observe prior to conducting the observation. Usually, researchers remain removed from the situation they are observing and avoid interaction with the participants. The researchers instead choose an inconspicuous location and proceed to take notes about observed behaviors in order to draw conclusions in the future. By keeping their presence discreet, researchers can avoid the possibility of **reactivity**, which occurs when people being observed act differently than they usually would simply because they know that they are being observed.

An example of naturalistic observation would be a researcher observing children in a classroom during school. You can see how a child being observed for behavioral problems might try to be on his best behavior if he knows the reason for the observer's presence. Alternatively, he might act out even more or in different ways than he usually does, which would compromise the validity of the results obtained. Thus, it is often best to remain inconspicuous when conducting naturalistic observations (e.g., behind a one-way mirror, use of closed circuit cameras, use of concealed recording equipment).

Of course, there are times when remaining unobtrusive is just not possible. An example of this would be a researcher seeking to study a child's interactions with his parents or siblings in the child's own home environment. Obviously, the child will notice the researcher's presence in his or her own home, so in situations like these it may be better for the researcher to spend time in the child's home prior to the study so the child can become used to the researcher's presence and behave more naturally when the study is conducted.

The benefits of naturalistic observation are evident. Naturalistic observation provides the clearest picture of how people actually behave in everyday situations. It also provides detail and depth not possible in more structured experiments. Naturalistic observation is very useful for studying populations that lack the capacity to provide reliable self-reports. Young children may lack the verbal skills to adequately express their thoughts, feelings, and behaviors. By observing them researchers glean important information that might otherwise be unobtainable. Using naturalistic observation could also provide more honest accounts of the behaviors of those who may try to hide maladaptive behaviors, such as persons with addictions, or those who cannot accurately recall their behaviors, like those suffering from Alzheimer's disease.

Unfortunately, there are limitations to naturalistic observations as well. The most problematic limitation is that the possibility always exists that people will behave differently as a result of being observed. For example, children may act especially silly or show off for a new adult audience. The researcher may also bias the behavior of the participants, either accidentally or purposefully. The researcher must be aware of his own personal biases, assumptions, and expectations before the study begins. Time can also pose an obstacle, as extensive amounts of time are often spent waiting for the target behavior to be presented. Studying rare or unpredictable behaviors is thus less feasible. Finally, although naturalistic observations can have strong explanatory power for the specific participants being studied, the lack of experimental control results in the researcher's inability to pinpoint the causes of the observed behaviors.

Structured observation addresses some of these limitations by allowing researchers to design situations or stimuli to elicit the behaviors of interest. This allows researchers to increase internal validity and study more rare and unpredictable events. For example, Latane and Darley (1968) were able to test how participants reacted to a room filling with smoke when alone, with unworried confederates, or in groups of three. They found that people were much more likely to report the emergency when alone and least likely to report it when with passive others. This study of the "bystander effect" would not have been possible without staging the smoke-filling room. As a result, external validity may have been compromised because the results obtained in these structured observations may not transfer to the real world. The possibility exists that the participants behaved a certain way as a function of the experimental setting or due to reactivity, and thus their behavior may not generalize to the real world. Therefore, it is essential that the researcher strive to make the structured setting as realistic as possible in order to obtain generalizable results. In the final analysis, it is up to the researcher to choose either naturalistic observation or structured observation.

Case Study

A **case study** is an open-ended, in-depth examination of a "unit," such as a single individual, family, or small group. Information gathered in a case study can include interviews with the subject of the case study or known associates, observation, testing, or examination of the subject's personal materials, such as a diary. A researcher typically conducts a case study to learn more about a person with a rare condition or disorder in order to better understand how the condition or disorder may affect other individuals. The long-term nature of case studies provides researchers with ample time to gain a complete picture and rich detail, but the researcher must work to maintain objectivity. Unfortunately, because a case study focuses solely on one unit (e.g., person, group, family, class, community), it is difficult to generalize the observed responses to an entire population. However, the depth and elaboration provided by a case study enables researchers to gain knowledge about rare phenomena and make predictions about human development. Case studies are more useful as sources of rich detail and inspiration for further study than scientific explanations of causality, since any inferences about the reasons behind developmental paths taken are merely conjecture.

There are some conditions that would be unethical to inflict upon people in the name of research. However, when these conditions are naturally occurring, they present an opportunity for scientists to research the effects of these rare, harmful conditions on human development. An example of this would be the case study of Genie, a 16-year-old girl who suffered from extreme social isolation and environmental deprivation for the majority of her life. As a result, her language development was severely impaired and she had difficulty attempting to learn language at such a late age (Fromkin, 1974). Clearly, researchers could never legally or ethically keep a child in social isolation and deprivation for any period of time, but Genie's case presented a unique opportunity to learn about language acquisition after the early-childhood sensitive period for language.

Phineas Gage was also ideal for a case study. Phineas suffered trauma to his brain that resulted in changes in personality and functioning. Phineas went from a well-liked, temperate man to a man described as fitful, profane, and impatient, although the accuracy of these descriptions has been contested (Macmillan, 2000). By examining how Phineas Gage changed from before to after his accident, researchers were able to make predictions about the functions of the brain area that suffered trauma. So his accident provided a rare opportunity for researchers to learn more about individuals who survive severe brain trauma and to gain understanding about the functions of specific areas of the brain.

Thus, individuals with unique conditions that set them apart from the norm are the best candidates for case studies. However, as a careful consumer of information, keep in mind that case studies are not usually generalizable to a population and are subject to the researcher's personal biases. Furthermore, those who conduct case studies rarely corroborate their conclusions by eliciting the opinions of other professionals (Stake, 2010).

Self-Report

Self-report is another useful way of obtaining information about participants' attitudes, thoughts, feelings, and behaviors. Researchers can use a variety of methods, such as questionnaires, checklists, or interviews, to get participants to report various data about themselves. Interviews or surveys can be conducted in person, online, by telephone, or by mail. Researchers must be aware of age and cultural differences in comprehension and reading ability when administering written instruments. It is imperative that researchers design clear, unbiased survey or interview questions that adequately tap all aspects of the construct being studied. For example, a researcher attempting to learn more about a participant's self-esteem would want to assess how the person thinks, feels, and behaves in various situations with various people. It is the researcher's choice whether to follow a structured, standardized format or to use an open-ended format in which the questions flow more naturally from each other. While structured formats are useful for ensuring that every participant experiences the same interview or survey questions, open-ended formats provide the opportunity for elaboration and exploration of interesting information that arises during the interview.

Self-reporting is an advantageous data collection method because it allows researchers to collect a great deal of data in much less time than observational methods require. However, there are a few drawbacks to self-reporting that researchers must be aware of. First, using surveys or questionnaires with set responses may prove too limiting to accurately capture the span of possible responses, leading to a restricted range of data. For example, if a participant is forced to choose among four options, none of which truly apply, he will likely choose the closest possible answer. However, the researcher will not know the difference between this participant's choice of a close answer and another participant's choice of a definite answer, meaning each response will incorrectly be treated equally. Additionally, participants may choose not to respond to some questions, which makes data analysis more difficult. To guard against response bias, researchers should design short surveys with less time-consuming formats such as checklists instead of open-ended questions.

Another drawback of using surveys is that for sensitive topics on which participants may be embarrassed or ashamed to report honestly, the possibility exists that the data obtained will not accurately reflect how participants truly feel or behave. The tendency of participants to report socially desirable, rather than truthful, answers is a major problem with surveys in general, but especially with surveys around sensitive topics (Tourangeau & Yan, 2007). For example, in a study evaluating the drinking behaviors of adolescents, some adolescents may skew reality for a host of reasons, including, but not limited to, the desire to make themselves look better (i.e., social desirability), to help what they perceive to be the researcher's purpose, and even because they may not accurately recall correct information. Reducing the presence of the researcher and increasing the participant's motivation to be honest, through methods such as private data collection, assurance of confidentiality, survey self-administration, and priming of honesty, can reduce social desirability bias.

A good way to guard against untruthful responses is to include a social desirability measure, such as the Marlowe–Crowne Social Desirability Scale (Crowne & Marlowe, 1960). Items include statements like "I have never intensely disliked anyone," where people attempting to put on their best face would answer "true" even though that is not actually the case for most people. A high score on this measure indicates a high level of social desirability bias, and perhaps a need to discount a participant's data due to lack of truthful answers. Additional ways to guard against inaccurate responses are to ensure that questions are worded unambiguously and anonymity is assured. Finally, asking the same question in different ways will alert you to any inconsistencies in the responses.

Self-report data can be extremely useful because researchers gain participants' insights and evaluations of their own thoughts, feelings, and behaviors. While self-report is not always appropriate or practical, when researchers are able to use self-report, it is quite informative and time and cost effective.

Research Designs Most Commonly Used in Human Development Research

Data collection and research designs are intimately linked, since research designs inform data collection methods chosen and the data collection methods available limit the potential research designs that can be used. Various research designs, including correlational methods and experimental methods, are commonly reviewed in research courses; the reader is referred to Erford (2015) for expansions on these common designs. This section will focus on designs specific to human development research, such as longitudinal, cross-sectional, sequential, and time-lag designs. Finally, cross-cultural research will be highlighted. There are costs and benefits associated with using each of these methods.

Longitudinal Designs

When using **longitudinal designs**, researchers follow one group, or cohort, of participants over an extended period of time in order to repeatedly measure different aspects of development. A cohort is defined as a group of individuals born at about the same time who experience similar cultural and historical events as they grow up. By following the same group of participants over time, researchers are able to eliminate sources of individual variability in data collection. In other words, because researchers are evaluating the development of the same individuals over time, rather than different groups of individuals at the same time (as in cross-sectional research, which will be discussed next), researchers can be confident that the changes observed are the result of the passage of time rather than individual differences.

Researchers may choose to use longitudinal designs for various reasons. Longitudinal designs are often used to chart developmental trajectories, which illuminate developmental patterns over time. Thus, if a researcher is interested in determining at what age most children seem to develop various cognitive capacities, he could evaluate the same children at various intervals to pinpoint when these cognitive abilities, on average, begin to emerge. A researcher would also likely choose a longitudinal design if she wanted to examine the stability of personality traits or abilities over time. Finally, longitudinal designs are useful for tracking long-term effects of events experienced in early childhood. Najman et al. (2010) tracked a large cohort of participants over 21 years to determine the effects of poverty on anxiety and depression at different points throughout the lifespan. They found that the experience of poverty in late childhood and adolescence was a predictor of adolescent depression and anxiety. More frequent, recurrent exposure to poverty also increased the risk of children becoming anxious or depressed in adolescence. They were able to determine the cumulative effects of poverty by using a longitudinal design.

Thus, longitudinal designs are advantageous because they afford researchers the opportunity to chart developmental trajectories, track the stability of traits and abilities, and measure long-term effects. Furthermore, the use of the same participants over time eliminates individual differences and allows the researcher to be confident that observed changes are due to increases in age rather than differences among individuals. However, there are some limitations to longitudinal designs. Longitudinal designs are by nature extremely time consuming and expensive. In addition, **mortality** or **attrition** is a potential problem; that is, researchers may lose participants due to death, relocation, or a loss of interest in such a long-term undertaking. This introduces bias, because participants who choose to drop out or are forced to drop out due to relocation or death may be inherently different from participants who are able to remain in the study. For instance, those who drop out may be less reliable, less worried about pleasing others, or less economically privileged. In addition to the loss of motivation that may occur after repeated evaluations, the results of participants may become contaminated as a result of continued exposure to the independent variable over time.

Longitudinal designs are also problematic because the researcher cannot be sure that the observed changes will generalize to other age cohorts. The various historical events and cultural milieu experienced by one generation may affect their development so greatly that any results obtained from that cohort would not be comparable to other cohorts. For example, imagine that researchers were studying the prevalence of anxiety and post-traumatic stress disorder (PTSD) among today's generation of adolescents as they progress into young adulthood. It is quite likely that war and a poor economy may have effects on the mental health of this age cohort that would not necessarily be observed in the age cohort prior to, or following, the current cohort. Thus, anxiety and PTSD may be observed not as a result of simply getting older, but as a result of reaching young adulthood during such an unstable and stressful time. Some of these limitations of longitudinal designs can be addressed by using cross-sectional designs. An outstanding example of the complex principles that can be discerned from longitudinal designs is evident in the 30-year longitudinal attachment study conducted by Sroufe, Egeland, Carlson, and Collins (2005).

Cross-Sectional Designs

Instead of measuring the same individuals at multiple points across time as in longitudinal designs, researchers using **cross-sectional designs** measure individuals of different ages at a single point in time. This approach allows researchers the opportunity to determine the average behaviors and characteristics of people of a certain age, but no conclusions can be reached about the continuity of development. Researchers using the cross-sectional method compare different cohorts of participants at different times in their lives, but there is no measure of whether the groups were equal to start with. This approach assumes that older people in the study were similar to younger people in the study when the older people were younger, but in reality the disparate formative experiences shared by members of a younger or older generation may shape their development very differently. For example, older adults may be more politically active not because they are older *per se* but because they grew up during a time when political activism was valued more than it is today. Cross-sectional designs are quite susceptible to these **cohort effects**, which occur when observed differences may be due to shared experiences rather than maturation. Matching groups to ensure similarity prior to beginning the study is one way to minimize cohort effects. In general, it is good practice to always keep in mind that cohort effects can paint a misleading picture of human development.

There are, however, numerous advantages to using cross-sectional designs. To begin with, they are much less costly than longitudinal designs and can provide immediate results. There is no possibility of participant attrition or mortality since the study is performed in one shot. Additionally, unlike longitudinal designs, cross-sectional designs cannot suffer from practice effects from repeated testing. It is evident that longitudinal and cross-sectional methods seem to complement each other's limitations. The sequential method combines the cross-sectional and longitudinal designs to provide the best of both worlds.

Sequential Methods

As implied by the combination of longitudinal and cross-sectional methods, **sequential methods** measure multiple age cohorts at multiple intervals over time. This effectively allows researchers to pinpoint which observed differences are due to maturation, and which are due to shared historical or generational experiences. Sequential methods also enhance the generalizability of the results obtained. Thus, sequential designs are extremely advantageous. However, they are also tremendously time consuming, complex, and expensive to conduct.

Archambault, Eccles, and Vida (2010) provide an excellent example of a sequential study. They tracked first, second, and fourth graders from 10 different elementary schools over an 8-year period to assess their perceptions of ability and task importance in regard to literacy. The three groups of children were retested at five different intervals over the 8-year period. The researchers' use of a sequential design enabled them to track children's ability, self-concept, and subjective task value over the entire K–12 timespan. Although many children followed diverse patterns of decline, the vast majority of children experienced an overall decline in literary motivation. Perceptions of competence and task value seemed to vary together. These results cannot be deemed cohort effects because the research design included three different cohorts. Thus, it seems that the decline in literacy competence perceptions and motivation was likely due to common developmental or environmental factors. This study has significant implications for the importance of fostering competence and engagement in elementary school and maintaining it throughout high school.

Time-Lag Designs

Time-lag designs, also known as **cohort-sequential studies**, are replications of previous studies. By using the same age groups and parameters as researchers from a previous era, researchers from the current era can determine if dated findings still apply today or have changed in some way. For example, a study of self-esteem in adolescents conducted in the 1970s could be replicated to see if the self-esteem of adolescents today is similar to or different from the self-esteem of adolescents in the 1970s. The time-lag design clearly appears quite similar to the cross-sectional design. The difference lies in the fact that the different groups tested are of the same age at the time of the study but are separated by a number of years in history. In the cross-sectional design, the different groups tested are of varying ages at the time of the study and the study occurs at a single point in time. The time-lag design is by nature subject to the cohort effect, but this is viewed positively in this case because it allows researchers to make comparisons across generations.

Cross-Cultural Research

Cross-cultural research is conducted in order to illuminate the differences and similarities among various people of diverse cultures. The American Counseling Association recognizes that various facets of culture include age, disability, ethnicity, race, religion, spirituality, gender, gender identity, sexual orientation, marital status or partnership, language preference, or socioeconomic status (Herlihy & Corey, 2006). Because the majority of published research has been conducted mainly on middle-class Europeans or Americans, the account of human development across the lifespan lacks accuracy and specificity (Patterson & Hastings, 2007). There is a dearth of information pertaining to whether current theories and findings apply to people of other cultures or whether aspects of their development are characterized by entirely different processes and outcomes. Researchers thus use cross-cultural methods to compare data from two or more cultures. Finding commonalities extends the applicability of that specific domain of research to other cultures, while finding differences highlights variance in human development as a result of culture.

The first step in conducting cross-cultural research is to define the cultural group or subgroup being studied. Researchers may elect to study people of varying socioeconomic statuses or ethnic groups. Comparing people based on their country of residence is an interesting way to highlight broad cross-cultural differences. However, readers are cautioned to keep in mind that wide individual variation exists among members of a certain nationality. The concept of within-group variation is equally important when studying smaller subsets of a population, like Mexican-Americans or Americans living below the poverty line.

It is crucial for researchers studying other cultures to define the constructs to be examined with cultural sensitivity. For example, it is likely that depression will appear quite different in America than it will in a more traditional Eastern society like Japan. The Japanese culture, which is more collectivistic, discourages adults' expression of negative emotions that might negatively affect the harmony of the group (Safdar et al., 2009). However, in preschool, the expression of sadness is viewed positively because it enhances social interactions (Hayashi, Karasawa, & Tobin, 2009). Then, once close relationships have been established, older children cannot express sadness within these close relationships because it could upset the social harmony of the relationship. Thus, older Japanese children and adolescents are likely to mask negative emotions and may internalize depression by presenting with somatic complaints. Therefore, a survey instrument determining the prevalence of depression in America and Japan would need to account for the possible cultural differences in symptom presentation and willingness to share depression with others. Researchers must also be aware of the developmental changes likely to occur in symptom presentation. Researchers must be ever-cognizant of their own cultural assumptions and avoid imposing on others their perceptions of what is "right" or "natural."

An interesting example of cross-cultural research comes from St. James-Roberts and colleagues' (2006) investigation of different parental caregiving styles in London and Copenhagen. One group of London parents used the least physical contact and responsiveness to crying with their infants. The group of Copenhagen parents displayed more care and contact with their infants than the first group of London parents. A second group of London parents, termed proximal care parents, held their babies for the majority of the day, responded immediately to infant distress, and co-slept with their infants more than the other groups. Infants in the proximal care parenting group cried less daily overall but woke and cried more frequently at night at 12 weeks of age. London infants in the first group woke less frequently throughout the night but cried more overall. Copenhagen parents, whose parenting style represented a middle ground between the infant-response style of proximal caregiving and the traditional Western style of London parenting, had the best outcomes. The Copenhagen parents both minimized their infants' crying and maximized their infants' frequency of sleeping through the night, possibly due to their sleeping arrangement of having the baby in the room with them at night, but on a separate cot.

This cross-cultural research focused on examining differences and similarities across cultures by taking an etic approach. It would be helpful for future researchers to examine the macrosystem cultural values inherent in the cultures of London and Copenhagen to illuminate why most parents subscribed to these parenting practices. This article also high-lights the importance of recognizing subgroups within a culture rather than treating all the people as one homogenous group. Differences in cultural values likely exist for the subset of proximal care parents, driving their different style of caregiving.

The Ethics of Human Development Research

Researchers must take care when conducting any type of research, but research regarding human development presents special challenges. Because the participants involved are humans, and often children, researchers must be especially cautious in protecting the rights of their participants. It is necessary to obtain approval from Institutional Review Boards (IRBs) before beginning research. Various organizations, including the American Counseling Association (2014), have set forth ethical standards for conducting research with humans. The ethical principles of autonomy, nonmaleficence, and beneficence are of the utmost importance. **Nonmaleficence** means doing no harm, while **beneficence** means promoting the welfare of those involved. Research participants have the right to **autonomy**, meaning that they have the ability to make their own well-informed decisions. They should not be coerced or forced into participation in research. This principle ties in with the importance of informed consent.

Informed consent is necessary for participation in human development research. This means that a participant must have full knowledge of the potential risks, benefits, procedures, and purpose of the study. Participants must also be made aware that they are free to withdraw their participation at any time during the study, and without penalty. Children and those with cognitive limitations are not deemed able to provide informed consent, so researchers should obtain written consent from their parents or guardians. Researchers should still strive to provide information about the study to the child in vocabulary that the child can understand and to seek assent from the child participant.

However, what if you were conducting a study where giving away the purpose of the study at the beginning would influence or bias the results? This was the case in Bucciol and Piovesan's (2011) investigation into the relationship between honesty and age. Children aged 5 to 15 years tossed a fair white and black coin in private, then reported their results. Children were only rewarded for their white outcomes. Bucciol and Piovesan found that the probability of cheating was not related to age. They would not have been able to conduct this study if they had informed children at the outset of the study that they were study-ing cheating, because children likely would have behaved differently. When the research-ers performed the same experiment again but first told children not to cheat, the results were in fact different—children were less likely to inflate their reports of the prize-winning outcome.

Deception is therefore justified when the potential benefits outweigh the risks and there is no alternative way to achieve the desired results. When using deception, it is essen-tial for the researcher to explain the nature and purpose of the deception immediately after the study concludes. This explanation of the study's purpose, called **debriefing**, is necessary in all studies, but is especially important in studies where deception is used. The researcher should also use this time to ensure that the participant has not sustained any physical or psychological harm as a result of participation in the study.

Deciding whether it is appropriate to use deception falls under the overall umbrella of the principles of beneficence and nonmaleficence mentioned earlier. Again, beneficence refers to the responsibility of the researcher to uphold the best interests of the participant, while nonmaleficence refers to doing no harm. Taken together, these principles imply that the researcher must do everything possible to protect research participants from physical and psychological harm. Sometimes some level of risk or harm is unavoidable in the study.

For instance, it is likely that adolescents will feel embarrassed when asked about their sexual experiences, but if the benefits of the study outweigh this risk, the researcher can handle the situation by electing to conduct the study in a private setting, ensuring confidentiality, and taking steps to help the adolescent feel more comfortable at the conclusion of the study. Weighing the benefits of the study for the participants and humanity in general against the risks for the participants is the best way to determine whether the study is ethical. If the benefits greatly outweigh the risks and there is no less-invasive procedure, the study is deemed ethical. In the United States, children can only participate in research that poses greater than minimal risk if there is a direct benefit to the child or if the research produces knowledge about a condition that is generalizable to future children (Blake, Joffe, & Kodish, 2011).

Confidentiality is not just guaranteed in some studies; it is a necessary component of all ethically sound research. Researchers must take steps to safeguard the confidentiality of the information gained by blinding or disguising the identity of participants in coding and reporting. If a researcher wishes to identify a research participant in a subsequent publication, the researcher must first gain explicit written permission from the participant to do so. Sometimes situations will arise in which a researcher learns confidential information that he feels should be shared. For instance, upon finding out that an adolescent participant has HIV, the researcher would likely want to ensure that the adolescent receives appropriate help and treatment. The best way to go about this would be to encourage the child to disclose this information himself and provide the child with resources and support. There has been much debate about whether researchers should report suspected maltreatment of children participating in their studies. Allen (2009) examined both sides of the ethical debate and concluded that researchers should be mandated reporters of child maltreatment, just as many other teaching and counseling professionals are. He feels that the importance of protecting vulnerable populations overrides the importance of protecting the integrity of scientific studies.

It is important to keep in mind that all of these guidelines of informed consent, protection from harm, and confidentiality are just that—guidelines. It is the responsibility of the researcher to determine how these guidelines best apply to their studies. The researcher must take necessary steps to appropriately uphold these guidelines. It is incumbent on the researcher to continually evaluate the ethics of the study throughout the experiment in order to make adjustments if necessary. For example, if children with PTSD are showing incredible gains through the experimental treatment, it would be unethical to continue to withhold treatment from the control group.

Finally, researchers must bear in mind the importance of cultural sensitivity. This means that researchers must obtain informed consent in culturally appropriate ways to ensure that diverse participants understand what is being asked of them. Researchers must also choose culturally appropriate designs and tests, and refrain from using tests which have not been shown to yield valid scores for the multicultural population in question. Furthermore, it is the responsibility of the researcher to acquire culturally sensitive knowledge and attitudes. The researcher needs to understand which aspects of human development are universal and which are culture-specific to appropriately design and interpret the results of studies. Being aware of and avoiding ethnocentric biases and overgeneralizations of within-group homogeneity are important requirements for conducting culturally sensitive research. Finally, researchers should strive to include members of various minority groups in their samples to broaden the applicability of their findings to various groups. Unfortunately, the majority of research has been performed on White, middle-class Americans, so remember that the findings do not necessarily apply to all multicultural groups. Counselors strive to conduct studies to determine whether the findings are in fact corroborated or differentiated.

In conclusion, remember that while maintaining the integrity of research designs and the pursuit of knowledge is important, counseling researchers must always balance these benefits with the personal rights and privacy of the individual participants. Research with

REFLECTION **1.2** A QUICK EXAMPLE OF DESIGN CONSIDERATIONS
IN RESEARCH

Part of my scholarly research agenda includes the development and norming of psycho-edu-cational instruments, which are used to assess diverse samples of children, adolescents, and adults. When developing a standardized test, such as a behavior rating scale to assess hyper-activity in children and adults, I need to consider design and ethical implications. Because I usually attempt to establish score validity of instruments, I sometimes administer the instru-ment being developed (instrument 1) along with several other previously developed instru-ments (instruments 2 and 3). I do this in a counterbalanced sequence to be sure to correct for order effects. Thus, about one-sixth of the sample is administered the scales in the following orders: 123, 321, 213, 312, 132, and 231. When I am finished collecting a large sample of protocols, I determine intergroup differences and construct the norms accordingly by computing averages across various age groups (e.g., ages 6–8, 9–11, 12–14, 15–17, 18+). These intergroup differences demonstrate that differences in hyperactivity do exist across the child, adolescent, and adult samples, and usually stabilizes after 18 years of age. Thus, as children grow older, they become less active.

Many ethical implications must also be considered and addressed. First, the study needed to be approved by an institutional review board. Participants also needed to sign informed consent forms. In this study, most of the participants were under the age of 18 and therefore were not of legal age to offer their consent. Thus, I needed to secure informed con-sent from the parent or guardian of each participant under 18, and then attain assent from each minor child to be sure each participant understood the purpose of the study and their right to withdraw from the study at any time. [~BTE]

human participants can be challenging to conduct in ways that do not harm the partici-pants, but one must strive to meet this challenge to both gain new knowledge and protect the participants that help us gain it.

A final ethical issue pertains to the importance of keeping abreast of new information in the field of lifespan development. Practitioners must be aware of new knowledge and techniques in order to be competent service providers. It is the ethical responsibility of counselors to stay up to date on new information in order to provide the best possible ser-vices to their clients. By providing evidence-based, effective practices for clients, counselors are both minimizing risks for clients and promoting the good of clients (Barsky, 2009). Counselors should use these best practices as guidance, using professional discretion rather than strict adherence to guidelines. In this way, the counselor uses empirically based, evi-dence-based, or research-based practices while also taking into account the client's culture and preferences.

Summary

This introductory chapter lays the groundwork for the study of lifespan development by providing a comprehensive summary of the basic characteristics of development and debates occurring in the field of developmental science. It began with a brief overview of the stages of development and aging processes. Next, development was described as cumulative, variable, cyclical, and repetitive, and characterized by cultural differences, individual differences, and both stability and change.

Numerous important issues and principles in devel-opment were elaborated, including discontinuous versus continuous development, nature versus nurture, predict-able and historical changes, critical periods versus flex-ibility/plasticity, and active versus passive development. Special attention was paid to the nature versus nurture issue. Genetic contributions, environmental contributions, and the interactions between the two were highlighted. It was stressed that most of the dichotomous variables discussed may be better viewed as ends of a continuum because some measure of both variables is often important.

The three main types of developmental theories were then described, including stage theories, incremental theories, and multidimensional theories. Various data collection methods and research designs were also reviewed. Data collection methods were described, including standardized testing, naturalistic and structured observations, case studies, and self-report. Research methods described included correlational, experimental, longitudinal, cross-sectional, sequential, time-lag, and cross-cultural methods.

The next section was devoted to the importance of garnering appropriate knowledge to frame situations from a normal developmental perspective. Nosological systems of problem identification and intervention selection, namely the current edition of the DSM, were reviewed and critiqued. Recent emphasis on wellness and positive psychology models was reviewed as well.

The chapter concluded with an overview of ethical principles important in developmental research, namely nonmaleficence, beneficence, autonomy, informed consent, confidentiality, and cultural sensitivity. It was stressed that while maintaining the integrity of research designs and the pursuit of knowledge is important, we must always balance these benefits with the personal rights and privacy of the individual participants.

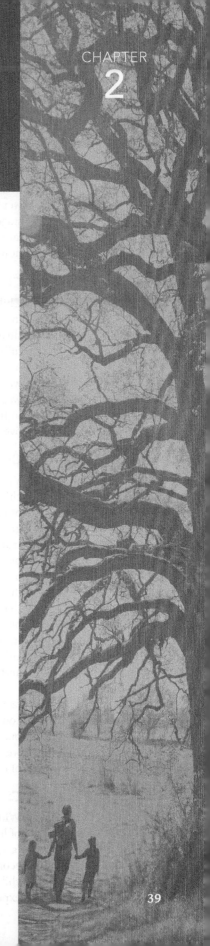

Theories of Human Development: Psychosocial, Sociocultural, Multicultural, Biological, and Learning Theories

By Caroline O'Hara, Lindy K. Parker, and Catherine Y. Chang

Human development is influenced by multiple factors (e.g., biology, society, culture, environment), and many theorists over the years have attempted to explain how humans grow and develop. In this and the next chapter, brief overviews of the major theories of human development are provided. More specifically in this chapter, human development is explored from historical, psychosocial, sociocultural, and multicultural perspectives. Biological and learning theories are also examined. While this chapter serves as an introduction and overview of the myriad theories attempting to explain human development, many of these theories will be discussed in later chapters in the context of the appropriate life stage.

Historical Perspectives

Over the years there have been varied views of childhood, adolescence, and adulthood. Today in modern Western cultures, a prominent belief is that children are innocent and entitled to nurturance and protection. Further, children are believed to be fundamentally different from adults. This concept of childhood as a distinct phase of life did not develop in Western culture until the 16th and 17th centuries (Aries, 1962). A review of how children were portrayed over the years clearly demonstrates that childhood is more than a biological stage of development. Childhood is influenced by attitudes, beliefs, and values of a particular society at a particular point of time. In this section, we will provide a brief overview of how our conceptualization of childhood has evolved over the centuries.

Childhood in the Middle Ages

Children in the Middle Ages were viewed as miniature adults. This is evident in paintings from the 15th and 16th centuries, where children in family portraits are depicted as shrunken replicas of their parents. Children during this period were expected to participate fully in all aspects of social life. By age 7, children were expected to enter the workplace, and by age 12 most girls were married (Barr, 2009). This perspective on childhood most likely was related to the life expectancy at the time. Before the 17th century, the average life span was between 30 and 40 years. Infant mortality rates and fatal diseases were extremely high in the Middle Ages, and therefore, parents were less likely to allow themselves to become overly attached to a child whose chances of survival were limited (Aries, 1962).

Children in the 18th and 19th Centuries

Views on childhood began to change in the 18th century with the growing perception that children are innocent and in need of adult protection and discipline. With the development of industry, commerce, and city dwelling, the idea of education for children also began to grow. Prior to this period, children were sent off to work at an early age; this was especially true for children in rural areas. The 18th century also saw the spread of the Puritan view of human development. According to religious leaders during the Puritan era, children were born into original sin and it was the responsibility of parents and adults to provide strict discipline for the children (Barr, 2009). **Original sin** is a Christian doctrine that states that all infants are born with the hereditary stain left behind from Adam's sin. Because of Adam's sin, we have inherited the propensity to sin. The belief that children were born into sin began to change with the work of John Locke (1632–1704), who believed that a child was a **tabula rasa**, a blank slate. Locke asserted that we are born without innate ideas and that knowledge is determined by experience and perception (Locke, 1689/1996).

With the spread of the Industrial Revolution in the 1800s and the growing number of factories came the need for increased numbers of workers. Children as young as 4 and 5 could be found working long hours in factories as well as in coal mines, often under dangerous conditions. In some cases, child labor was preferred over adult labor because children were more docile and cheaper to employ. Slowly this began to change with the introduction of child labor laws (Cunningham, 1995).

Childhood in the 20th Century

With the Industrial Revolution firmly established and the passage of a growing number of laws restricting child labor, children were no longer viewed as economic necessities. In fact, Zelizer (1994) described the period from 1870s to 1930s as "the emergence of this economically 'worthless' but emotionally 'priceless' child . . ." (p. 3). She explained that children from a strict economic perspective are worthless; in fact, children are quite expensive. According to the U.S. Department of Agriculture (USDA), estimates of annual child-rearing expenses range from $11,880 to $13,830 for a child in a two-child, married-couple family (Lino, 2011). In return for this expense, children are expected to provide "love, smiles, and emotional satisfaction" (Zelizer, 1994, p. 3). Having children fulfills a desire for love and affection and promotes a feeling of being a family. Thus, this contemporary view of children is based on a society that values children not for their economic worth but for their emotional connection.

Childhood in the 21st Century

Children in the 21st century continue to be viewed as valuable and entitled to protection from harm. Additionally, children are viewed as deserving a life full of good emotional, mental, and physical health (Kehily, 2004). Organizations like the United Nations International Children's Emergency Fund (UNICEF, 2014) and the Office of the Child Advocate (2013) continue to advocate for the well-being of children and view the protection of children as a priority for the well-being of society.

Think About It **2.1**

Reflect on the various perspectives on childhood over the ages. What is your perspective on childhood? What messages about childhood did you receive from your parents? From school? From society?

Psychosocial Theories

The historical roots, perspectives, and philosophies undergirding theories of human development are vast and varied. The following section covers some major psychosocial theories of development over the lifespan. As one develops a theoretical orientation, it will be important to consider the fundamental assumptions that these theories hold. To what extent are people bound to their childhood experiences? How much influence do sociopolitical and environmental factors have on development? Where is the presumed locus of control and responsibility? How do systems affect clients? How does change occur and how is it measured?

Sigmund Freud (1856–1939)

Much has been written about Sigmund Freud, as he is credited with being one of the most influential forces in shaping the trajectory of psychology, counseling, and "talk therapy." Today, the very mention of Freud can be polarizing: Some professional counselors want to discard what they believe to be antiquated or misogynistic ideas, while others see value in reworking his principles that explain human behavior so coherently. Either way, it is clear that professional counseling would not be where it is today without him. For instance, before Freud, irregularities in human development or variations in the expression of the human experience were viewed as demonic possessions or moral deficits (Bankart, 1997). "Treatment" involved exorcisms, witch-hunting, imprisonment, or involuntary commitment to an asylum. Freud's revolution came not only from his theoretical ideas about personality and early childhood experiences, but also in the radical shift to the idea that talking with someone in a private setting on a regular basis could be curative.

Freud founded psychoanalytic theory, which is an intrapsychic, deterministic theory focusing on early childhood experiences, characterological change, the unconscious, and insight (Bankart, 1997). Freud believed that personality structure consists of the **id** (governed by pleasure and instinct—the **pleasure principle**), **ego** (governed by reality and logic—the **reality principle**), and **superego** (governed by society and morality—the **morality principle**). There is an assumption that people have inherent pathologies, spurred by unconscious drives, which they need to address and overcome.

Freud believed that the first few years of life determined how personality forms. He created a model with five **psychosexual stages** (i.e., oral, anal, phallic, latent, and genital) that speak to the importance of early childhood. The **oral stage** lasts from birth to 18 months and centers on the pleasure of sucking and eating. Trust and security are major concerns. The **anal stage**, from 18 months to 3 years, focuses on pleasure received from controlling one's excretory functions. The **phallic stage** ranges from 3 to 5 years and attends to children's fascination with their genitalia and other bodily functions. During this stage, Freud theorized that children deal with unconscious sexual desires for their caregivers: Girls unconsciously yearn for their fathers (i.e., the Electra complex) and boys unconsciously yearn for their mothers (i.e., the Oedipal complex) (Corey, 2009). The **latent stage** lasts from age 5 until puberty begins and is marked by calm after the torment of the earlier years. Finally, the **genital stage** begins at puberty and lasts through the remainder of the person's life. During the genital stage, conscious and unconscious behaviors manifest as a result of the culmination of early childhood experiences.

Fundamental to psychoanalysis are the **defense mechanisms** that people employ to protect themselves from unwanted anxiety, experiences, or pain. When the ego cannot keep the id and superego in balance, anxiety develops and people employ these defense mechanisms (see Table 2.1). Examples include repression, denial, sublimation, projection, reaction formation, displacement, rationalization, introjection, compensation, acting out, and splitting (Corey, 2012). The goal of psychoanalysis is to make the unconscious conscious by gaining insight into current patterns with the goal of changing personality, resolving underlying conflicts, and attaining freedom from the past.

> **Think About It   2.2** Sigmund Freud and Psychoanalysis
>
> Where might helping professions be at this time without the influence of Sigmund Freud? How would you apply his theory to a child currently living through these stages? How useful is Freud's theory for a diverse clientele? What defense mechanisms do you typically use?

TABLE 2.1 ✦ COMMON DEFENSE MECHANISMS

Defense Mechanism	Example
Repression—to push aside unwanted or painful thoughts, feelings, or experiences involuntarily. Repression operates on a primarily unconscious level.	People who may have experienced trauma may repress memories in order to cope with the horror.
Denial—to ignore, turn away from, or refuse to acknowledge painful realities that others can detect. Denial may occur at preconscious or conscious levels as well.	A doctor has become addicted to alcohol and other drugs. Although she is late for work or absent regularly and she has been performing poorly, she does not see a problem.
Sublimation—to channel energy from unwanted or unacceptable impulses into more socially appropriate avenues.	People engage in sports or physical activities to discharge aggressive urges.
Projection—to attribute one's own unacceptable desires, behaviors, thoughts, feelings, etc. to others and not to oneself.	One may criticize coworkers for being stingy with a lunch bill but then fail to chip in regularly or consistently tip poorly.
Reaction Formation—to express the opposite impulse in an effort to conceal one's true stance. This commonly occurs with repression.	People may devote their lives to promoting the sanctity of marriage, but then engage in multiple extramarital affairs.
Displacement—to redirect one's feelings or responses from one object toward a safer target when the original object is inaccessible.	Before work, a man has a fight with his partner. When he arrives, he yells at his subordinate.
Rationalization—to make excuses for one's impulses to provide reassurance and offer incorrect explanations.	In order to cope with not getting the desired grade on an assignment, a student starts to believe that the teacher is unfair and that the grade does not matter.
Introjection—to accept the values and standards of others without question, critique, or analysis.	A child may espouse and articulate a caregiver's exact political beliefs.
Compensation—to conceal perceived limitations by developing strengths elsewhere.	Individuals who may not possess physical characteristics deemed "ideal" by society may focus on and excel at academics and school.
Acting Out—to deal with emotional conflicts with actions rather than by reflecting or being open to feelings.	Children may throw or break things when their caregivers are fighting.
Splitting—to fail to integrate positive and negative aspects of self or others, resulting in imbalanced vacillation between polar opposites.	People may view others as "all good" or "all bad" but then go back and forth between idealizing others and devaluing them.

Neo-Freudians

The neo-Freudians include some contemporaries and followers of Freud as well as those who extended and expanded upon his ideas in the years after Freud's death. One of the main differences for these theorists was that they began to emphasize *interactions* and *interpersonal* relationships, not simply intrapsychic events. However, despite the shift, it should be noted that these theoretical perspectives are also insight-oriented, are primarily deterministic, and still focus a great deal of attention on intrapsychic disturbances.

Carl G. Jung (1875–1961)

Carl Jung was a student and friend of Freud who eventually branched from his mentor to found analytical psychology. Instead of focusing exclusively on early childhood, Jung focused on the later years of an adult's life (Corey, 2012). The primary goal of Jung's theory was for clients to achieve **individuation**, a balanced integration and expression of one's conscious and unconscious (Jung, 1961). His approach uses myth, legend, religion, symbols, dreams, and archetypes to understand the unconscious. Some of the most important archetypes include the persona, shadow, anima, and animus.

Alfred Adler (1870–1937)

Alfred Adler was a contemporary of Freud who eventually founded individual psychology. Some of Adler's key concepts include social interest, purposeful behavior, and belonging. Adler's approach is considered **teleological** (i.e., goal-directed). One of Adler's major contributions was the shift to an egalitarian relationship between counselor and client (Bankart, 1997). In addition, his work with clients focused more on the conscious than the unconscious. Adler believed that each individual has a unique **private logic** that consists of core assumptions, beliefs, and philosophies about life (Adler, 1970). He theorized that, by examining faulty conclusions that clients make about private logic, clients would be able to overcome feelings of inferiority and live more meaningful lives. Popular methods he created to understand clients include the examination of birth order, sibling relationships, and early recollections.

Karen Horney (1885–1952)

It is easy to notice that this section is full of male theorists. However, Karen Horney was a pioneering female analyst who broadened the field of psychoanalysis to include alternatives to androcentric perspectives and to be more responsive to gender dynamics (Bankart, 1997). For example, she reworked and reframed Freud's notion of "penis envy" to suggest that instead of envying male anatomy, women in fact seek the privilege, power, respect, control, and esteem traditionally offered to men. Horney (1950) proposed that individuals employ three **coping strategies** (postures) to protect themselves and provide safety from anxiety. People are (1) helpless, compliantly moving toward others; (2) aggressive, moving against others to dominate them; or (3) detached, moving away to avoid hurt or abandonment.

Harry Stack Sullivan (1892–1949)

Credited with founding interpersonal therapy, Harry Stack Sullivan believed that the relationships between and among people served to form the personality and were both the cause and the cure of psychological problems (Yalom & Leszcz, 2005). He asserted that each person's core self consists of "reflected appraisals" that are constructed through interpersonal relationships. Similar to transference, Sullivan used the term **parataxic distortions** to describe the patterns of skewed or irrational perceptions people have regarding others' perceptions of them. These beliefs are based upon childhood experiences that linger and that people superimpose upon others in their current lives. One of the dangers of parataxic distortions is that they tend to yield "self-fulfilling prophecies," which is similar to the idea of projective identification. Basically, a person will have a deeply embedded belief about the world or others and unknowingly, yet repetitively, act in certain ways that elicit from others the very behavior that they expect. This only serves to confirm suspicions about others, usually in a negative or unhealthy manner. For these reasons, Sullivan championed the use of interpersonal relationships and group counseling settings to explore and reassess early experiences and the meanings they currently hold.

Erik Erikson (1902–1994)

One of Erik Erikson's primary contributions to counseling and human development was his focus away from childhood toward adulthood. He proposed that people encounter eight sequential **psychosocial stages** over the course of their lives, each presenting a unique challenge or crisis (Erikson, 1963). Those who successfully address these central goals or conflicts move forward in a healthy and fulfilled manner. Those who do not are at risk for remaining stuck or regressing backward. Erikson's approach is psychosocial in nature and focuses on interpersonal relationships as well as the individual's capacity to navigate the obstacles of each stage. His stages are as follows:

1. *Infancy*—**trust vs. mistrust**. Infants develop trust with secure caregiver relationships when their basic needs are met. If physical and emotional needs are not me, the child may develop a mistrusting attitude toward others.
2. *Early childhood (toddlerhood)*—**autonomy vs. shame and doubt**. From about ages 1 to 3 years, children explore the world and experiment. If parents or caregivers do not promote autonomy, children may lack self-reliance as they develop.
3. *Preschool age*—**initiative vs. guilt**. Between ages 3 and 6, the focus is a basic sense of competence. If others monopolize decision making on behalf of these children, then they become guilty and reluctant to make their own decisions.
4. *School age*—**industry vs. inferiority**. With children ages 6–12, the focus is on goal-setting and achievement. Without success at this task, feelings of inadequacy may develop.
5. *Adolescence*—**identity vs. role confusion**. During adolescence and puberty, individuals explore limits, boundaries, meaning, identity, and goals. Failure to achieve a coherent identity may yield confusion.
6. *Young adulthood*—**intimacy vs. isolation**. For individuals ages 18 to 35, the major task is the development of and security within intimate relationships. Without these, alienation and isolation may persist.
7. *Middle age*—**generativity vs. stagnation**. With adults ages 35 to 60, the focus is on transcending self and family and focusing on the next generation. People in this stage must reconcile differences between their aspirations/dreams and their actual accomplishments.
8. *Later life*—**integrity vs. despair**. For those over age 60, this stage deals with coming to terms with one's life. People look back either with a sense of pride and contentment, or perhaps with feelings of failure, guilt, and despair.

Jane Loevinger (1918–2008)

Jane Loevinger (1976) developed a theory of personality and **ego development** that examines interpersonal, cognitive, and moral development across the lifespan. Her theory proposes that individuals experience a sequential progression through nine possible stages. These stages include (1) presocial, (2) impulsive, (3) self-protective, (4) conformist, (5) self-aware, (6) conscientious, (7) individualistic, (8) autonomous, and (9) integrated. Her view holds that growth and development relate to how individuals respond to new information or environmental interactions. The further people progress through the stages, the more they are able to integrate complexity, incongruity, and conflict, each of which yields the capacity for nuanced perceptions and meaning-making.

Arthur W. Chickering (1887–1974)

Arthur W. Chickering proposed a theory of identity development that he generated by studying traditionally aged college students (Chickering, 1969; Chickering & Reisser, 1993). Chickering's theory consists of **seven vectors** or areas that individuals navigate as they grow and develop, with particular attention to those aged 18–22 years. Overlap and similarities to Erikson's theory are evident. Unlike Erikson, however, Chickering's vectors are not sequential, and people may negotiate multiple vectors simultaneously or revisit vectors over time. The seven vectors are as follows: (1) developing competence, (2) managing emotions, (3) moving through autonomy to interdependence, (4) establishing identity, (5) developing mature interpersonal relationships, (6) developing purpose, and (7) developing integrity. As with other previously mentioned theories, limitations to Chickering's approach may include the emphasis on the universal instead of the impact of specific sociocultural factors on development (e.g., sexual identity, race, ability, gender, age) and the intersection of these characteristics.

➤ CASE EXAMPLE **2.1**   BIANCA.

Unfortunately, when working in mental health agencies or hospitals, there is sometimes a tendency to refer to clients by their diagnosis instead of by their names—a distancing and dehumanizing practice. This is often the case with individuals diagnosed with borderline personality disorder. People with borderline features are very commonly trauma survivors (e.g., emotional/physical/sexual abuse, natural disasters, war, terrorism). They may have difficulties regulating their emotions and maintaining interpersonal relationships. Often, they feel empty and suicidal. They may engage in many of the defense mechanisms listed in Table 2.1 as a means of coping with adverse or unspeakable life experiences.

Take Bianca, for example, who was referred to a local psychiatric hospital after attempting suicide. She is 15 years old and lives with her mother and stepfather (who has been emotionally and sexually abusing her for years). Bianca displays behavior that is labeled as "defiant," "unruly," or "oppositional." She sneaks out of the home, smokes cigarettes and cannabis, and often gets into fights at school. She states that she is a horrible person and wants to die. Instead of focusing on her defense mechanisms (e.g., introjections, acting out, splitting), professional counselors are in a unique position to screen for trauma history and promote recovery by addressing what may be hidden and shameful. Hopefully, professional counselors can continue to promote wellness by focusing on recovery and growth rather than pathology.

Sociocultural Theories

The following section elaborates upon several theories that emphasize people's environments, interactions, and systems in which they are embedded. These theories continue to lean toward viewing clients in context and conceptualizing clients in dynamic, interactional terms.

Lev Vygotsky (1896–1934)

In order to understand how people develop, Lev Vygotsky proposed the examination of the social processes occurring around children. He proposed the idea of the **zone of proximal development**, which is the difference or distance between what children can achieve individually versus what they can achieve with adult guidance and support (Vygotsky, 1978). Vygotsky also introduced the concept of **scaffolding**, which is the process that helps children move from a position of an inability to complete challenging tasks to a position where they can eventually complete the tasks independently. This is done with assistance from helpful others such as parents, caregivers, coaches, and teachers who build support structures. In addition, Vygotsky also described a concept called **private speech**, whereby an individual talks aloud to oneself and not to others for the purposes of self-guidance. The idea is that private speech aids in mental processing of challenging tasks. Vygotsky theorized that developmental problems occur when external support is insufficient or lacking altogether. Thus, social interactions promote cognitive development and learning.

Murray Bowen (1913–1990)

Murray Bowen, a **multigenerational family systems** theorist, argued that previous generations greatly affect the development of future generations' egos (Goldberg & Goldberg, 2013). One of his main goals for family counseling is the **differentiation of self**, a process that includes separating oneself from one's family of origin and distinguishing one's emotions from one's cognitions. The goal for Bowen (1978) was to have each member of the family differentiate as much as possible from the others to avoid the fusion of individuals with one another and the fusion of each member's thoughts and feelings in order to avoid developmental impasse or stagnation. Thus, members can eventually free themselves from unresolved emotional attachments stemming from their family of origin (Goldberg & Goldberg, 2013). A limitation of Bowen's theory is the prioritization of autonomy, which may not be appropriate or encouraged by various cultures or for different genders.

Family Lifecycle Development

Betty Carter and Monica McGoldrick have collaborated on a number of texts elaborating on family processes and the family lifecycle (see Carter & McGoldrick, 2005). This approach often uses **genograms**, which are pictorial, symbolic representations that elucidate the structure and processes of multiple generations within a family system. The family lifecycle perspective suggests that families navigate developmental and unexpected transitions over time by completing specific tasks. These tasks can be relatively universal (e.g., attachment, role shifts) or more culture-specific (e.g., identity development, community engagement, survival skills; Goldberg & Goldberg, 2013). The stages are as follows:

1. *Leaving home/Young adulthood.* Individuals accept emotional and financial responsibility for themselves as individuals.
2. *Joining of families/New couple.* The couple becomes a new system and there is a realignment from the identity of an individual to the identity of a committed partner.
3. *Childbirth/Childrearing.* New members are accepted and incorporated into the system. Parenting and grandparenting roles are incorporated.
4. *Middle marriage/Families with adolescents.* Need for more flexible boundaries as adolescents experiment with independence.
5. *Launching children/Moving on.* Marital dyad must be renegotiated. Focus returns to the couple and may also expand to attend to aging parents.
6. *Later life.* Acceptance of new generational roles. Dealing with loss of partner and other peers.

Think About It   2.3

How well do Carter and McGoldrick's family life-cycle development stages fit diverse populations and lifestyles? What impact might challenging economic times have on the various stages? How well do the stages apply to nontraditional families (e.g., LGBTQIQ, single parent/caregiver)?

By examining clients within this framework, professional counselors can help conceptualize growth, obstacles, and change. It is important to note that a multitude of factors (e.g., socioeconomic status, gender, race, culture, political context) and the intersection of these factors impact development; professional counselors need to attend to these factors in the families they serve and examine these factors within themselves as well.

Uri Bronfenbrenner (1917–2005)

As discussed in Chapter 1, Uri Bronfenbrenner proposed that the processes that occur between people and their environments are best conceptualized using a type of systems perspective called a bioecological model. His **ecological model of child development**

> focuses on the progressive accommodation, throughout the life span, between the growing human organism and the changing environments in which it actually lives and grows. The latter include not only the immediate settings containing the developing person but also the larger social contexts, both formal and informal, in which these settings are embedded. (Bronfenbrenner, 1977, p. 513)

Bronfenbrenner's theory (1978) holds that individuals exist not in a vacuum, but in a vast, complex, interwoven net of social structures including families, communities, local and global economies, political organizations, and historical eras. The different systemic levels include the microsystem, mesosystem, exosystem, macrosystem, and chronosystem. Consider the circumstances in which Marcus is embedded in Case Example 2.2.

➤ CASE EXAMPLE **2.2** MARCUS.

In order to serve our clients, it is helpful to see them in an ecological context and to understand where they are embedded. For example, when discipline problems occur in the classroom, professional counselors in the schools often want to observe the classroom environment in action in order to gain a better understanding of the student's context. Taking that a step further, we can examine the case of Marcus, age 9 years. Marcus's mother died when he was very young, and he currently lives with his father and 15-year-old brother. Marcus has been increasingly agitated at school and his teacher is growing more concerned. Marcus is growing more isolated and detached from other students, even his close friends. Upon further investigation, the teacher discovers that Marcus's father has lost his job and his older brother has been working more hours to help support the family financially. Marcus misses playing with his brother and having him around the house. As a result, Marcus has felt less like himself and says he often feels "down." The changes in his family's interactional patterns (microsystem) resulting from the changes in the economy of the country (exosystem) have affected Marcus directly. By connecting Marcus and his family to resources and by addressing larger, contextual concerns, professional school counselors can serve as advocates for Marcus and his family.

Multicultural Theories of Development

Many of the earlier theories discussed in this chapter were designed by, studied on, and applied to people in the dominant sociocultural majority (e.g., European-Americans, males, people with stable and secure financial status). It is important to note that all theories of helping and change exist within a cultural context, whether they overtly address culture or not (Ivey, D'Andrea, Ivey, & Simek-Morgan, 2007). The advantage of multicultural theories is that they help attend to real differences that may exist among individuals and groups. In addition, these theories strive to assist professional counselors in being more effective, respectful, and ethical with clients from diverse backgrounds.

The theories discussed in this section are primarily stage (discontinuous) models. The idea is that an individual can progress through each stage over time depending on a variety of internal and external factors and experiences. In addition, some people may remain at the first stage or in any subsequent stage without moving into the following stage(s). In general, stage models delineate transformations from

Think About It **2.4**

What are some of the sociocultural identities that are part of your identity? Which identities come to mind that put you in a position of power and privilege or a position of marginalization? What identities would you like to know more about (and what can you do to learn more)?

positions of unawareness to positions of positive awareness and synthesis of the constructs at hand. Over the last few decades, theorists and practitioners have proposed dozens of identity development models concerning racial identity, sexual identity (Cass, 1979; Sullivan, 1998; Troiden, 1989), feminist identity (Downing & Roush, 1985), racial/cultural identity (Sue & Sue, 1990), and multitudes of other identities. Some models focus on dominant sociocultural identities, while others focus on marginalized identities. Four models of identity development were selected for further discussion.

White Racial Identity Development

The work of Janet Helms (1984, 1990) has been essential in conceptualizing the racial identity, attitudes, psychosocial development, and levels of race salience for many groups of people. However, because European-Americans are a dominant and privileged group in the United States and because they outnumber other racial and ethnic groups, it is common for European-Americans to experience their lives oblivious to issues of their own racial identities and race privilege. The work of Peggy McIntosh serves as a primer for understanding race privilege and unearned advantages and power conferred on European-Americans (see McIntosh, 1989). Helms' model (1990) of **White racial identity development** (WRID) includes the following statuses that demonstrate an evolution in abandoning racism and developing a positive identity:

1. *Contact*—Individuals are oblivious to issues of race and racial identity; they maintain the status quo. They are unaware of privileges and think that race does not matter.
2. *Disintegration*—Questioning of beliefs causes cognitive dissonance, conflict, anxiety, and/or guilt.
3. *Reintegration*—May actively or passively/covertly believe in White superiority and dominance. Racial identity is acknowledged.
4. *Pseudoindependence*—This is the beginning of defining a positive White racial identity, with an emphasis on intellectual understanding.
5. *Immersion/emersion*—Individuals replace old misinformation and stereotypes with accurate information. The goal shifts from changing marginalized individuals to changing Whites.
6. *Autonomy*—Whites are able to continue commitment to understanding and acknowledging racism and privilege. Individuals exhibit the ability to understand complexities of race (and other systems of oppression) and welcome cross-racial interactions.

Black Racial Identity Development

William Cross' Nigrescence model was one of the first theories of **Black racial identity development** (Cross, 1971, 1995; Cross, Parham, & Helms, 1991) and has served as a template for other models including the WRID model discussed previously. Although Cross and his colleagues have adjusted the model over the years, it consists of the following stages:

1. *Preencounter*—Whites are the primary reference group; race is not very salient. People here have limited awareness of racial oppression.
2. *Encounter*—An event helps a person reflect on race and racial identity; new views are inconsistent with old views.
3. *Immersion-emersion*—Immersion consists of dichotomous thinking that rejects Whiteness and fervently embraces Black identity. Emersion represents a lessening of rigidity and reactivity.
4. *Internalization*—Black identity is based on appreciation, flexibility, and love instead of a hatred or rejection of others. Individuals are secure in their identities and open to those who are different.
5. *Internalization-commitment*—Increasing levels of social and political commitment against singular or multiple forms of oppression.

Biracial Identity Development

Poston (1990) developed a **biracial identity development model** that is more suited to individuals who identify as biracial. In this model, **biracial** indicates a person conceived by people of different races. The model attempts to address some of the complexities associated with being biracial; it consists of the five following stages:

1. *Personal identity*—relates to self-esteem, internalization of values and prejudices, and identification with reference groups.
2. *Choice of group categorization*—the push to identify with a particular group, often accompanied by alienation and crisis for the individual.
3. *Enmeshment/denial*—often yields confusion and guilt about choosing a group to which to belong, which may not fully encompass one's identity or heritage.
4. *Appreciation*—valuing and learning more about multiple identities.
5. *Integration*—the development of a secure, stable, integrated identity.

Multiple Heritage Identity Development

The work of Henriksen and Paladino (2009) has yielded the multiple heritage identity development (MHID) model. One of the unique aspects of this model is that it integrates many facets of a person's identity. Not only is the focus on individuals who may have parents/caregivers of multiple or different races; the focus is also on other aspects of identity such as socioeconomic status, gender, religion, language, national origin, and sexual identity. This approach, which incorporates "multiple dimensions to [clients'] backgrounds," may better reflect the intersectionality of people's identities and the nuances of their lived experiences (Henriksen & Paladino, 2009, p. xiii).

> **Think About It   2.5**
>
> What are the counseling implications for clients and professional counselors who may be mismatched in their identity development? For example, what would be the potential consequences if a client were at a later identity development stage or status than the professional counselor? Vice versa?

REFLECTION   2.1   MY OWN RACIAL IDENTITY DEVELOPMENT

On personal reflection, it has been quite an experience as I journey through various stages of my own racial identity development. I remember being very young, maybe 6 years old, when my mother taught me about discrimination and prejudice. I remember thinking they were bad things and that I did not want to engage in those behaviors. It was so simple—so cut and dried. However, it was not until college that I actually examined my own Whiteness. Before I took Psychology of Racism in college, I knew that people in the racial and ethnic minority were marginalized, and I did not like it. But it was so external to me, so removed. I wanted to help *them* with *their* problem. However, only after intensely exploring the flip side of oppression (privilege) over time did I begin my journey in earnest. I had to examine *myself* and my assumptions about the world including *my* unearned advantages and power.

As I reflect on my journey, I believe that the factors that contributed to a positive identity for me included surrounding myself with others who are also engaging, struggling, and actively learning about these ideas. I try to stretch myself to experience discomfort and take risks to explore and enrich my understanding of my privileges and of the many ways that people are marginalized based on race and a multitude of other social identities. I try to maintain an open, humble stance that allows for active reflections on myself and my role as well as the roles of others in these matters. In addition, I find that engaging in anti-racist activities (e.g., interventions against slurs or hate speech, legislative efforts, privilege-awareness discussions) helps me feel connected to something positive. I have had to get in touch with many emotions such as anger, guilt, fear, and confusion. Thankfully, many of those difficult emotions have been replaced with hope, pride, and fulfillment over time. ~CO

Biological Theories of Human Development

Biological theories of human development integrate physiological and biological aspects of development. Central to biological theories is the belief that behavior and mental processes can be explained by examining human physiology and anatomy.

Darwin (1809–1882)

Charles Darwin, a British naturalist, developed the **theory of evolution** based on his assertion that all living species have descended over time from common ancestry. His theory emphasized the principle of natural selection. **Natural selection** refers to differential reproduction or the process whereby certain traits or characteristics of a species that are more adaptable to the environment survive. Over time this process can result in the emergence of a new species uniquely situated for the given environment. Conversely, traits and characteristics within species that do not promote survival within the environment result in the extinction of that species (Darwin, 1869). Darwin believed that observing children could provide important information related to the evolution of the human species; thus, he and other scientists at the time kept detailed records of their own children's development. These were considered the first organized studies of human development (Charlesworth, 1992).

Ethological Theory

Ethology is the study of the adaptive and evolutionary basis of animal behavior; it is concerned with studying the behaviors of species that promote their survival. According to ethological theory, species have inborn or instinctual responses which are shared by all members of that species, and these instinctual responses guide individuals to similar developmental paths. The origins of ethology applied to human development can be traced back to Darwin and his theory of natural selection (Hinde, 1989). Ethology offered psychologists a methodology (i.e., study in natural settings and laboratories) for studying human behavior and a theory to explain instinctive behavior (Salzen, 2010). Building on ethological theory, Bowlby (1969) and Ainsworth, Blehar, Waters, and Wall (1978) developed a theory of infant–caregiver attachment.

Attachment Theory

Attachment is an emotional connection with important people in one's life. Attachment leads to a sense of security and gives people pleasure as they interact with other people to whom they are attached. Bowlby (1969) was the first to apply the concepts of ethology to the infant–caregiver relationship. Later, Ainsworth et al. (1978) studied the interactions of mothers and children using attachment theory as a foundation.

John Bowlby (1907–1990)

Bowlby began to develop his theory of attachment while working in a home for maladjusted boys. He observed that disruptions in the mother–child relationship could lead to later psychopathology in the offspring (Cassidy, 1999). According to Bowlby's (1969) attachment theory, infants are pre-adapted to respond to their caregiver and to exhibit behaviors that enhance the infants' chances of survival. This pre-adapted attachment to the caregiver promotes close proximity, and therefore safety for the child. This early mother–child attachment affects not only the individuals as children but also in future relationships.

The attachment behavioral system includes a cognitive component whereby individuals construct, at the subconscious level, mental representations of the attachment figure, the self, and the environment. Bowlby (1969) postulated four phases of infant attachment:

1. *Phase 1: Non-focused responsiveness* (birth to 3 months). During this phase, the infants cry, smile, and make eye contact with anyone with whom they come into contact.

These behaviors sustain the attention of others, and therefore, their proximity to the infant.

2. *Phase 2: Discriminating attention* (3 to 6 months). Babies begin to focus their social responsiveness to fewer people and become less responsive to unfamiliar people. A primary attachment figure begins to emerge.
3. *Phase 3: Proximity-seeking behavior* (6 to 24 months). The attached figure becomes a base for the infant/toddler to explore; therefore, the infant/toddler will display proximity-seeking behaviors such as following the caregiver or calling out for them.
4. *Phase 4: Reciprocal relationship* (24 months and beyond). During this stage, the child begins to develop an internal model of the attachment relationship. For example, the child begins to understand parental intent and can envision the parent's behavior during separation. This child is more willing to separate from parents.

Bowlby (1969) also believed that these attachment relationships have a **sensitive period**, between 6 months and 24 months, when the attachment relationship will develop more readily. After this period, attachment relationships can form but with more difficulty.

Mary Ainsworth (1913–1999)

Using attachment theory as a framework, Ainsworth and her colleagues conducted naturalistic studies on mothers and infants (Ainsworth et. al., 1978). Like Bowlby, Ainsworth et al. (1978) believed that when individuals feel a strong attachment to each other, a proximity seeking system engages and individuals will want to be with the attachment object no matter the cost. Ainsworth and colleagues developed the Strange Situation where they recorded how children responded to their mother after a period of separation. The children were observed for 20 minutes while their mother and a stranger entered and left the room. Based on their observations, Ainsworth and Bell (1970) and Ainsworth et al. (1978) postulated three attachment categories (a fourth one based on their observations was added later):

1. **Secure attachment**. Although the child demonstrates signs of missing the parent, the child easily separates from the mother and becomes engaged in exploration. When the parent returns, the child greets parent actively and then returns to play. The child demonstrates a clear preference for the mother over the stranger.
2. **Insecure: Anxious-avoidant attachment**. The child does not cry at separation but rather continues to play. When the parent returns, the infant actively avoids and ignores the parent but does not resist the mother's efforts at contact. The child demonstrates no preference for the mother over the stranger.
3. **Insecure: Anxious-ambivalent attachment**. The child is preoccupied with the parent throughout the procedure. The child demonstrates little exploration and is wary of the stranger. The child both seeks and resists contact with the mother. The child resists both comfort and contact with the stranger.
4. **Insecure: Disorganized-disoriented attachment**. The child appears confused and displays contradictory behaviors in the presence of the parent. For example, the child may cry unexpectedly after having settled down or display odd postures (Main & Solomon, 1990).

Researchers found that these patterns of attachment can be both stable and changeable. Children who experience fairly stable environments are more likely to maintain their attachment patterns than children who experience some major environmental or familial change. Attachment patterns were more secure and stable for infants in middle SES and in favorable life conditions, and for babies who moved from insecure attachment to secure attachment. Children from lower-SES families either moved from secure attachment to insecure attachment or changed from one insecure attachment pattern to another (Fish, 2004; Thompson, 2003). In addition to SES levels, marital status, caregiver's emotional responsiveness, and mental health of the caregiver have been associated with attachment patterns. Researchers have also examined the cultural variations of attachment patterns and have found some evidence for both the universality of the attachment patterns and some variations (see Posada et al., 1995; van Ijzendoorn & Krooneberg, 1988).

Maturation Theory

Maturation theorists believe that human development is biological and that development happens automatically and in predictable, sequential stages with few individual differences. **Maturation theory** was first introduced by Arnold Gesell (1880–1961), an American pediatrician and child psychologist. Gesell (1929) believed that heredity was largely responsible for child development and that parental influence had limited impact on the development of the child. Children mature following an inherited timetable and develop skills and abilities in a preordained sequence. Gesell described developmental milestones in the areas of: motor characteristics, personal hygiene, emotional expression, fears and dreams, self and sex, interpersonal relations, play and pastimes, school life, ethical sense, and philosophic outlook.

Through observations of hundreds of children, Gesell et al. (1974) developed these age norms, which they described as milestones:

1. Birth to 16 weeks—newborn gains control of muscles and nerves in their faces.
2. 16 to 28 weeks—the baby gains control over his head and neck and begins to reach out for objects.
3. 28 to 40 weeks—the baby gains control over her trunk and hands, and begins to grasp at objects.
4. 40 to 52 weeks—the baby gains control over legs and feet and begins to talk.
5. 2nd year—toddler learns to walk and run; language is developing with some words and phrases; the baby gains control over bladder and bowel moments; and the baby begins to develop a sense of personal identity and personal possessions.
6. 3rd year—the child speaks clearly using words as tools for thinking; he begins to control his environment.
7. 4th year—the child asks questions and begins to grasp concepts.
8. 5th year—the child is mature in large motor development; can jump and skip. The child can now tell stories. The child is self-assured in the home environment.

Although many quickly rejected Gesell's theory of maturation for Piaget, behavioralism, and cognitive development theories, his contribution to human development is important and continues to influence our thinking today. He pioneered the scientific observation of infants and children. The developmental norms that he outlined for child development are still the basis for early assessment of childhood functioning (Thelen & Adolph, 1992).

Learning Theories

Learning theorists believe that development can be described in terms of behaviors learned through interactions with the environment. **Learning theories** stress the role of external influences on behavior. According to learning theories, all behavior is learned and the basic principles of learning are the same regardless of who is learning and what they are learning.

Behavioralism

Behavioralism operates on the principle of "stimulus–response." All behavior is a direct response to environmental stimuli. From this perspective, learning is a passive experience, with the learner simply responding to external stimuli. Behavioralism has emphasized two primary types of learning: classical (respondent conditioning) and operant (instrumental conditioning). In this section, the work of Thorndike is also discussed. Thorndike helped to build the bridge between classical and operant conditioning.

Classical Conditioning

Classical conditioning was first described by Ivan Pavlov (1849–1936), a Russian physiologist who worked with animals; later, the concept was studied in infants by John Watson (1878–1958). Pavlov, in his famous experiments with dogs, demonstrated how he could train dogs to salivate at the sound of a bell after that bell was repeatedly presented to the dog immediately before the meat powder. Salivating is an **unconditioned response (UCR)** to meat powder, which is an **unconditioned stimulus (UCS)**. The sound of the bell is a neutral stimulus until the dog learns to associate the sound of the bell with food. Then the sound of the bell becomes a **conditioned stimulus (CS)**, which produces the **conditioned response (CR)** of salivation (Pavlov, 1927).

John Watson extended the work of Pavlov and applied it to human behavior. In his famous experiment with "Little Albert," Watson conditioned Albert, an infant, to develop a fear of a white laboratory rat by pairing a white rat with a very loud noise. Prior to the experiment, Albert displayed no fear of the laboratory rat. In pairing the loud noise (UCS) with the white rat (neutral stimulus changed to CS), Albert developed a fear (CR) of white rats. In this experiment, Watson introduced a loud noise (UCS), which lead to a fear response (a natural response). He paired the rat (neutral stimulus) with the loud noise (UCS), which resulted in fear (UCR). After several pairings, presenting just the rat (CS) resulted in fear (CR); thus, Albert learned to fear the rat. The rat evoked fear in Albert the same way that the loud noise evoked fear in him (Watson & Rayner, 1920). Watson and Rayner demonstrated that some phobias in humans could be caused by classical conditioning.

Thorndike's Law of Effect

Another influential American psychologist who helped promote behavioralism and the study of learning was Edward Thorndike (1874–1949). Thorndike developed the **law of effect** while studying how cats learned to escape from puzzle boxes. Thorndike's theory represents the behavioral stimulus–response framework. According to Thorndike (1932), learning results from associating stimuli and responses. These associations become strengthened or weakened depending on the nature and frequency of the S-R pairing. More specifically, individuals' responses are more likely to be connected to situations that are followed by a satisfactory outcome compared to those situations followed by discomfort or an unsatisfactory outcome. Those responses associated with a satisfactory outcome are more likely to be repeated, and those responses associated with unsatisfactory outcomes are less likely to occur again. For example, in the cat experiments, the cat learned to escape from the puzzle box by associating the pressing of the lever (S) with the door opening (R). This S-R relationship was established because it resulted in a satisfactory outcome (law of effect).

Operant Conditioning

Unlike classical conditioning, operant conditioning refers to behaviors that are learned not by association with stimuli but as a result of previous consequences. In **operant conditioning**, a term first coined by B. F. Skinner (1904–1990), individuals learn by associating a consequence with a behavior. Skinner believed that all behaviors could be explained by examining external, observable causes of human behavior. Central concepts in operant conditioning are reinforcements and punishments (see Figure 2.1). **Reinforcements** are consequences that strengthen or increase the frequency of the behavior that they follow, while **punishments** are adverse events that decrease the frequency of the behavior they follow

Goal	Increase Behavior	Decrease Behavior
Stimulus applied	Positive reinforcement (rewards: stickers, praise)	Punishment (stimulus applied) (spanking, extra chores)
Stimulus withdrawn	Negative reinforcement (relief: chair returned, noise off)	Punishment (stimulus withdrawn) (privileges removed, "grounded")

Figure 2.1 Operant conditioning concepts.

(Skinner, 1953). Reinforcements can be either positive or negative. **Positive reinforcements** (reinforcement, stimulus applied) are favorable events or outcomes (rewards) that follow a behavior with the goal of increasing the frequency of occurrence of that behavior. **Negative reinforcement** (reinforcement, stimulus withdrawn) involves the removal of an unfavorable event or outcome (i.e., relief) after a behavior with the goal of increasing the frequency of that behavior. In either case, the behavior is strengthened; the goal is to increase the frequency of the behavioral display. Examples of positive reinforcement are praise and rewards. An example of a negative reinforcement is when a parent stops nagging a child to clean their room once the child cleans the room. The removal of the nagging (negative reinforcement) leads to an increase in the child cleaning the room. Like reinforcements, punishments can either be positive or negative. **Positive punishment** (punishment, stimulus applied) involves the presentation of an adverse event, while **negative punishment** (punishment, stimulus withdrawn) involves the removal or withholding of a pleasant event. For example, a parent may choose to nag (positive punishment) his daughter for hitting her brother or he may choose to take away electronic games for the day (negative punishment). In either case, the intention is to decrease the behavior of hitting her brother. Importantly, punishment only decreases, but does not extinguish a behavior. To extinguish a behavior completely, one must also reinforce the competing positive behavior. For example, punishing an adolescent for smoking does not extinguish the smoking, unless the adolescent is also rewarded for avoiding cigarettes. Figure 2.1 summarizes these four operant conditioning concepts, upon which numerous counseling interventions are based.

In addition to understanding the different types of reinforcements, one must also understand different reinforcement schedules. **Reinforcement schedules** refer to how and when reinforcements are applied. Reinforcements can be applied every time the behavior occurs (continuous schedule), or they can be applied on an irregular or partial basis (variable schedules). There are four types of reinforcement schedules: (1) fixed ratio; (2) fixed interval; (3) variable ratio; and (4) variable interval. In ratio schedules, the reinforcement is based on the number of behaviors, whereas in interval schedules, the reinforcement is based on the passage of time. **Fixed ratio** involves applying the reinforcement after a specific number of behaviors. For example, a mother tells her son to stop hitting his sister. After the third time, she puts him in timeout. The son quickly learns that he can get away with the first two requests before he has to listen to his mother. **Fixed interval** involves applying the reinforcement after a specific amount of time. An example of fixed interval is getting a bonus at the end of the year. This schedule can lead to individuals improving their performance at the end of the year to look good before the bonus is distributed. In **variable ratio**, reinforcements are given following a variable number of responses. Gambling and lotteries are examples of a variable ratio because one does not know how many times one has to gamble or purchase lottery tickets before winning. In **variable intervals**, reinforcements are distributed following a variable amount of time. Imagine that a boss comes by the office periodically during the week, but the time and day she stops by changes weekly. This is an example of variable intervals because one does not know when she is stopping by. Therefore, one is more likely to be productive at all times so that one is prepared no matter when the boss stops by. The type of reinforcement schedule implemented is dependent on the behavior reinforced.

REFLECTION 2.2 NEGATIVE REINFORCEMENT, PUNISHMENT, AND SISTER RITA

We have all seen reinforcements and punishments in action. Every time a parent uses praise, a special activity, or a favorite treat to gain behavioral compliance, the parent is using positive reinforcement. Every time the parent tries to get a child to stop doing something annoying or dangerous by yelling at, spanking, or taking a privilege away from the child, the parent is using a punishment. Or is she? Sometimes it is not so clear, until you understand the goal of the parent. You see, whenever a parent is trying to increase the frequency of a child's behavior, she is using reinforcement; whenever she is trying to decrease the frequency of a child's behavior, she is using punishment. You and I might find yelling to be punishing, and it may result in our decreasing some undesirable behavior; some people view yelling as a positive reward and will actually *increase* the frequency of some behavior to elicit more yelling—which these children view as attention from the adult. (Some children—and adults—crave attention of any kind.)

Take the example of young Bradley as a first grade student in Sister Rita's class. Young Bradley was quite a live wire and frequently left his seat without Sister Rita's permission, let alone her blessing. Sister Rita attempted to modify young Bradley's behavior by taking his chair away and making him stand at his desk for a half hour. Was this a reinforcement or punishment? Well, that would depend upon Sister Rita's intention (goal) (and young Bradley's reaction). If Sister intended to decrease the frequency of young Bradley's "out-of-seat behavior," then her intervention was a punishment (stimulus applied); Bradley's legs would tire, serving as a deterrent to future out-of-seat transgressions. However, if Sister Rita's goal was to increase young Bradley's in-seat behavior, then Sister was actually using negative reinforcement (relief given by returning the chair to reduce fatigue and encourage in-seat behavior). We may never know Sister's intentions regarding increasing in-seat (reinforcement) or decreasing out-of-seat behaviors (punishment), but we do know that Bradley adhered to Sister's "bottoms on the chair" rule with only a few applications!

As an aside, parents and teachers (and partners) will always have a long list of things they want others to do less of (i.e., decrease). Interventions aimed at decreasing the frequency of behaviors will, by definition, require punishment. However, the wise professional counselor (parent, teacher, partner, etc.) knows that every negative behavior has at least one competing positive behavior—which will lead to a reinforcement intervention. You accomplish this by asking, "What would you like him to be doing instead of [insert negative behavior here]?" Once the alternative competing behavior is identified, start reinforcing it and the negative behavior usually decreases on its own. ~BTE

In general, for new behaviors counselors may want to begin with continuous reinforcement and then switch to partial reinforcements (Fester & Skinner, 1957).

Social Learning Theory

Social learning theory, developed by Albert Bandura (b. 1925) and others, helped to fill the gap left behind by behaviorists. Social learning theory helped to explain the sudden appearance of complex behaviors. According to social learning theory, learning occurs through observation, imitation, or modeling, and the following conditions must be present in order for modeling (i.e., observational learning) to occur: (1) attention (one must pay attention to the behavior you are learning), (2) retention (one has to remember what was observed), (3) reproduction (one must translate what was observed into actual behavior), and (4) motivation (one must have some reason for imitating that behavior). Bandura believed in **reciprocal determinism**—the relationship between an individual and the environment. Unlike behaviorists, Bandura (1977, 1986) believed in the mutual influences between the psychological processes of the individual, the environment, and the behavior. In the now famous "**Bobo doll**" experiment, Bandura, Ross, and Ross (1961) examined the effects of models of aggression on preschool children's aggressive behavior. Preschool children were exposed to scenarios where models would display aggression toward a Bobo doll. The children exposed to the aggressive scenarios were more likely to act in physically aggressive ways than those in the control group. This demonstrated that aggressive behaviors may be acquired through observational learning.

Associated with Bandura's social learning theory is the concept of **self-efficacy**. As children receive feedback about their behaviors, they become more selective of their behaviors, and they begin to develop beliefs about their capabilities and their ability to influence events that affect their lives. This belief in their capabilities is self-efficacy. Self-efficacy determines how we feel and think, and it motivates us to behave (Bandura, 1994). Bandura's updated version of social learning theory is the social cognitive theory. This change in name reflects a greater emphasis on one's cognitive processes (Bandura, 1989) as a part of one's development. **Social cognitive theory** can be seen as a bridge between behaviorist and cognitive theory in that it includes attention, memory, and motivation, and because it emphasizes the active role of the individual's psychological processing in the learning process. Following is a discussion of psychoanalytic learning theory; cognitive and intellectual development will be explored in Chapter 3.

Psychoanalytic Learning Theory

Dollard and Miller (1950) developed **psychoanalytic learning theory** as a translation of psychoanalytic theory. They adapted psychoanalytic constructs for operationalization and testing in a laboratory setting. According to Dollard and Miller, drive, cue, response, and reinforcement combine to form the foundation of learning. **Drive** in this theory refers to a need that impels people to action. **Cues** determine when, where, and how people will behave. Cues are the discriminative stimuli that people notice at the time of the behavior. **Response** refers to behaviors. **Reinforcements** are the consequences of people's responses; they are connected to drives. According to Dollard and Miller, people continue to try different responses until they find the reinforcement that reduces or satisfies the drive. When attempts to reduce drives are blocked or prevented, frustration occurs. And when frustration becomes severe, it becomes conflict.

Think About It 2.6

Considering the four types of Dollard and Miller's conflicts and provide an example of each.

According to Dollard and Miller's theory, conflict is related to incompatible responses or to one's inability to respond to the drive that has been triggered. Dollard and Miller identified four types of conflicts:

- **Approach-avoidance conflict** occurs when the same behavior produces feelings of approach and avoidance.
- **Avoidance-avoidance conflict** occurs when one is forced to choose between two equally undesirable options.
- **Approach-approach conflict** refers to situations when one has to choose between two desirable things.
- **Double approach-avoidance conflict** occurs when one is faced with two choices that have both desirable and undesirable aspects.

Summary

Human development is cumulative, complex, and multi-faceted. No one theory can adequately describe or explain how we grow and develop. In this chapter, a brief overview of some of the major human development theories was presented. Although these theories were grouped in broad categories, there are some overlaps among the theories. In this chapter, human development theories were covered that viewed human development from a strictly biological stance to theories of human development that were more sociocultural in nature.

More specifically, this chapter began by examining human development from a historical context. Over the years, there has been a shift in how society views childhood and adolescence. In modern Western cultures, children are viewed as innocent and entitled to nurturance and protection. Additionally, children are viewed as fundamentally distinct from adults. This was not always the case. During the Middle Ages, children were viewed as miniature adults. In the 18th and 19th centuries, children were viewed as innocent and in need of adult protection and discipline. With the spread of the Industrial Revolution and the growing need for workers, children began to be viewed as part of the workforce and an economic necessity. This view of children as laborers shifted with the emergence of child labor laws and the growing perspective that children are to be valued and fulfill our need for love.

The psychosocial theories of human development are based on the belief that human development is influenced by our unique life history, including our early developmental years and sociopolitical and environmental factors. The psychosocial theories explored in this chapter include: Freud's psychosexual theory, the theories of neo-Freudians (Carl Jung, Alfred Adler, Karen Horney, and Harry Stack Sullivan), Erikson's psychosocial stages, Loevinger's theory of personality and ego development, and Chickering's theory of identity development. Psychosocial theories are especially appealing since they emphasize the importance of understanding each individual's unique life history.

Sociocultural theories of human development emphasize the important role of the environment, interactions, and systems on the development of the individual. The sociocultural theories examined in this chapter were Vygotsky's zone of proximal development, Bowen's multigenerational family systems, theories which address the development of the family lifecycle (i.e. Carter and McGoldrick), and Bronfenbrenner's ecological model of child development. These theories view individuals within a contextual framework and support conceptualizing individuals in a dynamic, interactional manner.

Similar to sociocultural theories of human development, multicultural theories of development emphasize the importance of context. What distinguishes this group of theories is that they were developed to address the needs of diverse individuals in an effective, respectful manner. Multicultural theories addressed in this chapter include the White racial identity development model, the Black racial identity development model, the biracial identity development model, and the multiple heritage identity development model. It was also noted that there are many more identity development models in the literature that focus on other marginalized minority groups.

Biological theories of human development include Darwin's theory of evolution, ethological theory, attachment theory, and maturation theory. Central to these theories is the belief that all behavior and mental processes can be explained by examining the human physiology and anatomy.

In contrast to the biological view of human development, learning theories propose that behaviors are learned through interactions with the environment. Learning theorists emphasize the influence of external factors on behavior. Learning theories explored in this chapter include behavioralism, social learning theory, and psychoanalytic learning theory. The major behavioral theories include classical conditioning, Thorndike's law of effect, and operant conditioning. In the next chapter, we will continue to explore theories of human development.

Theories of Human Development: Cognitions, Morality and Faith, and the Human Experience

By Lindy K. Parker, Caroline O'Hara, and Catherine Y. Chang

In this chapter, the exploration of theories of human development continues by examining theories of cognitive and intellectual development, moral development, humanism, and faith development. Finally, the chapter ends with a brief introduction to adult development theories, with a special focus on developmental theories of womanhood.

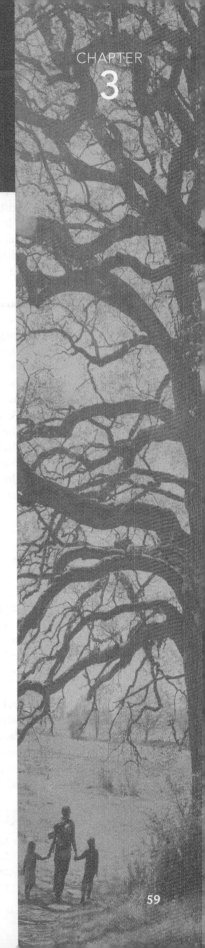

Theories of Cognitive and Intellectual Development

Theories of cognitive and intellectual development focus on the development of the thought process and the construction of knowledge.

Piaget's Stages of Development

Jean Piaget (1896–1980) was a Swiss researcher, trained as both a biologist and psychologist, who spent most of his career studying how people come to know what they know. He invested a great deal of time researching specifically how children learn. Though he ultimately defined himself as a genetic epistemologist, his constructivist theory of cognitive development has been influential in multiple disciplines, and continues to prompt writings and research today.

Piaget's theory begins with the process of **adaptation**, or how the human mind constructs knowledge (Piaget, 1970). As humans encounter new things (by experiencing them, hearing them, etc.) they **assimilate** this new information, fitting it into the already existing cognitive structures, so that it can be learned and understood in context along with everything else the person already knows. Still, the new information does affect a person, and the addition of this information may require that more sophisticated cognitive structures be formed and organized. This process is called **accommodation** (Piaget, 1970). Together, assimilation and accommodation are referred to as adaptation (Singer & Revenson, 1996). As the cognitive structures become more and more sophisticated and organized, so does the thinking of the individual. Piaget saw this cognitive development occurring within children in four general stages: sensorimotor (birth to 2 years), preoperational (2 to 7 years), concrete operational (7 to 11 years), and formal operational (12 years and older). Each of these stages of Piaget's theory of cognitive development will be discussed in more detail in later chapters.

Intelligence, Genetics, and Environment

While Piaget's theory is rather uniform and inclusive, other theorists have focused on the differences among people, specifically differences in race, environment, and SES, and how the intersection of these characteristics affects a person's intelligence. One of the most controversial researchers in the field, Arthur R. Jensen, has theorized that differences in intelligence can largely be attributed to a person's genetics. Thorndike stated that the chief determining factor is heredity and the goal of life is not to get ahead but to get ahead of someone else (Jensen, 1969). Jensen claimed in his research that those with lighter skin colors had higher intelligence than those with darker skin tones, ultimately due to their inherited genetics, with little due to their environment.

More recently, psychologist Richard J. Herrnstein and political scientist Charles Murray published their 1994 book *The Bell Curve: Intelligence and Class Structure in American Life*, which argues that a person's intelligence is determined by both genetic and environmental factors. They, too, bring up the connection between race and intelligence by stating: "It seems highly likely to us that both genes and the environment have something to do with racial differences," yet they say that more evidence is needed in order to understand the relationship (Herrnstein & Murray, 1994, p. 311).

Think About It   **3.1**   Multiculturalism

Some readers may remember the release of the 1994 book *The Bell Curve: Intelligence and Class Structure in American Life*, simply because of the media coverage surrounding both the criticism and support for the book. If not, please read it now. What are your own reactions to the connection the book makes between race and intelligence?

Intelligence and Age

Cognitive psychologist John L. Horn (1929–2006) thought of intelligence as having two parts: fluid intelligence and crystallized intelligence (Horn, 1968; Horn & Cattell, 1963). Working with Raymond B. Cattell (1905–1998), the crystallized and fluid theory of intelligence emerged. The theory considers the things learned from facts and experiences to be crystallized intelligence. *Crystallized intelligence* is less likely to decrease with age—in fact, it can even increase into old age. On the other hand, fluid intelligence is what we draw upon to complete tasks and to solve puzzles and other problems. *Fluid intelligence* can begin to decline in adulthood, just as the speed of completing tasks often slows as people age (Horn & Cattell, 1963).

Identifying Intelligence

Alfred Binet (1867–1911), a French psychologist, and his collaborator Theodore Simon (1872–1961) are often credited with creating the first measurement of intelligence, or what is called Intelligence Quotient (IQ) tests today. In their book, Binet and Simon (1916) recount their purpose in developing such a test: "In October, 1904, the Minister of Public Instruction [in Paris] named a commission which was charged with the study of measures to be taken for insuring the benefits of instruction to defective children" (p. 9). Ultimately, the charge was to find a way to predict which children would struggle with and even fail in traditional school, due to impaired or delayed intelligence. In order to do that, Binet had to first determine what intelligence was, and then decide how it could be measured. Dacey, Travers, and Fiore (2009) detail the three elements of Binet's view of intelligence:

1. There is direction in our mental processes; they're directed toward the achievement of a particular goal and the discovery of adequate means of attaining the goal. In the preparation of a term paper, for example, you select a suitable topic and the books and journals necessary to complete it.
2. We possess the ability to *adapt* by the use of tentative solutions—that is, we select and utilize some stimuli and test their relevance as we proceed toward our goal. Before writing the term paper, for example, you may make a field trip to the area you're researching, or to save time, you may decide to use relevant sources on the Internet or library resources.
3. We also possess the ability *to make judgments* and to criticize solutions. Frequently called *autocriticism,* this implies an objective evaluation of solutions. You may, for example, complete a paper, reread it, decide that one topic included is irrelevant, and eliminate it. This is autocriticism at work. (p. 242)

With this view of intelligence in mind, the Binet–Simon scale—considered the first IQ test—was created in 1905 (Binet & Simon, 1916). In 1916, the Stanford psychologist Lewis M. Terman revised the Binet–Simon scale, and his revised version is called the Stanford–Binet (Terman, 1916). Today, the Stanford–Binet is currently in its the fifth revision—the Stanford–Binet 5.

Information Processing: Wechsler (1896–1981)

Like Binet, David Wechsler developed a measurement of intelligence. Wechsler's work was highly influenced by his time spent as chief psychologist at the famous Bellevue Psychiatric Hospital (1932–1967) in New York City. Wechsler (1958) famously wrote, "intelligence is the aggregate or global capacity of the individual to act purposefully, to think rationally and to deal effectively with his environment" (p. 7).

As such, Wechsler's adult exam generally measures intelligence in four main areas: verbal comprehension, perceptual reasoning, working memory, and processing speed.

Wechsler also created two popular intelligence tests for children. Notably, Wechsler's tests did not use the ratio quotient scores used in IQ tests at the time, but instead used deviation quotient (DQ) scoring, or deviation IQ scores.

Multiple Intelligences: Gardner (b. 1943) and Goleman (b. 1946)

Also dissatisfied with the emerging assessments that provided only a single measure for intelligence, Howard E. Gardner proposed his **theory of multiple intelligences**. Gardner (1996) stated that his view "is a pluralistic view of mind, recognizing many different and discrete facets of cognition, acknowledging that people have different cognitive strengths and contrasting cognitive styles" (p. 6). Gardner goes on to specifically define intelligence as "the ability to solve problems, or to fashion products, that are valued in one or more cultural or community setting" (p. 7). He clarifies this by explaining that a culture of sailors might define a member of their society as being intelligent if he had great navigational ability, even though he might not, say, be familiar with the seminal works of English literature.

Through his research, Gardner (1999, 1983/2003) has been able to identify eight types of intelligence: linguistic, logical-mathematical, spatial, musical, bodily-kinesthetic, interpersonal, intrapersonal, and naturalist. He does emphasize that this list is only preliminary and not exhaustive—its main use is to explain that multiple intelligences do in fact exist (Gardner, 1996). Gardner has expressed hope that schools will take a student's unique intelligences into account for curriculum development and career training, rather than focusing on increasing a single universal intelligence score that does not accurately capture the student's unique intelligence. He suggests that many of the careers that students will enter will only require intelligence in some areas, not all.

Daniel J. Goleman believes that, in addition to cognitive intelligence, there is also emotional intelligence. Goleman (2001) says that emotional intelligence refers to the ability "to recognize and regulate emotions in ourselves and in others" (p. 14). In his research, he specifically emphasizes the importance of increasing emotional competencies for success in the workplace.

William G. Perry, Jr.: *Forms of Intellectual and Ethical Development in the College Years*

Harvard University professor and psychologist William G. Perry (1913–1998) studied the way intellectual and cognitive abilities developed in college-age students, and ultimately published his theory in 1970 as *Forms of Intellectual and Ethical Development in the College Years*. Perry's scheme, as it is referred to, includes three phases of development: dualism modified (sometimes referred to as dualism and multiplicity), relativism discovered, and commitment in relativism developed (Perry, 1970).

In **dualism modified**, a college-age student transitions from thinking that facts are facts, and professors must impart these facts to her, to realizing that even these teachers admit they do not know all the answers, and that there are differences in opinion and uncertainties among these authority figures (Perry, 1981). As the student progresses through **relativism discovered**, she begins to value opinions that can be strongly supported by facts; most knowledge is contextual, the world is complex, and Truth is not always clearly available (Kloss, 1994). Finally, in **commitment in relativism developed**, the student learns that everyone, including oneself, commits to a set of chosen values and beliefs without knowing, definitively, if they are *right* or *true,* and will have to do so throughout life (Perry, 1981).

Robert Kegan: The Constructive-Developmental Approach

Also a psychologist and professor at Harvard University, Robert Kegan (1980) developed what he called "constructive developmental psychology—the study of the *development* of

Think About It   3.2

What career did you want to pursue as an adolescent or young adult? Was it a career that was important to your parents or teachers, or highly regarded by the public? As you became more self-aware of your own skills, the available job market, and even the *meaning* you derive from your job each day, did your career aspirations change or evolve in any way, and if so, why?

our *constructing* or meaning-making activity" (p. 373). Influenced by the work of Jean Piaget, Kegan (1980) emphasized that his developmental approach applied not just to an individual's development during childhood or traditional college-age years, but throughout an entire lifespan. Kegan (1982) described his constructive-developmental framework as studying the "evolution of meaning" (p. 15). While Kegan (1980) broke the framework into several stages (i.e., incorporative, impulsive, imperial, interpersonal, institutional, and inter-individual), he stressed that the stages are "only a way of marking developments in a process. And it is this process that is fundamental to the framework, the process of restless, creative *activity* of personality, which is first of all about the making of meaning" (p. 374). Kegan's work has been applied to all areas of adult development, including the areas of professional and career development.

Cognitive Behavioral Theories

In the 20th century, the hypothesis that individuals hold greater control over the development of their own thoughts and feelings than earlier psychoanalytic theories described gained greater acceptance. Notable researchers and clinical practitioners created theoretical models of counseling and psychotherapy based on these newer ideas of development, and their theories are still studied and practiced by professional counselors today.

Rational Emotive Behavior Therapy

Albert Ellis (1913–2007), the developer of rational emotive behavior therapy (REBT), wrote, "there are a number of very common irrational, unrealistic, grandiose, self-defeating beliefs that people in our culture and in most other cultures have; and when they strongly believe these ideas they frequently, though not always, produce dysfunctional emotions and behaviors" (2003, p. 222). Ellis thought that people are born natural philosophers—of varying degrees—and have the tendency to think both rationally and irrationally (Ellis, 1980). By changing problematic personal philosophies or cognitions, a person could alter both his behavior and his emotions, and ultimately his life.

Ellis developed his ABC model to explain that an activating event (A) provoked a person to draw upon past beliefs and even form new beliefs (B) about potential and actual consequences (C) of this event (Ellis, 1991). By further examining the beliefs a person has drawn upon or formed and determining if they are rational or irrational beliefs, or if they can be positively altered, a person can control or create a better outcome. If the belief is irrational and leads to a negative consequence or emotional state, the client can dispute the belief (D) and then evaluate (E) the results to determine whether the altered belief led to a better consequence or emotional outcome. Ellis's views on cognition, emotion, and behavior greatly affected the field of psychotherapy, and his rational emotive behavior therapy is still popular today.

Cognitive Therapy: Aaron T. Beck (b. 1921)

Psychiatrist Aaron T. Beck and his associate Marjorie E. Weishaar (2000) claimed that infants are born with the ability to process information, and that they continue to process information throughout their development in order to survive. Understandably, the information processing begins very primitively—touch, taste, sound—and gradually develops into more sophisticated cognitions over time. Beck (1996) explains the developing cognitive functioning of the mind, specifically the expression of personality, in terms of schemas, systems, and modes. **Schemas** can be described as the framework or building blocks of the mind, and they consist of five basic **systems**: cognitive (or information processing), affective (or emotional), behavioral, motivational, and physiological. A **mode** is the integration of these systems and the many schemas that make up each system that is being integrated; and mode in turn activates a person's response.

Professional counselors continue to study and explore Beck's theory and research. In 1994, the Beck Institute was founded in Pennsylvania by Beck and his daughter, Judith Beck; it offers mental health professionals training and supervision in the practice of Beck's therapeutic model.

➤ CASE EXAMPLE **3.1** JUDY.

Judy originally came to counseling to address her difficulty with weight loss. After working with a cognitively oriented counselor to address Judy's susceptibility to salty and fatty foods and her negative thoughts about exercise, Judy's resolve to make better food and exercise choices was strengthened. Judy lost her extra weight and was successfully maintaining her healthy lifestyle.

Feeling more confident and happy with herself, Judy asked her counselor if they could now work on her parenting relationship with her two children, 7-year-old Max and 13-year-old Melissa. Judy told her counselor that Max was very loud, rambunctious, and difficult to calm down. Judy described Melissa as being very emotional and materialistic, always in search of new clothes to impress her friends.

The counselor knew Judy deeply loved her two children, but also noticed all the negative labels and descriptions Judy was using to describe them. The counselor asked Judy what might happen if she thought of Max as being energetic and confident, rather than loud and rambunctious. Judy said those more positive terms did describe Max, but she rarely used them. The counselor asked Judy what positive terms might be used to describe Melissa, and they came up with sensitive, caring, and fashionable.

The counselor challenged Judy to not only use those new positive terms when thinking about her children, but to also use them out loud when talking with Max and Melissa. With this new awareness, Judy became aware of all the times she used negative labels for her children in her thoughts and her discussions. As she began to use the more positive terms, her children began to soften and become much happier around Judy. Just a small shift in thoughts and language created big positive changes in the family dynamics.

Choice Theory: William Glasser (1925–2012)

According to **choice theory**, developed by William Glasser, all humans are born with five basic needs that they continually seek to fulfill: survival, love/belonging, power, fun/learning, and freedom. When Glasser writes about cognition, he often includes what he calls the **quality world** picture album each person holds in her mind, made up or remembered pictures of the person fulfilling their needs. Glasser (1998) states that pictures in this album are of "the people we most want to be with; the things we most want to own or experience; and the ideas or systems of belief that govern much of our behavior" (p. 45). As we and our environments grow and change, pictures can be removed or replaced with newer and more fulfilling pictures. Unfortunately, a person may choose to hold on to a picture that no longer satisfies or fulfills her needs, which could then lead one to choose behaviors that are ineffective and maladaptive. This can be seen, for instance, in a person who has lost a job that previously offered him belonging, power, and fun. He may choose to hold on to the picture of this job that is no longer available, and be unable to fulfill those needs for belonging, power, and fun, at least until he is willing to choose another picture.

Think About It **3.3**

What pictures in your own "quality world" album show your needs being fulfilled? Are there any pictures you are still holding on to that may not be able to provide you with the fulfillment they once did?

Moral Development

A shared morality, of course, is vital to the humane functioning of any society. Many forms of behavior are personally advantageous but are detrimental to others or infringe on their rights. Without some consensual moral codes people would disregard each other's rights and welfare whenever their desires come into social conflict. (Bandura, 1991, p. 45)

But how do we arrive at these moral codes? And when does moral development begin?

Locke's Tabula Rasa

John Locke (1632–1704), a 17th-century philosopher, felt that morals were learned by the teaching and observations of others, as well as by one's own experiences. His epistemological theory is often referred to as the **tabula rasa**, a Latin term that translates as "blank slate." Locke (1689/1996) explained that the mind is like a piece of white paper, void of any knowledge or understanding—including ideas of morality—and only comes to this knowledge or understanding through experience. Because we possess no innate tendencies and all differences among us can be attributed to experience, we can mold children to be and believe what we want them to.

Rousseau and Innate Goodness

Jean-Jacques Rousseau (1712–1778) was an 18th-century philosopher and writer who felt that we are born innately good, with a primitive sort of morality, but that society in fact corrupts man, evoking feelings of greed and jealousy. Proper morality can only come to man through formalized education (Rousseau, 1749/1964).

The Psychoanalytic, Social Learning, and Behavioral Perspectives

From the psychoanalytic perspective, moral development occurs as a child struggles to balance his instinctual drives and the expectations of his external authority. The child quickly learns that fulfilling his instinctual drives often results in punishment from the authority figure. As Freud explained, the child begins to identify with his same-sex parent—an external authority figure—and his superego begins to form (Freud, 1971). This superego serves as the moral regulator of his drives and instincts, and helps the child resist these urges and in turn avoid punishment.

From the social learning perspective, a child develops morals by learning what is and is not accepted by society and its members (Bandura, 1991). The social institutions that model this acceptable behavior can include members of the family, teachers at school, or any authority figure the child encounters or observes.

The behavioral perspective sees moral development as occurring in a controlled environment that conditions good, moral behavior. While some behaviorists might say that moral development also occurs through the punishment of bad behavior, in Skinner's (1962) utopia a child's positive behavior, and ultimately their moral code, is shaped only through reinforcement.

Piaget's Theory of Moral Development

While observing children of various ages engage in games of marbles, and after interviewing the children about concepts such as justice and ethics, Piaget constructed his theory of moral development of children (Piaget, 1932). His theory consists of three stages through which children pass when developing their own morality:

1. **Premoral**: From birth to around 4 years of age, children are not concerned with rules and have little to no sense of morality. During this time, the child moves through a purely motor period of simply handling the marbles as he pleases at a given moment, to an egocentric period of appropriately playing with the marbles, but on his own, without regard to other players in the game or being a part of the game itself.

2. **Heteronomous Morality**: From around 5 to 8 years of age, children adopt rules from authorities without question. In order to avoid punishment, these absolute rules must be obeyed. A period of cooperation emerges, in which the children play the game of marbles against one another to win, following the rules as they understand them.

3. **Autonomous Morality**: From around 8 to 12 years of age, children learn that the rules are set by society, including their peers, in a cooperative fashion. A codification of rules period occurs, during which the child learns the common and set rules of the game of marbles. Justice is delivered fairly, and that fairness can be adjusted based on the intent of the violator and the general agreement of society.

Kohlberg's (1927–1987) Theory of Moral Development

One of the most well-known theories of moral development was developed by Lawrence Kohlberg (1971, 1975). Almost as well known as the theory itself are the moral dilemmas Kohlberg used to develop his theory. In one particularly popular dilemma, Kohlberg (1975) explains

> the issue of stealing a drug to save a dying woman. The inventor of the drug is selling it for 10 times what it costs him to make it. The woman's husband cannot raise the money, and the seller refuses to lower the price or wait for payment. What should the husband do? (p. 671)

A study participant is then forced to decide the husband's best course of action: steal the drug and save a life, or follow the law and allow the wife to die. Then the participant must defend the choice with moral reasoning. The interesting facets of these dilemmas lie less in whether you decide one course or another, but *why*; what is the reasoning behind the decision?

Kohlberg's theory consists of three levels (preconventional, conventional, and postconventional), with each of the three levels having two stages (Kohlberg, 1971).

Level 1: Preconventional Level

Stage 1: *Punishment and obedience orientation*. Children obey the rules simply to avoid punishment, and they obey those in power simply because they are in power. The morality behind the rules and those enforcing them is not important or considered. It is only important to follow those rules made by the unquestioned authority so as not to be punished. Responding to the Kohlberg dilemma above, children might tell the researcher that stealing the drug is wrong because stealing is bad and a person will be punished for doing something bad like stealing (Kohlberg, 1984).

Stage 2: *Instrumental relativist orientation*. Children obey the rules, but only for self-satisfaction. Kohlberg (1971, p. 87) writes, "Reciprocity is a matter of 'you scratch my back and I'll scratch yours,' not loyalty, gratitude, or justice." There appears to be a shift from focusing on avoiding punishment to seeking self-satisfaction in one's own interest (Colby & Kohlberg, 1987). There is also a recognition that a reward for one person might not be a reward for another. At this stage, a child may suggest stealing the drug to save the wife, so the husband will be happy and his wife will be saved, but the child will recognize that stealing the drug is not the best thing for the seller of the drug and his perspective (Kohlberg, 1984).

Level II: Conventional Level

Stage 3: *Interpersonal concordance or "good boy–nice girl" orientation*. Children or teens seek the approval of society, and begin to appreciate good intentions. A sense of caring for humanity emerges, and actions motivated by empathy and caring, rather than individual greed, are valued (Kohlberg, 1981). Research participants classified in this stage may state that since the husband is stealing the drug to save a life, he should be forgiven or only punished lightly.

Stage 4: *"Law and order" orientation.* Children begin to value good behavior for the sake of social order. Laws must be obeyed so that the system can go on functioning; moreover, all must be mindful of what is best for the system. Responses to the dilemma at this stage can include "Exceptions to the law cannot be given. This would lead to totally subjective decisions on the part of law enforcers," which can lead to chaos in a society (Colby & Kohlberg, 1987, p. 43). Yet this stage can also include responses such as "Did the druggist have the right to charge that much? No, for him to make that much profit is ignoring his responsibility to people" (Colby & Kohlberg, 1987, p. 43).

Level III: Postconventional (or Autonomous, or Principled) Level

Stage 5: *Social-contract legalistic orientation (generally with utilitarian overtones).* The laws in place reflect the best values of society as well as the individual rights of each member within the society. If a law does not properly serve society, that law should be changed by the society. Specifically, Kohlberg (1984, p. 191) states that a response in this stage should demonstrate that "one recognizes that in this situation the wife's *right to life* comes before the druggist's right to property. There is some obligation to steal for anyone dying; everyone has a right to live and to be saved."

Stage 6: *Universal ethical-principle orientation.* A conscience of universal justice and respect for humanity decides what is right, and this conscience is above the law. Each individual and his dignity is respected, valued, and taken into account when seeking justice. Kohlberg (1981) provided an example of a response at this stage:

> Q: Should the husband steal the drug to save his wife? How about for someone he just knows?
>
> Richard (age 25 years): Yes. A human life takes precedence over any other moral or legal value, whoever it is. A human life has inherent value whether or not it is valued by a particular individual.
>
> Q: Why is that?
>
> Richard: The inherent worth of the individual human being is the central value in a set of values where the principles of justice and love are normative for all human relationships. (p. 120)

Carol Gilligan (b. 1936)

While Kohlberg's theory is well known, it has not gone unchallenged. Carol Gilligan (1982), using Kohlberg's own moral dilemmas in her research, argued that the autonomous thinking that comes along at Kohlberg's Postconventional level is encouraged more in boys, and perhaps even discouraged in girls. That is not to say that girls do not reach the same

---

Think About It **3.4**

What would your response be to the following Kohlberg (1984) dilemma and why?

> There was a woman who had a very bad cancer, and there was no treatment known to medicine that would save her. Her doctor, Doctor Jefferson, knew that she had only about six months to live. She was in terrible pain, but she was so weak that a good dose of painkiller like morphine would make her die sooner. She was delirious and almost crazy with pain, but in her calm periods, she would ask Dr. Jefferson to give her enough morphine to kill her. She said she couldn't stand the pain and she was going to die in a few months anyway. Although he knows that mercy-killing is against the law, the doctor thinks about granting her request. (p. 644)

Within which stage would your response likely fall according to Kohlberg's theory?

level of moral development as boys, but they might display their development in a different way. Gilligan and Attanucci (1988) refer to this different way as a **care perspective**—having concern for those in need, being mindful of relationships—as opposed to a **justice perspective**—having concern for fairness and focusing on what is right. In the famous Kohlberg dilemma that deals with stealing an unaffordable drug to save a dying wife, some girls might suggest pleading to the druggist for a discount or payment plan, or reaching out to friends and family for a loan. Boys, on the other hand, are inclined to do what they see as just, and make the case for stealing the drug to save an irreplaceable life. Still, the morality of caring is not reserved for girls alone. Gilligan and Attanucci (1988) saw the care perspective in boys as well, just as the morality of justice appeared in girls, when the researchers presented more real-life moral dilemmas.

Humanistic Theories of Development

Humanistic theories are rooted in the philosophies of existentialism and phenomenology; they embrace a holistic, positive approach to human existence. Humanistic psychology focuses on the individual's potential and stresses the importance of growth and self-actualization. Maslow (1962) described humanistic psychology as the "third force" in psychology, following psychoanalysis (first) and behaviorism (second). Humanist theories of human development include Maslow's hierarchy of needs, Rogers' personal growth, Buhler's developmental phase theory, and Johada's positive mental health.

Maslow's Hierarchy of Needs

> What a man can be, he must be. This need we may call self-actualization. . . . It refers to the desire for self-fulfillment, namely, to the tendency for him to become actualized in what he is potentially. This tendency might be phrased as the desire to become more and more what one is, to become everything that one is capable of becoming. (Maslow, 1943, p. 383)

Abraham Maslow (1908–1970), a founder and driving force behind humanistic psychology, is best known for developing the theories of hierarchy of needs and self-actualization. Fundamental to these concepts is a belief in the positive sides of mental health. As opposed to focusing on abnormalities and mental illness, Maslow focused on human potential and mental health through personal growth and development (Maslow, 1954/1987, 1962).

According to Maslow's **hierarchy of needs**, human beings have basic needs that must be met before we can meet other developmental needs. The hierarchy of needs is most commonly depicted as a pyramid (see Figure 3.1), with the lowest levels constituting our fundamental needs and more complex needs situated higher up on the pyramid (Maslow, 1954/1987). We must first satisfy our fundamental needs before we can progress through the more complex needs. There are five different levels, which can be divided into three main needs categories. The fundamental needs include both physiological needs and security needs. The first level, **physiological needs**, includes the basic needs for survival—water, air, food, and sleep. Our basic physiological needs are instinctive, and all other needs become secondary until these are met. Level two, **security needs**, include our need for safety and security. We all have a need to feel safe and out of danger. A sense of belonging (level 3) and esteem needs (level 4) make up the psychological needs. We are social beings and have a **need for belonging**, love, and acceptance. This is accomplished through our relationships with family and friends and our involvement in social groups. **Esteem needs** refer to our need for self-esteem, personal worth, and social recognition. The final category and level is **self-actualization**, which involves fulfillment of one's potential.

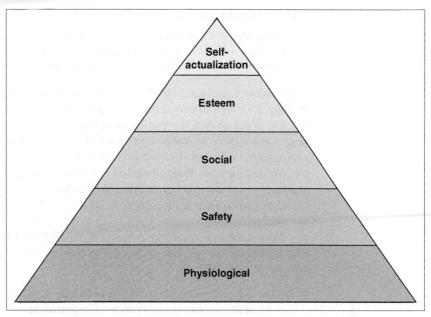

Figure 3.1 Maslow's hierarchy of needs.

According to Maslow (1954/1987), a self-actualized person has the following characteristics:

- Acceptance of self and others.
- Problem-centered and not self-centered.
- Spontaneity—self-actualized persons may conform to the social norms and expectations and still remain open and unconventional.
- Autonomous—self-actualized persons have a need for privacy and independence.
- Sense of appreciation for the world.
- Peak experience—self-actualized persons experience moments of intense joy, wonder, and awe.

Maslow's hierarchy of needs and his theory of self-actualization have been criticized for lack of empirical support for the individual-specific levels as well as lack of support for the hierarchical structure of the levels (Wahba & Bridwell, 1976). Despite these criticisms, Maslow's theories represent an important shift in psychology—a shift from abnormal development to a focus on the development of a healthy individual.

REFLECTION 3.1 MASLOW'S HIERARCHY OF NEEDS

Anyone who knows me knows that I am a big fan of zombie media (e.g., *The Walking Dead*, *28 Days Later*). These movies, television shows, and comics showcase an endless number of dire scenarios where survival and basic needs are emphasized. However, when considering Maslow's hierarchy of needs in the context of the zombie apocalypse, I may offer a challenge to the order of the hierarchy. From my perspective, if you are not safe and secure from rampaging zombies then it does not matter if you can sleep or find food or water. These musings underscore three important ideas when studying theories. First, theories may not align precisely with practice for each client (as they often do in textbooks). Second, examining and clarifying theories is a crucial critical thinking skill in the counseling profession. Third, consider the specific context of your client(s) when applying a theory. Although your clients may not be struggling to outpace zombies, each person's circumstances are unique! [~CO]

Rogers' Fully Functioning Person

> This process of the good life is not, I am convinced, a life for the faint-hearted. It involves the stretching and growing of becoming more and more of one's potentialities. It involves the courage to be. It means launching oneself fully into the stream of life. (Rogers 1961, p. 196)

Like Maslow, Carl Rogers (1902–1987) is considered one of the founders of humanistic psychology. Although Rogers is best known for developing client-centered (person-centered) therapy, which shifted the therapist-led psychotherapy toward a client-centered practice, Rogers also applied his belief in the uniqueness of each person and his belief, that given the appropriate conditions we all will gravitate toward psychological health, into a theory of personality development. Rogers believed that human beings were dynamic and ever-changing and that the self was in progress. Also, like Maslow, Rogers (1959) believed that humans had a tendency toward self-actualization. According to Rogers, we become self-actualized when our ideal self (who we want to be) is congruent with our actual behavior (self-image).

The outcome of successful personality development is the **fully functioning person**, who is striving for self-actualization. The characteristics of the fully functioning person include (Rogers, 1961):

1. *Openness to experiences.* The fully functioning person is free from threat, and therefore free from defensiveness and open to all experiences.
2. *Existential mode of living.* Fully functioning persons trust and accept themselves. There is recognition that each experience is new and that one cannot have complete control over experiences; therefore, life is approached with flexibility and adaptability and fully appreciated in the moment.
3. *Trust in one's organism.* Trust in one's organism involves trusting one's self-evaluation as a guide to satisfying behavior. The fully functioning person recognizes that they have the authority over their own lives, and this trust in one's authority is based on data gathered from past experience.

Rogers viewed these three characteristics as a process rather than an end product; therefore, in order to develop into a fully functioning person, one also has to have a willingness to be in the "process of becoming" (Rogers, 1961, p. 119).

Bühler's Developmental Theory

> It is becoming clearer that we in youth psychology, as in psychology in general, cannot proceed from single investigations, but must ask ourselves: how does the growing person gradually gain his relationships to the world, its laws, tasks and possibilities? (Buhler, 1929, p. 186)

Charlotte Bühler (1893–1974) was also instrumental in the development of humanistic psychology. Bühler espoused a holistic view of human development, emphasizing the end goal of human fulfillment. She believed that we find personal fulfillment through fully realizing our potential (Bühler & Allen, 1972). We all have four basic human tendencies and a core self:

1. The tendency to strive for physical and personal satisfaction (e.g., water, food, love, ego recognition);
2. The tendency toward self-limiting adaptation; these needs include our need to adjust and adapt to our environment for the purpose of fitting in, belonging, and gaining a sense of security in the world;
3. The tendency toward creative self-expression and accomplishments; this need includes our desire for authority and leadership as well as our need to be industrious, enterprising, and self-expressive; and
4. The tendency toward integration or order-upholding involves our desire for congruency and unity in our personality.

The **core self** is what integrates and directs the four tendencies, and it is the source of our unique personality patterns. Because the core self is unique, we each strive toward our tendencies in a unique manner. Bühler believed that although the need for integration remains active throughout one's lifespan, the first three tendencies correspond to infancy (primary tendency), childhood (self-limiting tendency), and adolescence (creative tendency), respectively. Bühler is best known for advancing her theories of child and adolescent development (Derobertis, 2006).

Jahoda's Positive Mental Health

> . . . the absence of disease may constitute a necessary, but not a sufficient, criterion for mental health. (Jahoda, 1958, p. 15)

Marie Jahoda (1907–2001) developed "**positive psychology**" by focusing on the mental health of individuals rather than mental disease. She believed that psychologists were not giving enough attention to mental health and well-being. She identified five characteristics of a healthy person: (1) time management, (2) meaningful social relationships, (3) ability to work effectively with others, (4) high self-esteem, and (5) regular activity.

Jahoda (1958) described six major approaches to defining positive mental health:

1. *Attitude toward self.* An important indicator of positive mental health is one's attitude toward oneself. Self-confidence, self-reliance, independence, initiative, and self-esteem are all indicators of positive mental health. Individuals who have a clear understanding of their own strengths and limitations, coupled with a belief that their positive attributes outweigh their negative attributes, are more likely to experience positive mental health.
2. *Growth, development, and self-actualization.* In contrast to the first category, this category is concerned with what an individual does over time. Similar to Maslow's concept of self-actualization, this aspect of positive psychology is concerned with developing toward a higher goal, one that is concerned with other people and one's environment.
3. *Integration.* Integration "refers to the relatedness of all processes and attributes in an individual" (p. 36). Individuals with positive mental health have a balanced, unified outlook on life, and a tolerance for tension, ambiguity, and frustration.
4. *Autonomy.* Individuals with positive mental health are self-determined, self-directed, and self-controlled.
5. *Perception of reality.* Individuals who are mentally healthy perceive the world free from distortions and with empathy.
6. *Environmental mastery.* This category refers to an individual's achievements in some significant areas of living and one's ability to adapt to their environment. Jahoda (1958) further delineates this dimension into these forms of human functioning: "(1) the ability to love; (2) adequacy in love, work, and play; (3) adequacy in interpersonal relationship; (4) efficiency in meeting situational requirements; (5) capacity for adaption and adjustment; and (6) efficiency in problem-solving" (p. 53).

Since the work of Jahoda, others have formulated their own views on positive psychology. Specifically, Jourard and Landsman (1980) proposed the following criteria for positive psychology: positive self-regard, ability to care about others, ability to care about the natural world, openness to new ideas and to people, creativity, ability to work productively, ability to love, and realistic perception of self. Additionally, consistent with Jahoda's six criteria, Jensen and Bergin (1988) identified eight themes for a positive, mentally healthy lifestyle:

> (1) competent perception and expression of feelings (sensitivity, honesty, openness with others); (2) freedom/autonomy/responsibility (self-control, appropriate feelings of guilt, responsibility for one's actions, increasing one's alternatives at a choice point); (3) integration, coping, and work (effective coping strategies, work satisfaction, striving to achieve); (4) self-awareness/growth (awareness of potential, self-discipline); (5) human relatedness/interpersonal and family

commitment (ability to give and receive affection, faithfulness in marriage, commitment to family needs, self-sacrifice); (6) self-maintenance/physical fitness (healthful habits, self-discipline in use of alcohol, drugs, tobacco); (7) mature values (purpose for living, having principles and ideals); and (8) forgiveness (making restitution, forgiving others). (Jensen & Bergin, 1988, p. 292)

Character Strengths and Positive Psychology

Originally known for his work on learned helplessness, Martin Seligman branched out to explore, define, and expand the knowledge base of the field of positive psychology. Working with Christopher Peterson, he developed a catalog of strengths and virtues (Peterson & Seligman, 2004), a direct challenge to the pathology and deficit foci of the *Diagnostic and Statistical Manual of Mental Disorders* (APA, 2013). The six character virtues include courage, humanity, justice, temperance, transcendence, and wisdom/knowledge. Within each virtue are several subfactors (strengths). For example, the factor of wisdom/knowledge includes the strengths of creativity, curiosity, judgment, love of learning, and perspective. See http://www.authentichappiness.sas.upenn.edu/ for links to many resources and assessment tools related to the character strengths and virtues.

Faith Development

James Fowler introduced his **faith development theory** almost four decades ago; Fowler and Dell (2006) defined faith development theory as

> a framework for understanding the evolution of how human beings conceptualize God, or a Higher Being, and how the influence of that Higher Being has an impact on core values, beliefs, and meanings in their personal lives and in their relationships with others. (p. 34)

Fowler and Dell (2006) further define faith with the following:

> Understood in this more inclusive sense, faith may be characterized as an integral, centering process, underlying the formation of beliefs, values, and meanings that:
> 1. Give coherence and direction to persons' lives;
> 2. Link them in shared trusts and loyalties with others;
> 3. Ground their personal stances and communal loyalties in a sense of relatedness to a larger frame of reference; and
> 4. Enable them to face and deal with the challenges of human life and death, relying on that which has the quality of ultimacy in their lives. (p. 36)

While the stages of faith development are generally associated with certain age groups, it is not guaranteed that all will move along the stages of faith development as they age. Or others may progress through the stages more rapidly. Still, most of the stages of faith development, particularly the four earliest stages of faith development, rely on and occur in concert with the stages of biological and emotional development (Fowler, 1974, 1995). The four earliest stages of faith development (referred to as stage 0, stage 1, stage 2, and stage 3) are:

- Stage 0—*Primal Faith* (infancy to age 2): This stage focuses on the infant receiving (or not receiving) everything necessary for healthy and normal growth and development, including proper nutrition and nurturing from a caregiver to whom the infant has a healthy attachment. Not only are these basic needs crucial to healthy brain and body functioning; they also allow the infant to develop a sense of trust in his or her surroundings, world, and perhaps even the divine (Erikson, 1963; Fowler & Dell, 2006).
- Stage 1—*Intuitive-Projective Faith* (toddlerhood and early childhood): The introduction of words and symbolic thought allows children to imagine and construct ideas beyond

what they experience within their immediate reality. Questions about death can arise, as well as a fascination with fantasy stories and tales of good versus evil (Bettelheim, 2010; Fowler & Dell, 2006).

- Stage 2—*Mythic-Literal Faith* (middle childhood and beyond): The notion of cause-and-effect becomes clearer, and the concept of justice becomes important. Fowler and Dell (2006) state that "the child believes that goodness is rewarded and badness is punished" (p. 39); in turn, rulings meted out by a higher power are done so in fairness.
- Stage 3—*Synthetic-Conventional Faith* (adolescence and beyond): As thought processes become more sophisticated, so do ideas and reflections about faith. Still, thoughts of the divine are largely influenced by the thoughts of those surrounding the individual, and one often conforms to the beliefs of the important figures in his life.

The final three stages of faith development (stages 4, 5, and 6) are mainly intended to be descriptions of phases in which one might find oneself along the spiritual journey; that is, they are *not* measures to identify a "better" spiritual life. Fowler and Dell (2006) stated that the later stages are simply attempts "to describe patterns of knowing and relating through assessing cognitive, moral, and other forms of development that constitute a person's relationship to the transcendent or the Higher Being of a particular religious tradition and relationships with other humans, both inside and outside a person's particular faith community" (p. 40). The three later stages of faith development are:

- Stage 4—*Individuative-Reflective Faith*: During this stage, a person begins to reflect on and even question what one believes and why one believes it. One explores self-awareness and personal identity, and the beliefs that remain at the conclusion of this exploration become more personal to the individual.
- Stage 5—*Conjunctive Faith*: This stage is rarely encountered before midlife, and when a person is in this stage the person begins to accept that there may be multiple truths. Paradoxes do exist and cannot always be reasoned away; rather, they might be embraced (Fowler & Dell, 2006).
- Stage 6—*Universalizing Faith*: Fowler and Dell (2006) state that for persons in this stage, "evil of all kinds is opposed nonviolently, leading to activism that attempts to change adverse social conditions as an expression of that universal regard for all life that emanates from God's love and justice" (p. 41).

While it is rare for a person to encounter this last stage, many of us can recognize the names of those who have likely experienced this stage of faith development: Mohandas Gandhi, the Reverend Dr. Martin Luther King Jr., and Mother Teresa (Fowler, 1995). These people, along with others in this stage, are inspired to act because of their beliefs, yet their actions seem inclusive and to the benefit of all humanity and not just those who subscribe to their way of believing, thinking, or faith.

Oser's Religious Judgments

Professor of education and educational psychology at the University of Fribourg, Switzerland, Fritz K. Oser (1994) addressed moral, religious, and faith development in terms of **religious judgment** that were centered around a person's religious understanding. Religious judgment does not refer to the judgment that God (or a higher power, ultimate being, etc.) might make on humanity; rather, it refers to the human "reasoning that relates reality as experienced to something beyond reality and that serves to provide meaning and direction beyond learned content" (p. 376).

For example, imagine something tragic has happened to a client—perhaps a client has been in a terrible motorcycle accident that has left him partially paralyzed and seeking the assistance of a rehabilitation counselor. Or suppose a student is experiencing

Think About It   3.5

Think about the last time you experienced a tragedy or crisis. Did you wonder about the involvement of God or an Ultimate Being in that event or its aftermath? How might you work with a client who is experiencing a tragedy or crisis and making these religious judgments during a counseling session?

grief over the accidental death of a teacher, and the student goes to visit her school counselor. Often in these counseling sessions, discussions can occur around how God was involved in the tragedy, or even perhaps how God appeared *uninvolved*. Clients may ask why God *allowed* these events to happen. Oser (1994) might say these discussions and "assessments of the accident involved religious judgments made in the light of their conceptions of how God and they are related" (p. 376).

Through his research, Oser identified stages of religious judgment. At stage 1, an incomprehensible God is seen as simply acting upon the world uninfluenced by people, while at stage 2 these actions by God can be influenced by a person's good or bad deeds (Hood, Hill, & Spilka, 2009). Stage 3 focuses on the realization that God is separate or distinct from the autonomous human world, whereas stage 4 considers freedom stemming from God's ultimate and divine plan that gives meaning to a person's life. Finally, in stage 5 God is seen as intertwined in human action that takes place in the world, including love and kindness.

Adult Development Theories

Adult development theories are concerned with examining the development of individuals in their adult years. Adult development theorists typically divide adult development into three periods [i.e., young adulthood (see Chapters 13–14), middle adulthood (see Chapters 15–16), and later adulthood/old age (see Chapters 17–18)], each of which you will read more about later in this book. In this section, we will provide a brief overview of some of the theories that examine how we develop throughout our adulthood.

Gould's Phases of Adult Life

Roger Gould (b. 1935) developed a theory of adult development based largely on the work of Erik Erikson. According to Gould (1978), we progress through a series of age-defined life phases in which we attempt to give up the illusions and myths of our childhood, with the goal of establishing a personal identity. Gould's stages include:

- *Leaving the Parents' World* (16 to 22 years old): The goal of this stage is to break away from parental control while maintaining a sense of safety and belonging.
- *Entering the Adult World* (22 to 28 years old) (aka: I'm nobody's baby now!): This stage is full of optimism and determination. During this stage, we pursue our career aspirations but with very little introspection.
- *Questioning and Reexamination* (28–34 years old): The individual becomes disillusioned and begins soul searching.
- *Midlife Decade* (35–45 years old): The individual becomes aware that time is running out and encounters the finite nature of life.
- *Reconciliation and Mellowing* (45–50 years old): The individual begins to settle down and turns more introspective.
- *Stability and Acceptance* (50 years and over): In this stage, the individual experiences an increased level of consciousness and acceptance of accomplishments.

Levinson's Seasons of Life

Daniel Levinson (1920–1994), an American psychologist, developed a comprehensive theory of adult development based on intensive interviews with men and later with women (Levinson, Darrow, Klein, Levinson, & McKee, 1978). Central to this theory is the concept of **life structure**—the underlying pattern of a person's life. Your life structure is shaped primarily through your interactions with individuals, groups, and institutions. According to Levinson, development is a sequence of distinct eras or stages, each beginning with a transition and then followed by a period of stability. The four eras (with overlapping age ranges to account for developmental variations) include:

1. *Childhood and Adolescence* (age 0–22 years): This was considered the era of preadulthood. During this era, the individual begins to make preliminary choices for adulthood.
2. *Early Adulthood* (17–45 years): This era involves important decisions related to work, marriage, children, and lifestyle. During this era, individuals may construct a dream or image of their adulthood that guides their decision making. As this era ends, one enters middle adulthood, begins to question the meaning in life, and becomes increasingly aware of mortality. Based on one's desire to leave a legacy, a new life structure may be created.
3. *Middle Adulthood* (40–65 years): During middle adulthood, one is committed to the new life structure. This new life structure is based on a major life review, which may include a readjustment of priorities and aspirations that were constructed during early adulthood.
4. *Late Adulthood* (60 years and older): The final era is late adulthood, during which, similar to Erikson's stage of ego integrity versus despair, one is focused on reflecting on past achievements and regrets.

Each era has distinctive and unifying qualities which take into account biological, psychological, and social aspects.

Havighurst's Theory of Human Development and Developmental Tasks

Robert J. Havighurst (1900–1991) developed a theory of human development based on accomplishing a series of developmental tasks. **Developmental tasks** refer to both problems and life adjustments that individuals must accomplish. Successful resolution of these developmental tasks results in happiness and success with future tasks, while unsuccessful resolution can lead to unhappiness and difficulty with future tasks. Havighurst (1973) believed that the tasks for each developmental stage are contingent on the individual and the individual's society; therefore, his theory can be seen as bio-psycho-social. There are developmental tasks associated with physical maturation (bio), those which arise from personal values (psycho), and those related to societal expectations (social). He also believed that certain developmental tasks were universal (e.g., learning to walk), while others were socially or culturally bounded (e.g., the age when individuals leave home). Following are the developmental stages and the developmental tasks associated with each specific stage (Havighurst, 1973):

1. *Infancy and Early Childhood* (birth to 6 years old): The developmental tasks include learning to crawl, walk, eat solid foods, talk, control bodily functions, and begin formulating concepts related to social and physical reality.
2. *Middle Childhood* (6–12 years old): The developmental tasks include getting along with peers, developing concepts necessary for everyday living, developing a conscience and values, achieving independence, and developing attitudes about social groups and institutions.
3. *Adolescence* (13–18 years old): The developmental tasks associated with this stage include developing masculine or feminine social roles, enhancing mature relations with peers, achieving emotional independence from parents and other adults, preparing for marriage, establishing a set of values to guide behavior, and working toward socially responsible behavior.

4. *Early Adulthood* (19–29 years old): The developmental tasks include finding a life partner, starting a family, raising children, establishing an occupation, finding a social group, and taking on civic responsibility.
5. *Middle Age* (30–60 years old): The developmental tasks include adjusting to teenage children and aging parents, reaching satisfactory performance in one's occupation, developing adult leisure activities, relating to one's partner as a person, and accepting the physiological changes associated with middle age.
6. *Later Maturity* (60 years and older): Tasks include adjusting to failing health, retirement, death of a spouse, and adapting to more flexible social roles and a satisfactory living situation.

Vaillant's Adaptation to Life

George Vaillant (b. 1934), like Levinson, proposed a model of adult development based on a longitudinal study in which he followed approximately 250 men born in the 1920s. He later interviewed them at ages 47, 60, and 70 about work, family, and physical and mental health. He was primarily interested in examining the traits that either enhanced or prevented success and happiness in these men (Vaillant, 1977). Like Levinson, Vaillant also interviewed women later in his career. Vaillant's **adaptation of life theory** is similar to Levinson's seasons of life, although his stages do not follow a strict age-related sequence like Levinson's. Also, Vaillant's theory confirms and expands on Erikson's stages. According to Vaillant, adult development follows this sequence: intimacy, career consolidation (early adulthood), generativity, keeper of meaning (middle adulthood), and ego integrity (late adulthood). Vaillant used the Freudian concept of defense mechanisms to interpret his results. According to Vaillant, defense mechanisms range from psychotic mechanisms to mature mechanisms, with immature and neurotic mechanisms in between. The more immature mechanisms may be pathological and can result in socially unacceptable behavior, while the more mature mechanisms tend to produce positive side effects.

Vaillant and Mukamal (2001) identified six functional domains that lead to well-being in late adulthood: (1) objectively assessed physical health; (2) subjectively assessed physical health; (3) length of time participants were active; (4) objectively measured mental health; (5) subjective measure of mental health and life satisfaction; and (6) objectively measured social support (Nolan & Kadavil, 2003).

Sheehy's Passages

Gail Sheehy (b. 1937) is best known for her book *Passages* (1976/2004), where she described the external (e.g., influence of culture) and internal (e.g., our perception of external events) forces that influence individuals as they journey through adulthood. Like others, Sheehy based her description of adult development on in-depth interviews. Central to Sheehy's description of adult passages are the constructs of marker events and life accidents. **Marker events** are those concrete events in our lives (e.g., graduation, marriage, childbirth). These marker events do not define our developmental stages but may accentuate our need to change. **Life accidents** are those events that people are powerless to prevent (e.g., war, economic decline, death of a family member) and, like marker events, may influence how we resolve our life passage.

Sheehy (1976/2004) described life passages or developmental ladders that each of us will experience, as follows:

- *Pulling Up Roots:* The task in this passage is to begin developing social connections so that we can begin the process of leaving home.

- *The Trying Twenties:* The task in this passage is to prepare for life work and to form the capacity for intimacy.
- *The Catch-30s:* This passage involves reevaluating the choices made in the twenties and either forming new dreams or converting an old dream into a more realistic one.
- *The Deadline Decade:* As one reaches the halfway mark to the lifespan, one must reexamine one's purpose and reevaluate resources. This passage can be a time of danger and opportunity. This passage is marked with darkness and great hope as one learns to disassemble and renew oneself.
- *Renewal or Resignation:* As one approaches the mid-forties, one achieves a new stability and views life with satisfaction if she has successfully embraced the midlife transition. Conversely, if one has refused to engage in the midlife transition, one will experience resignation.

In Sheehy's original writings, the age range for her passages included 18 years of age to the 50s. Later she (Sheehy, 1995) extended the age range and renamed her passages to: provisional adulthood (from age 18 to 30 years), first adulthood (from 30 to 45 years), second adulthood (from 45 to 75 years), and third adulthood (from 75 years on).

Duvall's Life Course Transition

Evelyn Duvall was concerned with adult development as it related to the **family lifecycle**, the patterned stages of family composition and changes that affect family members' behavior over time. Duvall proposed the following stages of the family lifecycle based on changes in family size, the developmental stage of the eldest child, and the work status of the breadwinner (Duvall, 1957, 1977):

- *Stage 1: Married couples without children:* In this stage, the couple is newly married and childless, and the major task involves the couple being committed to each other.
- *Stage 2: Childbearing families* (oldest child, birth to 30 months): With the birth of the oldest child, the parents must begin to develop their parent roles.
- *Stage 3: Families with preschool-aged children* (oldest child 30 months to 6 years): As the oldest child enters the preschool age, the parents are learning to accept the child's personality.
- *Stage 4: Families with school-aged children* (oldest child 6–13 years): During this stage, the parents begin to introduce their child(ren) to institutions including school, churches, and sports groups.
- *Stage 5: Families with teenagers* (oldest child 13–20 years): At this stage, the parents must begin to accept their growing adolescent(s) and adapt to the social and sexual role changes of their child. As the children grow, parents must also adapt to their child(ren) experimenting with independence.
- *Stage 6: Families as launching centers* (first to last child leaves home): This stage begins with the oldest child leaving home and involves the parents' acceptance of their child's independent adult role.
- *Stage 7: Middle-aged parents* (empty nest to retirement): In this stage, parents learn to let go of their children and begin to refocus on each other.
- *Stage 8: Aging family members* (retirement to death of both spouses): This stage involves retirement and accepting old age.

Duvall's life course development is based on the assumption that families are interrelated and that as members enter and exit the family and as the eldest child transitions into the next developmental stage, all family members must redefine their roles in relation to each other. There is also an underlying assumption that success in one stage leads to success in the next stage, and that failure in one stage could lead to difficulties in the next stage.

Peck's Theory of Adult Development

Robert Peck, building on Erikson's lifespan theory, expanded on the life tasks of older adults. He suggested that older adults progress through three major tasks. They are (Peck, 1968):

1. *Ego development vs. work-role preoccupation:* The task is to develop satisfaction in oneself that is not constructed through one's occupation or work role.
2. *Body transcendence vs. body preoccupation:* The task is to learn to derive pleasures psychologically rather than be absorbed with the health issues associated with the aging process. This task involves coping with the physical changes associated with aging.
3. *Ego transcendence vs. ego preoccupation:* The task is to find satisfaction in reminiscing about life rather than obsessing on impeding death.

Peck suggested that development occurs sequentially; however, development may vary among individuals. According to Peck (1968), older adults who successfully achieve the identified tasks will feel a sense of satisfaction and a vision of a world beyond themselves.

Butler's Life Review

Robert Butler (1927–2010), a gerontologist, pioneered the study of aging. He believed in the importance of **life review**, the process of reflecting on and reevaluating one's life. Butler (1968) suggested that life review is triggered by an increasing awareness of the inevitability of death and that older adults engage in the process of life review in order to attain ego integrity.

Developmental Theories (Perspectives) of Womanhood

> **Think About It   3.6**
>
> What is gender? How does it contrast with one's sex? In what ways has gender been an organizing principle in your life, with your family, and in your activities? What do you know about transgender people, experiences, and identities? If you could spend a day as another gender, what would you do and why?

As you may have noticed, European or European-American males have developed the vast majority of the theories discussed up to this point in the book, many by studying males exclusively. Although that is not a reason to discard or dismiss an idea, it is important to acknowledge that unless professional counselors actively address issues around gender, sex, and gender identity, the potential to do harm to clients (regardless of sex or gender) is a very real possibility. As multicultural counseling theories have broadened the perspectives of traditional theories to consider diverse populations, several pioneers have also addressed women's perspectives, challenges, and strengths. The following theories serve to examine power imbalances based on gender and to acknowledge the systemic, contextual, and cultural influences on all people. These perspectives can integrate naturally into the wellness model within which professional counselors work because the approaches are strengths-based and developmentally attentive. Furthermore, these theories acknowledge the multidimensional and dynamic nature of human development.

Jean Baker Miller (1927–2006)

In her groundbreaking book *Toward a New Psychology of Women* (1976), Jean Baker Miller spoke to the social, economic, and political changes that were sweeping the United States. She offered new perspectives in understanding people in context and in identifying the strengths and challenges that women face from systems of sexism and patriarchy, systems which damage all people regardless of sex, gender, or gender identity. Her central thesis holds that **connectedness** in relationships is central to the promotion of growth and development. Conversely, disconnection is the source of psychological ills and obstacles to wellness. Instead of focusing on independence, autonomy, and individualism, Miller and other feminists of the time advocated for connection and interdependence as means to achieve optimal growth and development (Ivey et al., 2007). In addition, she recognized that women are socialized to suppress anger, particularly in interpersonal relationship conflicts. The results can be damaging to wellness and may lead to psychological and physical distress. Miller also found that women tend to devalue womanhood as a result of contextual forces of power imbalances, male privilege, and sexism. Miller is one of the scholars who provided a theoretical foundation for **relational-cultural theory**.

Harriet Lerner (b. 1944)

The Dance of Intimacy (1989) by Harriet Lerner focused on how to define intimacy and how to enhance genuine closeness without sacrificing one's self or another's self in the process. Her body of work asserts that distance, intensity, and pain can serve to inhibit true and lasting intimacy. Lerner has often employed the use of genograms to help elucidate family and relationship patterns and processes. Throughout her career, Lerner has infused principles of feminism and family systems theories in her work and publications, with attention to culture, sexual identity, gender, and other social identities.

Carol Tavris (b. 1944)

Carol Tavris's *The Mismeasure of Woman* (1992) furthered the exploration of the impact of using a male standard to judge women. She suggests a shift away from the scientific inquiry of differences between males and females, as females usually end up in an inferior position, and argues against biological reductionism. She also challenges essentialist ideas that women are innately more nurturing, caring, and connected to others; she suggests instead that it is external political and social forces that encourage women to fulfill these roles. In addition, Tavris draws attention not only to the double standard in judging women, but also to the double standards within these debates (e.g., multiple races or ethnicities are often unrepresented in dialogues about women).

Carol Gilligan (b. 1936)

The work of Carol Gilligan has been highly incisive in broadening theories of mental health, wellness, growth, and development for women or for those not in the male majority. She and others have been tireless in challenging, questioning, and critiquing traditional theories of "normal" or "healthy" development as they point out that these theories are embedded with androcentric assumptions about humanity. For example, many theories of development equate maturity with qualities typically associated with males or masculinity. Her book *In a Different Voice* (1982) spoke to these concerns, including specific themes that contrast with the work of Lawrence Kohlberg on moral development.

➤ CASE EXAMPLE **3.2**   THE CASE OF BINDU.

Bindu is a young adult woman who is about to graduate from college. Her family originally hailed from Liberia. She is struggling with the transition as she does not have a job secured and her father is pressuring her to attend graduate school. Bindu also does not know where she will live after graduation. Her parents have indicated that she could stay with them, but she knows that if she lives with them she will feel additional pressure from them as to how to live her life. However, since she has limited financial resources, Bindu may have to return to live with her parents, at least temporarily.

 Several issues arise with Bindu. One might initially think of traditional theories of development such as Erikson, for example, or one might consider theories of the family lifecycle. The primary tasks for Bindu might include forming intimate relationships and separating from her family of origin. However, when we consider the perspectives of Miller, Lerner, Tavris, and Gilligan, the situation may not be so clear. Bindu not only wants to express more individuality and autonomy to her parents, but also does not want to disrespect them. Her culture of origin and the culture of her family system is more collectivist in nature. So a professional counselor who pushes Bindu to practice assertiveness training or anger expression techniques may not be properly attending to her relational and cultural context. As a Liberian-American woman, Bindu may value the family unit over her own individualism. However, given that she may be more acculturated than her parents, she may feel a pull toward "American" culture as well. When working with Bindu, it will be important to understand her frame of reference with respect to herself, her gender, her family, and her culture, and to not incorrectly pathologize or overpathologize her expressions of distress, coping mechanisms, and help-seeking behaviors.

Summary

This chapter examined human development theories that explain cognitive and intellectual development, humanistic perspectives, morality, faith, and womanhood. Several theories attempt to explain cognitive and intellectual development, including Piaget's stages of development, multiple theories on development of intelligence, and cognitive development. Intelligence theorists have attempted to define and measure intelligence (e.g., Binet, Wechsler). Others (e.g., Gardner, Goleman) have focused on multiple intelligences and on the connection between intelligence and ethical development (e.g., Perry). More from a counseling perspective, Ellis, Beck, and Glasser developed theories of cognitive development to explain how cognitions affect behaviors.

In addition to intelligence and cognition, theorists as far back as Locke in the 17th century have attempted to explain moral and faith development. Locke believed that humans are born as a tabula rasa and that humans develop morals through observation and interaction with others. And Rousseau believed in the innate goodness of all people. More current views on moral development include Piaget's theory of moral development, Kohlberg's theory of moral development, and Gilligan's theory focusing on the development of morality in girls. Faith development theory was first introduced by Fowler in an attempt to understand the evolution of how we conceptualize God or a supreme being, while Oser addressed the religious judgments made around a person's religious understanding.

Humanist theories of development are based on the philosophies of existentialism and phenomenology. Believing in a holistic, positive approach to human existence, humanistic theories focus on the individual's potential and stress the importance of growth and self-actualization. The major humanistic theories of human development include Maslow's hierarchy of needs, Rogers' personal growth, Buhler's developmental phase theory, and Johada's positive mental health.

While most of the previously mentioned theories begin at childhood, some cover the entire lifespan. Still others specifically examine adult development; these include Gould's phases of adult life, Levinson's seasons of life, Havighurst's theory of human development and developmental tasks, Vaillant's adaptation of life, Sheehy's passages, Duvall's life course transition, and Peck's theory of adult development. These theories are all concerned with examining the development of individuals in their adult years; they typically divide adult development into three periods: young adulthood, middle adulthood, and later adulthood.

Recognizing that the majority of human development theories were created by European or European-American males examining males exclusively, several theorists have attempted to present human development models from the perspectives of womanhood. These include works by Miller, Learner, Tavris, and Gilligan. These theories examine the role of power imbalances based on gender, acknowledging the systemic, contextual, and cultural influences on all people.

As you progress through the rest of this book and journey along the lifespan, the reader will be reintroduced to some of the theories presented in Chapters 2 and 3. Continually examine how the various theories personally relate to growth and development. What parts of the theories resonate with you and which parts appear in contrast with your own experiences?

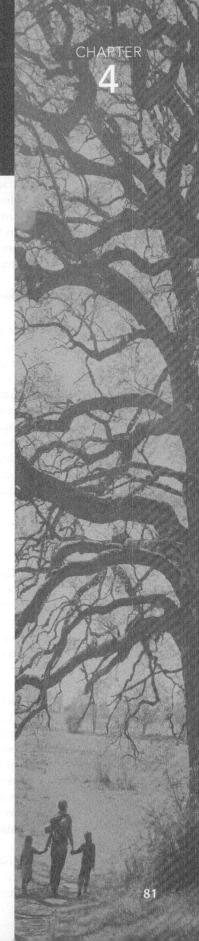

Genetics, Heredity, Environment, and Prenatal Development

By Taryn Richards and Bradley T. Erford

Human beings are complex creatures whose similarities and individualities are determined in large part by genetics and heritability. From conception, a person's physical and cognitive development unfolds in a predictable manner according to information encoded in DNA. As the embryo or fetus develops, environmental influences become more important, and trauma in the prenatal environment can have significant long-term effects—and can even result in death. This chapter reviews the importance of genetics and heritability to the developing human being, and normal and abnormal developmental processes throughout the prenatal period, which begins at conception and culminates in the birth of a new living, breathing human being just waiting to embark on a lifespan odyssey!

Genetics and Heredity

Genetics is the field of study of how inheritance operates. When people hear the word inheritance, they think of possessions and wealth that are passed down from parents to heirs at the end of the parents' lives. Well, in the genetic sense, inheritance operates very similarly, except that the transfer happens at the beginning of the heir's life. **Inheritance** involves the transmission of (genetic) characteristics from parents to offspring. Because parents possess diverse physical, cognitive, social, and emotional characteristics, when the sperm and egg from the parents combine, each parent passes along many of these diverse characteristics to the child. Variations are the differences in characteristics between parents and their offspring. Genetics is a fascinating field of study, but before diving into the genetic pool, let's explore a few components of the human cell and the important structures found therein.

The Cell and Its Makeup

A **cell** is the smallest independent, yet interdependent structure in the human body. It is enclosed by the cellular membrane or cell wall. The cell wall is kept from collapsing by **cytoplasm** or cellular fluid. Within the cytoplasm is the cell's **nucleus**, which is like a command or activity control center, and which houses the chromosomes. The nucleus, enclosed by a nuclear membrane and the walls of the nucleus, are kept from collapsing by **nucleoplasm**, or fluid within the nucleus. Both nucleoplasm and cytoplasm are types of **protoplasm**, or bodily fluids. When it is said that most of the human body is made up of water, this is true primarily because much of the body's cells are composed of protoplasm. As will be explained in more detail in the next section, chromosomes contain the directions that help the cell to function properly. Another important type of structure within the cell, but outside of the nucleus, are the **ribosomes**, which are small particles in the cytoplasm that help produce products necessary for cellular functions, such as cellular replication. This has been a very brief and simplistic introduction to the human cell, but it serves as a jumping off point for further exploration of genetics and the prenatal period.

Genes, Chromosomes, DNA, and Replication

The construction of a human from a zygote to an adult involves about 100 trillion cells, each of which carries all the genetic information needed to guide one's development (Mattick, 2007). The miraculous accuracy of genetic coding is seen in identical twins, in whom the genetic information is replicated to produce nearly indistinguishable physical and psychological characteristics. All of the genes in the body taken together are called the human genome (National Human Genome Research Institute, 2010a), and a great deal has been discovered over the past few decades about the genetic makeup of human beings.

Genetic information is contained in the form of the double helix of **deoxyribonucleic acid (DNA)**. Each DNA strand is made up of four bases: adenine (A), thymine (T), guanine (G), and cytosine (C). Importantly, adenine bonds only with thymine and guanine bonds only with cytosine. The sequences of these bases create directions for the cell to construct proteins and to perform other duties. Chromosomes consist of protein and a single strand of DNA, which contains the genes. The Human Genome Project estimated that there are approximately 20,500 human genes. The genome includes specific instructions to create human cells, which guide the development of biological characteristics. The information from the gene is then copied to the **messenger ribonucleic acid (messenger RNA)**, and the instructions are transmitted by proteins (Mattick, 2007).

The human nucleus contains 23 pairs of chromosomes (46 total chromosomes) (National Human Genome Research Institute, 2010b). A copy of one-half of each chromosome is inherited from the mother and one-half from the father to form a new human being's genetic makeup. Cells divide through two processes. **Somatic cells**, which are virtually all of the cells which make up the human body, divide through a process called mitosis. **Germ cells**, or sex cells, which are the cells used to procreate new organisms, divide through a process called meiosis. During **mitosis**, a somatic cell divides and duplicates itself into two new cells with replicated genetic information. Thus, a parent cell in the **diploid state** (having the full complement of chromosomes) divides into two daughter cells that are identical to the parent cell (i.e., also in the diploid state). During **meiosis**, the sex cells (germ cells) are divided into a **haploid state** (half chromosomes), so that when the sperm from the male (in a haploid state) and egg from the female (also in the haploid state) genetically recombine, each resulting fertilized egg cell will contain 23 complete pairs of chromosomes.

Simplistically speaking, sex is determined by the 23rd pair of chromosomes, with one haploid contribution each from the mother and the father (National Human Genome Research Institute, 2010c). The mother, whose 23rd chromosome is XX, always contributes an X chromosome to the offspring, while the father, whose 23rd chromosome is almost always XY, may contribute either an X or a Y chromosome to the offspring. When the 23rd pair contributed to the genetic sequence is an X chromosome from the mother and an X from the father, the sex of the baby will be a female (XX). When the 23rd pair contains an X chromosome from the mother and a Y from the father, the sex of the offspring will be a male (XY). Thus, the male's sperm determines the sex of the offspring. Complications can arise if an extra X is contributed or missing, which can result in physical or mental disorders such as Klinefelter's syndrome in men and Turner's syndrome in women. These and other anomalies are discussed below under Heredity Disorders.

Multiple Births

In the vast majority of cases, a human female gives birth to only one offspring at a time. However, a small percentage of births involve the carrying of more than one baby to term simultaneously. In almost all of these multiple births, twins are the result. The terms monozygotic twins or dizygotic twins refer to the mode by which multiple conception occurred. **Monozygotic twins** began as one egg, which was fertilized by one sperm and that split into two separate eggs that developed independently in the mother's womb (Lau et al., 2009). We refer to monozygotic twins as **identical twins** because they share identical copies of genetic information. In contrast, **dizygotic twins** began as two eggs, each fertilized separately by two different sperm cells. We refer to dizygotic twins as **fraternal twins**. Fraternal twins are as similar to one another as they would be to siblings born from the same parents at different times.

Influencing Traits

Genetic transmission is quite complex, but a few terms can sometimes help understand why some traits have a greater probability of being passed on, while others have a lower probability. The following explanation is an oversimplification of this complexity, but suffices for the present purpose. Genes consist of units called alleles, and it is these alleles that express characteristics that can be seen or determined (phenotypes). Genes are sometimes referred to as dominant genes and recessive genes. **Dominant genes** are generally expressed in a phenotype (and thus can be observed). **Recessive genes** are usually not expressed in a phenotype (and thus are not observed). As an example, let's take the very fictitious example of an allele that would determine whether a human would have one or two heads. Suppose H is used to indicate a dominant gene of one head and h is used to indicate a recessive gene. Looking around in society today, one observes that most people have one head. So most of the phenotypes are expressing H. But to understand phenotypes and probability more deeply, one must consider the alleles inherited from each parent. If both parents are HH, then all offspring will be HH, and all family members would have one head each. There is no other possibility (i.e., when one recombines the choices from splitting *HH* and combining it with the other split *HH*, one gets four *HH*s). Likewise, if both parents where *hh*, all offspring would be *hh* and each member of the entire family would have two heads. However, probability is quite different if both parents are *Hh*. You see that both parents will express the one-headed phenotype, but because each carries a recessive allele it is possible that a two-headed progeny could emerge (i.e., *Hh* and *Hh* yields possible recombinations of *HH*, *Hh*, *Hh*, and *hh*); indeed, the parents have a one-in-four chance of being the proud parents of a two-headed child! Genetic interactions are generally far more complex than explained here because the recombinations generally involve polygenetic inheritance.

Polygenic Inheritance

Polygenic inheritance is the concept that individual differences in biological characteristics are not traceable to one single gene (Mather, 1943). Polygenic traits are developed through multiple pairs of genes in combination with their interactions with the environment. Polygenetic traits are characteristics such as a person's height, weight, intelligence, or even mental state. The concept of polygenic inheritance can be seen in many psychiatric disorders. While an individual's susceptibility to a psychiatric illness or cognitive disorder sometimes can be predicted by single-gene inheritance, the inheritance of a disorder in one individual of an identical twin pair and not the other cannot be explained by single-gene inheritance (Rucker & McGuffi, 2010). This leads researchers to believe that many psychiatric disorders are polygenic traits. Multiple gene pairs contribute to cognitive impairments, and their interactions with the environment can lead to the development of a diagnosable disorder. The varying combinations of multiple genes and experiences also create wide ranges of differences in behaviors and symptoms across individuals with the same disorder.

Hereditary Disorders

Chromosomal abnormalities may occur through a number of problematic processes. Abnormalities occur through inherited errors in cell division or through a novel abnormality attributable to random error, maternal age, or environmental factors (National Human Genome Research Institute, 2010b). Abnormalities can result through an error in the number of chromosomes or in the structure of the chromosomes. Abnormalities may also occur through an error in the construction of chromosomes through deletion, duplication, translocation (i.e., a segment becomes unattached and reattached to another chromosome), inversion (i.e., a segment is turned upside down and reattached to the same chromosome), or a segment may become unattached and form a loop. These structural errors can result in physical or mental disorders or defects.

Some chromosomal disorders are called **sex chromosomal disorders** because they are caused by missing or extra chromosomes on the 23rd chromosomal pair, which is the sex-determining chromosome. Examples are Turner's syndrome and Klinefelter's syndrome. Others are called **autosomal disorders** because they involve anomalies on any of the other 22 chromosomal pairs. Down syndrome and sickle cell disease are well-known autosomal diseases. X-linked diseases involve genetic anomalies on the 23rd chromosomal pair due to defective genes (but not missing or added chromosomes), such as red-green color blindness.

It is important to place the following information in the appropriate sociocultural context. Even though individuals diagnosed with the genetic anomalies in the following sections face substantial challenges, most contribute to families and society in meaningful and productive ways and are certainly nurtured by loving, caring parents and guardians. In other words, hereditary disorders present challenges, but individual variations also allow the expression of strengths. All people, with or without visible or invisible disabilities, have gifts to offer our society.

Down Syndrome

There are many examples of chromosomal abnormalities that counselors should be aware of. **Down syndrome** is caused by an extra 21st chromosome, which results in cognitive delays and physical abnormalities seen in the facial region (Moldrich, Dauphinot, Laffaire, Rossier, & Potier, 2007). This chromosomal abnormality occurs in 1 out of 1000 births; however, by the time the mother's age reaches 40 years, the risk increases to 1 in 200 births. Individuals with Down syndrome often have facial irregularities such as a flattened face and slanted eyes, immune deficiencies, hearing and speech impairments, heart disease, and cognitive impairments. The intellectual disabilities of an individual with Down syndrome may vary; however, their cognitive function often declines with age and often results in the onset of Alzheimer's disease.

Turner's Syndrome

A chromosome missing from a chromosomal pair is called a monosomy. An example of chromosomal abnormality caused by a monosomy is **Turner's syndrome**, in which a female loses an X from the 23rd chromosomal pair. In the majority of Turner's syndrome cases, the X from the father is lost during meiosis (Ranke & Saenger, 2001). Thus, when the defective sperm fertilizes the intact egg, a chromosomal anomaly on the sex chromosome (#23) results. The prevalence rate of Turner's syndrome is one female for every 2000 live births. A female with Turner's syndrome has characteristic features such as shortened height, webbed neck, heart disease, and infertility.

Klinefelter's Syndrome

A chromosomal abnormality of one or more extra X chromosomes is called **Klinefelter's syndrome** in males, which is often undetected (Lanfranco, Kamischke, Zitman, & Nieschlag, 2004). Males with this syndrome may display characteristic physical features such as long legs, above average height, small and firm testes, and sterility. Cognitive deficits are also thought to exist in language and executive functioning ability among individuals with Klinefelter's syndrome.

Fragile-X Syndrome

The most common cause of intellectual disability is fragile-X syndrome (Garber, Visootsak, & Warren, 2008). Fragile-X syndrome is an X-linked chromosomal abnormality caused by repeats in genetic coding. Features of the syndrome include cognitive disabilities ranging from learning disabilities to autistic behaviors. Males with fragile-X syndrome are affected more severely with intellectual disability than females, who are more likely to have developmental delays. Physical features of the syndrome include flattened feet, a long and narrow face, and a prominent forehead and ears.

Huntington's Disease

Huntington's disease is caused by the gene huntingtin (HTT), in which the protein is abnormally expanded and misfolded (Ross & Tabrizi, 2011). The disease is autosomal dominant, which means that only one parent needs to have the gene HTT for an individual to inherit it, and the parent most likely also has the disease. Huntington's disease is a terminal, progressive neurodegenerative disorder in which the neurons lose their structure and function over time, eventually resulting in death. Onset of the disease usually begins around the age of 40 with symptoms of motor impairment, intellectual decline, and disturbances in mental health. After onset, an individual likely has only 15 to 20 years left to live.

Phenylketonuria (PKU)

Phenylketonuria (PKU) is caused by a gene mutation in which the enzyme phenylalanine hydroxylase (PAH) is not properly metabolized into the amino acid tyrosine (Widaman, 2009). The prevalence of PKU is 1 in 10,000 to 15,000 births in the United States. The effects of PKU depend on the interaction between genes and the environment. PKU is a recessive trait, which means that both parents would have to pass on a defective phenylalanine gene to the infant in order for the infant to have PKU. If only one parent passes a defective gene for PKU, the infant will be a carrier of PKU but will show no indications. However, if a pregnant mother has PKU and her diet introduces large amounts of phenylalanine into her bloodstream, it can cause irreversible damage to the fetus, regardless of whether the father is a carrier of PKU.

If a pregnant mother has PKU, it is imperative that she maintain a low-phenylalanine diet to prevent damage to the prenatal embryo or fetus. If the infant is diagnosed with PKU acquired from both parents, changing the environment through a low-phenylalanine diet can prevent serious harm. The diet supplements the infant with a phenylalanine-free formula drink to substitute for the mother's breast milk. The diet also includes fruits, vegetables, and a regulated intake of high-protein foods. An unregulated diet can cause severe damage to the infant's brain, which can lead to permanent alteration in the infant's IQ or an irreversible intellectual disability. In addition, those who maintain a low-phenylalanine diet until they become adults have a higher IQ than those who stopped the diet at a young age. Currently, there is no known correction for this gene mutation. However, the Guthrie screening test can identify PKU early in an infant's development and a change in the infant's environment involving a restricted diet can eliminate all severe damage caused by PKU.

Sickle Cell Disease

Sickle cell disease is an autosomal recessive disease that requires an individual to inherit two copies of the abnormal sickle hemoglobin (Hb S) gene to develop the disease (Elagouz, Jyothi, Gupta, & Sivaprasa, 2010). Sickle cell disease is one of the most common inherited disorders in the world, with about 250,000 infants each year born with it. An interesting fact about sickle cell disease is that those who carry the abnormal Hb S gene are resistant to malaria. It is possible that this evolutionary survival trait led to the high rate of sickle cell disease in African and Mediterranean populations. Manifestations of sickle cell disease can involve the eye, such as lesions and spots on the retina. Key symptoms of sickle cell disease include episodic occurrences of extreme pain throughout the body (Platt et al., 1991).

Twin and Adoption Studies

The argument of the opposing views in the nature versus nurture debate is generally seen as an outdated concept, as many theorists accept that both nature and nurture play a role in development. Still, behaviorists argue that nurture plays the dominant role, while many biologists argue that nature is the prime factor guiding development. In the end, it is commonly acknowledged that individuals both influence and are influenced by their environment. This is seen in many twin studies, in which two infants with similar genetic makeup (identical twins) are raised in separate environments, yet share similar personality, intelligence, and behavioral traits. Recent advances in technology have also pointed toward a new view of epigenetics. This field argues that twins' genetic makeup is not as identical as we once thought due to DNA alterations that affect the expression of genes (Haque, Gottesman, & Wong, 2009). Epigeneticists argue that differences in phenotypic traits in twins are not due to environments but rather to genomic imprinting, in which one twin may express certain gene alleles, while the other may not.

Numerous studies conducted with identical twins who either share environments or identical twins who were reared apart have come to similar conclusions about the role of nature and nurture. The Minnesota Study of Twins Reared Apart, which began in 1979, examined the role of genetics in twins' personality, temperament, intelligence, and a variety of other psychological measures (Bouchard, Lykken, McGue, Sesal, & Tellejen, 1990). The study found that identical twins raised in separate environments were highly similar on these characteristics, and that this was attributable to their genetic coding for these phenotypes. The study concluded that twins' genetic makeup affected their interaction with their environment, resulting in similar characteristics despite different nurtured experiences. A more recent study of twin adolescents and their behavioral display of ADHD symptoms found that nature played a large role in the development of hyperactivity and impulsivity despite a shared or non-shared environment (Greven, Rijsdijk, & Plomin, 2011). Twins' innate ability to recognize facial expressions have also been found to be highly similar between monozygotic twin pairs, with significant differences seen only in different sex pairs (in which females were more accurate) (Lau et al., 2009).

Along with these previous studies' conclusions of the interplay of genetic influence on interactions with the environment (Bouchard et al., 1990; Greven et al., 2011; Lau et al., 2009), a recent emerging view of epigenetics has come into the picture. Epigenetics involves the role of DNA alterations that modify the expression of phenotypes (Haque et al., 2009). This has been studied by examining alterations in the identical genes of monozygotic (identical) twins. In addition to the argument of nature versus nurture, epigenetics considers the sequence of DNA, modifications, and their interaction with gene expression of phenotypes. In monozygotic twins with psychiatric illnesses such as schizophrenia, rates of diagnosis have been known to be discordant between pairs. While this may be attributable to non-shared environments, epigeneticists argue that differences are due to inactivation of the X chromosome in female identical twins, genomic imprinting, or differences in DNA methylation. Genomic imprinting involves the random inclination of allele expression from one parent rather than the other. Studies of identical twins in which only one individual was diagnosed with a disorder have found evidence of genomic imprinting in the diagnosed twin. While the field of epigenetics is an emerging area of research, it is important to consider that there is far more to the argument than the simple juxtaposition of nature versus nurture.

Genetics and Behavior

Genetics are largely responsible for the development of an individual's temperament. **Temperament** involves unique behavioral dispositions that are stable over time (Henderson & Wachs, 2007). An infant's temperament can be observed in children as young as newborns, who can display negative affect, calmness, or awareness. While some infants may lie relatively still with little vocal expression, other infants may shriek and move their limbs around excessively. A common instrument used to measure infants' temperament is the Infant Behavior Record, which asks for parental ratings of activity, task orientation, and affect-extraversion (Saudino, 2005). In school-aged children, the Colorado Child Temperament Inventory is often used to assess emotionality, sociability, shyness, and attention/persistence. Heritability of temperament accounts for 20 to 60% of an individual's temperament, while the remaining percentage is contributed by the environment. With identical twins, temperament measures are highly correlated, while the temperaments of fraternal twins are rather discordant. Possible explanations for differences in temperaments may lie within the environment of the family structures rather than across families. Parents may display different parenting styles from one child to the next, or mothers may develop differing attachments with their children.

As an infant develops over time, temperament will typically stay the same across similar situations (Henderson & Wachs, 2007). For example, a child may always act calm or reserved in school and yet act in a boisterous manner at home. Infants' temperaments usually follow them throughout childhood and into adolescence, which can aid in predicting the occurrence of likely problem behaviors. In a recent study, infants who were high in emotionality were more likely to display anxious or depressive symptoms as a teenager (Saudino, 2005). In general theories of temperament, two opposing facets, reactivity and self-regulation, are used to measure one's temperament (Henderson & Wachs, 2007). **Reactivity** relates to the individual's positive or negative response to arousal. **Self-regulation** refers to the ability to sooth oneself or control one's behavior to avoid negative stimuli. Ivan Pavlov contributed to temperament theory with his work in classical conditioning. Pavlov thought that individuals and animals have an excitatory and an inhibitory response to stimuli triggered by the central nervous system (CNS). Pavlov also believed that the environment influenced reactions of the CNS. He theorized that each individual has a behavioral-approach activation system (BAS) that relates to reactivity, and a behavioral inhibition system (BIS) that relates to self-regulation. The BAS responds to positive stimuli and evokes happy feelings, whereas the BIS responds to negative stimuli and creates feelings of fear or anxiety. These two systems influence an individual's temperament. If an individual is high in BAS or BIS, it is likely that the individual will have a negative affect.

Behavioral Traits

Researchers often study individuals with mental disorders to examine the role of genetics and the environment in the development of psychiatric illness. A recent study examined individuals with conduct disorder in childhood and antisocial behavior disorder in adulthood. The researchers found that genetics, shared environments, and non-shared environments contributed equally to the variability exhibited in childhood conduct disorder (Meier, Slutske, Heath, & Martin, 2011). The study also concluded that genetic influence accounted for a majority of the variability in adult antisocial behavior but not childhood conduct disorder, possibly because adults can establish greater control over their environments.

Recent advances in neuroimaging have allowed researchers to locate brain regions in which personality and temperament are active (Hariri, 2010). Anxiety reactions originate in the amygdalae, and increased consistent activity in this region may be related to trait anxiety. Individuals with trait anxiety are more likely to interpret situations as intimidating or threatening, and they are at risk for developing anxiety disorders or depression. With the use of an fMRI (functional magnetic resonance imaging), researchers are learning more about which locations in the brain are related to personality, behavior traits, and mental disorders. With knowledge of the brain locations, advances can be made in mental health treatments.

Attitudes and Social Behaviors

The genetic influence of attitudes and social behaviors are thought to account for about half of the variability in individuals, with the rest attributable to environmental influences. Some theorists suggest that different attitudes have heritability ranges from low in heritability to high in heritability. Research has examined the high heritability of attitudes such as altruism, aggression, and political attitudes, to name only a few (Tesser & Crelia, 1994). Attitudes high in heritability are thought to be resistant to change or social influences, while attitudes low in heritability are malleable. The niche theory suggests that those with highly heritable attitudes seek out environments which support their attitude and therefore rein-force their attitude by creating a niche with like attitudes. Still, it is important to remember that genes do not cause behavior.

Intelligence

Genetics play a large role in the development of an individual's intelligence. Intelligence is a steady and enduring trait that involves the ability to comprehend stimuli from one's environment using logic and reason to solve problems and produce abstract ideas (Deary, Spinath, & Bates, 2006). IQ tests such as the Wechsler Intelligence Scale for Children (5th edition) are administered to youth as a considerably accurate measure of their cognitive capability. Researchers have found through the use of IQ tests that the heritability of intelli-gence is around 50%. In twin studies, high correlations between intelligence measurements in monozygotic twins have been reported for inheritance of verbal and spatial intelligence as well as memory. In a review of adoption studies and intelligence, it was concluded that an adopted child's IQ is highly correlated with their biological parents' IQ rather than their adoptive parents' when assessed as an adolescent. As a young child, the influence of the environment on intelligence is great; however, as the child moves through middle child-hood to adolescence, the environment has little effect on the development of their cogni-tion. This is seen in studies of children in poverty. As younger children are removed from poverty, they are better able to break through the barrier and reach their true genetic poten-tial for intelligence.

Genotype and Phenotype

An individual's **genotype** is the genetic makeup which comprises the inheritance from both parents. A **phenotype** is the expression of their genotypes given an individual's environment. An example of this interrelationship can be seen in those with genetic syndromes such as Down syndrome. Behavioral phenotypes involve genetic traits that appear only in individuals with the behavioral syndrome and not in those without it (Tunnicliffe & Oliver, 2011). This recent review of studies on the expression of behavior in those with genetic syndromes sought to examine the degree to which the genotypic syndrome behavior is influenced by the environment or how the phenotype is expressed. The review found that within genetic syndromes in which individuals are intellectually disabled, there are phenotypic behaviors that are likely to be exhibited. In reaction with the environment, these behaviors are often conditioned to continue and therefore are repeated by the individual.

Canalization refers to the large influence of genes on the expression of pheno-types early on in development (Gottlieb, 1991). **Canalization** is an individual's innate, expected developmental trajectory (Boersma & Wit, 1997). This predictable path is highly evident in the early years of development, but becomes less noticeable through adolescence as growth slows and environmental interactions are prominent. However, if the impact of an adverse environmental event interrupts the canalization process in the early years of development, it is difficult to reach one's true genetic potential. On the other hand, environmental impact later on in development (e.g., young adulthood, middle adulthood) is not as detrimental, as the individual has had the opportunity to reach full genetic potential. For example, if an otherwise normal individual experiences a debilitating condition in infancy or early childhood, their canalization process is dis-turbed and they may never recover to their true cognitive or physical capability. How-ever, if the same debilitating condition were to occur in adolescence, the individual would not be as greatly affected, as their canalization process had had the opportunity to take its course earlier in life.

REFLECTION   4.1 HANNAH AND CANALIZATION

I met Hannah when she was almost 3 years old. Her development was normal up until about 10 months of age, and she was even beginning to stand and walk. Then came the onset of juvenile rheumatoid arthritis (JRA). She regressed physically (neither walking nor crawling) and began displaying significant cognitive delays. When I evaluated her at that time, although the JRA had subsided, she qualified for preschool special educational services because of her developmental delays. Her cognitive abilities at that time were in the moderate to mild range (a standard score of 55). I tried to prepare the parents as best I could for the realities of raising a child with special needs. But Hannah's mother, Julia, would have none of that. Julia also had JRA, which began between 13 and 14 years of age, and although short in stature and walking with the aid of a cane and sometimes a wheelchair, she was one of the most verbally brilliant people I have ever met. Julia could talk circles around me! She knew that Hannah would be all right because she was all right. But there is a huge difference in the disruption of the canalized developmental path between onset at 13 years of age and at 10 months of age. The cognitive structures that needed to develop in an infant and toddler cannot be "regrown" as a 4- or 5-year-old. Hannah was bumped off her canalized trajectory and never got back on, whereas Julia had the benefit of having stayed on her canalized trajectory for more than 13 years. When I reevaluated Hannah three years later, Julia had processed the situation and her grief, so the fact that Hannah's IQ was still in the moderate to mild range of intellectual ability was readily accepted and services continued. And Hannah grew up in one of the most loving and supportive families with which I have had the privilege of working. [~BTE]

Think About It   **4.1**

Many of the clients seen by counselors have disorders with a genetic or partially genetic basis. What would be the implications for these clients in society if nondiscrimination laws did not exist or if employers, educational institutions, or other organizations used loopholes? How can counselors continue to advocate for social justice and equity for these individuals?

Molecular Genetics: The Human Genome Project

The Human Genome Project, supported by the U.S. Department of Energy and the National Institutes of Health, began in 1990 and was completed in 2003 (see Human Genome Project Information at genomics.energy.gov). The project located 20,000 to 20,500 human genes, discovered the sequences of 3.2 billion bases of human DNA, and organized this information into databases for further research. The knowledge of the exact gene sequences involved in diseases and disorders has great implications for genetic testing and diagnosis, gene therapy, and pharmacogenomics. The Human Genome Project has provided databases for pharmacogenomics to examine an individual's genetic predisposition to responses to medicine, which can help improve treatment outcomes. But the discovery of personal genetic information is accompanied by ethical and legal issues surrounding use of this sensitive material. In 2008, the Genetic Information Nondiscrimination Act was enacted to prevent discrimination by health or insurance providers or employers based on an individual's genetic coding. For example, knowing about the genetic coding information of potential employees could lead to discriminatory hiring practices. And knowing information about an individual's genetic anomalies could lead insurance providers to deny coverage because of "pre-existing conditions." The Act was meant to prevent these forms of discrimination.

Genetic Counseling

Genetic counseling is recommended for families that plan to conceive but have a family history of abnormalities or disorders. Women of older maternal age are normally recommended for counseling and often referred for screening, as the probability of fetal abnormalities increases with rising age. A genetic counselor aims to educate the family and help them learn to cope with and adjust to the demands of a child with hereditary diseases and disorders (Bjorvan, Eide, Hanestad, & Havik, 2008). Women may receive genetic counseling prior to gestation or during their pregnancy. Counseling prior to conception is suggested; however, counseling during pregnancy is beneficial in terms of receiving information about possible abnormalities. Genetic counselors will obtain an extensive family history to look for hereditary disorders that are known to exist (Hafen, Hulinsky, Simonssen, Wilder, & Rose, 2009). The American College of Obstetrics' standards state that all women should receive genetic counseling and should be knowledgeable about the options of diagnostic testing and noninvasive screening. If a high risk for abnormalities is suspected, the doctor will provide a screening, which usually involves an ultrasound to identify a potential condition (Tapon, 2010). Women may also be offered blood tests to determine the status of their fetus regarding inheritance of maternal diseases and fetal abnormalities. In the case of sickle cell anemia and thalassemia, a blood screening tests for the presence of the condition in the mother's genes (Reed, 2009). If the gene is present, the father will be tested as well. If the father is a carrier of the gene, then the child will have a 25% chance of diagnosis. If the father is not a carrier of the gene, the child will not acquire the disorder.

If it is likely that any possible condition exists, the health care provider may recommend amniocentesis or chorionic villus sampling (CVS). **Amniocentesis** involves the extraction of amniotic fluid from the mother to examine the cells of the fetus during the second trimester, or at about 15 weeks (Medda, Donati, Spinelli, & DiRenzo, 2003; Tapon, 2010). These cells are examined to look for chromosomal or genetic defects. CVS occurs at 11 to 14 weeks of pregnancy and involves the removal of placental tissue to diagnose a disorder (Tapon, 2010). Possible risk factors are associated with these invasive procedures, such as loss of the fetus. A recent study found that of the women referred for diagnostic testing involving amniocentesis, 10–43% had a hereditary history of structural abnormalities (Hafen et al., 2009). The goal of genetic testing for chromosomal abnormalities is to provide the parents with substantial information about the disorder so that they can prepare themselves for three main decisions (Tapon, 2010). Parents may choose to learn more about the condition so that they are prepared to give birth to and raise a child with a disability, or they may wish to learn more information about giving up their child for adoption or terminating the pregnancy.

Fetal Medicine

In the case of a high-risk pregnancy, the health care provider may refer the mother to a maternal fetal medicine (MFM) specialist for consultation or care (Sisson, Witcher, & Stubsten, 2004). The MFM specialist acts as a team member with other health care providers to assist with critical aspects of a high-risk pregnancy. MFM specialists have extensive training and knowledge in complicated pregnancies such as maternal medical complications or diseases and fetal abnormalities. MFM specialists also have knowledge of the role genetics play in disease and fetal development; they often perform diagnostic procedures similar to a genetic counselor. The MFM provider's role in care may be to consult with the mother about the best medicine for the fetus in treatment of the disorder or disease, increased observation of the fetus, and consultation about mode or time of delivery based on fetal development or maternal health. The MFM specialist is also trained in surgical intervention procedures to ensure the best outcomes for both the mother and the fetus.

➤ CASE EXAMPLE **4.1**   AL AND SHARYA.

Al and Sharya are a happily married African-American couple who are thinking about starting a family. But they are very concerned about a few things. Al has sickle cell disease and attention-deficit hyperactivity disorder. Sharya has juvenile rheumatoid arthritis, one family member with Down syndrome, and a family history replete with depression and anxiety disorders. She even has a cousin diagnosed with schizo-affective disorder. As their counselor, what recommendations would you make regarding genetic counseling or tests? To whom would you refer them in your broader community to help them gain information and make informed decisions?

Reproductive Technologies

Contraception

Half of all pregnancies in the United States are reported as accidental (Centers for Disease Control and Prevention, 2011g). A majority of these accidental pregnancies result from the adolescent population as the United States continues to have the highest teen birth rate among developed countries (Wingo, Smith, Tevendale, & Ferre, 2011). In 2008, this rate was on the rise, with African-American and Hispanic populations having the highest birth rates for ages 10 to 19 years. Among the teenage population, 24–27% of pregnancies are terminated through induced abortion. However, there are a variety of contraceptive methods available in private doctors' offices as well as in government-funded family planning programs to prevent unwanted pregnancy.

The most commonly used methods that are readily available and reversible are oral birth control and male condoms. However, the effectiveness of these methods depends on the user's commitment to use them correctly. In the United States, lack of perfect adherence to oral birth control results in a 7% failure rate (Cleland et al., 2006). In the case of failed contraception or lack of use, emergency contraception (otherwise known as the "morning-after pill") can be taken within five days of intercourse to prevent pregnancy. Lack of oral contraceptive use can also be explained by the presence of female medical conditions, which may prevent women from using oral contraception due to the hormone dosage. However, other contraceptive methods are rarely advertised and are lesser-known alternatives to oral birth control or condoms. Long-acting reversible contraceptives (LARCs), such as an IUD (intrauterine device) or a vaginal implant, are available as modes of protection that last for a prolonged period of time. Reports from adolescents about their lack of use of contraception reveal unrealistic perceptions about the inability to conceive later on after use of long-acting contraceptives (Barnha, 2011). This suggests the need for enhanced education about the benefits and drawbacks of reversible and irreversible modes of contraception in young teenagers and adults.

In the case of preventing pregnancy most effectively and for a prolonged period of time, female and male sterilization is a viable option (Shiha, Turokb, & Parkerc, 2011). While female sterilization or tubal ligation is often seen as a health risk, it is more often relied on than male sterilization, or vasectomy, which is a simpler process and more cost-effective. However, one aspect often overlooked is that female tubal ligation is effective immediately, while a vasectomy is not. Both female and male sterilization are meant for long-term contraception but can be reversed through surgery. After sterilizations are reversed, pregnancy success rates range from 40 to 70%.

Infertility and Assisted Reproductive Technology

On the other end of the continuum of preventing unwanted pregnancy, many hopeful parents experience **infertility**, the inability to conceive a child after one year of sexual intercourse without the use of contraception. The causes of infertility vary from female or male reproductive abnormalities to the age of the couple. Common reasons for infertility in women include ovulation dysfunction, sexually transmitted diseases, and abnormalities in the uterus or fallopian tubes that prevent transmission or implantation (Ledger, 2009). STDs are often undetected and can lead to complications, which may result in tubal disease in women, which prevents transmission of the embryo to the uterus. Women may also suffer from endometriosis (a deterioration of the cellular membrane enclosing the egg), which has been correlated with low pregnancy rates due to difficulties with implantation (O'Flynn O'Brien, Varghese, & Agarwal, 2010).

Male infertility is most likely due to chromosomal abnormalities that result in the absence of sperm, lack of sperm quality, or sterile sperm. Also, in the past decade it has become more common for men and women to pursue career and educational attainment prior to starting a family. As parents wait longer to conceive, the quality of oocytes and sperm decreases with rising age (Ledger, 2009). This results in "unexplained" infertility in older couples. Despite the hardship of failed conception attempts, infertility is treatable in most cases, although the cause is most often unknown.

Couples may turn to fertility treatments to induce ovulation and attempt to conceive naturally. If fertility treatments fail, advancements in technology have made it possible for infertile couples to conceive a child with their genetic contribution, or at least one parent's genetic makeup. **Assistive reproductive technology (ART)** involves several different ways of achieving fertilization. The most common solution to male infertility was once **artificial insemination (AI)**, in which sperm is injected into the uterus (Richards, 2008). Today, AI is often used with anonymous donors in single females or lesbian couples who wish to conceive. In couples with an infertile male partner, a recent technology called intracytoplasmic sperm injection (ICSI) gives the male an opportunity to reproduce despite his infertility as the sperm is injected directly into the egg. Current studies are looking into the possibility of increased chromosomal abnormalities and birth defects due to this mode of conception (Barnha, 2011).

ART for female infertility most frequently involves *in vitro* fertilization, in which the woman's egg is removed from her uterus and fertilized with the sperm in a Petri dish (O'Flynn O'Brien et al., 2010). Once fertilization occurs, the egg is implanted into the uterus. The first birth through *in vitro* fertilization (IVF) occurred in 1978, and the procedure has been on the rise ever since, with 1 in 80 infants conceived through IVF today (McDonald et al., 2009). Pregnancy rates of IVF may depend on whether the embryo is fresh or frozen and how many embryos are implanted in the uterus. IVF may involve multiple cycles until a healthy pregnancy and a live birth are achieved. Unfortunately, each cycle is known to be an extremely costly process with little coverage by health insurance. A recent study of 8500 women in Australia from 1993 to 2002 examined the effectiveness of IVF and found the success rate for live births was 47%, with an average of three cycles (Stewart et al., 2011). While the pregnancy rates with ART are relatively high, the outcomes for the infants may result in disadvantages compared to natural birth. Recent studies of single infants born through ART found that they were more likely to have a low birth weight or be delivered preterm than naturally conceived births (Gibbons, Cedars, & Ness, 2011; McDonald et al., 2009). ART is also more likely to result in multiple births, which increases the risk for low birth weight, preterm birth, and infant mortality as well as health risks for the mother (Lynch et al., 2001).

If the woman is unable to physically carry a child to term, but the couple wishes to have a child with one or both of their genetic contributions, they may opt to use a surrogate mother. The surrogate mother's own egg may be artificially inseminated with the potential father's sperm. It is also an option for the potential mother's egg and the father's sperm to be fertilized *in vitro* prior to implantation into the surrogate mother (Bhatia, Martindale, Rustamov, & Nysenbaum, 2009). For many mothers, the thought of having their child share genetic information with their partner and another female is undesirable; therefore, many choose to use IVF with a surrogate.

Think About It 4.2

Teenage and adult clients often seek counseling to deal with pregnancy, childbirth, and child-rearing issues. How can counselors prepare themselves for the breadth and depth of issues encountered related to these topics?

Motivations for Parenthood

Motivations and timing for parenthood have changed over the past decade. While teen birth rates for the most part have been steady, there has been a recent trend for first-time planned pregnancies to occur with parents in their late 20s to early 30s, rather than in their early 20s, as in the past (Van Balen, 2005). In 2002, 28% of births were to parents age 30 and above. Possible explanations for this shift in age are due to changing college motivations and career aspirations. In a survey of first-time parents in Europe, the most common motivations for parenthood were to achieve happiness and to strengthen their identity. This survey also reported that older first-time parents were more likely to have attended college and were interested in strengthening their personal growth and identity as well financial stability prior to beginning parenthood. The study found that younger parents reported a stronger desire to have children than older parents. This strong wish for parenthood may have resulted in younger parents forgoing their personal development prior to having children. Similar motivations were found in a survey of college students in Portugal aged 17 to 37 who reported personal fulfillment as the number one motivation for parenthood (Franco-Borges, Vaz-Rebelo, & Kourkoutas, 2010). Men and women also reported significantly different motivations for parenthood. Women were more likely to indicate strengthening their identity and passing on their legacy as motivators. Key motivations in avoiding parenthood were reported as maintaining leisure time and focusing on career achievement.

Family Planning

Family planning programs began in developing countries in the 1960s as a movement to slow population growth (Cleland et al., 2006). Today, family planning programs are widely accessible in hospitals, health centers, and community-based centers such as Planned Parenthood (see www.plannedparenthood.org). Planned Parenthood focuses on prevention of unwanted pregnancies through providing education and access to contraception. Health centers also provide reproductive health care, sexually transmitted infection education and testing, and abortion services. While family planning programs are active in developing countries, there is a need for advocacy of these programs in poorer countries. Family planning has reduced poverty and increased health benefits. Families with many children are more likely to be poor, and their individual children are less likely to receive quality education than families with fewer children. Family planning programs aimed at prevention can also help reduce abortion rates and maternal death rates from unwanted pregnancies.

Adoption

Individuals who wish to experience the joys of parenthood yet are unable to conceive due to infertility or failed assisted reproductive procedures may turn to adoption. Each year, numerous children are unable to be adequately cared for by their biological parents. These parents may voluntarily give up their children for adoption because they are aware of their inability to provide care, or their children may be involuntarily removed from their care by state agencies charged with ensuring the proper care of all children. Biological parents who place their child for adoption voluntarily may wish to search for the ideal parent for their child. Parents looking to adopt must go through an extensive screening process that assesses their strengths and weaknesses and ability to provide sufficient care. Infants and children up for adoption often come from unstable home environments with parents who are unable to provide quality care. Adoptive parents are often socially and economically stable and can act as a viable substitute for the adopted child's previous home life (Johnson, 2002). Adopted children have better outcomes and develop more positively in their adoptive homes than if they had remained in their unstable environments.

In the past, the most common form of adoption was a closed adoption, in which records were sealed and the adopted child's former life was virtually erased. However, with a closed adoption today, it is easier for adopted children to locate their birth parents through the Internet or investigators who specialize in identity searches. Today, it is becoming more commonplace for biological parents to request an open adoption. This involves the active communication between the biological parents and the adoptive parents. An open adoption may involve a range of levels of communication or contact, as requested by the biological parent.

Prenatal Development

The prenatal stage of development begins with conception and ends with birth. This section will begin with an overview of pregnancy detection, miscarriages, and abortions; it will review the physical development of the zygote, embryo, and fetus, and then conclude with a discussion of factors that influence the prenatal environment.

Detecting Pregnancy

"Am I pregnant?" There are signs of pregnancy that occur early on, but each such sign or symptom could be caused by conditions other than pregnancy. For example, spotting and cramping could indicate pregnancy, but could also stem from the onset of menstruation, an abrasion from sex, or a change in birth control medication. Breasts may become sore or swollen beginning a week or two after conception, but this could also be the result of premenstrual syndrome or a change in birth control pills. Fatigue and nausea are common signs of pregnancy, but are also common occurrences when one is ill, stressed, or depressed. Missing a period is often a significant sign that a woman is pregnant, but women can also miss a period because of recent weight gain or loss, hormonal surges, competitive sports, stress, and fatigue. Other symptoms may include dizziness or fainting, back pain, frequent urination, and mood swings, but again, none of these symptoms are exclusively related to pregnancy.

To answer the question definitively, a woman should get a pregnancy test, which is designed to determine if urine or blood contains human chorionic gonadotropin (hCG), a hormone produced after a fertilized egg attaches to the wall of the uterus, ordinarily about six days after conception. There are two main types of pregnancy tests: urine and blood tests. Urine tests are private and convenient; they can be purchased over the counter and conducted at home or in a doctor's office. They are about 97% accurate, so long as the instructions are followed properly and one waits at least 10 days after a missed period. Home testing products vary but usually cost less than $20. Usually the test strip is held in the urine stream or dipped in a urine specimen, and results are evident in minutes. If a positive result is found, pregnancy is indicated, no matter how pronounced the indicator is. In a small percentage of cases a false positive test result is indicated (you are not pregnant but the test says you are), but this is usually because blood, protein, or certain drugs (e.g., anticonvulsants, hypnotics, tranquilizers) are present in the urine.

If a positive pregnancy test results, one should confirm this qualitative result with a quantitative blood test, which must be conducted at a medical facility. A blood test can actually determine the amount of hCG present (quantitative result) rather than the mere presence or absence of hCG. A blood test can be conducted as soon as six to eight days after ovulation, and so are far more accurate earlier in one's pregnancy. However, the results of a blood test usually are processed at a lab, so the expectant mother may need to wait days to weeks for the results.

➤ CASE EXAMPLE **4.2**   EMILY AND MARK.

Emily and Mark have been trying to have a baby for more than a year. Both extended families are very excited about the impending arrival of grandchildren and many conversations have taken place outlining future plans. But as each month passes, Emily has become more and more depressed over an inability to conceive a child. She has sought counseling to help deal with the situation and her emotional reactions. As Emily's counselor, what are the primary issues you would need to consider and how would you construct a treatment plan or plan of action?

Miscarriage and Abortion

While most women have the opportunity to conceive a child and safely carry that child to term, many women experience the spontaneous death of a fetus, otherwise known as a **miscarriage**. In the United States, approximately 15% of pregnancies end in miscarriage (Ljunger et al., 2011). In a population-based study of women in the United Kingdom, it was reported that women who had miscarried often wished to know the cause of death to ease their guilt (Simmons, Singh, Maconochie, Doyle, & Green, 2006). However, the causes of miscarriages are unidentified in about half of all cases. If a miscarriage was attributable to an unpreventable, medical cause, women described feeling more at ease than those who were left wondering if they had personally contributed to their miscarriage. Many women also reported a lack of emotional support from health care providers after the miscarriage had occurred. Women who have miscarried had fostered a connection with their unborn baby that was taken away from them suddenly. They are in need of extra support such as loss and bereavement counseling or a support group with other mothers who have miscarried. The causes of **spontaneous recurrent abortions (SRAs)** or repeated miscarriages are often unknown. The most common risks of miscarriage include increased maternal age and chromosomal abnormalities in the fetus. Japanese women with two or more spontaneous abortions were examined to understand the causes. Most common causes were found to be abnormalities in the uterus followed by tubal infection, cervical failure, endocrine system dysfunction, chromosome abnormalities, or autoimmune deficiencies (Morikawa et al., 2003). With increasing numbers of repeated miscarriages, the chances for a healthy live birth decreased.

As stated earlier, about 50% of all pregnancies in the United States are either accidental or unwanted (Centers for Disease Control and Prevention, 2011g). Abortion of an unwanted pregnancy or abnormal fetus may be the resolution for some mothers. The 1973 U.S. Supreme Court decision in *Roe v. Wade* upheld the legality of a woman's right to terminate her pregnancy. Since this decision, abortion has been legalized across the United States. However, barriers still exist to carrying out an abortion, such as minor consent laws and gestational age restrictions. Depending on the state where an abortion is sought, minors may need parental consent or simply parental notification to carry out the procedure. The reasons for choosing to have an abortion are many. The decision to terminate a pregnancy may result from inability to care for a child, risk for maternal death, fetal abnormalities, or ill timing of conception.

Despite women's personal and private decisions to end their pregnancies, unlike the involuntary decision of miscarriage, emotional support is needed for women who have had an abortion. Studies have reported that women tend to report elevated levels of anxiety for several weeks following the abortion (Bradshaw & Slade, 2003). However, whether this anxiety is higher or abnormal compared to women who give birth at the end of an unwanted pregnancy is questionable. It is possible that women who have an abortion are dealing with the added emotions of guilt as well as the stress of keeping the procedure hidden from those around them due to the social stigma involved (Upadhyay, Cockrill, & Freedman, 2010). It is recommended that all women who seek an abortion participate in abortion counseling to help identify coping mechanisms, social supports, and so that health professionals can recognize women who may be at risk for more severe mental health issues post-abortion. Recent trends in abortion counseling include peer counseling, Internet-based support, telephone support, and workbooks aimed at increasing self-awareness.

Physical Development

Prenatal development begins at conception. The average full-term pregnancy lasts about 280 days, which is 40 weeks, or a bit more than nine months. The information provided in this section is derived from numerous commonly accepted formal and informal sources. The prenatal developmental period is generally demarcated by trimesters.

The First Trimester

The point in time when the sperm fertilizes the egg is called **conception**, and the two haploid cells (i.e., sperm and egg) become a single zygote cell with the full complement of 23 pairs of chromosomes (the diploid state). This marks the onset of the **zygotic period** of development. The single-celled **zygote** immediately undergoes mitosis, the process of somatic cell division discussed earlier in this chapter. Mitotic replications continue throughout prenatal development, but the first 14 days are referred to as the **period of the ovum**. The developing zygote travels down the fallopian tube and implants onto the blood- and nutrient-rich uterine wall. This implantation is necessary for the zygote to become a viable embryo within the mother's womb. Development throughout the prenatal period is highly canalized, pointing to an unfolding genetically programmed sequence.

The 14th day after conception begins the **embryonic period**, which lasts until the end of the second month. The embryonic period is a time of rapid cell division and specialization—which also makes it a precarious and dangerous period because traumatic insults and the introduction of teratogens can lead to spontaneous abortion or irreversible birth defects. For example, the heart begins to form on the 18th day after conception, and a crack binge or other insult at this time could lead to a malformed heart, and end the embryo's lifecycle, a very sad result given that many pregnant females may not know they are pregnant at two to three weeks after conception. During the embryonic period, support structures such as the umbilical cord, amniotic sac, and placenta form. The **amniotic sac** encloses the embryo, except where the umbilical cord passes through to the placenta. The amniotic sac contains amniotic fluid, which protects the embryo from being injured by internal pressures and bumps—sort of like floating about in a water balloon. The amniotic fluid also provides a temperature-controlled environment for the embryo, and later for the fetus, an important support since at this point the developing organism cannot self-regulate temperature. The **umbilical cord** carries oxygenated blood from the placenta to the fetus and carries away deoxygenated blood and waste products from the embryo or fetus.

Key developments during the embryonic period include the appearance of heart cells on day 18, resulting in a functional heart by three weeks. The backbone begins to develop, a structure that encloses and protects the spinal cord. Various internal organs form, including the lungs, liver, kidneys, and endocrine glands. The digestive system also forms. Small arm buds develop on day 24, leg buds on day 28, then shoulders, arms, and hands on day 31. Fingers develop on day 33 and the thumbs develop a few days later. By the end of eight weeks, when the embryo is about an inch long and weighs only one-thirtieth of an ounce, the neck and facial features begin to develop. The start of the ninth week marks the beginning of the fetal period, and by the end of the first trimester, a highly complex organism is on full display.

The Second Trimester

A rapid increase in growth occurs during the second trimester. During the fourth month after conception, the fetus grows to approximately seven inches in length and weighs about four ounces; that's right, after nearly four months of development the fetus still only weighs about a quarter of a pound. During the fifth month after conception the fetus will grow to almost a foot in length and between one-half and one pound—virtually doubling in length and tripling in weight in just one month. All of this growth requires additional resources, so the fetus substantially increases its intake of oxygen, food, and water. Excellent maternal nutrition and health habits are critical to fetal development. Bones continue to form and harden, a process known as **ossification**.

A downy growth of hair, called **lanugo**, now covers the entire body of the fetus, and the skin is covered with a waxy substance, **vernix caseosa**, to protect the fetus's skin from constant exposure to amniotic fluid. Anyone who has ever taken a bath has seen how prunelike skin becomes after just 15–30 minutes of exposure to water; imagine how it might look after six or more months!

The Third Trimester

During the third trimester the fetus will increase in length by another 50% and gain an additional six pounds, resulting in average birth lengths of 16–20 inches and average birth weights of 7 to 9 pounds. Reflexes and other central nervous system structures mature during the seventh month, and most of the fetus's organs are mature enough to allow the fetus to function properly outside of the prenatal environment, if necessary, as is the case in premature births. However, the final weeks and months of gestation are critical for further maturation of the brainstem. In a short time the fetus will be ready for delivery, and will immediately graduate to a neonate when delivery is accomplished!

Factors Affecting the Prenatal Environment

Teratology involves the study of structural malformations in newborns (Kalter, 2003). Congenital (i.e., present at birth) malformations in infants occur in approximately 3% of live births. **Teratogens** are substances that may cause these abnormalities, but most can be avoided or prevented, or their negative effects can be mitigated. The combination of the properties of the teratogen, time of exposure to the fetus, and their reaction with the fetus's genotype creates a set of characteristic malformations that will occur in the case of exposure to certain teratogens.

Fetal Alcohol Syndrome (FAS) and Fetal Alcohol Effects (FAE)

Exposure to alcohol during the prenatal period can result in a variety of physical, cognitive, and behavioral impairments known as fetal alcohol spectrum disorders (FASD). Extreme levels of consistent maternal alcohol use can lead to fetal alcohol syndrome (FAS), which is characterized by impaired and delayed developmental and cognitive growth in both the womb and after birth (Hellemans, Sliwowska, Verma, & Weinberg, 2010). Diagnostic features of FAS can include low birth weight, inability to maintain weight, abnormally small skull size, flattened facial features, brain structure abnormalities, or neurological deficits such as learning impairments or even intellectual disability.

Recent research has linked FASD with additional issues in mental health such as depression and anxiety disorders that may occur in childhood and adulthood. Depression and anxiety may stem from environmental factors of family alcohol abuse, which may pair with cognitive dysfunction from prenatal alcohol exposure. A child exposed to any substantial quantity of alcohol in the prenatal period will most likely struggle with academic issues of attention and memory, behavioral issues such as impulsivity and hyperactivity, and social deficits (Kalter, 2003). Social difficulties may include an inability to reason about the effects of their actions, recognize social cues, or communicate effectively in social situations (Mooney & Varlinskaya, 2011).

Cocaine

Prenatal exposure to cocaine can cause physical and behavioral problems in children. Infants exposed to cocaine are more likely to have a low birth weight, shorter body length, and smaller head circumference than non-exposed infants (Lumeng, Cabral, Gannon, Heeren, & Frank, 2007). In a recent study on teacher and parent ratings of children with behavioral issues, inattention, and impulsivity, children with prenatal cocaine exposure (PCE) were rated higher than their non-exposed peers on all measures (Bada et al., 2011). Prenatal exposure to cocaine can also result in learning deficits in reading comprehension during pre-adolescence (Lewis et al., 2011). One study found that children with prenatal exposure to cocaine had difficulty with syntax, semantics, and phonological processing that was likely to continue into adolescence. Additional factors included the caregivers' vocabulary, as prenatally exposed children who were kept apart from the caretaker who abused cocaine had better outcomes in reading comprehension tests. In addition to physical and cognitive effects, maternal cocaine use and prenatal cocaine exposure can affect mother-infant interactions (Eiden, Schuetze, & Coles, 2011). One study found that mothers who abused cocaine were indifferent, hostile, and less engaged with their infant, who was in turn less responsive than non-exposed infants. Prenatally exposed children were also found to be more impulsive and to react with frustration as they developed into toddlers.

Cigarettes

Prenatal exposure to tobacco smoke can cause permanent deficits in cognition and behavior as well as pose serious health risks. In underweight and average weight women, smoking during pregnancy greatly increased the risk for a low birth weight infant and the risk for sudden infant death syndrome (SIDS) (Dwyer, McQuown, & Leslie, 2009; La Merrill, Stein, Landrigan, Engel, & Savitz, 2011). Infants exposed prenatally to cigarettes were more irritable and had an increased negative affect in comparison to infants who had not been exposed (Schuetze & Eiden, 2007). Infants exposed to cigarettes maintained a negative affect when observed later on at seven months. This may give insight into possible connections between prenatal cigarette exposure and oppositional and defiant behavior in adolescence. Mothers who smoke are also more likely to drink alcohol during pregnancy, so tobacco effects could be combined with the effects of alcohol (Willford, Chandler, Gold, Schmidt, & Day, 2010). Prenatal tobacco exposure is linked to poor motor performance, visual perception, memory, verbal learning, and auditory functioning. Individuals who were prenatally exposed to tobacco and later smoked in adolescence experienced enhanced effects of slowed processing speed and impaired memory.

Caffeine

Caffeine consumption during pregnancy is associated with high risk for miscarriage, stillbirth, and fetal death (Weng, Oduli, & Li, 2008). Mothers who consumed 0 to 200 milligrams of caffeine a day were at increased risk for miscarriage compared to mothers who refrained from caffeine consumption. For mothers who consumed more than 200 milligrams a day, the risk for miscarriage doubled. The study also found that the increased risk for miscarriage was directly associated with caffeine in any form, regardless of whether it was coffee, cola, tea, or chocolate. In light of the high risk of fetal death or miscarriage, it is recommended that mothers steer clear of caffeine intake.

Antidepressants Including SSRIs

A considerable number of women are diagnosed with depression during pregnancy (Ellfolk & Malm, 2010), perhaps as many as 10%. In order to combat this prolonged negative affect, individuals are often prescribed antidepressants such as serotonin reuptake inhibitors (SSRIs). Recent research with animals has suggested that these drugs have caused malformations in fetal facial development. In humans, the studies have been small but have reached similar results. Many human studies have found SSRIs to be associated with cardiac malformations; however, more research is needed to draw confident conclusions. Lithium has also long been suspected of causing congenital malformations and should be avoided during pregnancy (Kalter, 2003).

AIDS

Today in the United States, the rates of transmission of HIV (human immunodeficiency virus) from mother to child have decreased significantly (Maiques, Garcia-Tejedor, Perales, Cordoba, & Esteban, 2003). Mothers with HIV should undergo treatment such as highly active antiretroviral therapy to break down the virus. With treatment, the risk of transmitting the virus to the fetus greatly decreases and the placenta may stop the virus from spreading to the fetus. A planned cesarean section can also protect the infant from obtaining the virus through vaginal birth. However, a cesarean section can put the mother's life at risk due to the low function of her immune system.

Nutrition/Malnutrition

Proper maternal nutrition is vital to the healthy development of the fetus. During pregnancy, mothers should strive to eat a variety of foods to ensure adequate intake of vitamins and nutrients. An acknowledged view in prenatal nutrition is the Barker hypothesis, which states that fetal nutrition can permanently affect the child's health into adulthood (Barger, 2010). An example of this is seen in obese mothers. Pre-pregnancy obesity can put the mother at risk for gestational diabetes mellitus, which may lead to poor outcomes for the infant, and a likely chance for obesity in their future development (Josefen, 2011). This is known as metabolic programming, which can have long-term effects on the child. Overnutrition during the prenatal period in rats metabolically programmed the fetus with increased levels of fat mass, glucose, insulin, leptin, and triglycerides. Excessive weight gain during pregnancy can also lead to adverse outcomes for the fetus including increased body fat, which has been linked to predisposition to obesity. Women who are obese should attempt to lose weight prior to conceiving a child and should receive individualized instruction for the proper amount of gestational weight gain.

In addition to obesity, lack of proper food or inadequate amounts of food can result in malnutrition for the infant and increase the risk of producing a low birth weight infant. Many mothers are aware that they should avoid certain foods and habits such as raw fish and meat, alcohol, nicotine, and caffeine (Josefen, 2011). However, mothers are less aware of what foods they should incorporate into their daily diet. A recent study examined a lack of protein intake during the prenatal period in rats and found that it significantly affected the development of the nervous system as it slowed down the rate of processing and decreased brain and body weight (Frias, Varela, Oropeza, Bisiacchi, & Álvarez, 2010). Recommendations for daily dietary intake include consumption of a variety of fruits, vegetables, whole grains, and protein (Barger, 2010). It is suggested that meal frequency should include three meals a day with two snacks to maintain levels of glucose and insulin. The diet should include adequate levels of iron, vitamin A, vitamin D, folic acid, calcium, and iodine. It is known that iron is involved in blood oxygenation and promotion of cell growth. A lack of iron intake can significantly affect fetal development (Hautvast, 1997). A sufficient amount of vitamin A is suggested; however, too much can result in birth defects, so avoidance of large amounts of chicken or beef liver is recommended (Barger, 2010). Folic acid intake is important during the critical period of neural tube development, and a lack of intake can result in defects. Lack of iodine in maternal diet has also been linked to cognitive deficits in the infant.

Radiation

Studies of the effects of radiation on the fetus and abnormalities in infants date back to the 1920s. Women who received X-rays of their pelvic region while pregnant were found to have infants with a smaller head circumference, known as microcephaly, as well as eye malformations such as cataracts (Kalter, 2003). Infants are diagnosed with microcephaly if their head circumference is more than two standard deviations below the mean for their developmental age and weight. The timing during the gestational age and the dosage of radiation factor into the degree of malformations created. A study of pregnant women in Japan in close proximity to the atomic radiation from the Hiroshima and Nagasaki bombings in 1945 revealed indications of microcephaly as well. The old fears of standing too close to the television or microwaves or radiation from an ultrasound have not been proven.

Mercury

Methyl mercury consumed in fish or shellfish has been shown to cause abnormalities and intellectual disability (Kalter, 2003). First discovered in the city of Minmata, Japan, it is known as Minmata disease. In addition to structural abnormalities, the victims were seen to have cerebral palsy-like symptomatic defects.

Marijuana

Studies of the effects of marijuana use on the fetus are uncommon, even though marijuana is the most frequently used illicit drug. A recent study found prenatal marijuana exposure was linked to deficits in visual problem solving and impaired attention span, learning, and memory (Willford et al., 2010)

Rh Factor

The rhesus blood system was first discovered in 1939 through a transfusion containing Rh factor which caused hemolytic disease in a newborn (Lurie, Rotmench, & Glezerman, 2001). Rh negative is more prevalent in the Caucasian population than in other racial groups. In the 1960s, prevention of Rh factor, Rh negative, and Rh positive became possible with an immune globulin (immunization). Mothers with a partial Rh antigen are encouraged to receive preventive treatment to decrease the risk of transmission to their fetus or newborn.

Maternal Emotions

Previous studies have concluded that maternal distress during prenatal development has possible links with irreversible damage to neural pathways in the fetus (Weinstock, 2008). However, recent research points to both adverse and advantageous outcomes depending on the timing of cortisol exposure in the gestational period. A recent study examined the role of cortisol exuded during maternal stress in 125 infants and measured their cognitive development through the Mental Developmental Index (MDI) measure (Davis & Sandman, 2010). Measures of cortisol exposure and MDI scores revealed that high cognitive functioning was related to low cortisol levels early on in gestation and high levels later in the gestational period. Thus, mothers-to-be should reduce their stress levels during the early critical period of development as high levels of stress can adversely affect the infant's cognitive development.

Infants born to a mother with a DSM diagnosis (mental disorder) before birth such as depression or anxiety disorders had higher cortisol levels (a reaction to stress) than infants born to a mother without a mental health disorder (Kaplan, Evans, & Monk, 2008). However, this effect can be combated with the mother's level of sensitivity. This study found that infants with a mother who displayed high sensitivity were more likely to be more responsive and engaged in play.

Maternal/Paternal Age

The risk for birth complications rises dramatically with increasing maternal age. Among these complications are the potential for miscarriage, stillbirth, and even death of the mother. A recent study in Scotland found that mothers older than 40 were more likely to have a perinatal death caused by anoxia (Pasupathy, Wood, Pell, Fleming, & Smith, 2010). In addition to high-risk delivery and birth outcomes, increased maternal age is associated with increased risk for chromosomal and nonchromosomal abnormalities (Hollier, Leveno, Kelly, McIntire, & Cunningham, 2000). Women aged 25 and older are at significantly greater risk of giving birth to an infant with malformations than women aged 20–24 years. At age 35, this risk is even higher, and at age 40 and over, the risk doubles. Specific birth defects have been found with women of older maternal age, such as heart defects, club foot, and diaphragmatic hernia.

Advanced paternal age can also result in negative outcomes for the fetus. With advancing age, DNA mutations and chromosomal aberrations increase greatly in males' sperm. The National Birth Defect Prevention Study gathered data from 1997 to 2004 on risks with increased paternal age and found high risk for miscarriage, birth defects, and genetic disorders (Green et al., 2010). Specific defects found to be associated with increasing paternal age were right ventricular outflow tract obstruction (RVOTO), pulmonary valve stenosis (PVS), diaphragmatic hernia, cleft palate, and a variety of other malformations.

Maternal Diseases

Rubella was discovered in 1941 by an ophthalmologist who recognized rare cases of malformed eyes with cataracts on the outer lens (Kalter, 2003). The ophthalmologist linked these infant cases back to the previous year's epidemic of the "German measles," which is now known as rubella. Infants exposed to this disease in the first or second month of pregnancy had cataracts, heart defects, deafness, and microcephaly (i.e., small head circumference). A later epidemic in 1964 affected 20,000 to 30,000 infants who displayed the characteristic malformations from rubella disease. Since this massive outbreak, immunizations for rubella were initiated, and so now the possibility of a fetus contracting the disease is rare.

Maternal insulin-dependent diabetes mellitus acts as a teratogen to the fetus (Kalter, 2003). This is separate from gestational diabetes, which is diagnosed late in pregnancy yet has no known teratogenic effects on the fetus. Type I diabetes may increase the risk of infant mortality, abnormally large birth weight, structural anomalies, spontaneous abortion, central nervous system disorders, and heart defects.

Parent Relationships

The intentions of a pregnancy on the part of both the mother and the father can affect the health status of the infant. The Early Childhood Longitudinal Study—Birth Cohort followed the experiences and relationships of mothers and fathers from conception to infancy (Hohmann-Marriott, 2009). The study found that those parents who had intended to have a child were more likely to receive prenatal care and had better birth outcomes than those who had not intended to become pregnant. Among parents whose pregnancy was unplanned, their infant was more likely to be preterm, which was most likely related to the stress of an accidental pregnancy. The chances for a preterm infant increased if neither the mother nor the father intended the pregnancy. In these parents, fathers who lacked communication with the mother were more likely to have an infant with a low birth weight. This is likely due to a lack of social support, which may increase distress, a result that research has associated with low birth weight. Stress and conflict are keys to the relationships of partners rearing a newborn, and the relationships among infant caregivers are critical risk and resiliency factors (see the section above on maternal emotions).

Importance of Prenatal Care

The benefits of prenatal care are indisputable. Prenatal care is essential to educate the mother on preventive health measures, assess risk factors and medical history, and check the current health status of the mother and fetus (Evans & Lien, 2005). Among the most important prenatal care measures is prenatal screening for maternal disease. Testing for diseases such as rubella, STDs, or HIV can alert health care providers to begin treatment and work to prevent transmission of the disease to the fetus. Without testing, maternal disease can go undetected and put the fetus at risk for mortality. Prenatal care also provides essential preventive advice for the mother, such as conveying the importance of smoking cessation. A prenatal care provider can emphasize to the expectant mother the need to refrain from tobacco, illicit drugs, and alcohol use during each visit. The American Medical Association recommends that women should attend about 14 prenatal care visits for a low-risk pregnancy. Prenatal care has been associated with better birth outcomes such as decreased risk for low birth weight and preterm birth. Pregnant women who fail to keep regular prenatal care appointments early on in their pregnancy are more likely to have poor outcomes and babies with lower birth weight. These individuals were also more likely to smoke, which was attributed to missing out on advice from their provider. It is not clear whether prenatal care later on in pregnancy is associated with better outcomes, but it is clear that early prenatal care is essential to the health of the mother and baby.

Birthing Methods

Parents-to-be have a number of options for how to bring a newborn into the world. The most common methods include natural or prepared childbirth, induced labor, and cesarean delivery, but a number of other lesser used options are still available.

Natural/Prepared Childbirth

Women's consideration of which birthing method to choose involves several factors. A woman's perception of the birthing process and how they believe it should look may vary. While some may believe that it is a natural process that women are equipped to handle, others perceive it is as a dangerous and risky event (Wilson & Sirois, 2010). Based on these perceptions, the selection of allowing another caregiver to attend to the process and mode of delivery depends on the fit with the mother's beliefs. Women who believe it is a natural life process may wish to choose a midwife rather than an obstetrician. A midwife will focus more on the mother's wishes and desires for how she would like the birth to occur. The midwife takes into account the social, emotional, and physical needs of the mother. Mothers who are more traditional or who perceive childbirth as a threatening situation may wish to have the baby delivered by a medical doctor, as medical doctors are better able to use medications or technological interventions such as cesarean sections.

Natural childbirth has many socially constructed definitions. It is most commonly referred to as childbirth without the use of medicine or obstetrical interventions (Mansfield, 2008). Most often women plan to have a natural childbirth; they should become informed about the birthing process, including the best options to reduce pain. A well-known approach to natural birth is the **Lamaze method** (Lamaze.org, 2013), which stresses that women should be educated and prepared for a safe, natural birth without medical intervention through support, relaxation, and optimal birth positions. Many women choose to use a variety of stress reduction and relaxation techniques to make the process less painful and decrease the anxiety involved with childbirth. When the mother is relaxed, natural endorphins can be released to ease the pain (Mallak, 2009). However, if the mother-to-be is extremely tense and anxiety ridden, the body will release adrenalin, which will override the pain-relieving capability of endorphins. Common stress management activities include coordinated breathing and massaging pressure points, especially the hands and feet. As contractions begin, the mother may also wish to stay active and move about to ease the pain.

Finally, women report that controlling their birthing environment can help them feel at ease and reduce the birth-related stress, which can hinder labor. Women may wish to specify who can support them in the room, playing of music, and lighting options. Some women may opt to have a home delivery as this is their most familiar and comfortable place to achieve optimal relaxation and reduce tension. With home delivery, the assistance of a midwife trained in the practices of child labor is usually present. Water birth in the home or a water birthing facility has also gained popularity recently (called the LeBoyer method). The warm water is aimed to relax the mother and birth the infant into an environment similar to that which the fetus is exiting for a smooth transition into the world.

Induced Labor

Women are most likely to be induced into labor for maternal or fetal medical issues, although in some cases a mother-to-be may request an elective induction (Grobman & Simon, 2007). The health care provider will perform an amniotomy, which tricks the uterus into thinking the membranes have ruptured, and it will begin contractions and start the birth process. After the amniotomy, the "latent phase" of labor begins as the cervix and uterus work together to move into the "active phase." The latent phase ends and the active phase begins when the mother is dilated to 5 centimeters or 4 centimeters with 80% efface- ment. If the mother stays in the latent phase for longer than 12 to 18 hours, the doctors will consider the induction to have failed and will begin a cesarean section.

Cesarean Delivery

Recently, there has been a rising trend toward planned cesarean births rather than natural births. A **cesarean section (C-section)** involves cutting an opening in the mother's stom- ach to remove the newborn. Often it is an emergency procedure, but lately there has been an increase in elective cesarean births. The World Health Organization (WHO) recom- mends that there should be a cesarean birth rate of 10 to 15%; in 2006, however, 31% of births were through a cesarean section in the United States (Chalmers et al., 2010). Women should be informed of the choice of a planned cesarean birth and should understand the expected consequences. A recent study called the Maternity Experiences Survey in Canada compared women's perceptions of their experiences of a planned cesarean birth with a planned natural birth. Women who had a cesarean birth were more likely to report a nega- tive or unsatisfying birth experience than mothers who had a natural birth. Several factors could explain the negative cesarean birth experience, as it is likely to involve a low birth weight infant, preterm birth, prolonged hospital stay, or having an infant placed in neonatal intensive care. Women also reported that the time between delivery and contact with their infant was longer than for a natural birth. This prolonged skin-to-skin contact can affect the infant-to-parent relationship if new parents are unable to establish the caregiver bond in a timely manner. However, despite the risks involved, there are cases in which a planned or emergency cesarean section may be the best option. Mothers with diabetes or high blood pressure may be advised to have a planned cesarean section (MacDorman, Declercq, & Zhang, 2010). The most common reasons for a planned or emergency C-section include older mothers, extremely high or low body mass index, birth weight, breech presentation, and the length of pregnancy (Neal et al., 2010).

Some mothers are "born to birth!" It seems so easy; labor starts, followed quickly by the birth. No problems, no worries. Such was not the case in our family. Both of my children apparently stayed in the womb a bit too long, so the OB-GYN decided the deliveries should be induced. This had some good points and some difficult points. On the upside, we were able to make convenient appointments for 6 am on Saturday mornings: at work on Friday, new parents on Saturday. On the downside, the Pitocin drip was like a 0–100 mph race car acceleration: at 6:30 am my partner was not in labor and at 7 am labor was at full throttle! We chose the birthing room option, a private, comfortable family-room environment while labor progressed, and were well prepared from our childbirth and Lamaze classes. But eventually the pain was too much and in between deep breaths my partner whispered that very important word: e-p-i-d-u-r-a-l! Having so many options available and such highly skilled medical personnel ready to swoop in should trouble arise was a very comforting reality during times when, for example, the fetal heart monitor flat-lined and it seemed (to us) as though a serious problem was at hand. Not at all. The nurse and OB-GYN shared a glance and then the doctor tugged on what was obviously just a detached filament. A minute later all was fine again. The quality of care in modern medicine and hospitals is magnificent! [~BTE]

Problem Pregnancies

Monitoring

During the activation of labor, close attention must be paid to the heart rate of the fetus to ensure a safe exit from the womb (Murphy, Halamek, Lyell, & Druzin, 2003). Electronic fetal monitoring (EFM) is used to track the fetal heart rate to indicate fetal distress and decrease the risk of mortality.

Medications

Today, it is common for women to receive medication to ease the sometimes excruciating pain of labor. The most common and perhaps most effective is epidural analgesia (Jain, Arya, Gopalan, & Jain, 2003). It blocks pain receptors from the mid-spine to the pelvic region. As this medication does not transmit through the placenta, it is seen as a safe method for the newborn. However, drawbacks of epidural analgesia include increased length of active labor and increased chance of instrumental intervention due to lack of feeling. Possible instrumental interventions conducted usually involve a vacuum suction on the head of the infant or the use of forceps (Roberts, 2002). Other pain sedatives used during birth include opioidism which transfer through the placenta to the fetus and risk potential adverse outcomes such as depressed breathing in the newborn (Mercer, Erickson, Owens, Graves, & Haley, 2007). Oxytocins are also given to help induce contractions in delayed or prolonged labor.

Oxygen Deprivation/Anoxia

During pregnancy, it is possible for the fetus to be cut off from oxygen supply, known as **anoxia**, or receive an insufficient amount of oxygen, known as **hypoxia**. Either condition is often caused by **asphyxia**, or choking (Martinez-Biarge et al., 2011). Common causes of asphyxia include an entangled umbilical cord, maternal medicine interfering with breathing, or the baby being in a **breech presentation** (feet first). In a breech presentation delivery, the risk for neonatal death is high, and an emergency cesarean section (C-section) may save the infant's life (Pasupathy, Wood, Pell, Fleming, & Smith, 2009). A recent study examined 19 years of data from 1985 to 2004 in Scotland seeking explanations for a dramatic decrease in neonatal deaths and stillbirths. The study concluded that the dramatic increase in planned or emergency cesarean sections in the case of a breech presentation were responsible for the decline in anoxia-related deaths.

The extent of damage caused by hypoxia or anoxia often varies. A recent study used a brain MRI on infants who suffered from perinatal hypoxia to discover affected brain regions and predict future outcomes (Martinez-Biarge et al., 2011). The MRI showed that infants who experienced hypoxia had central gray matter damage, which is associated with motor impairment, and which could later classify as cerebral palsy. Central gray matter damage or brainstem injuries were also associated with a high risk of mortality.

Low Birth Weight/Preterm

In the United States, the rate of preterm births has increased dramatically over the past decade. While the exact cause is unknown, it is an alarming health concern, as preterm infants are at increased risk for both death and handicapping conditions, particularly cognitive deficits (Deary et al., 2006). An infant born prior to 37 weeks of pregnancy is considered a preterm birth; prior to 32 weeks is called very preterm, 32–33 weeks is moderate preterm, and 34–36 weeks is late preterm (MacDorman et al., 2010). While the risks are great for a very preterm infant, consequences are also serious for moderate and late preterm births. While low birth weight may be associated with the age of gestation, it is possible for a full-term infant to be low birth weight as well. An infant who weighs in at below the 10th percentile for weight of children of similar age is considered low birth weight (La Merrill et al., 2011). Common measurements in grams for low birth weight are less than 2500, and a very low birth weight is considered to be 1500 grams or less (Mathews & MacDorman, 2010).

From 1991 to 2006, there was a 13% increase in late preterm births along with a 47% increase in cesarean births (La Merrill et al., 2011). Elective inductions have doubled since 1991. Due to the critical conditions and risks of mortality in preterm infants, it is important to consider whether these interventions are absolutely necessary. Health care providers will attempt to prevent labor or prolong the onset of labor prior to 34 weeks gestation. Once preterm labor risk is assessed, a few steps may be taken to ensure fetal survival (Reedy, 2007). First, the doctor will examine the mother for any infections and treat them. The fetus is monitored during the process to assess their level of distress and their heart rate. The health care provider will often conduct an ultrasound to assess the current development of the fetus and what needs to be done to ensure their survival outside the womb. Next, the doctor may give the mother steroids to accelerate the growth of the fetus and most importantly to develop their lungs for survival. Finally, the mother may be given tocolytics, medicine to delay labor, so that the steroids have time to work and increase the chances for the fetus's survival.

Three known medical explanations for preterm delivery and birth exist. The mother may have to be medically induced, the membranes of the uterus rupture early, or the mother enters into a spontaneous premature labor (Moutquin, 2003). A medical induction of labor prior to 37 weeks is usually associated with complications with the mother's health such as illness, or problems with the fetus's health such as stunted growth. While premature rupture of the membranes and spontaneous labor are most common, the exact cause for these is usually unknown. Possible risk factors for a premature rupture are thought to be due to maternal infection. The most frequent reason for spontaneous labor involves the birth of multiples, most commonly twins. Other risk factors associated with preterm birth have been linked to a prior preterm delivery, previous abortions, *in vitro* fertilization, the presence of multiple fetuses, medical complications, bleeding, smoking, and a low BMI, or being underweight

Post-Term Infants

Post-term pregnancies are considered to be past 42 weeks gestation. At this point, the infant is at high risk for mortality and morbidity and the mother is at risk for labor-related complications (Chanrachakul & Herabuya, 2003; Hermus, Verhoeven, Mol, de Wolf, & Fiedeldeij, 2009). Carrying the fetus past term can result in stillbirth, obstetrical interventions such as cesarean section, and risk for neonatal asphyxia. Many health care providers suggest induction of labor, while others prefer to closely monitor the fetus and the mother and wait for natural induction, which have been linked to similar birth outcomes.

Infant Mortality

In 2006, the Centers for Disease Control and Prevention released a United States–based national health statistic report on infant mortality (Mathews & MacDorman, 2010). The total infant mortality rate in the United States was 6.68 infant deaths for every 1000 births. Risk factors and likely causes for mortality were also recorded, with disparities between race and sex. Infants born to Black mothers had higher incidences of death compared with all other races, and male infants had higher death rates than female infants. The death rate among multiples was five times higher than that of single-birth infants. Important risk factors that likely increased the incidence of infant mortality included age of gestation, birth weight, and maternal age. Infants born prior to 32 weeks gestation accounted for nearly half of all infant deaths. Low birth weight (less than 2500 grams) rates were 55.38 deaths per 1000 births and very low birth weight (less than 1500 grams) rates were 240.44 for every 1000 births. Mothers under the age of 15 years and over the age of 40 years had the highest incidence of infant mortality. Protective factors included increased levels of maternal education, which likely is associated with increased socioeconomic status. The leading cause of infant death was birth defects, which accounted for 21% of infant deaths in 2006, followed by preterm and low birth weight, SIDS (sudden infant death syndrome), maternal complications, and accidental deaths.

Stillbirth

Stillbirth refers to an infant born after 28 weeks gestation with no vital signs (Lawn et al., 2009). It is estimated that approximately 1.02 million stillbirths take place yearly throughout the world. A majority of stillbirths occur in developing countries, where women lack access to proper health care, birthing facilities, and birth attendants. Stillbirths most often occur due to complications in the womb, most commonly hypoxia. Prevention of stillbirths involves advocacy for prenatal care to assess maternal health and disease, obstetrical interventions with high-risk pregnancies, resuscitation after delivery, and the presence of a trained birth attendant.

Childbirth

Childbirth ordinarily progresses through the phases of labor, dilation, effacement, delivery, and expulsion of the placenta.

Dealing with Labor

Today, a majority of women use an epidural to ease the pain of childbirth. An epidural is usually administered during the first stage of labor to ease the pain of contractions. While it may come with drawbacks such as a prolonged labor process, many health professionals believe it helps put the mother at ease to allow the fetus to smoothly enter the birth canal (Albers, Migliaccio, Bedrick, Teaf, & Peralta, 2007). To help ease the pain and guide the position of the fetus, the mother may also be instructed to move about to find an optimal birthing position. While the most advantageous position is unknown, anecdotal reports from mothers have been incorporated into practice. Sitting, squatting, or lying on one's side are most commonly used to encourage the fetus to move toward the birth canal (Roberts, 2002). Recently, rocking back and forth on one's hands and knees during the first stage of labor has also gained attention. Most women and health care providers recommend upright positioning to decrease duration of labor and reduce risk for instrumental interventions.

Dilation and Effacement

When the mother is ready to give birth, the first stage of labor, known as the "latent phase," begins as the cervix begins to efface, or thin (Roberts, 2002). Effacement is measured in percentages; for example, "90% effacement" refers to a very thin cervix lining as it is ready to begin dilation. The "active phase" of labor begins when the mother's uterus is contracting frequently and the cervix is dilated at 3 to 5 centimeters (Neal et al., 2010). There is no exactly defined rate of progression for dilation. Some health providers define the slowest acceptable rate to be 1 centimeter per hour. A woman who moves through the dilation phase slower than this rate, or who experiences a speed of dilation deemed abnormal by the health provider, may be diagnosed with **dystocia**—an unusually slow progression of dilation in labor. Women with dystocia will most likely have a cesarean section if attempted interventions to speed the labor fail. At 4 to 9 centimeters of dilation, the mother is at the "phase of maximum slope." At 9 to 10 centimeters, the mother is ready to progress to the second stage of labor.

Delivery

The delivery phase of childbirth begins when the mother's cervix is fully dilated at 10 centimeters (Roberts, 2002). At this point, the intensity of the contractions forces the fetus's head to rotate and align with the pelvis. As the fetus moves into optimal position, the mother feels an involuntary reflex emerge to bear down and has the urge to begin pushing. This is known as the "expulsive phase" in the second stage as the body is literally ready to expel the newborn. There is debate among health care providers over whether the practitioner should give directions to push when dilation reaches 10 centimeters or if pushing should wait until the mother feels the bearing-down reflex. Caregiver-directed pushing rather than waiting for the involuntary urge to push has been linked to pelvic trauma and increased risk for obstetrical interventions. Once the head begins to emerge from the birth canal, the second stage has progressed into the final phase of "transition." The newborn is delivered, cleaned off, and handed to the mother to begin a tactile connection and to look at her baby for the first time.

Expulsion of Placenta

After delivery of the baby, many women relax, thinking that the hard work is over; however, delivery of the placenta has yet to come. This third stage of labor generally lasts anywhere from 3 to 30 minutes (Bair & Williams, 2007). Duration exceeding 30 minutes places the mother at high risk for postpartum hemorrhage (PPH). PPH is a serious condition that can result in maternal mortality. During this third stage of labor, the health care provider may take a stance of expectant management, waiting for the placenta to deliver on its own, or active management, using medicine to induce contractions or manual stimulation. Through expectant management, the health care provider will look for signs of the placenta separating and may apply pressure to encourage delivery of the placenta. If delivery does not occur spontaneously, moving positions, having the mother empty her bladder, or nipple stimulation may help move the delivery along. If expulsion of the placenta still does not occur, the health care provider will physically remove the placenta. With active management, the risk for PPH is greatly decreased. The health care provider may supply the mother with uteronics after delivery of the baby, which is medicine to induce contractions to deliver the placenta. In addition to uteronics, controlled cord traction may be used, in which the health care provider presses down on the umbilical cord and applies pressure to the uterus simultaneously to speed up the expulsion process and prevent PPH.

Adaptation to the Environment and Physical Conditions

Routine procedures to help ease the newborn's transition from the womb to the new environment have been in place for many years. Upon delivery of the newborn, the umbilical cord is clamped and the air passages of the mouth and nose are suctioned for optimum oxygen intake prior to the cord being cut. Then the baby is cleaned, fully dried, and wrapped in a blanket. In order to regulate the infant's temperature, the newborn will be placed directly on the mother's skin, not only to absorb her natural warmth but also to establish their first bonding experience (Mercer et al., 2007). Infants with breathing issues, particularly preterm babies, may be given oxygen or resuscitated with room air if they cannot sustain breathing on their own. Breastfeeding following birth is promoted as a most favorable health practice for the infant. Breast milk contains vital nutrients for infant survival, antigens to fight disease, and also optimizes immune functioning (Davanzo, 2004). Breastfeeding also supports the infant's temperature regulation and enhances mother–infant bonding in the early hours of life.

For preterm and low birth weight infants, "kangaroo mother care" has recently been used to introduce skin-to-skin contact for early bonding (Davanzo, 2004). Kangaroo care involves placing the infant between the mother's bare breasts frequently throughout the day and continuously until the infant has reached full-term gestational age or weight. In addition to enhancing attachment, kangaroo care regulates the infant's breathing and temperature and steadies the heart rate. Kangaroo care is recommended in place of incubators for preterm or LBW infants in the neonatal intensive care unit (NICU). However, as this is a fairly new concept, it may take more time for all birthing facilities to incorporate this into their practice. Another method thought to stimulate weight gain is infant massage, in which the caregiver strokes the infant's body. Little scientific evidence has been collected on the benefits of infant massage, and more research is currently being conducted to establish its utility in promoting development.

Neonatal Procedures, Tests, and Adaptations

A number of tests and procedures are conducted just after birth. The **Apgar test** is given to an infant one minute after birth and again 5 minutes later (O'Reilly, 2009). After they are born, the first test assesses on a 1 to 10 scale, with 10 being optimal health, how well the infant did throughout the birth process. The second test, 5 minutes later, assesses how well the infant is adapting to their environment, also using a scale 1 to 10. The test observes and measures the infant's breathing, heart rate, muscle tone, reflexes, and skin color. Each category is rated with a 0, 1, or 2, with 2 being the healthiest. The five category scores are added together to create the total Apgar score. A healthy infant will normally have scores around 8 or 9. An infant with a score below 8 is in need of immediate medical attention. It is possible that an infant who has a low Apgar score at 1 minute after birth but advances to a normal level at 5 minutes may not have any lasting consequences.

Vitamin K is essential to humans to make the blood clot. The mother's milk contains a low dosage of vitamin K, and it has been shown that it is difficult for maternal vitamin K supplements to transfer through the placenta to the infant (Greer, 2010). Therefore, at birth, infants are given a vitamin K injection to prevent hemorrhagic disease, which involves the inability to control bleeding. Infants can also receive several vitamin K doses orally. If an infant is at high risk for vitamin K deficiency, the doctor may recommend additional formula supplements fortified with vitamin K.

Silver nitrate drops in the eye have been used for neonatal protection against conjunctivitis or opthalmia (inflammation in the eye) caused by chlamydia or gonorrhea (Zar, 2005). Recent research suggests that silver nitrate drops may irritate the eye and fail to protect against pneumonia in infected infants. Oral erythromycin is the recommended treatment for opthalmia, protecting against further eye irritation and pneumonia.

Circumcision

Throughout the world, the majority of males are uncircumcised; however, in the United States the practice has become routine. Neonatal circumcision is often a ritualistic practice for cultures or religions such as Islam and Judaism. Infants of Jewish decent are required by law to obtain a circumcision on their eighth day of life, and the circumcision is usually performed by a Jewish leader. The need for neonatal circumcision in the absence of religious practice is controversial. While the benefits of circumcision are reduced risk for urinary tract infections in infancy and HIV/STDs later in life, uncircumcised men tend to have similar positive medical outcomes (Lerman & Liao, 2001). Regardless of the reason for circumcision, the experience of the infant's pain and anesthesia for these practices has recently been brought into question; however, lack of availability of trained anesthesiologists in home rituals may prevent widespread use (Rosen, 2010).

Reflexes

Infants display normal reflexes involved in breastfeeding in the first couple of hours of life (Cadwell, 2007). The infant will use the stepping-crawling reflex to search for the mother's breast when placed in the breastfeeding position. Once the breast has been located, the infant should be able to latch onto the nipple and begin to suck the milk down for their first feeding. Once self-attached breastfeeding has occurred, the infant will use its rooting reflex to search for breast milk again.

Behavioral Assessment

The Brazelton Neonatal Behavioral Assessment Scale observes the behavioral, emotional, and social reactions and dispositions of the newborn (Brazelton & Nugent, 1995). The health care provider observes and measures basic developmental tasks, seeking to find their strengths and weakness and help them adapt to the necessary demands. The scale measures the infant's responses on 28 behavioral and 18 reflex items. The NBAS seeks to understand how infants are trying to communicate with its environment and people around them. The health care provider looks at the infant's ability to maintain and regulate breathing and temperature, motor control, state regulation and transition (from sleeping to crying), and social interaction (response). The provider will assess the infant's development and achievement in these areas and work with parents to suggest ways to best provide care and support for their infant. For example, if the infant is sensitive to light while sleeping and cannot block out the stimulation, the health care provider will suggest that the parents keep the room dark so that the infant can preserve energy.

Postpartum Depression

During pregnancy and after birth, 10% to 15% of women experience adverse psychological reactions referred to as perinatal depression (Sockol, Epperson, & Barber, 2011). The symptoms may be as mild as maternity blues or as severe as postpartum depression (Reck, Stehle, Reinig, & Mundt, 2009). Mothers with the "baby blues" may experience abnormal worry, crying, sadness, and varying moods. Maternity blues along with previous history of depression are important risk factors for an increased risk of developing postpartum depression.

It is estimated that 19% of women experience symptoms of postpartum depression (PPD) in the first year after childbirth (Gavin et al., 2005). This mental condition can have adverse social, emotional, and cognitive effects on the health of the mother, father, and the newborn child (Miyake, Keiko, Sasaki, & Hirota, 2011). The mother may experience symptoms involving feelings of insignificance, dejected mood, lack of interest in daily behavior, and a lack of vigor to perform usual duties (Iles, Slade, & Spiby, 2011). The mother may not be the only one to experience depression, as 24–50% of men whose partners have PPD indicate symptoms of PPD as well (Goodman, 2004). The relationship between the mother and father may be strained as unstable moods can emerge from either party. As the mother is distressed, this can affect her interactions with the child, leading to the development of a maladaptive attachment pattern (Sockol et al., 2011). This can be detrimental to the child, as it can stunt the child's cognitive growth and can lead to future behavioral issues.

One study looked at possible risk factors that contributed to the role of postpartum depression. The study found that young parents and first-time fathers were likely to have higher levels of depression, as they were unprepared or had unrealistic outlooks on the experience of parenthood (Iles et al., 2011). Individuals with anxiety or low self-esteem were also found to be more likely to be diagnosed with postpartum depression. The study found that couples were likely to experience depressive symptoms together; that is, it is more likely that the father will experience depressive symptoms if the mother experiences them as well. This may be attributed to the hypothesis that individuals may choose mates similar to themselves. The study found that attachment styles also played a role in the risk of developing depressive symptoms. Couples with insecure attachment were likely to experience depression, as it is possible that fear of abandonment or avoidance prevented them from discussing their distress. For men, frustration with their partner's support was the best predictor of elevated levels of depression.

Social and cultural aspects can act as protective factors in developing PPD. A study found that in Japanese women, mothers who were employed full-time in a professional or technical job were less likely to develop postpartum depression (Miyake et al., 2011). The study also found that there was no relationship between household income and postpartum depression. The study suggested that perhaps job satisfaction played a role in preventing the development of depressive symptoms.

Due to the severe effects on the mother, father, their relationship, and the child, it is important to prevent the onset of postpartum depression through early intervention. Health care providers should look for early symptoms of distress in the puerperal period, before it reaches the postpartum period. If the mother is depressed, the father is likely experiencing symptoms as well, and the health care professional should look into a family systems approach to address the contributing factors. Possible interventions focusing on combating irrational beliefs associated with maladaptive attachment styles could help mitigate the symptoms of depression in couples (Iles et al., 2011). Individuals or health professionals who are aware of these symptoms may recommend that the mother and father seek mental health care. Frequently used and effective treatments for postpartum depression include interpersonal psychotherapy (IPT) and cognitive-behavioral therapy (CBT) (Sockol et al., 2011). IPT focuses on interpersonal problems, disputes, and adjustment to roles and new transitions that relate directly to the experience of mothers. CBT focuses on cognitive restructuring along with behavioral applications.

Summary

This chapter highlighted the beginnings of lifespan development, from genetic inheritance to conception to the delivery of a new life. This chapter began with a summary of the basic mechanisms of genetics including the human cell, DNA, inherited traits, and hereditary disorders. The debate around nature versus nurture was highlighted in reference to twin and adoption studies as well as the role of epigenetics. Inheritance of characteristics such as temperament, intelligence, and attitude were also discussed. Then the theoretical models of gene and environment interaction were summarized. The discussion of genes came to a close as it connected heredity with special issues in parenthood including genetic counseling, reproductive technologies, adoption, and abortion.

Next, the importance of the prenatal environment for optimal fetal health was emphasized. The stages of physical development throughout the trimesters were summarized, followed by a description of the possible effects of several teratogens on the developing fetus.

Teratogenic substances and their effects range from alcohol and AIDS to maternal emotions and age. Next, the development of the fetal brain was highlighted.

The next section focused on practical issues in preparing for parenthood. The necessity of prenatal care as a preventive measure was discussed. Maternal options for birthing methods were summarized including natural, induced, and cesarean births. Complications in pregnancy were reviewed, including fetal monitoring/medicine, oxygen deprivation, preterm/post-term, low birth weight, and stillbirths/miscarriages.

Finally, the stages of labor and delivery were highlighted. The newborn's physical condition and adaptation to a new environment were discussed, including common neonatal procedures and tests to assess their developmental abilities. Newborn reflexes and states were also highlighted. The final section discussed the serious nature of postpartum depression, including symptoms, warning signs, risk factors, protective factors, and treatment options.

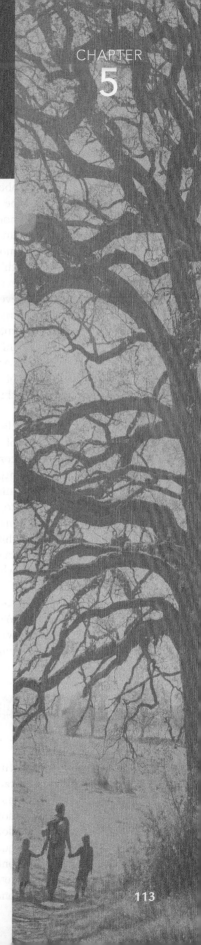

Physical and Cognitive Development in the Infancy and Toddlerhood Years

By Nadine E. Garner and Julia M. Dunn

The years from infancy through toddlerhood, spanning approximately birth through age 3 years, serve as a bridge between life in the womb and the more independent functioning of preschoolers. This chapter explores the tremendous changes that occur in the physical and cognitive domains of the infant and toddler. The rapid brain and body growth during this developmental period are highly context dependent, shaped by nutrition, sleep, parenting, the broader culture, and the child's own temperament. The child's unique pattern of development lays the groundwork for the continuing adventure across the lifespan.

Welcome to Infancy and Toddlerhood!

When you enter the world of infants and toddlers (children from birth to about 3 years), and their parents (used throughout this book to indicate any type of primary caregiver relationship), you are embarking on an extraordinary odyssey indeed! Parents have fears about their children's well-being, insecurities about their parenting techniques, strong opinions about their child-rearing preferences, and a fierce love for their children—all at once. So be prepared: When you walk up to a group of parents of infants and toddlers, there is not much information that is kept private, as parents seek to connect with each other and understand the bizarre journey of raising little people who seem to grow and develop a bit more each and every day. It is common conversation to talk about the intricacies of their children's bowel movements; any bodily function is fair game! Parents are on a continuous, ever-changing odyssey with their children, just as you—the counselor—are on an equally ever-changing odyssey when working with parents and their children. Forming a working alliance with families of children at this stage of development can be intense, often entertaining, and sometimes perplexing, but never boring. Navigating this journey through infancy and toddlerhood with parents requires an *extremely* open mind on the counselor's part, patience, diplomacy with delicate issues, and a willingness to be regaled with all kinds of amusing anecdotes about their children. There are contrasting views on many aspects of child rearing, as well as cultural considerations.

These years from birth to age 3 can be an emotionally charged time for parents, from elation at the thrill of parenting a child, to exhaustion when they are grappling with bouts of sleep deprivation from their child's night waking. It is not uncommon for parents to compare the development of their child to that of other children: When did your child begin to walk, use the potty, speak, hold a spoon? Counselors interacting with the parents of infants and toddlers will be exploring the uncharted territory of children's myriad physical, cognitive, emotional, and social changes that transpire magically before your very eyes. You may find yourself offering vital support and compassion to a parent like Linda, who went through the harrowing experience of watching her 8-month-old daughter, Shania, have her cardiovascular system shut down and put on a heart and lung machine to keep her alive, while surgeons corrected a life-threatening heart condition.

Counselors need to be sensitive to variations in approaches to parenting, including feeding issues, toileting, sleeping styles, and the choice of whether or not to vaccinate. While many well-meaning people may be offering their opinion and "expert advice" about what a parent *should* do, it is essential for the counselor to recognize that the parent is the ultimate decision maker for the child's welfare.

SECTION I: Physical Development

Body Size, Proportion, and Skeletal Age

The period of most rapid growth occurs from birth to 1 or 2 years (Doyle, 2009). The physical metamorphosis from newborn to toddler is nothing short of dramatic. Imagine beginning your semester at a certain weight, and by finals week your beginning weight has almost doubled! Shocking for adult growth, but normal for an infant, who, if 7.5 pounds at birth, doubles his birth weight by 5 months to 15 pounds, tripling it to 22 pounds by 1 year, and quadrupling it to 30 pounds by 2 years of age. Proportionally, a newborn's head takes up one-fourth of his body, compared to an adult head, which occupies about one-seventh of total body size. Body size for an infant who is too young to stand is measured in length; once the infant can stand it is measured in height. By 5 months the infant's length increases by 30%, and by 1 year height has increased by 50%. A boy toddler at 2 years of age has already grown to half of his adult height, and a girl toddler has grown to half of her adult height by 19 months.

A child who gains weight too rapidly during the first 2 years (a jump in 1 major centile band, such as from the 25th to the 50th percentile, or from the 50th to the 75th percentile) on a weight-for-age growth chart, doubles the risk of obesity compared to a child who has a more gradual weight gain, and this weight gain is also associated with insulin resistance in childhood (Demerath et al., 2009). Parents seeing conflicting charts for growth standards in their health care provider's office frequently become confused and worried that their child is growing at a rate that may be unhealthy. There are two different international **growth charts**—one published by the World Health Organization (WHO) and another published by the Centers for Disease Control and Prevention (CDC). For example, according to the WHO, a 1-month-old infant weighing 9 pounds 9 ounces is in the 57th percentile of body size, while the CDC puts that same-size infant in the 25–50th percentile. By 8 months, an infant weighing 15 pounds 11 ounces is in the 24th percentile according to WHO standards but is in the 5–10th percentile by CDC standards (Beck, 2012). One reason these charts differ is due to the differences in body sizes for infants who are breastfed (WHO chart statistics) or formula-fed (statistics predominantly on the CDC chart). The CDC (2010d) recommends that health care providers in the United States use the WHO growth standards to monitor infant and toddler growth from 0 to 2 years and the CDC growth charts for children 2 years and older.

The most accurate estimate of an infant's or toddler's physical maturity is obtained by determining **skeletal age**, often done by taking an X-ray of the child's hand and wrist and comparing the numerous bones in this area of the body to standards of bone growth on X-rays in an assessment atlas. The **epiphyses** (eh-PIF-i-sees), the active growing areas at the end of each growing bone, are examined to see how much soft cartilage has not yet turned to hardened bone (Haywood & Getchell, 2009). By calculating skeletal age, it becomes clearer whether or not the weight of an infant, paired with how quickly the infant is growing, is in a safe range (Demerath et al., 2009).

Fat Composition, Muscle Growth, and Teeth

The infant's **body fat** composition increases rapidly, from a proportion of 13% body fat at birth to 20–25% body fat by the first birthday, contributing to the chubby look of most babies and allowing them to maintain an even body temperature. After this peak, body fat declines steadily until preadolescence, when body fat returns to about 13% (Doyle, 2009). Unlike the fluctuations in body fat, **muscle growth** in a normally developing infant increases gradually throughout the first year (Sann, Durand, Picard, Lasne, & Bethenod, 1988) and continues slowly and steadily until adolescence. However, notable differences in muscularity occur in infants and toddlers who were born either small for gestational age (SGA, <10th percentile) or large for gestational age (LGA, >90th percentile) (Hediger et al., 1998). Determining muscularity by measuring the mid-upper arm circumference and mid-upper arm muscle area, infants and toddlers born SGA have a deficit in muscle but an increase in fat, and those born LGA have excess muscle but less surplus fat. Researchers are concerned that children born SGA may have experienced metabolic changes as fetuses, adapting to inadequate nutrition in the womb by developing fetal hypoglycemia to maximize the available glucose in the placenta. While this adaptation may have helped the fetus survive in the womb, in infants and toddlers the adaptation limits muscle growth, which may delay motor development and contribute to excess fat, thereby increasing the risk of developing coronary vascular disease, hypertensive disease, and diabetes as an adult.

An infant typically begins the **teething process** at 5–9 months, with the eruption of the first **baby teeth** (also called primary teeth or deciduous teeth), usually beginning with the lower central incisors (i.e., the two bottom front teeth) (Doyle, 2009). As the average teething process continues, the infant has 6 teeth by 12 months, 12 teeth by 18 months, 16 teeth by 2 years, and all 20 deciduous teeth by 2½ years. The great variability among children is largely due to genetic factors. For example, Cathryne was nearly 18 months old before she had four teeth, and Nadine startled her mother and disbelieving pediatrician when her bottom incisors emerged at 3 months. While for some families teething is a stressful time accompanied by the child's seemingly inconsolable crying and frustration at all hours of the day and night, some infants have a minimal response to teeth erupting through their gums and are able to sleep well through the process.

Reflexes

The infant adapts to his immediate setting through reflexes, automatic and hardwired responses to stimulation. Primitive reflexes are the reflexes we see in an early-developing infant (Schott & Rossor, 2003). When pressure is put on an infant's palm, he exhibits the **grasping reflex** by clenching his fingers around whatever is pressing on them, the reflex used when the infant holds onto someone's finger. Infants will also demonstrate the **sucking reflex** when something is placed inside their mouths (such as a nipple), and the **rooting reflex** when something is rubbed against an infant's cheek and he turns his mouth toward the object. Both of these reflexes are an integral part of survival if an infant is in need of food.

Reflexes are innate tools that allow the infant self-protection before developing the cognition to do so consciously. For example, an infant immersed in a pool of water exhibits the **diving reflex** by holding his breath and opening his eyes, allowing him to block off his airway and protect himself from inhaling water or other noxious substances (Pedroso, Riesgo, Gatiboni, & Rotta, 2012). The **blink reflex** is also used in situations that warrant protection. In a study by Richards (1998), infants were shown black-and-white images that did not elicit a raised heart rate, but when presented with a flash of a new visual stimulus, they blinked their eyes. This motion of blinking is not cultivated through experience; instead, infants are born with the instinct to protect their vulnerable spots—in this case, their eyes—by closing off contact with the environment.

Even when infants are not in immediate danger, their reflexes are still hard at work. A classic study by Sherman and Sherman (1925) sought to test the **Babinski reflex**, the extension and/or flexion of a newborn's toes when the bottom of the foot is stroked. The study showed that no matter how often the bottom of the infant's foot was stroked, the movement of the toes continued to take place, suggesting that there is little to no cognitive control over reflexive movement. A more elaborate reflex that causes an infant to extend is known as the **Moro reflex**, which allows the infant to stretch out his arms, legs, and fingers while elongating the neck muscles simultaneously when an infant is moved suddenly or hears a loud sound (Hunt & Landis, 1938).

While many infant reflexes are primal, and typically shared with other mammalian species, one reflex that is anomalous in humans (and apes) is the **postauricular reflex (PAR)**. As seen in many companion animals, when an animal feels attacked, it pins its ears against its head. This is a movement that is accessible to humans only as infants, but surprisingly, it is not used as a response to fear. Instead, infants have what is known as a positive PAR when they are breastfeeding. Instead of pulling back their ears in fear, infants use this reflex to signal that they are ready to feed, as well as to make themselves more comfortable during the process of nursing (Johnson, Valle-Inclán, Geary, & Hackley, 2012).

Infants also have reflexes that preclude movements they are not fully capable of making. One example of this is the locomotor reflex known as the **stepping reflex** (also called

walking reflex): When held above the floor, infants kick their legs in ways that simulate walking. The stepping reflex seems to grow more pronounced with practice (Cautilli & Dziewolska, 2006).

Nutrition and Malnutrition

According to the World Health Organization (WHO, 2013), a branch of the United Nations, **nutrition** is

> the intake of food, considered in relation to the body's dietary needs. Good nutrition—an adequate, well balanced diet combined with regular physical activity—is a cornerstone of good health. Poor nutrition can lead to reduced immunity, increased susceptibility to disease, impaired physical and mental development, and reduced productivity.

One of the major decisions of parenthood is whether to nourish the newborn and infant by breastfeeding or formula feeding. Human milk delivers the essential protein, sugar, and fat the newborn and infant need for optimal nutrition (American Academy of Pediatrics, 2012c). The position of the American Academy of Pediatrics (AAP) is to begin breastfeeding within the first hour after birth, continue breast milk as the *exclusive* source of an infant's nutrition for approximately 6 months, and then maintain breastfeeding in conjunction with solid foods until at least 12 months (AAP, 2012a).

The nutrients available to an infant via breast milk are capable of strengthening the immune system, minimizing the chance of having allergies later in life, and lessening the risk of developing diseases that are fatal to infants, such as sudden infant death syndrome (SIDS). Breastfeeding benefits the mother as well. Breastfeeding allows a release of oxytocin (a chemical that is associated with feelings of love and closeness) into the brain and is less expensive than buying formula. Breastfeeding makes feeding a baby outside of the home more convenient than formula feeding in terms of bringing along feeding supplies. It is also more environmentally sustainable since it does not generate waste from packaging materials. Situations where breastfeeding is not advised include those in which the mother is infected with HIV, is dependent on alcohol or illegal substances, or is undergoing chemotherapy (AAP, 2012b, 2012c, 2013).

Many mothers in the United States are attempting to follow the AAP's breastfeeding recommendations. More than half of the breastfeeding mothers in a study by Shealy, Scanlon, Labiner-Wolfe, Fein, and Grummer-Strawn (2008) fed their infants nothing but breast milk for the first four months. Comparing 1000 infants who were breastfed exclusively for at least three months with 1000 infants were who never breastfed, Ball and Wright (1999) discovered that never-breastfed infants suffered more lower respiratory tract illnesses, otitis media, and gastrointestinal illness than their breastfed peers during their first year, resulting in 2033 more office visits, 212 more days of hospitalization, and 609 more prescriptions, costing the managed health care system between $331 and $475 per never-breastfed infant.

Breastfeeding is an area requiring cultural sensitivity on the professional counselor's part. Some mothers will be capable of breastfeeding but choose to use formula instead. Others would welcome the chance to breastfeed but have situations that preclude them from nursing their babies. During your counseling career, you will likely work with mothers who have chosen to breastfeed their children well beyond the age of 1 year. It is more common for mothers in developing nations to continue breastfeeding children into toddlerhood and even preschool age, and the practice of extended breastfeeding is becoming more recognizable in the United States. If this style of parenting is not familiar to you, this counseling relationship may be an excellent opportunity to learn first-hand the philosophies of attachment parenting that undergird this choice in breastfeeding practice.

As babies move beyond breastfeeding, parents may be heartened to know that it is not as challenging to encourage infants and toddlers to eat a variety of foods as some parents might believe. Parents may have seen other adults employ bribing, rewarding, forcing, or tricking their children in the quest to provide nutritious food. These methods are not considered optimal in helping children develop a psychologically healthy relationship with food. However, parents who use early tasting exposures (see Taste and Smell below) and engage their children's mirror neurons find that their children willingly eat most foods. **Mirror neurons** are specialized cells in the brain that imitate the behaviors of what children see before they can actually perform the behavior themselves. An infant observes what adults eat by 4 months, when color vision is getting strong (Greene, 2009). Not only does the infant stare at what people eat, but also the infant remembers it and is more likely to eat a food the parents eat. Unfortunately, by 9 months, French fried potatoes have become the number three vegetable fed to children, and by 18 months, it is the number one vegetable! The ramifications of exposing infants and toddlers to healthy or unhealthy foods are lifelong; how a baby is fed early in life does not influence just the foods the infant is willing to eat. At a cellular level, specific genes that govern the quantity of food needed to satisfy an infant, metabolic rate, weight gain, how the body manages blood sugar and cholesterol, and diabetes or heart disease, are turned on and off.

Breastfeeding transmits the flavors of what the mother eats, serving as an opportunity for early, repeated tasting exposures. Strategies to help a toddler continue to acquire a taste for nutritious foods include allowing a "no thank you" taste, in which the infant has a right to refuse as long as the infant takes an initial taste (which, unbeknownst to the infant, counts as a tasting exposure to the brain); eating the food as a family; letting the infant/toddler help with a family garden; and letting the infant/toddler help prepare the food to the extent he or she is able.

An infant or toddler is diagnosed with **malnutrition** by comparing weight-for-height score with a healthy reference group's score. The most updated WHO international child growth standards, established in 2006, are based on a reference group of 8500 children from Brazil, Ghana, India, Norway, Oman, and the United States, who were studied from birth to 2 years between 1997 and 2003. These children had optimal nurturing from nonsmoking mothers who breastfed exclusively. An infant or toddler is diagnosed with *global acute malnutrition* (GAM) if the weight-for-height score is less than 80% of the reference group's median weight-for-height. *Severe acute malnutrition* (SAM) is the diagnosis given when the weight-for-height score is less than 70% of the reference group's median weight-for-height (Duggan, 2010). In 2011, 6.9 million children under the age of 5 died around the world, with over 70% of the deaths occurring in Africa and Southeast Asia. The majority of these deaths occurred in rural areas and in families who were poor and less educated. *One-third of these child deaths were linked to malnutrition* (WHO, 2012b).

Although infants and toddlers in the United States may not suffer malnutrition to the degree experienced by children in some developing nations, food insecurity is an ongoing problem for many American children and their families. While 85.1% (101.6 million) of U.S. households (including households with and without children) were **food secure** throughout 2011, meaning that they had continuous access to enough food for all household members to live healthily, the stark reality is that millions of children and their families suffer from food insecurity. **Food insecurity** means that at some time during the year, the household was either uncertain of having enough food to meet the needs of all the members or was unable to acquire enough food because of insufficient money or other resources for food (Economic Research Service, 2012).

In 2011, among U.S. households with children under age 18 years, 8.6 million children living in 3.9 million households (10% of households with children) experienced food insecurity for both children and adults. Many of these food-insecure households were able to employ coping strategies such as using federal food assistance programs, eating less varied diets, or receiving food from a food bank. This helped significantly reduce their eating pattern disruptions and food intake. However, 845,000 children (1.1% of U.S. children) living in 374,000 households (1% of households with children) lived in such food-insecure conditions that they experienced *reduced food intake* and *disrupted eating patterns* (Economic Research Service, 2012). Infants and toddlers living with food insecurity may develop **anemia**, a lack of iron in the bloodstream, which may persist even when the children are participating in federally funded programs to supplement their diet (Skalicky et al., 2006). Food insecurity also affects the social and emotional functioning of a family and children's early development. Mothers who live with food insecurity often suffer from depression and have less-nurturing parenting practices. In turn, their children who experienced food insecurity as 9-month-old infants were more likely to be insecurely attached to their mothers and had less advanced cognitive abilities when they grew into 24-month-old toddlers (Zaslow, 2009).

Health Concerns and Vaccinations

The adventure of parenting requires a great deal of personal fortitude, even when an infant or toddler has no major health issues. But what about a family who has just discovered that their child has a challenge that will change their lives forever? Counselors may enter a family's life during a time of crisis and despair, such as when their child is newly diagnosed with diabetes (see Case Example 5.1).

➤ CASE EXAMPLE **5.1** DIAGNOSIS OF DIABETES.

I still try to block most of it from my memory because it was such a horrible time. There is absolutely no feeling worse than the helplessness I felt as a parent unable to do anything for my baby. He was 2 years, 2 months, and 26 days old the day we took Zach to the emergency room because he'd been having trouble breathing the night before, all through the night actually. He had thrown up in his bed at bedtime, and as I put him in the bathtub, I noticed for the first time how skinny he looked, with all his ribs showing. He was so dehydrated. I remember the first time I had to give my 2-year-old a shot in the arm during our 6 days in the hospital. The nurses held him down in the bed, screaming, while I had tears streaming down my face and had to hurt my child so that he would live. I grabbed him as soon as I did it, and ran out of the room, down the halls of the hospital with him, determined that I would go find a cliff somewhere and jump off with him because I was sure there was no way I could do this to him every day, and it would be no way for him to live. Meanwhile, Henry, at 5 months old, was ignored from that point on for most of the first year of his life, while our lives revolved around coping with Zach's diagnosis and diabetes management. It got better when I was able to help other new parents going through the same thing with their newly diagnosed child by talking to them, and sharing our experience, and listening to theirs. We had also joined a support group in San Diego which met once a month at local parks where the kids could play and the parents could talk about issues related to diabetes. What variety of issues would a counselor need to address when helping this family through this major life event?

Michelle Probolus

Sudden Infant Death Syndrome

More than 4500 infants die suddenly and unexpectedly in the United States each year. Half of these deaths are attributed to **sudden infant death syndrome (SIDS)**, the spontaneous death of an infant 1–12 months old. African-American, Native-American and Alaska Native infants are the most susceptible to SIDS (CDC, 2012c). Since the American Academy of Pediatrics' (AAP) 1992 recommendation that babies be placed on their backs (the **supine** position) to sleep, there has been a significant decline in SIDS deaths; however, SIDS deaths continue to occur. The AAP launched the **Back to Sleep Campaign** to help parents adopt additional practices that have correlated with a reduction in SIDS, including the use of vaccines; avoiding smoking during pregnancy and after birth; using a firm sleeping surface; and eliminating blankets, pillows, wedges, and any other loose coverings in the crib (AAP, 2011).

Shaken Baby Syndrome

Each year in the United States between 1200 and 1400 infants and toddlers are victims of head injuries from abuse, and the majority of the children are under 1 year old (Bazelon, 2011). Some of these cases involve **shaken baby syndrome (SBS)**, which occurs when a parent becomes so frustrated with an infant's cries that the parent shakes the baby. About half of the infants who survive the violent shaking, which slams the brain against the skull, suffer from neurologic impairments that result in developmental and behavioral deficits. Of these victims, 13–30% die. These children may require custodial care for the rest of their lives, in addition to ongoing medical treatments and physical, occupational, speech, and educational therapies (Dias et al., 2005). SBS was more recently termed **abusive head trauma**, to include other abusive head injuries inflicted on an infant or toddler, such as with a blunt object. In some cases external symptoms of abuse, such as cuts, burns, or bruises may not have occurred, and the only medical evidence of SBS is by a brain scan that detects the internal symptoms of subdural and retinal hemorrhage, and brain swelling. In several court cases, adults who were imprisoned for committing SBS were later found to be innocent, as some infections and illnesses produce brain hemorrhaging and swelling that mimic the effects of SBS (Bazelon, 2011).

SBS is a form of child abuse and is punishable by law. SBS usually is not a premeditated act, and *anyone* could potentially shake a baby to death when frustrated: An infant's cries can provoke stress and anger in the listener, and when people become angry, extra blood is sent to the arms and hands. The majority of perpetrators of SBS are the baby's father or stepfather, or the mother's boyfriend, with mothers accounting for only 13% (Dias et al., 2005). A counselor is at the forefront of helping a parent who is frustrated by an infant's crying to recognize the parent's extreme agitation when their child cries; counselors can help parents remember to put the baby down, walk away, and call someone for support. Babysitting training programs for teenage babysitters often include SBS as part of the curriculum, and hospitals frequently require new parents to participate in educational programming about SBS before they are discharged with their newborn.

Vaccinations

Vaccines work to immunize the body against a particular disease by introducing a small-scale version of the pathogen into the body, usually by injection, causing the body to respond by producing antibodies as if it is really under attack. The body keeps a memory of this germ invasion so that in the event the body is exposed to the actual disease, the body will be able to identify the disease and neutralize it. Some vaccines use live, but weakened, viruses; others use a detoxified version, and some use only the components of the pathogen that cause an immune response (UNICEF, 2013). The Centers for Disease Control and Prevention publishes a recommended immunization schedule beginning at birth with a hepatitis B vaccine (CDC, 2011i).

The use of vaccines can be a controversial topic, as not all medical professionals unanimously endorse vaccines, and some parents consciously choose not to vaccinate their children for personal or religious reasons. As many as 21% of U.S. parents delay or refuse some or all of the recommended early childhood vaccines (Dell'Antonia, 2013). Whether personally for or against the use of vaccines, counselors will need to be sensitive to these diverse perspectives and separate their personal worldview from their work with clients. Parents who do not vaccinate their children have a minority status and are often marginalized by the majority culture. The parents may share with you the stress of being rejected as patients by pediatricians and the harsh criticism they have faced from others. They may hear that vaccines are mandatory before a child enters day care or school, although parents who choose not to vaccinate their children can complete exemption documents in most states. You may even work with a family that believes their child has been permanently harmed by a vaccination.

Motor Development

The Sequence of Motor Development

Although the motor development of infants and toddlers was traditionally viewed as a genetically determined, automatic process, contemporary researchers in child development such as Esther Thelen (1995) regard the sequence of motor development from a **dynamic systems perspective**, in which each new skill that the baby masters is influenced by both the baby and her environment. The baby and her environment create an intertwined, dynamic system that includes the *baby's factors* (her motivation, goals, and physical capabilities) and *environmental factors* (how her parents and physical structures around her either support or discourage the development of the skill).

Gross motor skills use large muscles that enable the infant and toddler to engage in **locomotion** (moving their bodies from place to place, such as rolling over, crawling, standing, and walking) as well as actions such as catching a ball. Ninety percent of infants and toddlers achieve typical gross motor skills between the following age ranges: holding head erect and steady when held upright (3 weeks–4 months); rolling from back to side (2–7 months); sitting alone (5–9 months); crawling (5–11 months); walking (9–17 months); and walking up stairs with help (12–23 months) (Bayley, 2005).

REFLECTION 5.1 CLIMBING TODDLERS

Around 2 years of age, identical twins Jack and Mason were running, jumping, and climbing on everything. We had to stack baby gates two high in the doorway of their bedroom to keep them safe while I took a 5-minute shower! Well, one day I came out of the bathroom and Jack had climbed to the top of the second gate, which means he was about 5 feet in the air. I had to take the bottom gate out and climb under the top one to get him down. I about had a heart attack and didn't trust leaving them in there for 5-minute showers any longer! [~Stephanie]

Stefanie Scarborough

REFLECTION 5.2 A LATER WALKER

My first daughter walked at 14 months old, so when my second daughter, Emma, was not walking by 15 months I became concerned. The pediatrician recommended that I have a physical therapist look at her. She checked out Emma's hips and legs and said she looked fine. Months 16, 17, and 18 came and went, and I was assured that she would walk soon and probably run very soon after that. I hoped so. I had visions of her crawling into kindergarten! The physical therapist said that when children are older they know they can fall and so are more tentative. At a younger age, they just start walking without a care. At 19 months, Emma finally started walking, and true to the physical therapist's word, she starting running just a few weeks later! [~Lisa]

Lisa Adams

Fine motor skills refer to the smaller bodily muscle movements, such as reaching and grasping, and those that often require eye-hand coordination. A newborn engages in **prereaching**, in which the infant swipes at an object but rarely reaches it. By 3–4 months, the infant reaches with an **ulnar grasp**, closing the fingers against the palm to grasp an object. By 4–5 months, the infant can transfer objects from hand to hand. At the average age of 9 months, the infant uses a **pincer grasp**, a precise movement that brings together the thumb and index finger, enabling the infant to pick up objects such as small pieces of cereal (Bayley, 2005).

The **dynamic systems perspective** is evident when considering studies that examine the interplay between babies and their environment. For example, conventional Western thinking is that a young infant's head and neck are muscularly weak and poorly controlled, resulting in parents paying special attention to protecting the head and neck, but not in providing activities to strengthen them during early infancy. However, Lee and Galloway (2012) discovered that the movement experiences to which an infant is exposed play a figural role in motor development. When caregivers of 1–4-month-old infants were enlisted to provide 20 minutes of daily, specially designed postural and movement activities for head control for four weeks, as well as carry the infants for another 20 minutes daily with a front carrier, the infants rapidly demonstrated advanced head control as early as 4 to 6 weeks old, far surpassing a control group that did not receive the special training. Mastery of head control in infancy is crucial to supporting other early behaviors, such as improved vision, oromotor skills, the use of the trunk and arms, and overall body control.

Cultural Variations

The dynamic systems perspective is also useful when considering how various cultures support early motor development. Numerous studies have demonstrated vast differences in gross motor development between sub-Saharan African and European-American infants (Lohaus et al., 2011). For example, Nigerian mothers place great importance on their babies becoming independent as early as possible. They expect their infants to sit by 4–5 months, crawl by 6–7 months, walk by 9–10 months, and walk without any assistance by 1 year. Nigerian babies are generally able to meet these goals in motor development, which are considerably earlier than the age ranges of their Western counterparts. Nigerian mothers support their infants' early motor development by using massages, motor games, and exercises, even helping their infants to stand on their legs at 2 months (Moscardino, Nwobu, & Axia, 2006). Comparing Cameroonian Nso farmer infants and German middle-class infants also highlights the accelerated gross motor development of the Cameroonian Nso infants (Lohaus et al., 2011). German mothers practice a distal parenting style, characterized by face-to-face contact and object play, with a de-emphasis on body contact and body stimulation. This style aligns with their socialization goal of developing psychological autonomy in their infants. Conversely, Cameroonian Nso mothers, whose socialization goal is to promote their infants' relational adaptation, emphasize close body contact and body stimulation, with children rarely lying on their back.

Sleep Cycle

Ask five parents about their infants' and toddlers' sleep cycles, and you will likely get five different answers, ranging from one parent who tells you that the child has such a predictable sleep pattern that the parent can set their clock by it, and another parent who answers, "What sleep cycle?" because they are sleep deprived from their child's unpredictable sleep pattern and frequent night waking. Although there are variations in sleep patterns, pediatric sleep experts believe that the drive to sleep is a powerful force in children, and that healthy, normal babies have the ability to sleep well (Ferber, 2006).

Sometimes infants have health issues or personal preferences that require parents to work harder to get a good night's sleep for everyone. When Kerry and Chris brought Colin home from the hospital, they were not able to go to bed until 6 am the next day. They were shocked to discover that Colin screamed every night for 4 hours at a time for the first 8 weeks of his life. From 7 to 11 pm every night, Colin would turn purple from screaming. Not knowing how to handle Colin or his screaming, they called Kerry's mom every single night asking what to do. Sleep deprived, exhausted, and anxious, Kerry and Chris met with a pediatrician who said, "Welcome to parenthood!" Colin was diagnosed with colic and acid reflux. Kerry says, "Everyone told us that we would forget what those long nights of screaming would be like. Our response was always, 'No we won't.' Now Colin is 3 months: His colic is gone and his acid reflux is controlled with medicine. Chris and I looked at each other the other night when Colin was asleep in his bed, and we both said we don't even remember what it was like when he was up all night screaming."

As an infant, Lori's third child, Anna, did not demand to sleep next to her mother, but on top of her! Lori would put a pillow on her chest, and the baby would fall asleep on the pillow. Lori would slide Anna and the pillow onto the bed once Anna was completely asleep, but when the baby awakened in the middle of the night, Lori would bring her right back up. This ritual continued until Anna became too heavy for Lori's internal organs. Finally, Lori and her husband used the Ferber sleep method and worked diligently to help Anna transition to a crib.

There are general sleeping and waking patterns from birth to 3 years, but don't be surprised or dismayed if you cannot find a child who fits this exact prototype. Newborns sleep about 16 hours a day, but usually no more than a few hours at a time. They ordinarily have seven sleeping/waking periods throughout the day, ranging from 20 minutes to 5–6 hours in length. By 3–4 months, infants sleep about 13 hours a day and have 4–5 regular and predictable sleep periods per day, with 2–3 of these sleep periods occurring at night. Their daytime sleep is often arranged in three nap patterns: midmorning, midafternoon, and early evening. Most infants have "settled" by this age, sleeping through most of the night (Ferber, 2006).

By 6 months, infants sleep about 12 hours per day, with almost all infants "settling" into a regular cycle. One change around the 6-month mark is that their continuous nighttime sleep is now longer (about 9¼ hours). By 1 year toddlers sleep 9–10 of their 12 total hours at night, with one nap around 12:30 pm or 1 pm. By 2 years, toddlers reduce their total sleep to around 11.5 hours, retaining the same night sleeping schedule and napping schedule (Ferber, 2006).

As a counselor, it will be important to recognize that parents have strong opinions about whether their infants and toddlers should ideally sleep in their own bed in their own room, or whether they should co-sleep (see Case Study 5.2). You may also serve as a facilitative voice to help parents adjust their thoughts and behaviors to accommodate their infant's individual traits, especially in situations where parents are puzzled and frustrated by their child's behavior. This is frequently apparent in families of multiple children, in which parents are not expecting the second-born child to be so radically different in personality from the first. In Think About It 5.1, consider how this mother attunes to her daughters' unique characteristics and the mindfulness that she puts into helping her daughters get their individual needs met.

Think About It   5.1   Sleeping Differences

Having two girls who are three years apart has been wonderful. It is so tempting to think that the second-born will be similar to the first, but that is not true in so many ways. This was evident with my daughters from day one. When we brought Sydney home from the hospital, we put her in a bassinet by our bed. She would stretch out as long as she could (she was 21½ inches long, so she was a long baby to start with!) and put her arms up above her head. At a week old, the bassinet seemed to hardly contain her, and I sensed that she felt cramped. We decided to put her in her crib one night even though it looked so big to us. She loved it! She stretched out and fell asleep quickly. At 7 weeks old, she was sleeping through the night. She has been a super sleeper ever since!

And then we had Emma! Emma could only fall asleep when she was swaddled as tightly as she could be. At night she would start crying, and I knew that she had gotten herself out of her "baby burrito." We swaddled her for months and months, and even then she was never a great sleeper like her sister. She still was waking up in the middle of the night at 4 years old and yelling "Mom!!" There was always some reason she would invent for waking me up, and it was very frustrating. Now at 5 years old she is finally doing better with sleeping through the night. While my girls are similar in some ways, they remind me daily that they are very much their own unique people. [~Lisa]

Lisa Adams

➤ CASE EXAMPLE **5.2**   CO-SLEEPING.

We started co-sleeping with Alex when he was 6 weeks old, as a means to support breastfeeding and get some rest. My son didn't sleep more than three hours in a row until he turned 2 years old, so co-sleeping was a wonderful way for me to breastfeed and comfort him at night without rousing too much. I came to realize that co-sleeping was a means of comfort for me, too. With my baby by my side I knew instantly when he was going to wake, cry, and need me. I take comfort in the fact that infants who sleep near their parents have more stable temperatures, and regular heart and breathing rhythms compared to babies who sleep alone. My son is now 3 years old, and we still co-sleep comfortably. He doesn't breastfeed any more, but when he wakes in the night a simple hand on his chest will comfort him back to sleep. [~Kylie]

Researchers have opposing views about the safety and efficacy of co-sleeping. Research this topic, describe the pros and cons of co-sleeping versus infants and toddlers sleeping independently, and discuss which method you would favor most and why.

Kylie Mohler

Perception

An infant engages in **sensation** (i.e., physically experiencing sensory stimulation) when his hands slide over his poodle's soft hair and when his eyes take in the color and curly pattern of the dog's coat; when he *organizes* and *interprets* this sensory stimulation, by recognizing that he is interacting with his family's companion animal, **perception** occurs. There are two types of stimulation, each playing a vital role in brain formation during an infant's and toddler's first three years: **exogenous stimulation**, which is external to the baby, and **endogenous stimulation**, which is *internal* to the baby (Marshall, 2011). Endogenous stimulation, beginning as the spontaneous firing of neural ganglion cells and leading to the creation of neural pathways, activates in infants during REM sleep (Graven & Browne, 2008). Endogenous stimulation can later come from the knowledge, memory, or expectation about an event (Sekuler, 1995). Both exogenous and endogenous stimulation transport neurons to clusters that eventually create six layers of cortex in the infant's brain (Marshall, 2011).

Vision

During infancy, the pathway from the eye to the brain develops, making this time period a critical one for the cells in the retina to differentiate and reorganize. The infant's neurons arrange themselves into specialized columns for specific visual functions, such as general ocular dominance, orientation, color, complex patterns, and disparities (Penn & Shatz, 2002).

Infants and toddlers who have sleep deprivation during their first 1 to 2 years may have diminished ability for the visual pathways to form correctly, resulting in visual gaps, or jumbled or reversed images. Visual development is so sensitive at this time that babies under 2 years who have experienced disrupted vision to just one of their eyes for even 1 to 2 weeks can permanently lose functional vision, as the wiring cannot be reversed.

If what the infant sees does not seem relevant, his brain will discard the information and not create a memory of it. The infant makes meaning—and therefore memories—from visual stimuli when parents connect what the infant sees to language, emotion, and loving touch (Penn & Shatz, 2002). The infant's visual focus begins as imprecise, and his attention is directed to faces and shapes; he begins seeing only in black and white, but by 4 months he develops color vision and also shifts his attention to hands and food (Greene, 2009).

Mini-video cameras placed on a toddler's forehead demonstrate that a toddler views the world quite differently from an adult (Smith, Yu, & Pereira, 2011). When playing together with toys, the adult takes in a broad and stable view of all of the objects in the visual field; a toddler tends to focus on a single dominating object that is close by, which then obscures other objects from sight. Individual objects go in and out of view, depending on where he is focusing. A toddler's short arms and use of his whole body when handling objects may contribute to his small visual-motor workspace (Smith, Yu, & Pereira, 2011). These findings are helpful for counselors and parents to consider as they structure the toddler's environment to maximize his attention and interest.

Although many parents and doctors do not consider screening an infant for visual problems, vision screening when the infant is a 1 year old can detect amblyopia, a lifelong vision impairment that is often preventable and treatable when detected early on (AAP, 2013). **Amblyopia**, or "lazy eye," is a disorder that only children can develop, and it affects 2 to 4% of the U.S. population, accounting for more vision loss in children than all other causes combined (American Association for Pediatric Ophthalmology and Strabismus, 2013). In amblyopia, one or both eyes send a blurry image to the brain; without treatment, it may cause permanent vision loss.

Hearing

An infant can learn 600 consonants and 200 vowels of the world's languages from 32 weeks gestation to 9 months, after which he discards auditory information that his brain does not consider necessary. As with vision, the sounds to which the infant gives meaning are those that are strengthened through the parent–child relationship (Kuhl, 2004), such as through the infant's native language. Some parents capitalize on this early critical time of auditory meaning-making by introducing their infant to additional languages, since infancy is the prime time to easily incorporate new sounds as useful and enduring.

REFLECTION 5.3 LEARNING A SECOND LANGUAGE

Nova and I moved to Honduras around the time he was 20 months old. At that time, he was just saying a few select words, such as daddy, but was showing a clear understanding of the English language. For example, when I asked him to get his cup, he would go find it for me. I could also tell that Nova was ready for something new and challenging. The situation in Honduras is nothing short of perfect. Nova attends day care at the same school I teach in with a couple of sweet Honduran women, who only speak Spanish. Besides day care, Nova hears Spanish from cartoons, the driver, the maids, and most other people we come into contact with on a regular basis. And everyone wants to talk to Nova! It was less than two months before Nova started saying: *agua* (never water!), *vamos* (while standing at the door), *mamá*, *adiof* (*adios*), and *hola*. But really, I might not even know if he says other things in Spanish because I know he´s going to know it better than I. His English is still strongly maintained, as most of his conversations outside of these activities are in English. [~Laura]

Infants would rather listen to **infant-directed speech** than adult-directed speech (Henning, Striano, & Lieven, 2005). Infant-directed speech (also referred to as child-directed speech (CDS), motherese, and parentese) is distinguished by its elongated, exaggerated vowels, use of high pitches, simple, repeated phrases, and its sing-song, lilting quality. As with vision, auditory development is highly influenced by sensory stimulation. Ideal conditions for auditory growth include REM sleep, alternating periods of sound and quiet, and exposure to interactive conversation with parents. Infants exposed to chronic background noise above 50 decibels are less able to differentiate changes in pitch, intensity, phonemes, and pattern (Marshall, 2011).

Taste and Smell

Like vision and hearing, **chemosensory** development (taste and smell) is not an automatic process that unfolds irrespective of the infant's sensory stimulation experiences. Instead, optimal development of taste and smell results from specific endogenous stimulation, such as sleep, and exogenous stimulation, such as exposure to a spectrum of smells and flavors. A fetus needs to detect a smell in his amniotic fluid in order to create an olfactory bulb, the precursor to specialized receptors that will develop throughout his first year. These specialized olfactory receptors, located in the throat and sinus cavity, enable the infant to detect four distinct types of smells: airborne smells, "flavors" in food, noxious smells, and flavors in blood (Browne, 2008; Schaal, Hummel, & Soussignan, 2004). The infant's throat and tongue respond to the five unique flavors: sweet, salty, sour, bitter, and umami (savory). Chemosensory development can be damaged by *lack* of exposure to odors in infants who experience chronic congestion, as well as by *overpowering* odors such as smoke, solvents, and perfumes (teratogens that directly impact brain functioning) (Browne, 2008).

Although the infant is hardwired to prefer a sweet taste and can recognize the flavors of his mother's milk, his taste buds can be trained in infancy to either like a wide variety of flavors or to become a picky eater with a limited flavor repertoire. Infancy is considered to be the period of **acquiring a taste for food**, and the early experiences with flavors shape which foods will later be preferred (Greene, 2009). Parents often do not realize the tremendous impact of tasting exposures on their infant's brain during this first year, and when infants initially reject a new food, parents may stop offering the food again, convinced that their infant must not like the new food. A counselor may be the one to help parents understand that it can take between 10 and 20 **tasting exposures** for the brain to accept the taste of a particular food. Maier, Chabanet, Schaal, Issanchou, and Leathwood (2007) discovered that something very surprising happened when mothers who had stopped feeding their 7-month-old infants a certain vegetable after the infants rejected it 2–3 times, agreed to offer the vegetable again every other day. After only 7–8 extra tasting exposures, over 70% of the infants not only *willingly* ate the vegetable but also consumed the same quantity as their favorite foods. Nine months later, more than 75% of the infants—who were now toddlers—ate the vegetable voluntarily. Unfortunately for some of the toddlers, 15% of the mothers never offered the vegetable again after the study was over.

Infancy is the key time to offer a child most of the foods that a parent is hoping the child will eat for the rest of his life, because by the time the child reaches toddlerhood, **neophobia** (the fear of something new—in this case, the fear of new foods) develops. A survival mechanism deeply embedded in the toddler's brain, neophobia keeps the toddler safe from foods that might be harmful, and the foods for which the toddler has not acquired a taste are ones that the toddler instinctively believes are harmful. Therefore, the foods that toddlers willingly eat become restricted to those they already trust (Greene, 2009).

Touch

During the infant's first year, the **somatosensory** system responds to stimulation by creating specialized receptors, linking the body site to the spinal column and brain (Blackwell, 2000). Three different **modalities of sensation** have their own unique pathways in the spinal cord, reaching different targets in the brain: (1) **discriminative touch**, sensations of touch, pressure, and vibration, allows the infant to perceive a stuffed animal in the dark that he can feel but not see; (2) **pain and temperature**, which includes the sensations of tickle and itch; and (3) **proprioception**, sensations that happen beneath the surface of the body, such as muscle stretch, joint position (Molavi, 2013), and feedback from the vestibular (balance) system (Bahrick & Lickliter, 2009). The 2–3-month-old infant knows the *orientation* and *direction* of his stuffed animal by feel alone, and by 6 months he can perceive its *surfaces, subtle vibrations, shape* and *form,* and *intensity of touch* (whether it is light, moderate, firm, or painful). The infant capitalizes on using his fingers and mouth, two key body sites that are especially wired for somatosensory information (Blackwell, 2000).

The level of pain that infants and toddlers experience during medical procedures or emergencies has historically been underestimated by professionals, resulting in inadequate pain control or sedation (Fein et al., 2012). Errors in understanding a child's level of pain occur when appropriate assessment tools are underutilized and the developmental stage of the child is not taken into account. Although baby boys used to be circumcised without analgesia, we now know that when newborns and older children receive insufficient pain control during medical procedures, they are likely to develop changes in the way they perceive and respond to painful experiences in the future. They may exhibit post-traumatic stress symptoms and have significantly higher pain scores when experiencing future painful procedures.

Intermodal Perception

The ability to perceive stimulation from events or objects by using multiple senses simultaneously is called **intermodal perception** (also referred to as intersensory or multimodal perception) (Bahrick & Lickliter, 2009). Although sensory stimulation travels along different pathways from the body sites to the brain, a newborn's senses work in concert to perceive objects and events in the environment as stable and unified. An infant can see, hear, and feel his hand clapping, but he recognizes it as one unified event instead of three fragmented ones. Multiple senses are also used to perceive **amodal information**, sensory information that is not tied to a specific sensory system. For example, while musical pitch is tied specifically to the auditory system, amodal information such as temporal synchrony, rhythm, duration, tempo, changes in intensity, shape, substance, size, and texture can be perceived by *more than one* sensory system. The infant can both see and feel the *texture* of his stuffed animal. **Intersensory redundancy** happens when identical amodal information— the texture of a stuffed animal—is perceived in synchrony by more than one sense modality (e.g., sight and feel).

Intermodal perception increases in precision throughout infancy. The infant at several weeks can move his eyes in the direction of a barking dog that he could not see at first, already synchronizing visual and auditory stimulation. At 3 months he uses his ability to coordinate sight and sound by matching facial and vocal expressions of happy, sad, and angry emotions. By 5 to 7 months, the infant focuses on someone's face while the person is talking to him, and by using this face–voice synchrony he can effectively separate what someone is saying from other background noise (Bahrick & Lickliter, 2009).

Toilet Training and Elimination Communication

REFLECTION 5.4 SIBLING MENTOR

A month before our son, Steven, turned 2 years old, we heard Hunter, his 4-year-old sister, talking in the bathroom. She was showing and explaining the steps of using the potty to her brother. Using what we had taught her, she shared how girls should wipe from front to back, how her brother wouldn't need to wipe "all" of the time, and, most importantly, how he would get to choose big-boy underpants once he wasn't wearing baby diapers. We couldn't begin to guess how many times our 4-year-old ran through her potty lesson, but we knew if Steven was showing interest in using the toilet, it was time for pull-ups and bringing out the portable baby potty. About a week before he turned 2 years old, Steven was letting us know he needed to use the bathroom on a regular basis and hadn't had an "accident." It was time for him to go pick out his big-boy underpants. [~Tracy]

Horror stories of parents desperately trying to get their toddlers to use the potty abound. Equally compelling stories of parents who say that their infants and toddlers transitioned easily out of diapers also exist. Depending on the temperaments of both the parent and child, and the method used, helping young children gain control of their bladder and bowels can range from being a source of intense challenge and frustration, to an easy-going part of the journey through infancy and toddlerhood for both child and parent. While most people are familiar with the concept of toilet training a child, many have not heard of elimination communication (EC), also known as infant potty training, or natural infant hygiene. People may be quite surprised to know that EC is a radically different way of helping children to gain control of their bladder and bowel movements. In this section, both perspectives are explored to help inform and culturally sensitize counselors.

Toilet training is the method endorsed by the American Academy of Pediatrics (AAP) to teach a toddler to transition from eliminating in a diaper to using the toilet independently. The AAP is a national organization of primary-care pediatricians, pediatric medical subspecialists, and pediatric surgical specialists. The AAP's position on children's physical readiness to control their bowel movements is mixed, with some authors within the organization stating that children under 12 months are *not likely* to be ready to control their bladder and bowels (Wolraich & Tippins, 2003), while others assert that they have *no control* before 12 months (AAP, 2009b). Parents using the toilet-training approach usually wait until their toddler is between 18 and 24 months, watching for signs that the child is ready to begin the process. Typical signs include: The toddler is able to stay dry for at least 2 hours at a time during the day or is dry after naps; bowel movements are becoming regular and predictable; the parent is able to tell when the child is about to urinate or have a bowel movement; the child can follow simple instructions, walk to the toilet independently, and help undress; the child is uncomfortable wearing soiled diapers, asks to be changed or to use the toilet or potty chair; and asks to wear "big-kid" underwear (AAP, 2009b). Parents using toilet training use verbal instruction and demonstration to teach the process and give rewards to mark successes. They encourage their child, monitor the process, use reminders, help the child set goals, and adapt their method to the child's style of learning (Wolraich & Tippins, 2003).

Elimination communication (EC), also referred to as infant potty training and natural infant hygiene, has been practiced for hundreds of years in cultures worldwide, and it is becoming more recognizable in the United States, especially among parents who practice attachment parenting. This method is based on the belief that the infant is not only aware of the elimination function from birth, but that the infant also has some measure of ability to control sphincter muscles from infancy. Parents using this method do not believe that they need to "train" their infant; instead, since the infant does not want to eliminate in his diapers and have the feeling of elimination against the skin from very early on, the infant will naturally "learn" to use a potty. The parent's job is to provide a sensitive and responsive environment for this natural connection to unfold (Bauer, 2001).

Parents use EC as a two-way communication process between parent and infant that may be initiated at birth. Parents who advocate for EC feel that waiting until toddlerhood before making direct connections to the toddler's elimination keeps him verbally, physically, and mentally disconnected from a natural process of which he is already aware. Parents using EC respond to the infant's cues from birth, observing the gestural and vocal cues that babies make when they are either eliminating or about to eliminate, such as grimacing and grunting. The parent responds by providing a receptacle in which the baby can have a bladder or bowel movement, often beginning within the first months of life or sooner. Parents will hold the infant over a sink or on their lap with a small bowl underneath the infant and use a sound like "ssss" to cue the infant that they are in an elimination location. Some parents set aside times during the day when the child is diaper free so that parent and child can be more attuned to the child's process. As with all methods, there is great variability in how parents practice EC regarding diaper use, age of initiating the process, and use of cues (Olson, 2011). Parents using this method often report that their children learn to eliminate on their own between 6 months and 2 years (Bauer, 2001). The online resource diaperfreebaby.org provides support groups and resources for parents who are using or contemplating using EC.

Toilet training and EC diverge in philosophy and technique in many ways. For example, proponents of toilet training believe that using a toilet is not an instinctive activity, but that the child will adopt the practice to imitate and please the parent (Wolraich & Tippins, 2003). Advocates of EC contend that even an infant is sensitive to eliminating on herself and enjoys the opportunity to have a place other than a diaper next to her skin to relieve herself (Bauer, 2001). The commonalities between approaches are that both seek to support what is best for the child's development, and children are able to successfully transition from eliminating in a diaper to using the toilet with both methods.

REFLECTION 5.5 USING EC

I learned about EC when Ruby was 6 months old, and I immediately ordered a baby potty, which arrived around the time she began sitting up. As I stabilized a wobbly infant on the potty, she relieved her bladder and laughed. Jim or I would carry Ruby to the potty and sit with her for a few moments every hour during the day, to help her make the connection that there was a place to go other than in her diaper. We would just say that we were going to the potty, but we didn't tell her that she needed to do anything. She would happily sit on her potty fiddling with a basket of trinkets, and we expressed excitement and interest when she had a movement. We kept diapers on her during the day and didn't use the diaper-free part of the toilet-learning approach. I taught her the sign for using the potty, and in a couple of weeks Ruby independently used the sign. Well before her first birthday, Ruby would give the sign that she needed to eliminate and could hold her bladder or bowels until someone placed her on the potty. We went through very few diapers. I would tell her that someday she would know when she never needed a diaper again, and that she would tell us. The week before her second birthday, Ruby said, "Mama, I have to go pee pee!" and from the way she said it, I knew that she was finished with daytime diapers. [~Nadine]

Structure of the Nervous System

Unlike many other types of animals, a human infant is not able to be independent from a parent for quite a long time. During infancy and the toddler years, the parent plays a critical role in providing stimulation in order for optimal brain development to occur. Stimulation can derive from any interaction, such as talking, playing, or presenting visual stimuli. The interaction of a mother rolling a ball across the floor to an infant prompts **neurons**, or nerve cells in the brain, to fire information back and forth, allowing the brain to develop a neural pathway, along which more information can travel as it presents itself in the future.

After the initial firing of the neurons, the infant processes the experience with the ball during REM sleep. During the processing stage, randomly positioned neurons in the brain will physically move to a distinct place in the brain to form a **cluster**. As the infant's mother continues to roll the ball during play times, eventually the neuron cluster will become the part of the brain dedicated to reacting to a ball being rolled toward the infant. Once the pathways are built to form these specialized areas of the brain, these pathways will lead to the **cerebral cortex**, the outer layer of the brain that controls the majority of our ability to understand and communicate (Marshall, 2011).

The **axon**, a tube-like part of the neuron that allows signals to be passed from one neuron to another, becomes coated in a sheath of a fatty substance called **myelin** as the infant grows. **Myelination**, the process of coating the neural fibers, is crucial to the development of the infant brain, as the myelin sheath facilitates "the rapid and synchronized information transfer required for coordinated movement, decision-making, and other higher order cognitive, behavioral, and emotive functions" (Deoni et al., 2011, p. 784).

Counselors working with parents of infants and toddlers are entrusted with playing a figural role in helping parents to more fully appreciate their direct impact on the miracle unfolding in their infant's brain. Brain development in the infant and toddler is dependent on the child's holistic experiences, the constant interplay of emotional, social, cognitive, and physical dynamics. From birth until age 2 years, the child's brain doubles in size. During this time of tremendous growth, hormones produced as a result of the social and emotional relationships that the child forms with a primary attachment figure actually *shape* the structures of the brain (Bowlby, 2007).

Until 30 months of age, the right hemisphere of the brain, which is responsible for the intuitive and emotional skills necessary for relationships including empathic understanding, develops more quickly and dominates more brain control than the left hemisphere. How the right hemisphere develops depends upon the quality of daily sensitive and responsive caregiving. Although children are unable to directly recall these experiences because they take place during the preverbal phase of development, the feelings and expectations generated from the relationship become mapped into the brain, influencing future personality (Schore, 1994). By 36 months, the toddler's brain has shifted dominance to the left hemisphere, which is responsible for complex speech, recalling past events, and anticipating future ones (Bowlby, 2007).

Sensorimotor Development

Jean Piaget (1896–1980) theorized that humans experience four stages of development: sensorimotor, preoperational, concrete operational, and formal operational. The **sensorimotor** stage, from birth to 2 years, is unlike the other three stages, in that it involves very little logical thinking. Instead, during the sensorimotor stage, the infant experiences the surrounding environment, learning information through the senses. Piaget believed that *knowledge* at this stage comes from the infant's perception of the world and actions stemming from these perceptions (Piaget, 1962). During this stage, however, the infant is not able to form abstract thought (Thelen, 2000).

From birth to 1 month the newborn relies on **reflexes** and changes behavior in response to environmental feedback (Piaget, 1962). When someone places a finger in an infant's mouth, the infant will engage the sucking reflex, but then, noticing that the finger is not producing any milk, the infant may instinctively attempt to push the finger back out of the mouth with the tongue. Between 1 to 4 months the infant accidentally notices interesting things about the *body,* beginning the process of **primary circular reactions**. The first time the infant accidentally discovers that she can pull her big toe up to her mouth and suck on it, she notices an interesting result, maybe thinking to herself, "Wow, this feels really amazing . . . I'm a circle!" Since she enjoyed the experience so much she will intentionally repeat this process many times, but never again accidentally. By 4 to 8 months the infant transfers the process of circular reactions to objects *outside of the body,* known as **secondary circular reactions**. So when Aunt Lulu, with her shiny, dangling gold necklaces, leans over the crib to see the infant, the first time that the infant pulls and yanks the chains off of Aunt Lulu's neck is accidental, but once the infant notices the interesting results of this action (e.g., gold chains in his little fist, a lot of commotion from a startled Aunt Lulu), the next time the infant sees Aunt Lulu wearing the chains, the grabbing and yanking will be goal directed.

By 8 to 12 months infants *coordinate* secondary circular reactions, which Piaget considered to be the first acts of true intelligence since these actions are intentional (Piaget, 1962). By now, Aunt Lulu has decided to stay far away from the chain-grabbing infant, but she is no match for the more ambulatory baby at this point: The infant is able to put together a series of secondary circular reactions, so that when she sees Aunt Lulu she intentionally *crawls* or *toddles* over to her, *climbs* up her lap, and *grabs* the chains. By 12 to 18 months the toddler has incorporated **tertiary circular reactions**. This spoon-dropping phase, in which the toddler engages in the physical experiments of dropping objects on purpose to see what will happen, may be a good time to limit restaurant visits, unless the parent has a lot of stamina! Physical experimentation leads to insight by 18 to 24 months, when the toddler invents new ways to achieve a goal through **mental combinations**. Parents are not sure what their toddler is thinking next, as in the time 2 year old Jason, still in his foot pajamas, ran up to the breakfast table one morning, and grabbing the entire bottle of Flintstones vitamins, ran through the house to his bedroom, where he locked the door behind him and shoved as many vitamins in his mouth as possible, until his frantic mother was able to break in.

A toddler also uses a higher level of strategic thinking to interact with another person when nearing the end of the sensorimotor stage. Toddlers who are 18 to 24 months old physically point at the correct location of an object before an adult is about to make a mistake and look in the wrong place, suggesting that the toddlers are using prediction and inference (Knudsen & Liszkowski, 2012).

For Piaget, **object permanence** is another concept that differentiates an infant mind from an adult mind. Object permanence is the understanding that when a previously seen object is no longer visible, it still exists. Piaget believed that this ability does not exist in infants until they are approximately 8 months old. A classic study by Piaget involves hiding a toy from an infant, allowing him to find it, and then re-hiding the object in a new location. Because of object permanence, the child is compelled to look for the item in the spot in which it was hidden the first time (Munakata, McClelland, Johnson, & Siegler, 1997). Object permanence is also the reason behind why playing peek-a-boo with young infants is so exciting for them—if they do not have object permanence they believe that once you are out of sight, you cease to exist. Object permanence correlates with Piaget's ideas of growth throughout the sensorimotor stage: Younger infants are only able to acknowledge what their senses are experiencing at the moment. As they grow into the higher stages, they are able to develop abstract thought processes, such as understanding that an object still exists when hidden behind a screen.

Although Piaget did not believe that infants have object permanence, Baillargeon and DeVos (1991) considered it to be an inborn ability, what they called *persistence*. The definitive answer is still not clear. Computer tracking software that follows and records 4-month-old infants' eye movements does seem to show that infants have a measure of object permanence, when they seem surprised and look longer at an object that violates an expectation of object permanence.

Information Processing

Infants and toddlers are constantly taking in their surroundings and making meaning out of the people, objects, and experiences in their environment. The **information processing** theory encompasses an infant's ability to categorize situations, create memories, and become familiar with reoccurring stimuli. Information processing researchers often use a computer model when considering this aspect of cognitive development. They believe that information enters the brain, is stored, and is then accessed in a precise sequence.

The ability to process information grows along with a child, but infants are capable of the three main components of information processing: encoding, storing, and retrieving information. **Encoding** is the process of making an experience relevant to one's life in order to access the information later. When infants and toddlers were asked to compare the length of a wooden rod to a similar rod they had seen previously, the children were not able to; however, they were able to point out similar-size rods when both were compared to a standardized object (such as a teddy bear). These results suggest that infants and toddlers are not able to encode information into their memory when a visible object stands alone; there must be a tangible comparison, such as the standardized object. Adults, however, are able to encode information without the presence of a comparable object, suggesting that with age comes a more developed encoding system (Huttenlocher, Duffy, & Levine, 2002).

Once information is encoded in the brain, it is stored there until the infant or toddler needs to access it, known as **retrieval**. A child's ability to retrieve information learned previously can be affected by how the information was encoded in the first place. Toddlers respond well to a multifaceted encoding process: Toddlers learned a new word for an object by being shown the object made out of Play-Doh and seeing an adult act out the item's function. The toddlers were successful at retrieving the word for the new object at a later time (Capone & McGregor, 2005). Infants and toddlers are capable of both **recognition** (noticing when a new object or event is the same/similar to one that was previously encountered) and **recall** (generating a mental image of a previously experienced object without the benefit of having something in the present moment to stimulate recognition of it).

REFLECTION 5.6 RECOGNITION

Sydney was 25 months old and we were in the car together. She asked me to turn on the radio. I did and a moment later she said, "The Beatles?" (her father's favorite band). It wasn't the Beatles but I asked her to repeat the word to make sure I had heard her correctly. She said, "The Beatles" loud and clear. I asked, "Who likes the Beatles?" and she got a big smile on her face and said, "Daddy!" Right after her second birthday, Sydney's father gave her a red MINI matchbox car similar to the one he drove fairly often. One day she picked it up, opened the side door, looked inside and said, "Hello Daddy!" When Sydney was about 2 years old, we were naming body parts and she pointed to her elbow and said, "Elmo!!!" [~Lisa]

Lisa Adams

Memories developed by infants and toddlers can be crucial to their learning process. One way in which **memory** can assist in a child's growth is through **deferred imitation**, the ability to remember an action performed by someone else and later reenact it. Infants are at a disadvantage in that they often see the same action, perhaps a mother brushing her hair, performed in many different contexts, which confuses their encoding process. However, an infant will retain a basic memory of the event and later act it out. Imitation allows an infant to learn how to interact in the world, which is beneficial if surrounded by people who model pro-social behavior (Jones & Herbert, 2006). Toddlers can demonstrate even more extensive deferred imitation, such as Lincoln's (who just turned 3 years old) ability to repeat almost an entire conversation that his parents may be having in another room.

Another way in which infants and toddlers learn about the world is through **object categorization**. This learning process enables them to think in categories (e.g., animals, colors, food) so that when they encounter something new, they can know general details about the new object based on category into which it fits, without specifically knowing the details of it (Bornstein & Arterberry, 2010). For example, a child may not be familiar with a rhinoceros, but by knowing it is an animal she can infer that it lives and breathes and could be found in a zoo.

Habituation occurs in infants and toddlers when they are shown a stimulus enough times that in each subsequent viewing the child looks at it for a shorter period of time. Toddlers and infants can become habituated in social situations to people's faces, which can contribute to the level of comfort with one's family and explain the anxiety some children have around strangers. Interestingly, toddlers with autism spectrum disorder (ASD) who showed deficits in social information processing had a more difficult time habituating to faces and pictures than typically developing toddlers (Webb et al., 2010).

Intelligence

Numerous researchers have proposed definitions of intelligence. Howard Gardner, a well-known pioneer in the field of multiple intelligences, offers the following definition: "An intelligence is the ability to solve problems, or to create products, that are valued within one or more cultural settings" (Gardner, 1983/2003). Assessing infant intelligence can be a tricky prospect, as the infant cannot verbally communicate with the examiner what the infant is thinking or feeling. When an infant doesn't respond to prompts on infant intelligence tests, is it truly a measure of cognitive functioning, or is the infant perhaps tired, bored, or something else? To capture a more accurate picture of an infant's cognitive ability, most assessments focus on observing motor and perceptual skills.

Infants and toddlers from 1 month to 3½ years can be assessed using the **Bayley-III**, the most recent version of the Bayley Scales of Infant Development (Bayley, 2005). This widely used test consists of three sections for the infant (Cognitive Scale, Language Scale, and Motor Scale). Examples of what an infant is prompted to do include looking for a fallen object, recognizing objects and people, following simple directions, naming objects and pictures, and stacking blocks. There are two sections for the parent to complete (Social-Emotional Scale and Adaptive Behavior Scale, where parents report their infant's abilities in areas such as ease of calming, imitation in play, and self-control), and an optional Behavior Rating Scale for the examiner to complete.

Like intelligence tests for adults, tests for infants and toddlers yield a score called an intelligence quotient (IQ). To distinguish these assessments from the type of tests given to older children and adults, the term **developmental quotient (DQ)** is used. Aside from two components of the Bayley-III, infant intelligence tests are not used to make predictions about future intelligence or achievement. However, the Cognitive and Language

Scales of the Bayley-III have been shown to predict mental test performance in preschool (Albers & Grieve, 2007). Assessments of infant intelligence are used mainly for screening purposes, as very low scores may predict later developmental problems. Infants who receive very low scores may then be observed further and provided with specialized interventions.

Living in poverty is correlated with poor intellectual development in children, and without interventions these children will likely have low socioeconomic status (SES) as adults (McLoyd, Aikens, & Burton, 2006). Children living in an economically disadvantaged environment may continue the cycle of poverty from one generation to the next, as poorly educated parents face challenges in providing the enriching experiences (Bradley, 2002) and verbal stimulation (Hoff, 2006) necessary for their children to achieve optimal intellectual development.

Early Interventions for At-Risk Infants and Toddlers

Early interventions are available for two groups of at-risk infants and toddlers: children who are economically disadvantaged and children who have special needs. For pregnant women and families with infants and toddlers up to age 3 years who live in economically disadvantaged homes, the **Early Head Start** program provides interventions in the form of child development and family support services. Early Head Start is governed by the U.S. Department of Health and Human Services' Administration for Children and Families. It is a federally funded, community-based program serving all 50 states, the District of Columbia, Puerto Rico, and the U.S. Virgin Islands. In 2011 it had 1027 programs serving over 147,000 children under the age of 3 (U.S. Department of Health and Human Services, 2012). Early Head Start was established in 1995 as an extension of the already well-established Head Start program.

Early Head Start provides center-based, home-based, and combination programs. Infants and toddlers receive early education services that support their physical, social, emotional, cognitive, and language development, as well as high-quality child care. Parents receive parenting education and support services. Early Head Start staff work with families to empower them to set goals for themselves and work toward self-sufficiency by co-designing **individualized family development plans** (U.S. Department of Health and Human Services, 2012). An evaluation of the Early Head Start program, which assessed parents and children when the children were 14, 24, and 36 months old, found that 3-year-olds who were completing the program had significantly better scores in cognitive, language, and social-emotional development than a randomly assigned control group. Their parents not only had significantly higher scores than control group parents in a number of components of home environment and parenting behavior; they had also improved their self-sufficiency (U.S. Department of Health and Human Services, 2006).

For infants and toddlers through age 2 who have special needs—developmental delays or diagnoses of physical or mental conditions with a high likelihood of resulting in developmental delays—an **Early Intervention Program** is available to help these children be ready to attend preschool and kindergarten (U.S. Department of Education, 2012). The U.S. Department of Education's Office of Special Education Programs (OSEP) oversees the Individuals with Disabilities Education Improvement Act (IDEA), a federal law regulating how early intervention, special education, and related services to children with disabilities are provided by state and public agencies. A recent major improvement to the IDEA is the 2011 release of final regulations for the early intervention program under Part C, the section of the IDEA that articulates important services to infants, toddlers, and their families. Part C is a $436 million program administered by the states, serving approximately 350,000 infants and toddlers.

Think About It   5.2   Early Intervention for Down Syndrome

Consider the challenges to all members of the family in Carley's situation. My brother, Spencer, was born with Down syndrome when I was 3 years old. A speech therapist would come to the house regularly to work with Spencer, and she tried to teach him some sign language. However, the only sign that really stuck with him was the sign for "more." He started speaking some words between ages 2 and 3, and he became more verbal when he began attending preschool. He went to preschool for two years, from ages 4 to 5. During those two years he went to an intermediate unit (IU) preschool for children with special needs and a general education preschool that my older brothers and I had attended. Spencer attended kindergarten in a general education classroom in a public school. While he was in kindergarten he began speaking in full sentences and continues speech therapy today as a young adult.

Carley Grab

➤ CASE EXAMPLE **5.3**   EARLY INTERVENTION FOR HEARING LOSS.

As you contemplate the case of Michelle and her son, Ryan, which issues surrounding this case would be helpful for a counselor to explore with Michelle?

It is an incredible advantage that newborn hearing screenings are now given in Pennsylvania hospitals, giving doctors the ability to diagnose hearing loss long before anyone would ever suspect it in a developing child. The one thing that we weren't prepared for was that our son, Ryan, would fail—repeatedly and in both ears. Before he turned 1 month old, he had gone through countless hearing tests to clarify his diagnosis of bilateral sensorineural hearing loss, and we had gone through more emotions than we ever thought possible in such a short period of time. We were elated to have our first child, who was so beautiful and otherwise healthy, but what did this mean? We didn't know of anyone in our families who was born with congenital hearing loss. Was this genetic? Was this somehow our fault? Was this part of a syndrome? How much can he hear? Who is going to help us with this? We didn't know anything about hearing loss! We learned that Ryan would get hearing aids in both ears. How will his life be different because of this? Hearing aids can't get wet. How would he hear in the bathtub or at the pool? I was terrified at the thought of taking him to the beach—sand AND water both damage hearing aids—and how would he hear us if he was in danger? Thinking of all the conversations he would miss out on in those instances, I grieved the loss of his normal childhood. I sobbed. I just never saw any of this coming and, although I knew I shouldn't, I felt so guilty!

In addition to the normal cuddles, smiles, and coos of the first few months, we were ruling out syndromes and getting second and third opinions from more doctors and audiologists across the state than we knew existed. It was such a humbling experience to realize that two parents, with graduate degrees in education and counseling, knew nothing about our son's needs. But at least we could learn—every chance we got. We were quickly connected with the Early Intervention Program and a hearing loss support group, two resources which provided us great relief. Ryan was seeing a speech therapist weekly by 4 months old and got his hearing aids at 5 months. Between regular visits to the audiologist and the careful vigilance of his speech therapist, we deduced that his right ear was over-amplified and went to Children's Hospital of Philadelphia for even more thorough testing at 10 months. Ryan had to be sedated for this test, instead of just asleep, like for all the others, which terrified me as well. However, we then got the best news that we never even imagined possible: that because of slight environmental interferences in his previous tests when he was asleep, it turned out that his right ear had been hearing in the normal range all along! His left ear's loss was more severe than we suspected, but we would happily take one good ear over anything else at this point. Ryan's speech remained delayed through his first year, but by the time he turned 2 he was speaking like a child who was almost 3! He still gets biweekly speech therapy, and there are gaps that still need to be filled, but after 2 years we finally feel that we have a handle on where he is and what he needs at this time in his life. We know where our resources are, and we feel confident that he will continue to experience successes in his life. We were extremely fortunate to learn that he had one normal ear—it really did make all the difference and was so close to what we had prayed for all along. But from that experience, as a parent and school counselor, I have such a better understanding of the range of feelings that other parents face as they learn how to best support their children with special needs—I will never forget what that first year was like for us!

Language Development

Laws of Language

An older toddler at a preschool was overheard telling another toddler, "Let's get the scissors so that we can *scissor* stuff!" Without even realizing it, the toddler was using the laws of language. Our communication system of symbols that we call **language** includes the four basic components of phonology, semantics, pragmatics, and syntax. Children use all four of these components on their journey toward effective communication (Gleason, 2005). **Phonology** is the study of a language's sounds. At this point in the child's development, he was in good command of phonology, being able to clearly articulate the sounds of the words. **Semantics** refers to the meaning of words. His semantic use of all of the words, except for his invented verb "scissor," did comply with the accepted meanings of those words in English. Even his use of "scissor" as a verb was creative and meaningful. **Pragmatics** is the way in which we use language to communicate with a specific listener. The boy's use of pragmatics was very effective, as he delivered his message in an enthusiastic way to persuade his friend to join in the fun. MJ, 2½ years old, however, was not using pragmatics when he calmly told his mother, "Mommy, Daddy is sleeping. Don't talk to him. Just shut up." **Syntax** is the grammatical component, how we put words in a specific order and change word forms, as in changing a verb from present to future tense. The humorous part of the first toddler's sentence was the syntax error, in which he created a verb form for the noun "scissor."

Comprehension vs. Production

Have you ever found yourself in this situation: You are listening to someone speak to you in another language, and you understand what the person is saying, but you find it very difficult, if nearly impossible, to produce the non-native words needed to respond to the person as well as you can understand him or her? If you can empathize with this example, you have a measure of compassion for what infants and toddlers experience: the great divide between comprehension and production. **Comprehension** refers to the ability to *understand* language, while **production** is the ability to actually *speak* it. Toddlers can comprehend 50 words by the time they are 13 months old, but it will generally take them until they are 18 months old before they can produce 50 words (Menyuk, Liebergott, & Schultz, 1995). In most stages of development, comprehension precedes production. When Liam was 9 to 10 months old, his mother began to recognize that he followed simple directions during bath time, such as, "we sit in the bathtub" versus standing in the tub. At 13½ months he could follow many more simple directions, such as "sit in the wagon," "in your mouth" versus throwing food on the floor, "go get your bear/toy," and "where's your foot?"

Think About It   5.3   Comprehension vs. Production

Think about how comprehension precedes production in the following example from the mother, Becca: Although he understands almost everything that is being spoken to him and says a few words, 14-month-old Canaan isn't significantly verbal. He is a shrieker (both his happy and angry noise) and has to be reminded to "speak nicely" often. He is also a mimicker of sound effects. Almost always he will say "cheeeeese" when he sees a camera, or when I get the clippers out to trim his hair he will make a "*zzzzzz*" noise. He copies people's sniffs, clicks, and lip vibrations, and prefers sound effects over words.

The Odyssey through Language Development

A human's amazing journey as a linguistic being begins in the womb. During the third trimester of pregnancy, a fetus responds to external sounds, as measured by changes in heart rate. A fetus not only responds to the mother's voice (Fifer & Moon, 1995), but also can distinguish between the words "babi" and "biba" played over a loudspeaker above the mother's abdomen (DeCasper, Lecanuet, Busnel, & Granier-Deferre, 1994).

Crying How would you enjoy signing up to participate in a research study where you were exposed to the sounds of a crying infant while trying to complete math problems? If this activity is not on your "bucket list," we think we know why. An infant's cry is an aversive sound, and research supports that adults find crying to be upsetting, distracting, or irritating (Chang & Thompson, 2011). The participants who did agree to sign up for Chang and Thompson's research study were significantly distracted from solving simple subtraction problems while listening to the sound of a crying infant, although they were not as distracted by the sound of neutral speech or the noise from a table saw. Trying to solve math problems uses working memory, simulating how parents might be distracted from whatever they were engaged in when their infant began crying.

A cry has distinctive acoustic characteristics: increased pitch, varied pitch contours, and slowed production (Chang & Thompson, 2011). Altogether, they make for a sound that is difficult to avoid, especially when infants use **hyperphonated cries**. While the pitch of an average infant cry is between 450–600 hertz (Hz), when infants decide to crank it into high gear, hyperphonated cries can average between 1000–2000 Hz! Hyperphonated cries result in high arousal in adults, as measured by skin conductance levels and changes in heart rate (Crowe & Zeskind, 1992).

From birth, infants are equipped to communicate their distress about physiological and emotional needs through crying. What purpose does this early stage in language acquisition serve, and why is it so useful to infants? Murray (1985) summarized three theories on crying: The *innate releaser model,* drawn from Bowlby's theory of mother–infant attachment, theorizes that an infant's cry is an innate releaser of caregiving responses in the listener that usually result in close physical contact. This biologically based mechanism in adults to detect infant crying and respond to it is so automatic that little or no cognitive processing is required. Another model, drawn from learning theory, uses the principle of *negative reinforcement:* the infant's crying (the stimulus) is so aversive that the parent responds by picking the infant up (the response). Since this is the response that the infant desires, she stops crying (providing the negative reinforcement). The infant shapes her parent's behavior, as the parent gets reinforced for picking up a crying baby, and the parent will continue to pick her up because picking up a crying baby eliminates the annoying stimulus of crying. Yet another theory comes from the idea of "sympathetic distress," in which the parent hearing the cry responds with sympathy and altruism.

More recently, Thompson, Dessureau, and Olson (1998) proposed a *respiratory drama hypothesis,* based on evolutionary psychology. An infant responds to his distress by crying in ways that mimic a respiratory emergency—gasping, choking, and panting. Infant crying is considered melodramatic: It is a distortion of reality. Unless the infant is really having a respiratory emergency, a cry that mimics extreme respiratory distress is a deception designed to prompt parents to attend to him immediately.

Cooing Infants between 2 and 4 months begin to make pleasing, vowel-like sounds ("ooh," "aah") when they are happy. The sound has been likened to the sound that doves make. They also begin to produce laughter (Menn & Stoel-Gammon, 2005). This stage enables infants to have a prelanguage conversational exchange with parents (Tamis-LeMonda, Cristofaro, Rodriguez, & Bornstein, 2006). Parents and infants can take turns vocalizing, the infant cooing and laughing, and the parent talking and laughing in response.

Babbling Between 5 and 9 months of age, most normally hearing infants begin to vocalize consonant–vowel combinations known as babbling. Reduplicated, well-formed syllables such as "dadadada" and "mamama" are often produced in long sequences. Babbling is a critical step in the language journey. It demonstrates vocal capability and readiness to produce sounds that can serve as words, as these syllables are the foundation for words in all spoken languages (Oller, Eilers, & Basinger, 2001). Although the infant may just be experimenting with her ability to babble and not intend the sound to mean any particular word, adults often give a specific meaning to what she is saying. Ruby's older sister, Brielle, was given the nickname "Baba" after Ruby began to babble "ba-ba-ba" when Brielle was visiting from college. Was Ruby really trying to say her sister's name, something else, or nothing at all? We'll never know, but the nickname has remained, and years later the whole family still calls her "Baba."

Parents are intuitively able to recognize when their children initiate babbling. More than being able to write down the first day that their infant babbles in a baby journal, parents are at the forefront of identifying **late-onset babbling** and seeking a professional assessment. Children who do not begin babbling until after 10 months, and who do not present any significant medical problems, are at extreme risk for hearing impairments and may be at risk for other language-related disorders such as phonological disorders, apraxia, dysarthria, specific language impairment, autism, and reading problems (Oller et al., 2001).

Gestures are intentional motor actions used to request and direct another's attention (Vallotton, 2008). No doubt everyone has observed an infant or toddler waving "hello" or "goodbye," or stretching her arms straight up in the air to signal that she would like to be picked up. Pointing is one of the earliest gestures. While some infants begin to point at 9 months, others do not start until 19 months (Hoff, 2006). Infants and toddlers naturally use nonverbal gestures as part of their everyday interactions between 10 and 24 months (Acredolo & Goodwyn, 1988). Gesturing has a number of uses, including *social interaction* (waving hello and goodbye), and *requests* (signaling to be picked up). The infant may also use gestures to symbolically *represent an object,* by waving her hand to indicate a butterfly, or *represent an action,* by panting to symbolize a dog.

Gesturing as an early step in language development is useful until the child's verbal abilities have developed further. Gesturing provides a mechanism for the child to more specifically communicate ideas and requests. It increases infant-directed speech by inviting more language-related responses from parents. If an infant gestures "bird," the parent is able to verbally confirm and then elaborate on what type of bird it is or what the bird is doing. An infant who uses gestures has increased control over the topic of conversation, by drawing attention to what he is interested in. An infant who gestures while he is still preverbal also allows him to experience the value of communication and his role in it. This was especially helpful in Lauren's family, when 9-month-old Christian began screaming and throwing himself on the ground when he wanted milk. Lauren was able to help Christian transform tantrums into using signs for "more," "please," "hungry," "all done," and "thank you."

A growing body of research indicates that giving infants and toddlers sign training can maximize communication between the children and their caregivers. Infants as young as 6 months can be taught simple signs (Thompson, Cotnoir-Bichelman, McKerchar, Tate, & Dancho, 2007). Vallotton (2008) discovered that preverbal infants and toddlers who were exposed to symbolic gestures were able to communicate their emotions as well as the emotions of others, for states such as anger, sadness, hurt, sleepiness, and fear. Thompson et al. (2007) found that 6–10-month-old infants who were given sign training were able to replace their crying and whining with a sign to help them communicate with their parents. The researchers hypothesized that sign training may help prevent behavior problems for at-risk children, especially those with developmental delays, language delays, and sensory impairments. Although some parents may be concerned that encouraging infants and toddlers to use symbolic gesturing may discourage them from articulating spoken words, Goodwyn, Acredolo, and Brown's (2000) longitudinal study discovered that infants trained to use symbolic gesturing actually had better language acquisition as toddlers. They used vocal language earlier and scored higher on measures of expressive language than infants who were not taught to pair a symbolic gesture with a spoken word.

Gesturing Using American Sign Language (ASL) Some parents and researchers, capitalizing on infants' and toddlers' abilities to gesture, teach them an organized system for communicating with gestures, such as **American Sign Language (ASL)**. Using an established signing system such as ASL allows the child to learn a language of gestures that is understood by people outside of the child's immediate circle, enabling the child to understand and be understood by a wider variety of people.

Some parents introduce sign language to their 6–9-month-old infants by demonstrating need-based and high-impact signs, such as the sign for "milk." Their intent is to foster infants' communication skills in their hands, since infants' hand muscles develop before they can speak (Start ASL, 2012). Parents notice that by 7–12 months, their baby often signs back to them. By the child's first birthday, parents introduce secondary signs; by 2 years the child may not only combine different signs but may also combine signs and speech. Using sign language while babies are preverbal facilitates their ability to communicate their needs and observations in many settings, including mealtimes, bath times, and bedtimes.

Parents and teachers who use sign language with infants and toddlers, whether they use ASL or another type of sign training, often remark that the communication between caregiver and child is easier and more accurate, that it fosters more positive interactions, and that it provides another tool for infants to use so that they do not have to cry in order to get their wants and needs met.

First Words A momentous day occurs for parents when they hear their toddlers produce first spoken words! Usually occurring around 13 months (Tamis-LeMonda et al., 2006), first words can be real or invented; usually they are single words that label familiar objects in the toddler's life, such as people, animals, foods, objects that move, and familiar actions (Hart, 2004). Of toddlers, 75% understand 150 words and can verbalize 50 of them by the time they are 18 months old (Kuhl, 2004). Toddlers also demonstrate their sensitivity to categories by engaging in an error known as **overextension**, in which the toddler applies a word to a wider range of objects than is accurate (MacWhitney, 2005), such as when Cole first identified their family dog as a "dog" but then extended the use of "dog" to horses and fish that he saw as well.

During a shift to verbal symbols, the toddler abandons gestures previously used. Vocalizations have distinct advantages over gestures: Unlike gestures, speech does not have to be seen by others to be understood, so that the toddler can be out of someone's direct line of vision and still communicate; speaking allows the toddlers to do other things with their hands while talking, and more people understand speech than gestures (Acredolo & Goodwyn, 1988).

Two-Word Phrases The next major linguistic milestone occurs when a toddler combines two words to express a single idea (e.g., "more milk"), which usually takes place between 18 and 24 months of age. During this time, a toddler produces one or two new words per day! The rate of word learning will increase steadily and continue through the early childhood years (Ganger & Brent, 2004). Toddlers sentences are referred to as **telegraphic speech**. Similar to the way people sent telegrams years ago when nonessential words were omitted because the sender of the message had to pay for each word, toddler speech is pared down to the basic elements (e.g., "more milk" instead of "I would like more milk").

Whining Do you remember those posters that simply say, "Whining" with a diagonal line striking through the word to indicate a "no whining zone"? Parents of toddlers have fantasies that their children will follow those directions! However, whining emerges in a toddler's growing collection of vocal abilities with the arrival of language. Children's use of whining is at its height between 2.5 and 4 years (Borba, 2003; Sears & Sears, 1995). Whining combines the acoustic features of cries (i.e., heightened pitch, exaggerated contours, slowed production) with speech, and the sound is considered to be even more annoying than infant cries (Sokol, Webster, Thompson, & Stevens, 2005). Studies show that whining elicits arousal in adults, as demonstrated by elevated skin conductance; adults are more distracted by whining than they are by crying (Chang & Thompson, 2010). Thompson et al. (1998) believed that whining, like crying, is an inborn deceptive feature that toddlers use to sound as if they are in more danger than they actually are, compelling adults to attend to them.

Theories of Language Development

The various theories of language development are as divergent as our profession's counseling theories! As each theory of counseling has its own way of explaining how people become stuck in unsuccessful patterns of thinking and behaving, and how they transform themselves to achieve greater mental health and personal success, each theory of language development offers a unique perspective on how humans end up successfully speaking the native language they experience in childhood.

The **behaviorist** perspective of B. F. Skinner (1957, 1991) proposes that language development is based on experience and shaped through **operant conditioning** (reinforcement). According to this theory, when an infant unintentionally babbles in a way that resembles words in his parents' language, his parents respond to the babbling behavior by smiling, praising, hugging, and giving other types of attention. Since the infant enjoys these responses, the babbling behavior has been **reinforced**, meaning that the infant is highly likely to babble more often in order to receive more enjoyable reactions from the parent.

On the other hand, Albert Bandura's (1986) theory, originally called social learning theory, maintains that an infant learns behaviors, such as language, by first observing others modeling the language and then by using **imitation**. Unlike behaviorism, the infant's learning does not take place because behaviors are being reinforced by his environment but rather because mirror neurons are actively practicing what is seen in the environment. Bandura (2001) later changed the name of his theory to **social cognitive theory**, removing the word "learning" because of its connection to the behaviorist concepts of learning through environmental conditioning, and to emphasize the role of children's own cognitions in their development. Although Bandura's and Skinner's ideas are not aligned with one another, the behaviorist and the social cognitive perspectives are often linked, with the idea that babies imitate the sounds modeled by their parents and then receive reinforcement for imitating them.

Noam Chomsky's (1968) **nativist** perspective focuses on the active role that the infant's brain plays in developing language. Chomsky believes that the human brain is innately wired for language by means of an inborn system called a **learning acquisition device (LAD)**. The LAD contains **universal grammar**, a set of grammatical rules shared by all languages and hardwired into an infant's brain before the infant even hears a word spoken. Hearing language triggers the infant's LAD mechanism, enabling the infant to understand and speak using these innate grammatical rules. The infant, therefore, does not need parents to supply intentional language training, making nativism quite different from the behaviorist perspective (Pinker, 1999).

Cognition and Language

The interplay of cognition and language can be seen in studies with young infants. Before an infant can learn words, the infant first needs to recognize that sounds are linked to objects and events. Gogate and Bahrick (2001) discovered that 7–8-month-old infants can learn to associate sounds with objects when they are synchronized. The researchers noticed that the infants learned to pair sounds and objects so well that the infants began to dishabituate when the word–object pairs were switched on them. As both cognition and language progress, infants will learn that words represent objects (Hollich, Hirsh-Pasek, & Golinkoff, 2000). Over time, the connections that the infant makes between words and objects will be strengthened if responsive parents make it a practice to pair words and objects.

Parental Influences

Infants babble, sometimes continuously. Distracted or busy parents might not realize that this babbling is purposeful, and that the investment they make in trying to figure out what their infant is communicating can have a significant effect on their child's early language development. Parents may be very interested to know that the way in which they respond to their infants' babbling may either facilitate later word learning or slow it down. An infant makes vocalizations called **object-directed vocalizations (ODVs)** when looking at an object that is either being held or within reach. These are vocalizations that are prelinguistic and are not crying. Far from being random vocalizations, ODVs are actually an indication of the child's readiness to learn (Goldstein, Schwade, Briesch, & Syal, 2010). For example, consider when the infant is sitting on his mother's lap, and, seeing a banana on the table, says, "na." Whether his mother consistently responds to these types of vocalizations by correctly identifying his object and saying "banana" (which connects sound and object) or whether she responds with an unrelated word, such as "nap," will make a big difference in infant vocabulary size in the months to come. Goldstein and Schwade (2010) found that when mothers of 9-month-old infants routinely labeled their children's object-directed vocalizations correctly, those children had larger vocabulary sizes at 15 months than did children whose mothers generally responded with a word that did not match what the child was looking at.

Parents sometimes wonder whether it might be helpful to teach their child a second language by exposing them to a televised or audio-recorded tutoring program. However, Kuhl and Rivera-Gaxiola (2008) demonstrated the importance of social interaction versus media instruction on language development. Nine-month-old American infants were exposed to native Mandarin speakers for 4 to 6 weeks. The Mandarin speakers regularly played with the infants and read to them in a laboratory setting. A control group of infants received the same Mandarin speech via television or audio programming. A month after the final exposure to Mandarin, all of the infants were given behavioral tests and brain scans; those who had received the personal interaction had learned and retained syllables in Mandarin that do not appear in English; however, the control group exposed to Mandarin via television or audio programming had not learned any more Mandarin than a second control group that was only exposed to English.

Cultural Variations

What may account for the interesting fact that while English has over 3000 words to describe colors, Berinmo, the language of a tribe in Papua New Guinea, has five words for colors (Roberson, Davidoff, Davies, & Shapiro, 2004)? Cultural variations in language usage are a reflection of what is considered useful in that culture. Similarly, infants' and toddlers' variations in language development are closely tied to what is valued and strengthened in their cultural environment. American mothers tend to label objects for their babies; as a result, nouns (i.e., object words) are a typical part of English-speaking toddlers' vocabulary. Conversely, Japanese, Chinese, and Korean mothers focus on words that describe actions and social routines with their babies; as one might expect, Asian toddlers have more words for social routines and verbs than their English-speaking peers (Choi & Gopnik, 1995; Fernald & Morikawa, 1993; Tardif, Gelman, & Xu, 1999).

The tremendous gap in American toddlers' language exposure, as correlated with socioeconomic status, was documented by Hart and Risley (1995). The researchers observed the everyday conversations of parents and their toddlers for 2½ years. The 42 families were either receiving public assistance or employed in working-class or professional jobs. Whereas parents with professional jobs used 2100 words per hour with their toddlers, parents on public assistance used only 600, and working-class parents used 1300. Toddlers of professional parents had a qualitatively different language experience in other ways as well: They not only received more parental responses to things that they said, but also those parental responses contained more encouraging statements than those made in the other groups. The cumulative effect of these types of behaviors was significant. By age 3, the children from professional families had been exposed to *8 million* more words than children whose families were receiving public assistance.

The counseling implications here are quite important, as counselors work with families from different socioeconomic groups. While counselors won't be able to change the parents' socioeconomic status (SES), counselors can be a valuable asset in helping parents from all SES groups to recognize the profound impact that seemingly simple, everyday interactions have on children over time. Parents from all walks of life can be encouraged to pay closer attention to what their children are saying, to expose them to rich language experiences that come from interactions with people, and to notice their frequency of responding to their children with affirmative, encouraging statements such as "What a great job!" compared to prohibitory statements such as "Stop doing that!"

Summary

The dramatic physical metamorphosis from newborn to toddler yields a human being who has quadrupled in birth weight by the second birthday and also significantly increased the proportion of body fat. However, weight gain that occurs too rapidly during this time period (a jump of 1 major centile band) puts the child at risk for obesity and insulin resistance. Parents and health care providers use the WHO and CDC international weight-for-age growth charts to monitor this pattern of development.

Breastfeeding, while not the preference of all new mothers and not an option for some mothers with specific medical conditions, is recommended by the American Academy of Pediatrics as the exclusive source of an infant's nutrition for his first six months. Breastfeeding supplies virtually complete nutrition to the infant, boosts immunity, minimizes allergies later in life, provides tasting exposures to the food that the mother is eating, is cost-effective, and requires few extra supplies when traveling with the infant. When solid food is introduced after 6 months, it is crucial for parents to provide healthy foods, as the feeding of healthy or unhealthy foods in infancy and toddlerhood triggers genetic mechanisms on a cellular level (metabolic rate, level of satiety, diabetes and heart disease risk) that will continue to activate throughout the lifespan.

While the number of infants and toddlers in the United States experiencing malnutrition is not nearly as high as in some developing nations, 8.6 million U.S. children struggle with food insecurity, ranging from eating less varied diets or receiving food from a food bank to suffering from reduced food intake or disrupted eating patterns. Long-term effects of food insecurity include anemia, lower cognitive ability, and insecure attachment. Two other major health concerns affecting infants and toddlers include spontaneous infant death, known as sudden infant death syndrome, and injury from abuse, known as shaken baby syndrome or abusive head trauma.

Gross and fine motor capacities progress rapidly during the first three years, transforming a physically helpless newborn into a child who can walk independently, pick up objects, and begin to dress. Early motor development can be considered from a dynamic systems perspective, in which the baby's personal attributes and her environment create an interactive system that either supports or discourages the development of each new skill. The dynamic systems perspective helps to explain the distinct differences in gross motor development between cultures: Sub-Saharan African infants often reach motor milestones far in advance of European-American infants, in part because sub-Saharan African mothers expect early motor independence, believe that their children are capable of it, and provide massages, motor games, and specific exercises shortly after birth.

Both exogenous stimulation (external to the baby) and endogenous stimulation (internal to the baby and first activated during REM sleep) play critical roles in brain formation and in allowing the baby to accurately perceive sensory events. The capacities for vision, hearing, taste, smell, and touch are dependent on both types of stimulation as well as adequate sleep.

There is great diversity in sleeping patterns and arrangements, the use of vaccinations, and the introduction of toileting. Although sleep is a powerful driving force in children, many infants and toddlers display their uniqueness by developing a sleeping/waking cycle that does not mirror textbook guidelines, requiring parents to have a flexible mind in accommodating a child's needs. Parents also differ in philosophy regarding whether a child should sleep in a separate room or share a bed or room with the parents. Toilet training and elimination communication (EC) are two effective, yet disparate, approaches to facilitating a young child to use a potty for elimination. While most toilet-training methods recommend waiting until the toddler is ambulatory and showing specific signs of potty readiness, parents who use EC may introduce their infant to a potty shortly after birth, focusing on the constant communication between parent and child. Regarding the use of vaccines, not all medical professionals and parents concur with the immunization schedule recommended by the Centers for Disease Control and Prevention, with approximately one-fifth of U.S. parents delaying or refusing some or all of the recommended early childhood vaccines. People generally have strong opinions for or against vaccine use, making this controversial topic an area for a counselor to navigate with cultural sensitivity.

Piaget's sensorimotor stage of cognitive development, from birth to 2 years, describes the process by which the infant experiences the world, learning information through senses and not by logic. The child progresses from the newborn stage of relying on reflexes, to accidentally noticing interesting things about the body and the world outside of the body, to experimentation and finally insight. Although Piaget did not believe that infants had object permanence (the ability to recognize

that an object still exists even when it is removed from view) until 8 months, Baillargeon's studies suggest that 4-month-old infants have this ability.

Information processing theory often uses a computer model to provide a framework for understanding how an infant categorizes situations, creates memories, and becomes familiar with reoccurring stimuli. An infant best encodes information when comparing it to another object.

Infants and toddlers are capable of retrieving stored information by using both recognition and recall. They make meaning out of the world by engaging in object categorization, grouping items into broad categories. They demonstrate that they have become habituated to stimuli by looking at a familiar object for a shorter amount of time than when the object was novel.

Assessing an infant's cognitive ability is typically done by observing motor and perceptual skills with a test such as the Bayley-III. Often used for screening purposes, the Bayley-III predicts mental test performance in preschool, with very low scores strongly signaling later developmental problems. Infants who receive very low scores are provided with specialized interventions, as are infants and toddlers who are considered to be at-risk due to living in poverty or those who are identified with special needs.

The odyssey through language development has many linguistic milestones, beginning with the newborn's crying, an innate prelinguistic vocalization that serves to alert parents when the infant is in distress. Cooing and laughing emerge between 2 and 4 months, leading to babbling beginning between 5 and 9 months. A toddler comprehends words well before actually verbally producing those words, and a preverbal infant or toddler frequently uses gestures to represent words that the infant is unable to articulate. Some parents capitalize on these gesturing abilities by exposing their child to sign language, thus increasing the communication between parent and child. The toddler usually produces first spoken word by 13 months and 2-word phrases between 18 and 24 months. Accompanying newfound speech is the ability to whine, an annoying amalgam of crying and speech.

Skinner's behaviorist perspective proposes that language development is dependent on experience and shaped through reinforcement. Bandura's social cognitive theory maintains that language is learned by first observing others modeling the language and then by using imitation. Chomsky's nativist perspective holds that the human brain is intrinsically wired for language with the learning acquisition device (LAD) system, a set of grammatical rules shared by all languages and hardwired into an infant's brain before she hears a spoken word. Parents can support their child's early language development by pairing words with objects, accurately tuning in to the infant's prelinguistic babbling, using social interaction instead of media to teach language, and by responding to their child with affirmative, encouraging statements.

Acknowledgments

The authors would like to thank all of the wonderful caregivers who so generously shared stories about their children, making the concepts from this chapter come to life, and Stefanie Moore, M.Ed., for her research assistance.

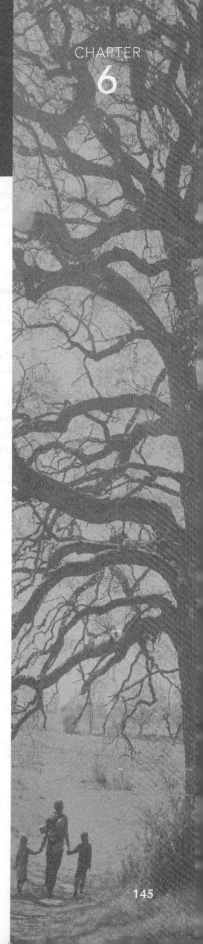

Emotional and Social Development in the Infancy and Toddlerhood Years

By Nadine E. Garner and Julia M. Dunn

This chapter explores the tremendous changes that occur in the emotional and social domains of the infant and toddler. The rapid changes during this developmental period are highly context dependent, shaped by the broader culture and the child's own temperament. The child's unique pattern of emotional and social development lays the groundwork for the continuing adventure throughout the lifespan.

The Function of Emotions

Emotions are brain-based impulses that motivate a person to act in a particular way (Goleman, 1995). Most parents would probably be interested to know that the seat of all emotional responses, in both themselves and their babies, comes from the **amygdala**, two almond-sized and -shaped structures, one on each side of the brain near the side of the head. The amygdala is tiny but mighty, to which anyone who has witnessed a child (or themselves) being overcome by intense fear or anger can attest!

The amygdala receives information from the senses directly and activates a response, before the neocortex has a chance to fully recognize the sensory input. From a survival perspective, this acting-before-thinking approach is useful in times of danger, as the quick reaction from the amygdala activates the flight, fight, or freeze response, so that we can swiftly manage perceived threats to our well-being. It helps us know when we might need to be angry or fearful. The challenge of being human is to know when you really are in danger and what to quickly do about it, or whether your neocortex needs to make a more rational decision and think through its actions first.

The **neocortex**, the large area of the brain responsible for rational thoughts such as strategizing and long-term planning, decides what it thinks about the feelings that were generated in the amygdala. So although the circuitry of these two minds is distinct from one another, the two minds cooperate by means of a web of connecting circuits from the emotional areas to the neocortex (Goleman, 1995). In this way, the emotional centers exert tremendous power to guide the thinking centers of the brain. We actually have two minds, what Goleman calls the emotional brain and the thinking brain. Goleman, an expert in the study of **emotional intelligence**, describes an emotionally intelligent person as one who has the ability to navigate the emotional brain/thinking brain system and develop "self-control, zeal and persistence, and the ability to motivate oneself" (1995, p. xii).

An emotionally intelligent person recognizes that the human brain is hardwired to have emotional responses in the amygdala first, and unless one is in danger (a flight, fight, or freeze response), those strong emotions need to be interpreted by the thinking brain so that the person knows what to rationally do about them. So how do parents begin this journey toward emotional intelligence with their infants and toddlers, to help their children balance emotion and reason? Parents have an enormous opportunity to help their children develop emotional intelligence: These opportunities lie in the fact that children are always noticing how their parents respond to them, how their parents model rational responses to their own emotions, and how parents respond in their relationships with other adults, especially their partners. As a counselor, you also have a tremendous potential to assist parents in this amazing emotional odyssey.

REFLECTION 6.1 EMOTIONAL BRAIN, THINKING BRAIN

Before Ruby was 2 years old, she was having a particularly noisy toddler tantrum, and, not exactly planning what to do but needing to get her out of the house (which sounded like an echo-chamber from her screaming), I scooped her up and took her outside, saying, "We need to go outside and talk about this." I held Ruby in my lap while we sat on a small, rough-hewn workbench made by my late father, which we called "Dan's bench." I started talking with her about the emotional brain and the thinking brain—how the emotional brain lets you know that something is wrong, and that the thinking brain helps you figure out what to do about it. I guessed what she was upset about and talked with her gently about how to resolve it, while she relaxed and looked at nature in the back yard. A few days later while Ruby was having another screaming episode, I asked, "What do we need to do about this?" I was shocked to hear my toddler say, "Sit on Dan's bench . . . talk about it," which we promptly did. Ruby is now 3½ years old and she has sat in my lap on Dan's bench dozens of times since then, all at her suggestion. She has responded so well to the idea that she has two brains and is able to verbalize from which brain she is operating that I have never had to give her a timeout or any type of punishment. She just takes me out to Dan's bench to talk about it, in any kind of weather or time of night. [~Nadine]

Emerging Emotions

Within the first year of life, an infant will display the basic emotions of happiness, anger, sadness, fear, surprise, interest, and disgust (Izard, 2007). To convey these emotions, infants use all of the communication methods that are at their disposal: crying, gestures, and movements (for more about crying and gestures, see Language Development in Chapter 5).

The basic emotions are deeply rooted in our neural circuitry, a sophisticated choreography of physiological events designed to keep us safe. When the infant or adult experiences **anger**, the brain directs more blood flow to the hands, preparing the person to defend against the strike of an opponent. The body also prepares for action by increasing the heart rate and flooding the body with hormones such as adrenaline (Goleman, 1995). **Fear** causes blood to be directed to the legs, preparing the body to make a quick getaway from whatever danger is causing the fear response. The body temporarily freezes, to help the person decide whether hiding is a better option. A hormonal rush puts the body on edge, so that it focuses its attention on the perceived threat. Infants and toddlers react to situations of uncertainty in the same way: Their motor activity is inhibited or temporarily stops. If infants and toddlers are unable to resolve the uncertain situation that they are in, they may cry or show other signs of distress (Kagan, Reznick, & Snidman, 1987). Two- to 3-year-olds react to uncertainty by stopping whatever they are playing with and whatever they are saying, and they immediately find a trusted person for security. Anyone who has seen a toddler happily walking alongside and chatting with a parent one minute in a grocery store, only to run hiding between her parent's legs the next, clutching the parent's pant legs like a wild animal, is familiar with this hardwired, biological response to an uncertain situation. Kagan et al. (1987) declare that the time period from 20–30 months is an important time for parents to notice whether their toddlers are tending toward inhibition or lack of inhibition to the unfamiliar. This topic will be discussed in more detail in the section on temperament later in this chapter.

Happiness quiets the areas of the brain that generate troubling thoughts, by activating the part of the brain that inhibits negative feelings. A quieted brain lets the body recover from the distressing emotions and gets the body ready and enthusiastic to strive toward goals (Goleman, 1995). **Sadness**, on the other hand, produces a decrease in energy or enthusiasm. It allows the brain to plan for the future by creating a time of mourning and reflection, which enables the person to transition from a loss to a new beginning. A characteristic look of **surprise** is a lifting of the eyebrows. This survival mechanism lets the person increase their visual field so that they can better appraise the surprising event and make a plan of action. The emotional response of **disgust** cannot be underestimated for its protective value: The action of curling the upper lip to the side while wrinkling the nose simultaneously closes the nostrils against an offensive odor and allows the person to spit out a poisonous food.

The Sequence of Emotional Development

As with the development of physical and cognitive capacities, there is a sequence to emotional development. A newborn begins an emotional kaleidoscope with two basic inborn states of arousal: showing attraction to pleasing stimuli and withdrawing from aversive stimuli (Camras, Oster, Campos, & Bakeman, 2003). However, not long after, during the first 6 months of the infant's life, the infant is able to express the recognizable emotions of happiness, joy, anger, sadness, fear, surprise, interest, and disgust (Izard, 2007). These are also known as the **primary emotions** (Lewis, 2000). Between 15 and 24 months, with the advent of the toddler's **self-awareness** (recognizing that his identity is separate and distinct from everyone and everything else), the **secondary emotions** appear. The secondary emotions have two stages. The first stage, **self-conscious emotions**, which are seen between 15 and 24 months, include embarrassment (the type that results from being the object of attention), envy, and empathy. By the time the toddler is between 2½ and 3 years old, he moves into the more advanced stage of secondary emotions. The infant has learned to incorporate society's rules and standards, leading to the expression of **self-evaluative emotions**, such as pride, guilt, shame, and embarrassment (i.e., an evaluative type of embarrassment that is a mild form of shame; Lewis, 2000).

➤ CASE EXAMPLE **6.1** PRIMARY AND SECONDARY EMOTIONS.

When Jacob was 2 years old he began to bite as a way of dealing with frustration. I realized this was a common response, but he would bite my shoulder and it would hurt. I researched the experts' opinions, and two common responses stood out. The first response was to bite the child back. I found this method to be distasteful because I did not understand how he would learn that biting was unacceptable if he was being bitten. The second response was to have the child bite a lemon immediately after he or she bit a person. This retort made sense and so I stocked up on lemons. I was so excited to try combating this issue, only to be met by a frustration of my own: The very next time my child bit me on the shoulder I responded immediately by popping a lemon wedge in his mouth. Rather than surprising him with the tart metaphorical bite, I was surprised because he actually liked the taste! We did ultimately break him of the habit, using patience and persistence, and I am proud to say that he now deals with the many frustrations of life appropriately. [~Lori]

What are your thoughts on how Lori handled her biting toddler?

Cultural Variations

The basic emotions an infant expresses in the first year seem to be demonstrated and understood in cultures worldwide (Izard, 2007). While the expression and interpretation of basic emotions may be hardwired from birth, the infant quickly learns to assimilate the **emotion schemas** of culture, the framework for how to conceptualize and show emotion. With new research demonstrating that infants only 3 months old are attuned to the emotional expressions of adults (Hoel, Wiese, & Striano, 2008), one can imagine that quite early on in a child's life, the brain is shaping its neural systems to align with the emotion schemas of culture.

Cross-cultural research on variations in emotion schemas often juxtaposes individualistic and collectivistic cultures (Trommsdorff, 2006). Individualistic, often Western, cultures tend to promote independence and personal accomplishment, whereas collectivistic, often Eastern, cultures tend to focus on interdependence and social relationships. These cultural values and tendencies inform the emotion schemas of their respective citizens. For example, people from collectivistic cultures, such as China, are acculturated to mask their emotions (believing that overt displays of emotion are disturbing), unlike people from individualistic cultures, such as the United States, who are taught to discuss their emotions (believing that revealing emotions is psychologically healthy and that masking them is harmful) (Wang, 2006a).

Bender, Spada, Rothe-Wulf, Traber, and Rauss (2012) investigated the differences in angry responses to the same event between people in Germany and Tonga, a small Polynesian kingdom. The researchers hypothesized that culture-specific values trigger different **attribution styles**, which then leads to differences in emotional responses. An attribution style is how a person cognitively appraises an event. Secondary school students in Germany and Tonga were given the same vignettes to read, consisting of events in which something went wrong. Study participants had to describe what their emotional response would be if they were in the situations they had just read about. The vignettes included scenarios such as "Peter and James want to meet up. However, James arrives almost one hour later than they have arranged"; "Tom has just bought a gift and is walking down the street with it. Suddenly he is pushed by a boy. The gift falls to the ground and breaks"; "Tom has just bought a gift and is walking down the street with it. Suddenly he stumbles. The gift falls to the ground and breaks"; "Jane has organized a big party outside to which she has invited many guests. Everything is prepared and festively decorated and all of the guests have arrived, when suddenly a storm breaks. The party falls through."

The study discovered that Tongans become more emotionally charged by the *outcome* of the event, by focusing on the damage caused, whereas Germans place more emotional emphasis on who or what was *responsible* for the problem. In addition, compared to Tongans, Germans more often or more intensely respond with anger, overall, and they appraised more damage and ascribed more responsibility to others in the same scenarios. Conversely, Tongans experienced more shame, guilt, and sadness in response to events, likely because they take more personal responsibility for the circumstances (Bender et al., 2012). As a culturally sensitive counselor, one can see what an adventure awaits, as one discovers the emotion schemas that underlie the cultures of the families.

Theoretical Perspectives

Freud

Sigmund Freud's (1856–1939) psychosexual stage theory focuses on the impact of the early parent–child relationship on emotional well-being and personality (Freud, 1938/1973). According to Freud, the relationship that parents create with their infants and toddlers, as they manage their child's sexual and aggressive drives in the first few years of life, has a life-long effect. Children have to resolve the personal and emotional crises that arise when their biological drives of sex and aggression (inborn urges to suck, defecate, experience pleasure, and avoid discomfort) come in conflict with the expectations of society. For Freud, parents have the task of figuring out how much or how little gratification to give their child's basic needs. The parents who are able to effectively balance gratifying their child's needs (i.e., not over-permitting or under-permitting) will raise well-adjusted children who will be able to satisfy their adult sexual needs while behaving appropriately as individuals within the fabric of society.

Erikson

Erik Erikson's (1902–1994) psychosocial stage theory examines society's influence on the person's emotional development and personality over the lifespan. His theory also recognizes that the relationships with caregivers in the early years of life provide the social influence on children during the infant and toddler periods (Erikson, 1982). During the **basic trust versus basic mistrust** stage, which lasts from infancy through about 18 months, babies develop a schema for how reliable people and things in their environment seem to be. Parents who are sensitive, responsive, and consistent in providing for their infant's feeding or other needs encourage a baby to develop a hopeful personality, one that trusts that desires

Cori Fetrow

REFLECTION 6.2 AUTONOMY

At the age of 3, my daughter's independence level seemed to take off overnight. I went from being able to dress her in my idea of a great outfit to having Aubrey tell me what I had picked out didn't match or she didn't like my idea of a great outfit. Now each night we have to pick out what she is going to wear for the next day so that we can smoothly get out of the house in the morning. Sometimes I just laugh and let her put on whatever she would like. The other day we were walking out of the house and she had on silver boots, white tights, a black skirt, and an orange polka dot sweatshirt. She looked more like a circus performer than a 3-year-old, but she was so proud of herself for picking out her clothes and getting herself dressed. If I even try to intervene and help I get met with "I can do it myself!" and a very determined little girl until she does get it. [~Cori]

will be met (as opposed to a mistrusting personality, one that sees the world as an unfriendly and unreliable place).

Erikson's second stage of personality development (from 18 months to 3 years) is known as **autonomy versus shame and doubt**. As toddlers begin to see that they can exert self-control over things that used to be controlled externally by caregivers, they will demand to feed themselves, handle new objects, and dress themselves. Hearing a toddler shout that she wants to do something "myself!" is a hallmark of this period of development.

Freud's and Erikson's theories can be contrasted in two distinct ways. Whereas Freud believed that one's personality and emotional development are determined in early childhood, Erikson viewed the development of these characteristics as a lifelong, continuous process—what he called a *cradle to grave* approach (Erikson, 1959). In addition, although both Freud and Erikson designed stage models of development—in which each stage presents a particular crisis or challenge that the individual must resolve—Freud's stages are psychosexual in nature, while Erikson's are psychosocial.

Attachment

Quality of Caregiver Relationship

Attachment is a mutual, sustainable bond that forms between two people, most notably between infant and parent. From the infant's perspective, the bond emerges based on how well the parent helps the infant to reduce distress. The brain is wired to perceive any type of distress as a potentially serious threat to our well-being, and for an infant, the experience of distress comes in many forms: hungry, tired, wet, gassy, hot, cold, the lights are too bright, there are startling noises, there is a scratchy tag inside a onesie, or overstimulation from too many people talking to or shaking a rattle in the infant's face.

Some parents spend a great deal of time outfitting their baby's nursery with all kinds of functional and decorative items to make taking care of the baby a more comfortable experience. In the end, the infant doesn't really care about the matching border around the wall, or the wipie warmer, but the infant *will* recognize how well the parent consistently provides a stable relationship, one in which the parent responds to needs and signals for comfort during times of distress, with close contact and loving touch.

When the brain's amygdala registers a perceived threat to the person's well-being (e.g., an infant who is being held by a visitor in such a way that arms and legs are dangling may perceive an imminent fall, even if the infant is in no danger of falling), the brain signals the adrenal glands—which sit atop the kidneys—to quickly release and circulate the steroid hormone **cortisol** throughout the brain and body. A measure of cortisol is necessary in infants and toddlers to give them the energy to respond to distress, to focus, and to learn new information (Gunnar, 1998). The cortisol prompts the infant to tense up and cry out in distress so that someone may come and save the infant from "falling." A responsive parent will remove the infant from the inexperienced visitor's arms and hold the infant's arms and legs close to the parent's body, allowing the infant to feel safe. With the threat of falling removed, cortisol levels, heart rate, breathing, muscle tension, and other physical processes return to an unthreatened state.

Although the body and brain systems are equipped to swing back and forth between distressed and relaxed states, Gunnar (2000) discovered that if threatening events happen too often or last for too long, the child may develop into a hyper-vigilant person, one who quickly responds to events with fear and anxiety and who has difficulty returning to a state of relaxation. This type of child may produce more cortisol more often each day to deal with the onslaught of perceived or real threats. In large amounts, cortisol has a toxic effect on the brain and body: It destroys neurons associated with the child's memory, emotional regulation, and the ability to adapt to stressful situations; it also causes problems with heart rate and digestion (Gunnar, 1998).

So how does attachment come into play? A parent who nurtures a secure attachment with their child in the early years of development can impact the child's ability to manage stress successfully. There is a direct connection between responsive caregiving and the development of the child's stress system (Gunnar, 1998; Gunnar & Cheatham, 2003). Megan R. Gunner, a leading stress researcher, posits that a child's stress regulation is "embedded in caregiver-infant interactions" (Gunnar, 2006, p. 106). Cozolino (2006) believes that as the child observes the parent modeling how to return to a relaxed state, she stores this process in her neural networks so that she can later replicate it for herself. Gunner and Cheatham (2003) discovered that securely attached children have normal cortisol levels even when they are distressed, unlike insecurely attached children, who have high levels. So imagine that the securely attached infant in the example above is now a 2½-year-old toddler, and two years later is being lifted up under her arms and held in the air with legs dangling, by the same annoying visitor. Although the child finds this position uncomfortable and threatening, because the infant has developed an emotional response system that can manage distressing situations effectively, the child will tell the visitor, "Please stop, please put me down!" instead of crying uncontrollably or cringing in fear when people try to pick the child up.

Models of Attachment

Psychoanalysts once believed that an infant forms an attachment to the mother because the mother satisfies a basic drive for food during the oral stage of psychosexual development. Directing one's emotional energy to a person or object (in this case the mother's breast or a bottle, and then to the mother) is known as **cathexis**, a term that psychoanalysts have used to mean attachment (Yates, 1991).

However, John Bowlby, a child psychiatrist trained in psychoanalysis and working at the Tavistock Clinic in London, deviated from the psychoanalytic explanation of attachment. As Bowlby observed the tremendous psychological distress of the children in the clinic, caused by their separation from their parents (Ainsworth & Bowlby, 1989), he believed that the psychoanalytic process of cathexis was not a sufficient explanation for attachment. Bowlby also gravitated to the work of Harry Harlow (1958), a researcher who took an ethological approach to the study of animal behavior. **Ethology** studies the distinctive adaptive behaviors in animals that will maximize the animal's chances of survival. Harlow's famous studies with baby monkeys who were separated from their mothers demonstrated that when the baby monkeys were distressed, they attached themselves to the surrogate monkey mothers that provided comfort, not food.

Reflecting on his own clinical work with distressed children, and his interest in Harlow's ethological research with animals, Bowlby applied ethological principles from Harlow's studies to human attachment. Bowlby perceived infants and caregivers as biologically predisposed to form attachments. An infant's attachment to a caregiver is an evolutionary survival mechanism, designed to protect the infant from predators. Whereas the young of many other animal species are able to follow adults shortly after birth, human infants rely exclusively on their caregivers for protection, nourishment, and comfort for an extended period of time. Human infants need to employ a variety of signals, such as crying, cooing, clinging, and smiling, to attract adults to keep them close by and take care of them. Infants will form attachments to those caregivers who best respond to their signals

(Bowlby, 1969). Bowlby developed his own **4-phase model for the development of infant-parent attachments**:

1. *Phase 1: Indiscriminate Social Responsiveness (birth to 2 months):* An infant sends signals to adults so that they will provide comfort and care. Crying prompts adults to come closer to the infant, and smiling ensures that the adult will remain close by.
2. *Phase 2: Discriminating Sociability (2–7 months):* The infant prefers to engage with familiar people, and so may smile widely at parents, but look warily or fearfully—or show other signs of hesitation—toward a stranger. This type of distressed behavior toward people the infant does not know is called **stranger wariness** or **stranger anxiety**.
3. *Phase 3: Attachments (7–24 months):* The infant or toddler, who is now more mobile, will initiate contact with parents by creeping, crawling, or walking to them. The child at this stage will seek out a parent especially when distressed, similar to the monkeys in Harlow's study. The parent acts as a secure base for exploration, so that the child can wander a short distance away to explore but visually checks back to make sure that the parent is there. It is during this phase that the child exhibits distressed behavior when the parent leaves, known as **separation protest** or **separation anxiety**. The child may cry and show other distressed behaviors, which are designed to signal a parent to return.
4. *Phase 4: Goal-Corrected Partnerships (2 years onward):* The child is able to realize that his parents sometimes need to do other activities before attending to his needs or wants. He is able to take his parents' needs into consideration when they engage with him.

Ainsworth and the Strange Situation

Mary Ainsworth, whose research interests included assessing and classifying emotional security, joined Bowlby's research team in 1950 (Ainsworth & Bowlby, 1989). Her naturalistic observations of infants and mothers in both Uganda and the United States led to the development of the **strange situation**, an experimental procedure that assesses the **security of attachments** in children 10–24 months old (Ainsworth & Bell, 1970; Ainsworth, Blehar, Waters, & Wall, 1978). The strange situation is a series of episodes providing an experience of increasing distress for the child (episodes 2–8 each last 3 minutes). The strange situation sequence incorporates the child, the mother, and a stranger:

1. Mother, child, and stranger enter a room equipped with a one-way mirror for observation, and the stranger immediately leaves.
2. Mother and child are alone in room.
3. Stranger enters. Mother leaves after 3 minutes.
4. Child and stranger are alone in room.
5. Mother returns, stranger leaves. Mother leaves after 3 minutes.
6. Child is alone for 3 minutes.
7. Stranger returns and is alone with child.
8. Mother returns.

Ainsworth and her research colleagues identified three patterns of attachment, based on their observations of 1-year-olds in their natural home settings and in the strange situation. These patterns are determined by the child's behavior when the caregiver *returns*, not necessarily when the caregiver leaves: **secure attachment**, and two types of **insecure attachment**: avoidant attachment and ambivalent (resistant) attachment. Although children with a secure attachment to their caregivers may cry and show other signs of distress when the caregiver leaves, when the caregiver returns they allow themselves to be comforted by the caregiver and enjoy the caregiver's return. Those with **avoidant attachment** seem unaffected by whether their caregiver leaves or returns, showing little distress or enjoyment either way. Children who form an **ambivalent (resistant) attachment** become distressed before the caregiver leaves and demonstrate even higher levels of distress when the caregiver is absent. However, when the caregiver returns the child simultaneously seeks comfort and resists it by wriggling or kicking.

Main and Solomon (1990) identified a fourth, and least secure, pattern of attachment, called **disorganized-disoriented attachment**. Children who form this type of bond use a confused response style: They may look to the stranger instead of the mother for comfort, appear to enjoy the mother's return but then turn away, or seek out the mother without making eye contact.

Attachment to Mothers and Fathers

An infant is biologically designed to seek and form attachment relationships. His attachments to his mother and father are the most prevalent, but as discussed in the section on Multiple Attachments, they do not have to be the only ones. However, a stable attachment relationship early on is essential for the infant's optimal development. The newborn is wired to recognize a mother, and by 6 months the infant already shows a preference for one person. The 9-month-old infant continues to strengthen his bond with the primary attachment (usually his mother), and he is now actively distinguishing familiar from unfamiliar people. By the time he is 12 to 14 months of age, the toddler has solidified his bond with the primary attachment caregiver. Researchers using the strange situation usually use children who are around 1 year old, so that they can assess the type of attachment relationship that has formed (Bowlby, 2007).

It is now well known that depriving a toddler of close contact with his parents can have damaging psychological results. In the 1950s the toddlers and children that Bowlby first observed when they were in a hospital or residential nursery setting received only brief visits from parents during their stays of 10 days or more. Although they were physically well tended, the children experienced very limited contact with a parent to comfort them in their distress. The separation produced such feelings of helplessness, hopelessness, fear, and danger in these children that the impact of this psychological trauma negatively influenced many of them into adulthood (Ainsworth & Bowlby, 1989; Bowlby, 2007).

Attunement is the term used by researcher and psychiatrist Daniel Stern (1987) to describe the process cultivated by a nurturing, responsive parent in the journey toward building an attachment bond with the infant. The process of attunement consists of millions of small, but continuously repeated, exchanges between the parent and infant. During these exchanges, the parent conveys that the infant's emotions are understood and accepted, allowing the infant to feel emotionally connected and safe. In the example above—in which the infant is feeling distressed while being held awkwardly by a visitor—the parent engages in attunement by removing the infant and holding the baby close to the parent's body, as if to say, "I understand what that must be like for you to feel like you are falling." Misattunement occurs if the unresponsive parent allows the infant to wail in distress in the arms of the visitor. There are countless ways in which a parent can attune to the infant's emotional world, such as through the voice and body language: An infant in her parent's arms squeals with delight to see a cardinal land on a branch right outside the window, and the parent hugs the infant, matches the high-pitched squeal, and moves them both closer to the window. Stern (1987) videotaped hours of mothers with their infants and discovered that empathic mothers engage in about one attunement episode *per minute* when interacting with their infants. Stern asserts that these infinitely occurring moments of attunement—or misattunement—in infancy are more powerful than later experiences in childhood in forming the brain's basic lessons of emotional life, and that they guide the emotional expectations that the infant will then bring to adult relationships.

It is important for counselors to avoid making sweeping generalizations that the infant's mother is the primary object of attachment, that fathers play a secondary role, or that fathers are generally not as present in their infant's and toddler's lives as mothers are.

You will notice over the course of your counseling career that these dynamics will vary widely from family to family. Indeed, you may witness more and more fathers choosing to work as stay-at-home fathers, or if they do work outside of the home, they may be devoting more time to caring for their children than fathers have done in past generations. Galinsky, Aumann, and Bond's (2011) 2008 national study found that employed fathers today, compared to three decades ago, spend significantly *more* time with their children under 13 years of age per workday. Fathers today spend an average of 3 hours with their children on workdays, an increase of an hour from the 2 hours they spent in the 1970s. When further dividing this group of fathers into age ranges, one can see the trend toward younger fathers spending even more time: Millennial fathers today spend an average of 4.1 hours per workday with their children, whereas Gen-X fathers spend an average of 3.1 hours per workday with theirs. Although employed mothers in each age group still spend more time with their children than the fathers in the same age group, this study shows a promising trend in fathers being more available to form significant attachments with their children.

Ching-Yun, Chich-Hsiu, Te-Fu, Ching-Hsuch, and Chien-Yu (2012) investigated the process of fathers beginning to develop a sense of attachment to their children during pregnancy. Fathers who perceived that they had marital intimacy and their partners' support during pregnancy were the fathers who reported feeling attached to their newborns shortly after childbirth. Fathers perceiving their partner's support also predicted father–infant attachment during the first postpartum week (Mercer & Ferketich, 1990). Fathers who felt supported in their work and their family had a secure father–son attachment during their sons' first 10 months, compared to fathers who had less support (Belsky, 1996).

Multiple Attachments

Siblings

The sibling relationship has the potential to be a complex and significant one, depending on birth order, differences in ages, gender, culture, parenting styles, and a host of interconnecting family dynamics; siblings may play the roles of rival, mentor, helper, confidant, friend, supporter, and possibly many others. In sibling relationships, it is not uncommon for one child to feel that another child is receiving more affection from their parents and to develop a long-standing jealously of the other child as a result. Interestingly, there is a long-term effect for this dynamic; both the sibling who feels the jealously and the sibling who is considered to be the favored one are highly likely to form problematic romantic relationships as young adults (Rauer & Volling, 2007). In one study, the single most significant predictor of an adult's adjustment in late life was the closeness that the person felt to siblings (Vaillant & Vaillant, 1990). Barnes and Austin (1995) concluded that an individual's perception of warmth between self and siblings, more than perceptions of maternal warmth and responsiveness, is an effective predictor of self-esteem.

A novel study by Donley and Likins (2010) used Bowen's family systems theory (Kerr & Bowen, 1988) to study interactional patterns across two generations of siblings. The transmission of generational conflicts was very apparent: Siblings whose parents had tense relationships with their siblings a generation before tended to replicate the same tense relationship with their own siblings, as opposed to siblings whose parents had developed calm relationships with their siblings. In addition, the siblings whose parents had the tense sibling relationships tended to have conflictual relationships with their parents.

> **REFLECTION   6.3**   SIBLING ATTACHMENT
>
> A problem that my brother, Spencer, who has Down syndrome, faced at birth (when I was 3 years old) was that he did not open his eyes for almost two days after he was born. I have been told the story hundreds of times how the doctors and my parents tried to get him to open his eyes, but he would not until my Dad first brought me and my brothers in to visit my mom and the baby for the first time. I went to Spencer and started talking to him, and he *immediately* opened his eyes and looked at me! I can't explain why he decided to open his eyes after he first heard me, but it was the beginning of a very special bond that we have shared forever. My older brothers get along well with Spencer, but we have always been especially close. Spencer has been the greatest thing to ever happen to me and my family. I love him more than anything. [~Carley]
>
> Carley Grab

➤ CASE EXAMPLE **6.2** THE UNIQUE ATTACHMENT OF TWINS.

As you consider the following cases, what themes seem to be consistent from case to case? My wife, Danielle, and I have been making efforts to keep twins Boden and Kellan (20 months) together since birth. But one day Danielle took Kellan to the mall while I took Boden to the store. We usually push them around the mall or store in their side-by-side double stroller. Danielle noticed that Kellan spent most of the time at the mall pointing to the other side of the stroller and seemed bothered that his brother was not with him. [~Steve]

From the time my twins were infants, I always noticed their need to know where the other one was through physical touch. I have numerous pictures of them as babies holding each other's hands or lying close together in one crib. Other pictures show them with arms casually around each other's waists as they looked out the window or posed for a photo. One of the most dramatic illustrations of this need occurred when they were about 10 months old, and my younger twin was hospitalized due to an allergic reaction from an antibiotic. At the hospital, my husband tried to console Marc and get him to settle down and go to sleep, but he refused to be comforted. The nurse suggested that maybe he was missing his brother, so I brought Eric in and the four of us tried to settle in as best we could in the hospital room. At one point during the night I woke up, and there was Marc, lying at the edge of the crib, with his arm sticking through the slats holding the hand of his brother. [~Cathy]

I have always heard of the special bond between twins and have enjoyed observing my boys connect in a way that only twins can. From their first days of life, they have soothed and calmed each other. The younger of the two, Holden, spent some time in the hospital nursery after delivery. He had some fluid in his lungs and was demonstrating a low oxygen saturation level in his blood. While he was being monitored, we had his twin brother, Porter, in our room. Porter seemed unable to rest comfortably so we walked him down to the nursery to visit his brother. As soon as their bassinets were side by side, Porter relaxed and fell asleep, while Holden's low blood oxygenation level slowly increased to a higher and more stable level. Since this first demonstration of their powerful twin bond, we watch with pure delight as they babble back and forth to one another, gaze at each other with huge smiles on their faces, and link arms automatically when laid down side by side. [~Meghan]

Steve Bubnis

Grandparents

In the United States, many children have the opportunity to form attachments with their grandparents because they live in the same home. According to U.S. Census Bureau data, 7.5 million children were living with a grandparent in 2010, accounting for 10% of all children in the United States. Of these children, 4.9 million lived in the grandparent's home. There were 6.7 million grandparents with grandchildren under 18 living with them in 2009. Of these grandparents, 40% (2.7 million) were responsible for their grandchildren's basic needs, such as food, shelter, and clothing (U.S. Census Bureau, 2012b). Parents' increasing issues such as teen pregnancy, AIDS, child abuse and neglect, mental and physical illness, drug use, divorce, and parental incarceration are prompting more grandparents to take the lead role in parenting their grandchildren (Bryson & Casper, 1999).

Grandparents who take over custodial care of their grandchildren will likely become the child's primary attachment figure. However, this adjustment is often complicated for both grandparents and grandchildren (Connor, 2006). Children whose primary attachment relationship to their parents becomes disrupted by separation due to the parents' problems (such as incarceration) may experience distress similar to what Bowlby (1973) observed in toddlers and young children who had prolonged separation from their parents. Bowlby noticed that children's reaction to parental separation involved moving through stages of **protest**, **despair**, and **detachment**. During the *protest* stage, distress, fear, angry protests, desperate efforts to find the missing parent, and hopefulness that the parent would return characterized the children's behavior from the first several hours through the first week or more following separation. However, as the separation continued, children *despaired* and became increasingly hopeless that the parent would return. Eventually, children experienced *detachment* and withdrew from interacting with their environment. You can imagine what a challenge the custodial grandparents have ahead of them as they help children gain trust in them as a new secure attachment figure, especially if the children's relationship with the separated parents was an insecure one. Milan and Pinderhughes (2000) observed that children who were abused by their parents before separation may be so familiar with the style of mistreatment that they may deny or ignore negative information about the abusive parent during the separation process.

Custodial grandparents experience mixed feelings regarding their attachment to their grandchildren. Sixty-one percent of the grandparents in Dolbin-MacNab and Keiley's (2006) study reported positive feelings, such as joy from positively affecting their grandchildren and witnessing the children's accomplishments, and love from their grandchildren. They also reported that positive attributes in the relationship included their ability to provide a secure environment and to help their grandchildren overcome challenges. Other studies show similar feelings of satisfaction, including grandparents experiencing a greater sense of purpose in their lives (Waldrop & Weber, 2001; Weber & Waldrop, 2000). At the same time, grandparents identify issues that interfere with creating an emotionally close relationship, namely grandchildren's emotional and behavioral problems (Dolbin-MacNab & Keiley, 2006).

Children certainly do not have to live with or be cared for by their grandparents in order to maintain close contact with them and develop attachment relationships. Many grandparents are embracing their roles as responsive attachment figures in their grandchildren's lives. There are resources for grandparents to navigate this attachment process, such as the website Grandparents.com. The site is designed for the public to recognize and become more informed about the important grandparent–grandchild relationship, with articles such as "Have you bonded with your grandchild?"

An infant or toddler may form a secure attachment with a **professional nonparental caregiver** when a parent is not available. Research indicates that there are a variety of conditions that improve the chances of infants and toddlers forming a secure bond with a caregiver who is not their primary source of attachment. Children between 6 and 30 months are likely to experience stress and anxiety in a day care setting, unless they have one professional caregiver who is reliably available to them (Bowlby, 2007). When children in this age range are separated from their parents and are simultaneously put in unfamiliar surroundings, their brains trigger an "attachment-seeking response," which causes distress. In order for their brains to stop this response, they need to have a responsive caregiver nearby.

Goossens and van IJzendoom's (1990) study showed that even though professional caregivers were responding to several infants simultaneously, the infants did not have any more insecure attachments to their caregivers than they did with their parents. In some cases, even when the infant had insecure attachments to parents, the infant had formed a secure attachment to the caregiver. Compared to caregivers with whom infants formed insecure relationships, caregivers who appeared to be younger and who were more sensitive to the infants during their free play were the most likely to form secure attachments with infants. Ahnert, Pinquart, and Lamb (2006) found that when comparing center-based to home-based settings, the children in the center-based settings formed secure attachments to their caregiver more often when the individual was able to display group-oriented sensitivity (which is a separate skill from responding to each child individually), rather than demonstrating sensitivity to individual children. Clasien De Schipper, Tavecchio, and Van IJzendoorn (2008) discovered that the frequency of sensitive caregiving (i.e., the number of sensitive caregiving events throughout the day) also plays a role in the formation of attachments between toddlers and young children and their caregivers.

Infants and toddlers can also form attachments to security objects. Keira was given a monkey blanket that she named "Boy Monk" and took everywhere. When she was 1 year old, Keira accidentally dropped Boy Monk off of a dock into the ocean, necessitating that her father frantically grab a net and save Boy Monk from drifting out to sea. Renee, who showed features of being a nervous, anxious toddler, carried a paintbrush in her hand at all times to feel secure; she would fall asleep with it in her hand, and her parents had to creep back into her room to remove it so that she would not poke herself. When Henry was a toddler, he became enamored with clothes dryer lint. He could often be seen carrying baseball-sized balls of lint around with him, and I (Nadine) saved our dryer lint to give him when he came to visit.

Cultural Variations

Researchers comparing how children from various cultures respond to the strange situation have found that the proportion of securely attached children is relatively stable from country to country, with approximately two-thirds of the children in one study considered to have secure attachment. The main differences between cultures lay in the proportion of children in the various insecure attachment classifications (Sagi, van IJzendoorn, & Koren-Karie, 1991; Svanberg, 1998; van IJzendoorn, Bakermans-Kranenburg, & Sagi-Schwartz, 2006).

However, when considering attachment issues in other cultures, counselors need to be aware of inadvertently taking an ethnocentric approach (e.g., viewing other cultures through an American lens). What constitutes a securely attached child, and what constitutes responsive parenting, varies widely from culture to culture. These differences reflect deeply held cultural beliefs, which are often intertwined with the historically significant experiences of those cultures. In your counseling work with parents from different cultures, you may find that you will be a more culturally sensitive counselor when you invite the family to teach you about their particular cultural beliefs. For example, how does the family's culture define a secure attachment? An American mother tends to perceive her child as secure if he displays autonomy and self-reliance, spending time away from his mother and involved in independent activities (Rothbaum, Kakinuma, Nagaoka, & Azuma, 2007). Similarly, German parents view a secure child as one who is independent and self-sufficient (Grossmann, Grossman, Spangler, Suess, & Unzer, 1985). However, a Japanese mother would consider her child to be secure if he is compliant and obedient, demonstrating an attempt to work in harmony with others (Rothbaum et al., 2007).

Employment, Day Care, and Attachment

People sometimes speculate that the attachment between infant and mother may tend to be an insecure one when the infant is placed in day care because the mother works outside of the home. However, a large, longitudinal research project from the National Institute of Child Health and Human Development (NICHD) showed other, interesting results (Belsky, 2005; NICHD Early Child Care Research Network, 1997). The research revealed that both insensitive mothering and *not* placing of the infant in nonmaternal care were correlated with an insecure attachment between the child and mother. In addition, the following three characteristics amplified the already negative effect of insensitive mothering: (1) The nonmaternal care that was provided was poor; (2) the infant spent more than 10 hours per week in nonmaternal care; or (3) the child had been in more than one nonmaternal care placement during the first 15 months of life.

Temperament Development

What is temperament? Let's begin by considering Angie's experiences with her two children.

Temperament is a concept for which many researchers have offered definitions. At a roundtable meeting of several well-known researchers in the field of temperament (i.e., Buss, Plomin, Thomas, Chess, Rothbart, Goldsmith), each with their own particular definition of temperament, a synthesis of their major elements was offered:

> Temperament consists of relatively consistent basic dispositions inherent in the person that underlie and modulate the expression of activity, reactivity, emotionality, and sociability. Major elements of temperament are present early in life, and those elements are likely to

be strongly influenced by biological factors. As development proceeds, the expression of temperament increasingly becomes more influenced by experience and context. (Goldsmith et al., 1987, p. 524)

Thomas and Chess (1977), in their classic New York Longitudinal Study (NYLS) of infant and childhood temperament in which they followed 141 infants in 1956 into their adult years, generated **nine categories of temperament**. Think of an infant or a toddler you know fairly well. Using Thomas and Chess' nine categories and constellations below as a guide, consider your impressions of that child in the following areas:

1. *Activity Level:* What proportion of time each day is the child active versus inactive?
2. *Rhythmicity (Regularity):* How predictable or unpredictable are the child's sleep–wake cycle, hunger, feeding pattern, and elimination schedule?
3. *Approach or Withdrawal:* How does the child respond to a new stimulus? Does the child have an approach response such as smiling, reaching for a new toy, moving toward an object, or swallowing a new food? Or does the child have a withdrawal response, such as crying, pushing a new toy away, spitting out a new food, or moving away from an object?
4. *Adaptability:* How easily does the child adjust to new situations?
5. *Threshold of Responsiveness:* How intense does the level of sensory, environmental, or social stimulation need to be in order for the child to make a response that you can observe?
6. *Intensity or Reaction:* When the child does respond to a stimulus, what is the energy level of the response?
7. *Quality of Mood:* What is the ratio of pleasant, joyful, and friendly behaviors to unpleasant, crying, or unfriendly behaviors?
8. *Distractibility:* How easily does the child allow irrelevant environmental stimuli to interfere with what the child is doing?
9. *Attention Span and Persistence:* For how long does the child involve himself or herself in a certain activity (attention span)? How well does the child continue a behavior, or continue to take steps to pursue an activity, when confronted with obstacles (persistence)?

The Stability of Temperament

Can a child's biologically based temperament be altered by experience, especially if it is a temperament that may lead to behavioral and adjustment problems? Or will a child's initially observed temperament remain stable throughout the course of the person's life? The answer: It depends. Change in the child's expression of temperament can occur if he is provided with specific nurturing experiences that will change the brain's synaptic connections over time. Without intervention on the part of counselors and parents, children who have been identified with a particular type of temperament at an early age tend to maintain that temperament as a stable characteristic for years to follow.

The developmental psychologist Jerome Kagan, who has researched temperament and stability extensively, identified four types of temperaments: timid, bold, upbeat, and melancholy, each type a result of different patterns of brain activity, based on inborn differences in brain circuitry (Goleman, 1995). A longitudinal study of two groups of toddlers who, when first observed at either 21 or 31 months, were categorized as either extremely cautious and shy (inhibited) or fearless and outgoing (uninhibited) showed that these temperaments remained consistent through their sixth year (Kagan et al., 1987).

> When the reticent toddlers were holding back from playing, heart rate monitors showed that their hearts were racing with anxiety. That easily aroused anxiety seems to underlie their lifelong timidity: they treat any new person or situation as though it were a potential threat. (Goleman, 1995, p. 217)

REFLECTION 6.4 STABILITY OF TEMPERAMENT

While my infant son appeared to enjoy the comfort and security of socializing with people, Emma's happiness seemed to come from her physical accomplishments. She reached all of her physical milestones early and became significantly happier with each newfound skill. She walked unexpectedly on her first attempt at 8 months and would perform unbelievable feats like balancing on a sewing machine case (sloped with a handle in the middle) with her eyes closed before her first birthday. In contrast, her brother Kadin reluctantly let go of the coffee table to walk at 13 months. These behaviors should not have been a surprise looking back on my pregnancies; my son moved like an active fish while my daughter moved like a cat-not-declawed performing martial arts inside of me. Needless to say, it is interesting to watch how their temperaments help shape their lives. [~Angie]

Angie Mahlandt

See Measuring Temperament for more about differences in these children's physiological functioning related to their brain's amygdalar responses.

Schwartz, Wright, Shin, Kagan, and Rauch (2003) demonstrated the stability of inhibited and uninhibited temperaments into adulthood and also showed how the brains of inhibited and uninhibited people work differently. Both inhibited and uninhibited adults, who years before had been categorized with their respective temperaments when they were toddlers in their second year, were tested with an fMRI (functional magnetic resonance imaging, a noninvasive scanning technique for measuring brain activity) to assess their brains' amygdalar responses to novel versus familiar faces. Inhibited adults showed a significantly greater response (fMRI signal increase) to novel faces in both their right and left amygdalae compared to uninhibited adults.

Remember Angie, the mother of children who displayed different early temperament traits? In Reflection 6.4, she describes her children's stability of temperament. Using Kagan's four types of temperaments, might we characterize her son as more "upbeat" and her daughter as more "bold"?

An important implication for counselors is that the signs of an inhibited temperament can be detected very early in life. If left untreated, it is highly probable that the child may develop shyness, social anxiety, and depression as she matures, even into adulthood (Moehler et al., 2008). Four-month-old infants who cried in response to novel visual and auditory stimuli presented in a laboratory setting developed into toddlers who were categorized as having an inhibited temperament at 14 months. The children were assessed for inhibition as toddlers (at 14 months) by exposure to situations that were novel but not frightening. Some of the novel situations to which the toddlers were exposed included asking the child to dunk her finger in small cups of water, red liquid, and black liquid; inviting the child to play with a large moving toy robot that made noise; and showing the child a puppet theatre where a friendly and an unfriendly puppet each spoke to the child. The correlation between the two assessments of the child was so strong that infant *crying reactivity* at 4 months old is a *significant predictor of behavioral inhibition* at 14 months (Moehler et al., 2008). The encouraging news is that even brief interventions with inhibited preschoolers have been effective in reducing their symptoms of inhibition and anxiety (Rapee, Kennedy, Ingram, Edwards, & Sweeney, 2005). Moehler et al.'s (2008) study is good evidence that if you work with a family that has an inhibited toddler, you may want to begin planning interventions with parents and the child during the toddler years and not wait until the child is approaching preschool age.

"Temperament is not destiny" (Goleman, 1995, p. 215). As a counselor, you play a vital role in helping parents to notice and identify patterns in their parenting style that may be reinforcing an inhibited child to remain inhibited. You are assisting parents in helping their child to literally reshape the wiring of their child's brain. The neural circuitry can be reformed over time, and while the emotional brain will always respond with a reaction to a perceived threat, the child can be taught to shorten the time it takes for the thinking brain to intervene with a message that is more functional, so that the child can maneuver confidently and competently in novel and social situations. When parents put "gentle pressure" on their timid children to encourage them to be more outgoing, it was found that the child's temperament could change over time; however, overprotective parenting maintains an inhibited child's response, since the child does not learn how to calm down when faced with unfamiliar situations. As Goleman (1995, p. 228) says, "Much psychotherapy is, in a sense, a remedial tutorial for what was skewed or missed completely earlier in life."

Measuring Temperament

Researchers measure temperament using a variety of assessments. Parents, day care providers, and preschool teachers can be asked to complete **surveys**, **questionnaires**, or **interviews** regarding their observations of the child's behaviors over time. One well-established parent questionnaire is the *Infant Behavior Questionnaire–Revised* (IBQ-R; Gartstein & Rothbart, 2003). The IBQ-R, based on Rothbart and Derryberry's definition of temperament, is a 191-item parent-report instrument. The IRB-R generates 14 scales that group into three overarching factors:

1. *Positive Emotionality/Surgency:* Activity Level, Smiling and Laughter, Vocal Reactivity, Approach, High Intensity Pleasure, and Perceptual Sensitivity.
2. *Negative Affectivity:* Fear, Distress to Limitations, Sadness, and negatively loading Falling Reactivity.
3. *Regulatory Capacity/Orienting:* Duration of Orienting, Soothability, Cuddliness/Affiliation, and Low Intensity Pleasure.

While using only a parent's report of their child to study temperament may seem biased or inaccurate, studies do show that parental reports of child temperament have superior predictive validity when substantiated by other sources of data about the child's temperament, such as structured observations (Hart, Field, & Roitfarb, 1999; Pauli-Pott, Mertesacker, & Beckmann, 2004).

➤ CASE EXAMPLE **6.3** MOTHERS' OBSERVATIONS OF CHILDREN'S TEMPERAMENT.

After reading the parent observations below, what are your initial impressions of each child's temperament from the mother's perspective?

Sienna: On weekend mornings my husband and I typically get our 2-year-old daughter, Sienna, out of her crib and then "gate" the stairway so she can play in her room as she pleases while we try to enjoy a bit more of our Saturday morning from our bed. This particular morning we must have forgotten to put the gate up, and once my husband and I noticed the unusual lull upstairs we quickly got up to investigate what mischief Sienna had gotten herself into. As I peered down the stairs I saw my daughter holding something that looked like poop. I immediately flew downstairs and found that she had gone into the refrigerator and helped herself to our doggie bag from the night before . . . and there she sat, on the floor watching TV, a fillet mignon in one hand and lobster ravioli in the other. The most unbelievable part of this story is that my child was actually eating something other than fruit or bread! Apparently the meals we had been offering her weren't fancy enough for her liking! [~Sharyn]

Owen: When Owen was 16 months old, he loved to talk, entertain, go to the store, and drop off his siblings at school. When anyone would pass by he would smile brightly and say "Hi!" At the library, Owen saw a cardboard cutout of a child reading. In his excitement, he ran past and shouted "Hi!" to the cutout. He quickly realized the child did not return a glance and he ran back to try again. When the cutout still did not move, Owen shrugged and ran off to find his story time club. [~Susanne]

Elijah: As an infant, Elijah would not be content to "be" on his own. He insisted on being nestled in the cloth baby sling slung over my body at every possible hour. As a toddler, he was given the nickname "my Velcro child," because it was as if he was velcroed to my hip at all hours of the day and night. [~Karen]

Keegan: My oldest son, who is now 15 years old, was and is a very strong, independent individual and has generally done things his own way. And yet he is and has been a sensitive individual. When he was just 18 months old we would look at photos together, but unfortunately he would just start crying even if it was a photo of the two of us. Of course, we stopped looking at photos because it upset him. We also had to lay down our standing picture frames because if he stopped to look at one of them he would again begin to cry. [~Karen]

Juliana: Simple explanations were rarely beneficial to Juliana. We have always had to do what seemed like over-explaining to appease her type-A personality. She just has that feeling of needing to understand the why of things. Subsequently, she also feels the need to constantly explain things and hasn't stopped for many breathers since. Her life is practically a musical. When she is playing she usually is narrating what she is doing in song. She craves structure and control. Potty training was done via a method of implementing a routine of when she was required to try to go, because that's what worked for her brain. She was trained before 2 years even though she never showed any initial signs of caring that she was wet or telling me on her own when she had to go. But once she got a hold of what was expected, that's just the way things were "supposed" to be, and so she operated by that. [~Becca]

Megan: Megan is very adventurous and would run immediately into any social situation without any hesitation. She is a risk-taker, and would slide down a sliding board headfirst at 2 years old. I was always a nervous wreck watching her, wondering what body part she was going to injure! Megan loves to get other people's reactions to her antics and if they laugh at her, that encourages her even more. [~Angi]

Joelle: As a toddler, Joelle took to any female and would instantly look to socialize with her. One day when she was about 3 years old, we were walking through the grocery store when she spotted two young girls around the ages of 8 and 10 years old. Without hesitation, she went running up to them and began to have a conversation as if she was their sister. Of course, the two girls were a bit confused, but my daughter was elated! [~Karen]

Temperament can also be measured in a laboratory setting. At the University of Melbourne, researchers used parent-completed questionnaires as well as **videotaped playroom observations** in the Social Development Laboratory. During the laboratory visits, 2-year-olds—in the company of their parents—were challenged with novel situations including the appearance of a clown, unusual and noisy toys, a brief separation from the parent, and playing with an unfamiliar child and his/her parent (Hemphill & Sanson, 2001).

Kagan et al. (1987) also used multiple measures in a laboratory setting to assess the differences between inhibited and uninhibited children. Researchers observed how children, beginning at 21 or 31 months (and reassessed a couple of years later), reacted to an unfamiliar female examiner and unfamiliar toys, a talking robot, and a temporary separation from the mother. Children were classified as inhibited if they avoided playing with the unfamiliar people and objects, stayed close to the mother, and stopped playing and vocalizing. The following **physiological responses** were also measured to assess the excitability of the child's amygdala under novel and potentially stressful situations: (1) *heart rate*—inhibited children show higher heart rates than uninhibited children, and their heart rate remains high compared with the fluctuations in heart rates for uninhibited children; (2) *pupillary dilation*—inhibited children have greater pupillary diameter than uninhibited children when they are asked to perform a cognitive task; (3) *norepinephrine level from a urine sample*—norepinephrine is a primary neurotransmitter in the sympathetic nervous system, and it appears in elevated levels in inhibited 4- and 5½-year-old children, but not significantly in inhibited toddlers; (4) *muscle tension*—assessed by measuring whether the child's voice has variability in pitch (a fearful child will have more muscle tension and less variability in vocal pitch); and (5) *cortisol*—some inhibited 5½-year-old children have higher levels of this stress hormone in their saliva than uninhibited children.

Temperament and Child Rearing

If you have ever watched the interaction between a toddler and her father and said to yourself, "Wow, those two really work well together!" you have had a glimpse of what Chess and Thomas (1996) called **goodness of fit**. Chess and Thomas, emphasizing the nature of the specific parent–child interactional process, described goodness of fit as a "two-way street, in which a child's temperament and other characteristics could influence the parent's attitude and behavior, as much as the parent's functioning could influence the child's behavior" (p. 52).

This doesn't mean that during your observation of father and daughter that both parties were always agreeing with what the other one was saying or doing, but rather that the parenting style was a good match for the child's temperament. For example, a toddler with an exuberant, adventurous temperament, one who enjoys novel situations and going outside to explore in all kinds of weather, would benefit from a parent who is willing to don waterproof gear and take her for a rain walk, reveling along with her to find the deepest puddles to jump in. "Goodness of fit results when the organism's capabilities, motivations, and style of behavior and the environmental demands and expectations are in accord" (Chess & Thomas, 1996, p. 52).

While working with children identified with behavioral disorders and their families from their New York Longitudinal Study (NYLS) of temperament, Chess and Thomas (1996) saw first-hand the consequences for children who were raised in an environment of consonance versus those who were raised in an environment of dissonance. **Consonance** ("goodness of fit," a good match) between the organism (the child) and the environment (parenting) supports the child's optimal positive development. However, **dissonance** ("poorness of fit," a mismatch) between the organism's capabilities and characteristics and the environment's opportunities and demands can result in maladaptive functioning and distorted development.

As a counselor, you will certainly witness numerous examples during your career of both consonance and dissonance in parent–child interactions. You will likely see unhealthy, dissonant parental responses to their children, which correlate to their children's behavioral disorders. You will be directly involved with parents in helping them to create a **parent guidance treatment program**. Counselors may echo Chess and Thomas' (1996) recommendations that it is essential to concretely identify the behavioral and attitudinal changes of the *parents* that will decrease unhealthy parent–child interactions while promoting healthy relationships. A treatment program would focus on changing parents' behavior and overtly expressed attitudes toward the child. The goal would be to change specific aspects of parents' *actual functioning* with their child, not necessarily the parents' own anxieties and conflicts. However, Chess and Thomas note that parents may end up making positive changes in their own personal anxieties and conflicts related to their child as a result of parent guidance.

What type of match between parent and child results in a goodness of fit or poorness of fit? Hemphill and Sanson (2001) conducted a longitudinal study, the Social Development Project, which investigated how the match between the toddler's temperament and the parent's style of parenting when the toddler was 2 years old related to the child's behavioral problems at 4 years. Pause for a moment to think about a child–parent relationship that you know, and then as you read on, relate how their interaction connects to the information in this section and to the findings of the study. The aspects of the *toddler's temperament* (Rothbart & Bates, 2006) under consideration were:

- *Negative reactivity:* Does the child display high-intensity negative reactions, such as irritability and whining?
- *Approach/inhibition:* Does the child approach novel situations and people or is the child wary of this type of stimulation and withdraw instead?
- *Persistence:* Does the child stay with an activity for a sustained amount of time?

The aspects of *parenting styles* under consideration were:

- *Parental warmth:* Does the parent display high parental warmth, verbally and physically showing affection, praise, and acceptance, or does the parent display low parental warmth, rejecting the child through criticism and disapproval?
- *Punishment:* Does the parent try to overpower the child with harsh, high-intensity discipline strategies such as physical punishments, direct commands, or threats?
- *Inductive reasoning:* Does the parent help the child to understand the child's behavior by explaining the consequences of misbehavior, setting limits, and giving the child input into disciplinary decisions?

Think About It 6.1 Goodness of Fit

What do you notice about the child's temperament, the parenting style, and the goodness of fit in the following scenario?

Chloe entered the world as a bubbly and gregarious baby. There were friends and family members who worried that prolonged nursing, constant holding, and "being there" 24/7 would bring about clinginess and over-dependence, but I knew that I was helping Chloe develop confidence, independence, and a sense of security with which to approach the world. In spite of people who thought she was too attached to me in those first two years of life, I knew we were building a bond of trust. She never suffered from separation anxiety when she began preschool at 2½ years. Instead, she was incredibly eager to meet new people and enjoy new experiences.

Chloe has been able to embrace new situations with confidence because of the trust she feels between us. This goes back to learning how to read her cues as an infant. Instead of putting her on our schedule, we sought to discover what her rhythms were. While my pediatrician and some family members thought her feedings were way too long, and "should" be accomplished within a specified time, I knew my daughter was a slow eater and there was no rushing her. While feeding her with a bottle would have been far more convenient, I knew the incredible benefits of nursing, and continued to do so until she was 16 months. Instead of seeing her crying as some sort of manipulation, we knew that she was trying to tell us something and it was our job to figure it out as best we could. Letting a baby "cry it out" never felt right to us. While I loved the idea of "wearing" her, unfortunately my back could not handle this after a C-section. But my husband would often put her in the carrier and hold her close to him. In spite of being unable to carry her close to me in a sling, my daughter accompanied me everywhere. From airplane trips to swim classes, library time to Music Together, she was constantly being exposed to new people and stimulating environments that were age appropriate and very hands-on. She adores people of all ages, and they are drawn to her. [~Lynn]

Lynn Donnavan

Parents and toddlers were videotaped in the Social Development Lab playroom to observe parents' interactions with their toddler (e.g., did they comfort, control, encourage, or play with their child?) and the toddler's interaction with the parent and other children (e.g., did the child stay close to the parent, disobey the parent, show persistence in activities, watch, join, or hurt other children) (Hemphill & Sanson, 2001)? A toddler whose temperament is high in **negative reactivity** is at the greatest risk for developing behavioral problems when the parent's style is either high in **punishment**, low in **parental warmth**, or low in **inductive reasoning**. An outgoing toddler whose temperament is high in **approach** behaviors is more likely than other children to have behavioral problems at 4 years of age if the parenting style is high in punishment; conversely, if a parent of a highly outgoing toddler channels the child's energy in positive directions, the child has a better chance of being well adjusted. A toddler with an **inhibited** temperament does not usually develop overt, "acting out" behavioral problems; however, a parenting style that is overprotective may result in an older child who is socially withdrawn, anxious, and fearful (Hemphill & Sanson, 2001).

Cultural Variations in Temperament

As we have seen, an infant's temperament has a biological component that is deeply rooted in his brain's stress-response system. But what could account for cross-cultural research on infant temperament? For example: (1) Taiwanese parents consider their infants to have higher levels of intensity and negative mood compared to the level that American parents consider their own infants to possess (Hsu, Soong, Stigler, Hong, & Liang, 1981); (2) American parents report more frequent examples of their infants' positive emotions compared to Russian parents, who report more frequent examples of negative ones

(Gartstein, Slobodskaya, & Kinsht, 2003); (3) researchers observed 4-month-old American infants demonstrate more motor activity and more distress than their Irish infant peers, but Chinese infants were less active and distressed than either their American or Irish age mates (Kagan et al., 1994). What accounts for these observations?

The culture in which an infant is raised, with values, practices, and socio-political issues that are different from another culture, influences which of the infant's temperament characteristics are reinforced or discouraged. Parents are the ambassadors of their culture, helping to shape their infant's temperament responses to the world, based on how well those responses will be received in their particular cultural setting.

When considering cross-cultural research, Super and Harkness (1986) developed a framework that took into account a variety of interrelating cultural influences: customs, settings available to the child, parents' attitudes, child-rearing practices, and perceptions of child temperament. Cross-cultural research on infant temperament often considers whether a culture has an individualistic or collectivistic orientation, and whether it is an Eastern or Western culture. **Individualistic** cultures tend to value the needs of the individual, are concerned with personal profit, and emphasize individual expression, whereas **collectivistic** cultures primarily consider the needs of the group, are concerned with responsibilities to the group, and have beliefs that are harmonious with others (Triandis, 1988).

Gartstein, Slobodskaya, Zylicz, Gosztyla, and Nakagawa (2010), using the Infant Behavior Questionnaire–Revised (IBQ-R) (described in the section Measuring Temperament), studied temperament among 3- to 12-month-old infants in United States (Western/individualistic), Polish (Western/mix of individualistic and collectivistic), Russian (Eastern/mix of individualistic and collectivistic), and Japanese (Eastern/collectivistic) cultures. Reliability and validity of scores on the IBQ-R has been substantiated from different cultural samples. The study yielded significant cultural differences. U.S. and Polish infants demonstrated the highest levels of Smiling and Laughing and High Intensity Pleasure. U.S. infants had significantly higher levels of Vocal Reactivity than Russian and Japanese infants. Japanese and Russian infants had the two highest levels of Fear compared to lower levels among U.S. and Polish infants.

Cross-cultural infant research from Gartstein et al. (2006), using an earlier form of the Infant Behavior Questionnaire (IBQ), measured temperament in 3-, 6-, 9-, and 12-month-old infants from the People's Republic of China (Eastern/collectivistic), the United States (Western/individualistic), and Spain (Western/collectivistic). Chinese infants were rated as significantly more fearful than U.S. infants. Compared to U.S. and Spanish infants, Chinese infants were also rated as most active, had the most distress to limitations, and had the highest scores on duration of orienting and soothability. Compared to the Spanish infants, U.S. infants had higher levels of stability for smiling and laughing over time. Infants from Spain demonstrated a greater stability for fear between 3 and 9 months than did their Chinese counterparts. The study yielded greater differences between cultures on the Eastern/Western distinction, rather than the collectivist/individualistic dimension.

SECTION II: Social Development

Developing the "Self System"

The infant's and toddler's odyssey through self-awareness, knowing that the child is a "differentiated and unique entity in the world" (Rochat, 2003, p. 717), begins at birth, and as with all developmental areas during this age span, it is a continually unfolding process. To develop this sense of self, the child needs to be consciously aware of her mental and bodily states, such as emotions, intentions for actions, perceptions, attitudes, and opinions

(Geangu, 2008). A newborn comes into the world with **implicit** awareness, meaning that she can demonstrate her sense of self by expressing her perceptions and actions, but she cannot yet use symbolic meaning—such as words—to convey self-awareness (Rochat, 2003). Rochat proposed five levels of awareness, from birth to age 4 or 5 years. A newborn has **Level 1 self-awareness (self-world differentiation)**; the infant can differentiate someone else's index finger touching the cheek from the infant's own hand touching her cheek (Rochat & Hespos, 1997). When an examiner touches the infant, the infant engages in more rooting responses (turning the head with the mouth open) than when the infant spontaneously touches herself. The newborn comes into the world predisposed to make a distinction between the world outside the infant and the infants own body and actions.

By the end of 2 months, the infant has added **Level 2 self-awareness (situated self)** to self–world differentiation ability. Now sensing how one's own body is situated in relation to other entities in the environment (Rochat, 2003), the infant systematically copies an adult who sticks out the tongue and pulls it to the left or the right (Meltzoff & Moore, 1992). The infant's ability to map her own bodily space to the bodily space of the adult shows that she is able to situate herself in relation to the other person (Rochat, 2003).

By 18 months, a toddler shows signs of beginning to use **explicit self-awareness**; the infant can now symbolically represent *self-recognition* of the infant's own body. In Amsterdam's (1972) classic rouge experiment, which has been replicated for 40 years, researchers secretly place a dot of rouge on the faces of 6–24-month-old infants, and then the infants are placed in front of a mirror. In similar studies, a yellow Post-it note is placed on the forehead (Povinelli, 1995). Unlike younger infants and toddlers, the 18-month-old will touch his face to access the rouge, or pull the Post-it sticker off of the forehead, neither of which can be seen unless the infant looks in the mirror. The toddler is demonstrating identification of the entity in the mirror as standing in for a representation of self. The toddler is now manifesting recognition of self, indicating the addition of **Level 3 self-awareness (identification)** development (Rochat, 2003).

By 20 to 24 months, the toddler begins to use the first-person pronouns "I," "Me," and "Mine," providing further evidence of her explicit self-awareness (Lewis, 1997). Between 24 and 28 months, and sometimes as young as 18 months, the toddler understands the concept of *ownership,* showing self-continuity and self-perception as a separate being from others. **Self-continuity** (also called the **extended self**) is a type of self-knowledge in which the toddler is self-aware of existing as a continuous being outside of the present moment, that the infant existed in the past, and that the infant will continue to exist into the future. Using the concept of ownership (being able to identify whether an item belongs to her or to someone else), the toddler is able to distinguish a toothbrush, book, block, shoe, and artwork from those that belong to other people (Fasig, 2000).

Effortful Control and Self-Regulation/Self-Control

Imagine observing two older toddlers who are sensing an itch inside their noses. One toddler immediately sticks his finger up his nose (much to the chagrin of adults watching!), and the other toddler runs to his father and asks for a tissue. What accounts for the difference between the first child's immediate reaction to use his finger to take care of the problem, and the second child using a different plan of action? Effortful control. Rothbart and Rueda (2005) define **effortful control** as "the ability to inhibit a dominant response to perform a subdominant response, to detect errors, and to engage in planning" (p. 3). In our example above, assuming that both children have been taught by their fathers to ask for a tissue when they feel something in their nose, toddler number 1 is not practicing effortful control, because he is not able to inhibit the *dominant response* (the overwhelming urge to stick his finger up his nose). Toddler number 2 also has the urge to perform the same action, but he performs a *subdominant response* (waiting to take care of the itch until his father can hand him a tissue to use instead of his finger). Toddler number 2 also engages in a measure of planning, knowing that he could run to his father and ask for a tissue, and then doing it.

Effortful control begins to emerge at the end of the toddler's first year and continues to develop throughout early childhood (Rothbart & Rueda, 2005). Infants and toddlers have to practice engaging in effortful control as a foundation for developing self-regulation. **Self-regulation** (or self-control) is the ability to control reactions to stress, maintain focused attention, and interpret mental states in oneself and others (Fonagy & Target, 2002). Self-regulation is of paramount importance because it affects the quality of children's social interactions, their capacity for learning, and the way that adults respond to them, as adults may respond negatively to children who do not make steady improvements in self-regulation as they mature (Eisenberg, 2012).

Researchers have evaluated five skills in children from 9 to 66 months that require suppressing a dominant response to perform a subdominant response. These skills consist of *delay*, such as waiting for candy that is sitting under a transparent cup; *slowing motor activity*, such as asking the child to draw a line slowly; *suppressing and initiating responses to changing signals*, like those used in "go-no-go" games; *effortful attention*, assessing whether the child can recognize small shapes hidden within a dominant large shape; and *lowering the voice* (Kochanska, Murray, & Coy, 1997; Kochanska, Murray, & Harlan, 2000; Kochanska, Murray, Jacques, Koenig, & Vandegeest, 1996). By 2½ years, a toddler's performance is consistent across the five skills, showing the level of control that the toddler is able to muster (Kochanska et al., 2000).

The encouraging news for counselors to share with parents is that while their child's initial level of effortful control has a biological basis, parents are at the forefront of helping their children improve this crucial skill. Research demonstrates the connection between nurturing experiences during the early years of life and higher levels of effortful control, as parenting style is a strong predictor of the child's level of effortful control. Children who receive warm, supportive parenting achieve higher levels of effortful control than children who experience cold, directive parenting (Eisenberg, 2012). **Positive parent–child relationships** that promote self-regulation positively affect children's ability to learn at school and simultaneously lower the child's risk of developing deviant behaviors or other adjustment problems (Vazsonyi & Huang, 2010).

When toddlers are upset and begin to show distress nonverbally, parents and teachers will often say, "Use your words" to express themselves. Vallotton and Ayoub (2010) discovered that this phrase has merit in the development of self-regulation. A longitudinal study of 120 toddlers, in which data was collected when the toddlers were 14, 24, and 36 months, revealed that a toddler's spoken vocabulary (not talkativeness) is a predictor of self-regulation growth in toddlers. Bridgett et al. (2010) demonstrated the value of self-regulation by following infants from 4 months until they were toddlers at 18 months. Mothers who themselves practiced a high level of effortful control spent more time in interactive caregiving activities with their infants, contributing to higher levels of effortful control in their toddlers.

Drawing on techniques taught to parents through the organization Resources for Infant Educarers (RIE), Elliot and Gonzalez-Mena (2011) offer the following strategies to foster positive parent–child relationships that may lead to improved self-regulation:

1. Provide predictability.
2. Help children develop awareness and acceptance of their feelings.
3. Encourage infants and toddlers to focus and pay attention by involving them in caregiving routines.
4. Help infants and toddlers understand perspectives other than their own.
5. Support infants and toddlers in handling prohibitions (explaining what they are allowed to do in addition to letting them know what they are not allowed to do).

Social Referencing

At some point in their development, infants begin to engage in **social referencing**, or using the emotional expressions of others to decipher unfamiliar events (Campos & Stenberg, 1981). An infant will look to the caregiver to decide how to feel and act, especially tuning in to whether the expressions from the caregiver are encouraging or discouraging. In the laboratory setting, the use of social referencing influences the behavior of infants during the **visual cliff** experiments: Infants who can already crawl look to their mothers' expressions for guidance as to whether or not to crawl over the visual cliff (Striano, Stahl, & Cleveland, 2009). In one study, when mothers standing at the opposite end of the cliff expressed joy, 75% of the infants willingly crossed the cliff; however, for the mothers who were asked to express fear, none of the infants crossed (Sorce, Emde, Campos, & Klinnert, 1985).

Although you might think that all infants would be attracted to a novel toy, when mothers show or voice disgust toward unusual toys, infants not only refuse to play with the toys in the moment but will still avoid them when they are presented again a few minutes later, even if the mothers display neutral or silent expressions the second time (Hornik, Risenhoover, & Gunnar, 1987). The counseling implications of social referencing are endless when considering how to help parents realize the power their expressions hold in guiding and shaping their children's attitudes and behavior. Consider the countless times that infants are interpreting their parents' expressions when reacting to strangers, trying new foods, entering an unfamiliar setting, or approaching unfamiliar pets!

When does social referencing begin? The answer is no longer clear. Research literature on social referencing has historically pointed to this development beginning between 7 and 9 months. However, a study by Hoel et al. (2008) shows that social referencing may begin as early as 3 months! The infants watched adults displaying either a fearful or a neutral face in response to looking at certain objects. An electroencephalogram (EEG) cap on the infants' heads detected that when 3-month-old infants saw adults make a fearful expression, their brain activity increased, and they looked more at the objects that provoked fear on the adult faces. Once again, the amygdala is hard at work, with a threat detection system that senses fearful expressions and also notices in what direction an angry or fearful face is looking.

Socialization

Socializing Emotions

"It takes a village to raise a child." This frequently-quoted proverb speaks to the social nature of infants' and toddlers' development, in that many social influences—not only those inside the home environment—will shape the child's understanding of how emotions and society intersect. As humans, we are emotionally hardwired beings who also need to figure out in our early years how to cognitively regulate our emotions to join the fabric of our society. In more good news for parents, Rothbart asserted:

> . . . people are not always at the mercy of affect. Using effortful control, people can more flexibly approach situations they fear and inhibit actions they desire. The efficiency of control, however, will depend on the strength of the emotional processes against which effort is exerted. (Rothbart & Rueda, 2005, p. 3)

Panksepp (2001) described how emotions are the foundations for social and cognitive abilities, and how emotions become socialized: As an infant projects his emotions out into the world, the cognitive structures of his brain provide feedback to regulate the emotional systems, based on how his responses were received by his environment. The emotional

REFLECTION 6.5 SOCIALIZING EMOTIONS

At 16 months, my daughter, Izzie, still doesn't fully understand how she affects others. She is in a hitting phase right now. One evening, she wanted to color. I told her that I needed to change her diaper first. As I laid her down on her changing table, she smacked me in the face. I took her hands and said, "Don't hit Mommy, it hurts." When I let go of her hands, she hit me again. I took her hands and said, "If you want to color, you need to be nice to Mommy." When I let go again, she stroked my face gently. She understands that she is not supposed to hit, but is not concerned about how it hurts others, only how it impacts her.

On the other hand, my son, MJ, is almost 2½ years old and has a much deeper understanding of how his actions affect other people. If he accidentally knocks his sister down, he will always ask her if she is okay. When Izzie hits him, he doesn't hit her back. He tells her, "No hit, Izzie! That's not nice. You hurt me!"

He is capable of generalizing his understanding beyond himself and other people too. I stepped on a bee on our porch. MJ looked at me and said, "Mommy! Don't hurt the bug! You stepped on it!!" He walked over and looked at the bee with such concern that it was very difficult for me not to laugh. [~Meghan]

Meghan Smith

systems then assign values to these environmental events. Over time, this relationship between emotions and cognitions organizes the psychic script for his life.

Socializing a toddler's emotions by helping the child to develop effortful control is an investment with visible results as the child matures. High levels of effortful control in 6–7-year-olds correlate with high levels of empathy and guilt and low levels of aggressiveness (Rothbart, Ahadi, & Hershey, 1994). **Empathy**, the ability to understand the feelings of others by interpreting signals of distress or pleasure, may be supported by effortful control. Watching a sad face activates the amygdala, but the child who has effortful control is able to attend to the thoughts and feelings of the other person without becoming overwhelmed by her own feelings of distress (Rothbart & Rueda, 2005). Effortful control may play a role in **guilt** by allowing the child to pay attention to the feelings of responsibility when actions have resulted in negative consequences (Derryberry & Reed, 1996).

Play and Social Skills

Harper and Rowan are playing hide and seek. Rowan, 2 years old, is the seeker. She says, "1, 2, 3, 5, 6, 18, 9, 10, 80. Weady not, I tome!" Infant and toddler play is a rapidly morphing landscape, marked by changes in the child's physical, cognitive, emotional, and social domains of development. Play simultaneously reflects the particular developmental stage of the child and provides stimulation to nurture the next frontier of development. An activity that is considered to be **play** has five essential elements: it is *intrinsically motivated,* done simply for the enjoyment of doing it; it is *freely chosen,* not assigned; it is *pleasurable;* it is *nonliteral,* often containing make-believe; and it *actively engages* the player, physically and/or psychologically (Rubin, Fein, & Vandenberg, 1983).

Infants engage in three forms of play: **sensorimotor** or practice play, when an infant accidentally discovers an enjoyable activity and repeats it continuously; **play with objects**, when an infant intentionally manipulates objects to observe the results; and **symbolic** or make-believe play, when an infant uses one object to represent another one, usually appearing around 12 or 13 months (Hughes, 2010).

The relationship between play and social skills begins in infancy. Play with infants usually involves experiences that provide sensory stimulation, such as with rattles, mobiles, and singing; research supports that **infant–parent play** contributes significantly to an infant's sensorimotor development. Psychologist Sibylle Escalona's (1968) classic study on the play behaviors of infants and their mothers demonstrated that infants who played with their mothers, as opposed to playing with the same objects by themselves, had more complex and more sustained sensorimotor play than infants who did not have play interactions with adults. Other research (Bigelow, MacLean, & Proctor, 2004; Stevenson, Leavitt, Thompson, & Roach, 1988) demonstrated that infant–parent play may set the stage for the child's later social interactions with others by encouraging self-confidence, exploration, social interaction, and attention to the social components of language.

With 2-year-olds' advances in gross motor development, language skills, and need for independence come changes in play materials and social interaction with peers. Two-year-olds can play effectively on swing sets and other playground equipment, continue to enjoy sensory play materials such as clay and finger paint, and begin to increase their social play with peers. In the 1930s, Parten (1932) found that 2-year-olds typically engage in three types of social play: **solitary play**, where the child is playing alone even in the presence of other children; **onlooker play**, where the child observes other children playing but does not participate; and **parallel play**, in which children are engaged in the same activity at the same time, but they are playing separately.

Beginning at around age 2, toddlers enter the **preoperational period**, the second stage in Piaget's (1983) theory of cognitive development. This period is characterized by a change in how children think, allowing them to engage in another type of play known as **pretend play**—also called imaginative play, fantasy play, or dramatic play—where not only can objects be used to symbolize or represent other objects, but children can take on dramatic roles as well. Two-year-olds use pretend play alone and in interactive play with other children. There are several benefits of interactive play in the development of social skills. For older infants and toddlers, interactive—or social—play is an opportunity for children to be exposed to **rules of behavior** that they can transfer to non-play interactions (Vygotsky, 1978). For inhibited or socially awkward children, manipulative materials—such as blocks—have been used successfully in social play to promote **social integration** with other children by allowing the children to converse and take part in a joint activity (Brassard & Boehm, 2007). Children who collaborate with one another in social play have the opportunity to practice moving out of their self-centered perspective, as social play requires the child to understand the **point of view** of others (Hughes, 2010).

➤ CASE EXAMPLE **6.4**   PRETEND PLAY AND SOCIAL PLAY.

In the following cases, describe the benefits that the children gain in engaging in these types of play.

For Keira's second birthday, she was given a toy cash register. She scans everything in the house (most things cost 6 cents). She asks you if you want to pay with your credit card, then she puts your purchases in a bag. One day while playing with her cash register, she scanned her favorite monkey blanket that she calls "Boy Monk." When I asked her how much her "Boy Monk" would cost, she said, "He is priceless." [~Kristina]

All the world's a stage. . . . William Shakespeare could not have more accurately described 3-year-old Tahlia's view of everyday life. From the moment she awakens until her head hits the pillow, she transforms herself into her favorite characters—changing her voice, appearance, and personality traits. Almost magically, she can convert her bedroom into a dance studio or a sandy beach. She will also assign a part to anyone who is willing to engage in imaginative play. As her mommy, I often play the role of Miss Lily, the dance instructor from one of her favorite shows, *Angelina Ballerina*. However, Tahlia's uncanny imagination has also led me to play a variety of roles, ranging from the complex role of Scar from *The Lion King* to the most simplistic role, that of a scoop of vanilla ice cream. Tahlia's vivid imagination allows her to create her own reality and to be someone other than herself. While I quickly return to Mommy, Tahlia continues to respond to me in ways that clearly communicate that she is not Tahlia. Instead, she is Angelina, Gracie, or Simba, and the world is her stage. [~Maya]

I love watching and listening to my 3-year-old daughter, Aubrey, engage in make-believe play. She loves her baby dolls and treats them as if they are real babies. She will hold them, rock them, feed them, change their diaper, give them baths, and soothe them when they cry. She will even show me when one has a "boo boo" and tell me it needs an ice pack and a bandage. I sit back and observe and listen to her call them "sweetie pie" and tell them "Shhhh, baby, it's okay, Mommy's here, don't cry." Then she'll very gently sit while putting the baby on her lap and pretend to pour tea for herself and another baby. She has one very large doll that she pretends is her sister, and she'll tell her to "Be careful, the tea is very hot!" After the tea party is over, one of Aubrey's favorite things to do is put her babies to bed. She will put numerous doll babies on the floor and carefully cover each one up with a small baby blanket. She'll pat their backs, read them stories, and tell them all that it is nap time. Sometimes she will even reprimand me if I am making too much noise, because her babies are trying to sleep. Aubrey loves being a mommy to her babies! [~Cori]

Linden and Mason's favorite accessory was a child-sized plastic shopping cart. They were 1½ and 3 years old at the time. I recall both boys shopping in our pantry every night while we did the dishes after supper. They would carefully sort and load the cart with items from the pantry each night and push the full cart around the kitchen. Frequently all of the canned goods and assorted boxes would be scattered on the floor of the pantry. When you opened the pantry door, it looked like an earthquake had shaken all of the food from the shelves. For the next two years we could never find a thing in our own cupboards. I personally love a neat, organized kitchen. This was torture for me, but it was worth it to see my young sons diligently working together to shop for groceries each night. [~Scott]

Interactive play is also strongly linked to peer group acceptance. It is helpful for counselors, parents, and teachers to carefully observe a toddler's social play for clues about his later ability to garner the acceptance of his peer group. A toddler who is not gradually developing socially useful behaviors such as taking turns, sharing, and making positive comments may grow into a preschooler who is rejected by his peers. Hazen and Black (1989) found that children who are disliked by other children are those who often make statements that do not relate to what is going on during social play, and they make critical or negative remarks about other children's play. Preschoolers who are destructive and disruptive during their play with peers in other ways—taking objects from others without asking, arguing, fighting, or walking away (Rubin, Coplin, Chen, Buskirk, & Wojslawowicz, 2005)—are often rejected by other preschoolers as well, further limiting their ability to practice successful social skills.

When you work with parents of toddlers who are demonstrating destructive and disruptive behaviors during social play, you may help to design a **social intervention program**. The **coaching** technique has been found to be the most effective type of social intervention program (Ladd, 2005), and the children who benefit from this technique showed improvements in socially useful behaviors and acceptance by their peer group. The coaching technique consists of a three-step process: (1) providing the child with *specific instruction* in how to perform certain social skills, (2) giving the opportunity to *rehearse* the skills, and (3) providing *feedback* regarding success in using those skills.

The Newborn in the Family Lifecycle

The arrival of a newborn in the family heralds an era of significant adjustment for all members of the family. Personally and relationally, parents have to negotiate their sense of identity, discovering what it means for them to now take on the roles of both parent and partner. Logistically, parents have to adjust their daily lives to the round-the-clock care and affection that a newborn requires. This may also mean changes in income level for all types of families. In a two-parent family, one parent may transition from the role of an employee outside of the home to a stay-at-home parent; in two-parent families where both parents will continue to work outside of the home, or in a single-parent family where the parent will continue to work outside of the home, parents may need to seek a paid child care arrangement in the form of a nanny or day care.

It is important for counselors to be cognizant of how the addition of a newborn also affects the family lifecycle for other members of the family, such as siblings and grandparents. For some siblings, this can be a time of confusion, as they figure out where they fit in the family. Simultaneously, the newborn provides older siblings with opportunities for bonding and caregiving, such as for Juliana, age 6, who does not enjoy extended time away from her 1-year-old brother, Cannan, and who always wants to make sure that Canann is all right. Lori, a mother of three children, who was intentional about building a team culture within her family, found a creative way for her older children to welcome a newborn into the family (see Think About It 6.2). Grandparents may consider the arrival of the newborn as a continuation of the family legacy, and for some grandparents it is also a chance to provide nurturing and support to another generation.

Think About It   6.2   Welcoming a Newborn to the Family

What is the impact of Lori's creative event on the individual family members? I have three children. When my middle daughter, Sophie, was born, my eldest son, Jacob, was 4 years and 5 months. As the pregnancy neared its end, my son and I shopped for all the fixings needed for a BIRTHday party at which we would all welcome our newest family member. We purchased plates, hats, noisemakers, and even a zero candle. Labor was long, but we were so happy our daughter was finally here and we wanted our son to meet her immediately. My husband helped Jacob set up the plates, gave out the party hats, and lit the candle. We all sang "Happy Birthday" to our Sophie Rose. After the candle was blown out, Jacob got to hold his new sister. I will never forget how he looked squarely in her eyes and said, "She's beautiful." Two years and eight months later we welcomed our youngest, Anna, with a BIRTHday party, this time at home. My older two sang with joy and warmly welcomed their little sister into the family. Including my children in welcoming our newest family members proved to be a very successful way to build a foundation of trust and caring. To this day our family has a strong bond, and together we welcomed our son's wife as a new daughter and sister. [~Lori]

Lori Taber

REFLECTION   6.6   THE GRANDPARENT–GRANDCHILD CONNECTION

I was born and raised in the 1950s in a rural conservative region, and during my upbringing I learned that generations of women helped each other, especially family members. When raising our children in the mid-1970s through mid-1990s, I received a lot of help with child care from my mother and mother-in-law, both of whom lived within 10 minutes or so from our home. So it was a natural thing for me that when our son and daughter-in-law had their first baby, Brandon, I was hoping to be involved in child care while my daughter-in-law was at work two days a week. I work part-time jobs but was able to fit in two days a week of child care. It means that on my days off from my "regular" jobs I do not always get much accomplished in my house and gardens. However, the benefits are so rewarding. It has given me an opportunity to revisit my own children's preschool years, forced me to realign my priorities, slow down a bit, and try once again to see life through the eyes of a 2-, 3-, or 4-year-old. I answer a lot of "why" questions (I do not always have the answers); I am able to show Brandon simple gardening principles and teach him where our food comes from; we play games together; we cook together in my kitchen; we read books; we work on projects together. I believe the simple things in life need to be appreciated in the fast-paced life we live, recognizing that his life will move even faster with all the technology he will live with. If I am able to give him memories of a great time with "nana," then I will have achieved my goal. Meanwhile, I get to enjoy a presence in my life that is extremely rewarding. [~Carol]

Carol Huber

Summary

A parent is the earliest nurturer of the infant's emotional intelligence, the ability to successfully navigate the emotional brain/thinking brain system. An infant within the first year generates the primary emotions of happiness, anger, sadness, fear, surprise, interest, and disgust, using crying, gestures, and movements to convey them. Toddlers begin to recognize secondary emotions, first self-conscious emotions and later self-evaluative emotions. An infant's culture plays a prominent role in how emotions are conceptualized and shown. An infant from a collectivistic culture will likely learn to mask emotions and place more emotional energy on the outcome of a negative event, whereas an infant from an individualistic culture will likely be shaped to express emotions freely and place more emotional energy on who was responsible for causing a negative event.

Freud and Erikson held contrasting views regarding emotional development. Freud believed that one's personality and emotional development are determined in early childhood, based on how well the parent was able to balance the child's basic needs without over- or under-gratifying them. For Erikson, the development of the personality and emotions is a lifelong, continuous process that he called a cradle-to-grave approach. Freud and Erikson both designed stage models of development; however, Freud's stages are psychosexual in nature, while Erikson's are psychosocial.

Attachment is the mutual, sustainable bond that forms between the infant and parent, and the type of attachment depends on how well the parent helps the infant to reduce her distress. A parent who consistently provides a stable relationship for the infant, one in which the parent responds to her needs and signals for comfort during times of distress, with close contact and loving touch, will teach the infant's brain to balance the quick, emotional responses of her amygdala with the more mindful, decision-making responses of the neocortex. Securely attached children learn to regulate their own levels of cortisol because they feel confident that they can manage distressing life situations.

Psychoanalysts viewed the infant's attachment as originating from the mother's ability to satisfy the infant's basic drive for food during the oral stage of psychosexual development, after which the infant directs emotional energy from the food to the mother, a process known as cathexis. However, Bowlby's theory of attachment, which diverged radically from the psychoanalytic explanation, held that infants are innately predisposed to form attachments and will attach most securely to parents who best respond to signals of distress. Bowlby created a four-phase model for the development of infant–parent attachments. Ainsworth, a colleague of Bowlby, developed an experimental procedure called the "strange situation" to assess the security of attachments in children 10–24 months old. Ainsworth and her research colleagues identified three patterns of attachment: secure attachment, and two types of insecure attachment [avoidant and ambivalent (resistant) attachment]. Main and Solomon later identified a fourth, and least secure, pattern of attachment known as disorganized-disoriented attachment. Infants and toddlers are able to form secure attachments with people in addition to the mother and father (such as siblings, grandparents, and professional caregivers) as long as those individuals provide a consistently stable relationship. Cultures differ in how a securely attached child is defined. Whereas American or German parents may view an independent child as one who is securely attached, a Japanese parent is more likely to consider a securely attached child as one who is obedient and compliant.

Temperament is a newborn brain's biological predisposition to interpret and respond to stimulation. Although temperament has a biological basis and tends to remain stable across the lifespan, the child's experiences and parental intervention are dominant influences in shaping the child's temperament. Thomas and Chess conducted a longitudinal study of infant and childhood temperament, identifying factors of temperament including activity level, approach or withdrawal to stimuli, adaptability, and attention span. Kagan's research on the differences in brain activity among children who were timid, bold, upbeat, and melancholy, based on inborn differences in brain circuitry, demonstrates the stability of temperament over time. An inhibited temperament can be detected in infants: If left untreated, the child is likely to develop shyness, social anxiety, and depression. However, parents and counselors can help to reform the neural circuitry with gentle and consistent challenges for the child to face. Temperament can be measured using surveys, questionnaires, and interviews. When a child's temperament and the parent's style of parenting match, this relationship is known as goodness of fit.

An infant or toddler who shows developmental delays in socialization and communication may be diagnosed with autism spectrum disorder (ASD). Parents can receive early interventions for their child, such as physical and behavioral therapy, and specialized educational programs, as well as support services for themselves.

Rochat's levels of self-awareness chart the increasing ability to differentiate the self as a unique being from all others. A newborn shows implicit self-awareness by distinguishing another person touching her cheek from her own hand touching her cheek. This native ability to self-differentiate matures steadily, so that the 18-month-old toddler can demonstrate explicit self-awareness during the classic rouge experiment. Around age 2 the infant is using the first person pronouns to self-identify.

The capacity to practice effortful control, stifling one's dominant response to a stimulus in favor of expressing a subdominant response, detecting errors, and engaging in planning, can be observed in a toddler by the end of the first year. This extremely important skill requires the toddler to engage physical, cognitive, emotional, and social abilities, as the infant must redirect cognitions and behaviors to those that would not have instinctively been a first choice but are required by culture to stay safe or to follow socially accepted practices. Children who have difficulty practicing effortful control have problems self-regulating, finding it challenging to control their reactions to stress, keep their attention focused, and decode their own and others' mental states. Early nurturing experiences, especially parenting style, correlate strongly with a child's well-developed ability for effortful control.

On the path of social development, infants and toddlers use social referencing, interpreting the facial and/or verbal emotional expressions of people they trust to make decisions about ambiguous events, such as whether to cross a visual cliff or touch a new toy. Although previous studies have placed the emergence of this important skill between 7 and 9 months, recent research indicates that infants as young as 3 months may use social referencing.

Parents and the larger culture help to socialize infants' and toddlers' emotions by providing continual feedback about how to join the fabric of their society. The brain of a child whose psychic script includes the regular practice of effortful control will activate empathy and guilt appropriately, helping the child to skillfully interact with others. While infants and young toddlers often play alone or with parents, by age 2 many toddlers engage in interactive play with other children, allowing them to practice taking others' points of view. Children who have difficulty gaining peer group acceptance because of deficits in skillful social interaction may benefit from specialized coaching interventions.

The addition of the newborn to the family requires all members to adjust their sense of identity, roles, and expectations. Aside from engaging in the continual care and affection required to nurture a newborn, parents who co-parent also navigate the dual roles of parent and partner, often making relational, financial, logistical, and employment changes. Siblings find themselves reorganizing their idea of where they fit in the family life cycle, and their responses can range from jealousy and confusion to bonding and caregiving. Grandparents have a unique opportunity to foster the development of the next generation.

The odyssey from birth to age 3 is a significant journey for all travelers involved: infants, toddlers, parents, family members, and counselors. For the infants and toddlers, how amazing it must be to embark at birth, and three years later be a person who is virtually indistinguishable in form, size, ability, communication style, and thought process from where one began. While the toddler's temperament may endure if not reshaped by specific intervention, the contextual elements of genetics, environment, stimulation, and relationships provide the raw materials for each child's brain to craft itself into a wholly unique being. For parents, there is no precisely laid-out treasure map to follow, as each child is wired differently and responds distinctively. However, we do know that optimal development emerges from a closely attached, relationship-dependent process, requiring parents to vigilantly monitor the minute-by-minute changes in their child's landscape and be willing to make course corrections in the way they interact with their child. Counselors are given a privileged invitation to accompany a family into the intimate world of raising children, with its attendant triumphs and struggles. Counselors have a special role, as parents share their vulnerabilities and look to shine a light into places that they themselves may not see. Counselors are a highly valued member of an expedition team that sets its sights on safe passage through the uncertain, but always fascinating, terrain of infant and toddler development.

Acknowledgments

The authors would like to thank all of the wonderful caregivers who so generously shared stories about their children, making the concepts from this chapter come to life, and Stefanie Moore, M.Ed., for her research assistance.

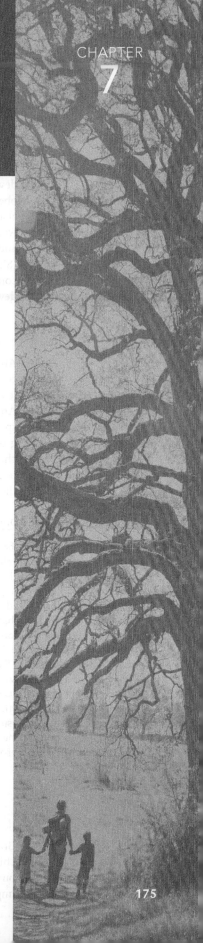

The Preschool Years: Early Childhood Physical and Cognitive Development

By Charlotte Daughhetee and Stephen Parker

In the odyssey of human development, the preschool years are a time of many momentous challenges and changes. This chapter provides an overview of both physical and cognitive development during the preschool or early childhood years (approximately ages 2 or 3 through 6 years), a time when children make substantial developmental advancements in their lifespan journey. Issues related to growth and health as well as the progression of cognitive processes will be explored. The preschool years are a time of tremendous growth for children, and healthy physical and cognitive growth and development are essential for well-being.

SECTION I: Physical Development

The early childhood years are a time of significant gains in motor skills and brain development, which provide the foundation for an individual's lifelong learning, growth, and health. Conversely, impediments to healthy development can set the stage for problematic developmental issues and health concerns across the lifespan. For example, childhood obesity is linked to adult health problems such as hypertension and heart disease (Brown et al., 2009). Additionally, environmental factors play a definitive role in brain development, with negative, deprived, or chemically toxic environments being linked to poor physical and mental health, subpar academic performance, and maladaptive emotional adjustment (Shonkoff, 2010). Therefore, the physical development of the preschool child, as well as the context of the child's development, are of major importance when considering the overall development along an individual's journey through the lifespan.

Individual Differences

After the rapid rate of growth during the infancy years, physical development slows down considerably during early childhood; rather than progressing in a steady constant mode, it continues in a start-and-stop manner (Steinberg, Bornstein, Vandell, & Rook, 2011). Anyone who has raised or taught a preschooler can attest to the on-again–off-again growth spurts: the times during growth spurts when preschoolers seem to eat all day and the non–growth spurt periods when one wonders if they are living merely on air. During this stage children's bodies become narrower, and they begin to lose their babyish appearance as their bodies take on more adult-like proportions (Papalia, Olds, & Feldman, 2009). According to the Centers for Disease Control and Prevention (CDC) growth charts, at the 50th percentile 3-year-old males are 37½ inches tall and weigh 32 pounds; by age 6, boys are approximately 45½ inches tall and weigh 46 pounds (Ogden et al., 2002). Three-year-old females at the 50th percentile are 37 inches tall and weigh 30 pounds; by age 6 years, females are 45½ inches tall and weigh 40 pounds. Across early childhood, boys tend to be slightly taller and heavier than girls the same age. While noting average rates of growth during the preschool years can provide a general idea of the typical expected developmental growth progression, it is important to remember that there is a great deal of variability among children in their physical growth and development.

As a clinical consideration, while taking into account recognition of variations, we do have standardized physical expectations for children of a certain age. Therefore, children who are physical outliers could be expected to have received social feedback that could well impact myriad psychological and emotional concerns.

> **REFLECTION 7.1 INDIVIDUAL DIFFERENCES**
>
> I can personally attest to the variability of children's growth patterns. My own children were quite illustrative of preschool growth variability. Throughout childhood, my middle son Jake was usually in the 15th percentile in height and weight, while my youngest son Michael (two and a half years younger) tended to be in the 90th percentile on height and weight. Jake at birth was 6 pounds and 12 ounces, and Michael at birth was 7 pounds and 5 ounces. When Jake was 5 years old and Michael was 3, Michael caught up to Jake in height and weight; in fact, they could wear the same clothes. This growth pattern continued until adolescence, when Michael suddenly grew much taller than his older brother; same parents, same environment, but vastly different growth patterns and body types. [~CD]

Brain Growth

Brain development is greatly affected by the environment and experiences of the young child. According to Shonkoff (2010), our genes determine the basic design of our brains, but environmental factors influence how the brain gets wired and how that design gets implemented. Positive environmental factors nurture the development of a sound foundation for learning across the lifespan, whereas negative experiences such as stress, abuse, and neglect can disturb optimal brain development and undermine future academic achievement and success. By age 3, the brain has attained 80% of its adult weight (Kail & Cavanaugh, 2010). Brain development in early childhood involves a significant increase in the number of dendrites and synapses, a process that is illustrated by increasing cognitive ability during these years (Dacey, Travers, & Fiore, 2009). During this stage of life, the brain develops more rapidly than any other organ (Rathus, 2012).

The human brain has the capacity for plasticity or flexible adaptive growth. Brain development generally proceeds according to an internal genetic blueprint (Shonkoff, 2010). However, if the brain should become damaged, it is possible for it to find alternate pathways for the development of abilities. Thompson et al. (2009) stated that, due to plasticity, injured brains in young children can compensate for problems associated with the injury and overcome early injuries. This plasticity of the brain is greatest during childhood; brain injury becomes much more difficult to overcome as humans age.

Brain lateralization refers to the fact that the two halves of the human brain house different functions. For instance, for a majority of people, speech tends to be housed predominantly in the left side of the brain. Similarly, 95% of right-handed people and 70% of left-handed people have left hemisphere language dominance (Sun & Walsh, 2006). The concept of being "left-brained" or "right-brained" has been over-generalized; it is important to remember that there is a great deal of function overlap and integration between the two brain hemispheres. Nevertheless, there are specific functions that are mainly associated with each hemisphere. Language and logical processing are mainly housed in the left hemisphere, while spatial recognition is contained in the right hemisphere. Emotional processing, specifically the recognition of facial emotional patterns, appears to be a right-brain function (Workman, Chilvers, Yeomans, & Taylor, 2006).

By age 3, most children have demonstrated a handedness preference. **Handedness** refers to one's preference for using the right or left hand. For generations in America, there was a strong social preference for right-handedness, and attempts were made to force left-handed children to switch to their right hands. Fortunately, today's left-handed children can write and draw without attempts to force handedness change. However, with the dominance of right-handedness, it is possible that parents and teachers may be unintentionally encouraging young children to use their right hands.

Think About It   7.1

Are you left-handed or do you know someone who is left-handed? What intentional or unintentional negative messages have you, or the left-handed person you know, received regarding handedness?

Motor Skills

Gross motor play that is lively, perhaps even rowdy, is a hallmark of the preschool years. As children age, while still active, their play will become calmer, more focused and cooperative. But from the toddler years up to age 5, children's play is active and high-spirited (Timmons, Naylor, & Pfeiffer, 2007). **Gross motor skills** developed in early childhood include hopping, skipping, throwing, catching, galloping, sliding, and riding a tricycle; movement patterns become goal driven and purposeful as children learn to play games (Williams et al., 2009). The gross motor skills enhanced through this physical activity will set the stage for later developmental physical advances.

While most people think of preschool children as being in nonstop action, the reality is surprisingly different. When physical activity is measured in preschools, most of the time the children were found to be sedentary (Oliver, Schofield, & Kolt, 2007). A sedentary school day coupled with an increasing tendency for children to engage in sedentary activities at home (e.g., watching television) is a contributing factor to an alarming increase in obesity among children in the United States. In order to instill lifelong healthy habits and offset the current societal tendency toward sedentary activities, teachers and parents should encourage and model more physical activity with preschool-aged children (Brown et al., 2009).

Timmons et al. (2007) state that physical activity not only enhances preschoolers' health, but can also increase self-esteem and social skills. Even as little as an additional 20 minutes of activity a day can positively influence psychosocial outcomes. Citing the Canadian National Association for Sports and Physical Education, the authors recommended that preschoolers should have 60 minutes of structured physical activity and at least 60 minutes or more of unstructured physical activity every day. Other than when they are asleep, preschoolers should not be sedentary for more than 60 minutes at any given time. They should develop competence in movement skills and have both indoor and outdoor areas for large-muscle activities. Parents, teachers, and caregivers should be cognizant of the importance of physical activity for preschool children. Large movement play is not only essential for gross motor development and physical health; it also contributes to social skill development and overall emotional well-being.

Think About It   7.2

Why do you think families are less physically active than in the past? What are some ways parents with preschoolers can incorporate more large movement play into the daily routine of the family?

Early childhood is a key time for development of the fine motor skills that are used for manipulation and control. **Fine motor skills** include being able to button and dress oneself, use a pencil and crayons, and master the use of scissors. Fine motor development across early childhood is evident in the advances in drawing skill that occurs from the toddler years to age 5. Toddlers merely scribble on paper, but by age 3 children can begin to draw shapes and designs, and by age 5 children begin to draw recognizable objects such as houses, people, and animals. Since fine motor skills are essential to learning, practice in these skills is very important for proper development of these abilities (Bergin & Bergin, 2012). Parents and preschool teachers should strive to incorporate fine motor activities into the daily schedule of children. Practice in cutting, holding a pencil, tracing, and drawing will be very beneficial in the refinement of fine motor skills. Rule and Stewart (2002) noted that children who are behind their classmates in the development of fine motor skills suffer ridicule and have lower self-esteem. Falling behind in fine motor skill development can also portend later behavioral problems and lower academic achievement (Losse et al., 1991). Conversely, early achievement in fine motor skills can predict higher achievement in literacy. Rule and Stewart (2002) recommended incorporation of fine motor activities into the preschool curriculum. Such activities would include children picking up pennies or practicing the **pincer grip** (which later leads to holding a pencil). The incorporation of fine motor activities into preschool settings significantly increases the fine motor development of children.

Health

The early childhood years are filled with sniffles and tummy aches. Children are exposed to more viruses because they are more likely to interact with other children (and consequently more germs) in preschool and kindergarten settings. These minor illnesses are to be expected, and children usually bounce back from most illness within a couple of days. More serious childhood illnesses such as measles and mumps are now, for the most part, controlled with **vaccines**. The Centers for Disease Control and Prevention (CDC, 2011i) recommend the following vaccines or booster vaccines for preschool age children: diphtheria, tetanus, pertussis (DTaP); pneumococcal (PPSV); inactivated poliovirus (IPV); measles, mumps, rubella (MMR); varicella; hepatitis A (HepA); meningococcal (MCVU); and influenza. In the United States, immunization coverage has reached most of the population; however, vaccine rates for minority children lag behind the general population (Chu, Barber, & Smith, 2004). There are a variety of reasons for the lower rates of immunization among minority children. Since minority families are over-represented in lower socioeconomic levels, they have less access to primary and preventive care. Moreover, they may also have a distrust of immunization. Community outreach and education have been found to be effective in closing the immunization gap.

The most common chronic disease in early childhood is dental decay or **caries** (Marrs, Trumbley, & Malik, 2011). This is alarming, especially when one considers that dental decay is a preventable disease. Dental problems interfere with children's social development since children may feel embarrassed about their appearance. Moreover, the pain from caries sometimes interferes with children's ability to function in school. Children from low socioeconomic status (SES) households are most at risk due to lack of preventive care. A child's first dental checkup should occur prior to the first birthday, but low-income families are unlikely to have dental insurance or be able to afford visits to the dentist. A poor diet high in sugar is another major contributing factor. Prevention strategies include supervised brushing with a fluoride toothpaste and fluoridated water, educational programs for families, proper diet, and access to health care for children. While there are some outreach programs that offer dental care to low-SES families, the need for more extensive intervention is apparent.

The most alarming health issue facing preschoolers is obesity (Ogden, Carroll, Curtin, Lamb, & Flegal, 2010). According to the Centers for Disease Control and Prevention (CDC, 2011h), childhood obesity has tripled in the last 30 years. The CDC defines obesity as a body mass index at or above the 95th percentile on growth charts. In 2007–2008, 10.4% of preschool-age children were obese (Ogden et al., 2010). The CDC recommends programs through child care settings that reach out to families to encourage healthy eating and physical activity. Such programs should include planned physical activities and information on healthy snacks, nutrition, and gardening. By intervening through school and child care programs and with the family, the CDC hopes that this alarming trend can be reversed.

The leading cause of death for preschool children is unintentional injury (Seattle. Gov, 2011). **Unintentional injuries** include injuries such as burns and scalds, poisoning, head injuries (e.g., lack of bike helmets), and pedestrian and street safety. According to Kendrick (2004), 77% of unintentional injuries occur at home. General home safety recommendations include home fire-appropriate installation of sprinkler systems, smoke alarms, and window locks, and safe storage of medicine, cleaning supplies, and sharp objects. Kendrick found that children from low-SES households were at the greatest risk due to the high cost of home safety measures and childproofing of the home. As a clinical consideration, the implications of low SES status on the physical health and development of significant numbers of children lead one to conclude that advocacy for social policies addressing these disparities is consistent with the professional obligations of the counselor.

Visual and Hearing Impairments

Vision impairment is rare among children. A recent CDC study conducted in the metropolitan Atlanta area found about 1 in 833 children had some type of vision impairment. **Vision impairment** can occur through damage to the eye, incorrect eye shape, or difficulties with brain processing of visual stimuli. While there is a genetic basis for some vision impairment, most vision impairment in children is the result of prenatal development problems, premature birth, and low birth weight. Vision impairment also tends to be co-morbid with other developmental disabilities.

During the preschool years, children undergo rapid development of speech, language, social, and emotional abilities (Yin, Bottnell, Clarke, Shacks, & Poulson, 2009). Additionally, this is the time when children are fostering foundational listening and literacy skills, as well as developing auditory-neural connections (Robinshaw, 2007). Therefore, screening and early diagnosis of hearing problems are essential to overall child development (Serpanos & Jarmel, 2007). About one in 1000 children have some type of hearing impairment. Effective screening methods are available for infants and young children, and considering the importance of hearing in child development, screening and early intervention are vital (Serpanos & Jarmel, 2007; Yin et al., 2009). Robinshaw (2007) recommended the following questions to assist parents, teachers, and physicians in noting the possibility of child hearing loss or difficulty:

- Is the child visibly frustrated or anxious?
- Does the child respond inconsistently or inappropriately to speech?
- Does the child need to visually track conversations?
- Does the child tend to turn a particular ear toward a speaker?
- Is the child easily distracted and disengaged from classroom activities?
- Can the child follow verbal messages without visual clues?
- Does the child look to others for confirmation of directions?
- Can the child keep up with playground games that are based on verbal arrangements?
- Does the child choose to sit near, or turn up the volume control, when using the radio or TV?
- How confident is the child at joining in classroom discussions?
- Does the child use strategies to request clarification? (p. 666)

Sleep Habits

Sleep is fundamental to healthy development, and the establishment of healthy sleep habits in infancy and early childhood will set the stage for lifelong beneficial sleep practices. A bedtime routine is very helpful in settling children down and helping them prepare for a restful night. For instance, if the child has a bath and bedtime story every evening, the child begins to associate these activities with settling down and going to sleep. Most preschool children have a security item, such as a blanket or stuffed animal, which becomes part of their self-soothing practices and can help them fall asleep (Hayes, Fukumizu, Troese, Sallinen, & Gilles, 2007). Attachment to security items is normal during early childhood and is not an indication of excessive anxiety. Ordinarily, as children age, the need for the security item fades.

According to the National Science Foundation, children ages 5 to 10 need 10 to 11 hours of sleep per night, but many children get far less than 10 hours of sleep. Sleep deprivation can cause depression, anxiety, irritability, inattention, and academic problems as children struggle to stay awake in school (Bergin & Bergin, 2012). In the United States, the problem of sleep deprivation is widespread across childhood and worsens as children enter adolescence. The formation of healthy sleeping habits in infancy and early childhood is crucial to overall health and well-being across the lifespan.

There are two main stages of sleep. **Non-rapid eye movement (NREM)** is a quieter type of sleep characterized by slower breathing, lower heart rate, and less brain activity. **Rapid eye movement (REM)** sleep is typified by breathing and heart rates similar to waking states, eye movement, and increased brain activity. REM sleep involves a light stage and a deeper stage, and dreaming occurs mainly during REM sleep. It is not uncommon for preschoolers to experience nightmares and sleep terrors. Nightmares are common and take place during the light REM period, whereas sleep terrors are less common and take place during deep REM sleep (Rathus, 2012). Sleep terrors are more frightening than nightmares and are usually associated with stressful times during a child's life, such as moving or beginning school. Once a child grows into adolescence, the likelihood of sleep terrors diminishes significantly.

Sleep disorders do occur in early childhood and are problematic for a child's overall well-being. Most commonly, **sleep disorders** involve difficulty falling asleep and frequent waking during the night with subsequent difficulties falling back asleep. Sleep disorders appear to be co-morbid with other childhood problems. For instance, Scher and Zuckerman (2005) found that difficulty falling asleep and staying asleep during infancy were linked to behavioral problems in early childhood. The existence of sleep disorders in infancy can alert parents, teachers, and physicians to be observant of potential behavior concerns and, therefore, prepared to initiate early intervention for behavioral issues.

Co-sleeping, the practice of children and parents sharing a bed, is a somewhat controversial issue, with strong opinions on both the pro and con sides of the argument. While co-sleeping is the norm in many parts of the world, in the United States it is generally frowned upon by most parenting advice books and pediatricians (Sobralske & Gruber, 2009). Proponents of co-sleeping see it as a way to increase bonding and sense of security, while those who advise against co-sleeping cite dangers to infants, such as smothering, and the inability of children to form self-soothing behaviors that enable them to fall asleep on their own. Disturbance to the intimacy of the parents is also noted as a problem with co-sleeping. Children who have difficulty sleeping in infancy are likely to continue to have sleep disturbances in early childhood, and if as infants these children co-slept with parents, the desire to sleep with parents continues across childhood (Hayes et al., 2007). It should be noted that there is no evidence that co-sleeping children are more dependent on their parents in general (Kail & Cavanaugh, 2010). It is important to recognize that the practice of co-sleeping may be culturally based and that it is considered a positive experience by many families (Sobralske & Gruber, 2009). The cultural underpinning of co-sleeping is evidenced by the fact that it is more common among collective cultures, whereas independent sleeping is more common among individualistic cultures (Kail & Cavanaugh, 2010).

➤ CASE EXAMPLE **7.1**   CO-SLEEPING.

You are seeing a couple in your counseling practice. They have a 4-year-old son who sleeps with them every night. One partner believes very strongly that co-sleeping is a positive child-rearing practice and is essential to the emotional well-being of the 4-year-old. The other partner does not believe in co-sleeping and has expressed anger and frustration at the disruption of the couple's intimacy. What are the pros and cons of each position? Could a compromise be negotiated? How might your personal beliefs on co-sleeping get in the way of your ability to be helpful regarding this impasse?

SECTION II: Cognitive Development

Of all the strands making up the complexity of the human odyssey, no particular area has received more attention than cognitive development. Thought and language are how we conceptualize ourselves and our world, and how we solve problems. Cognition is our steering mechanism throughout the odyssey of life.

Piaget's Preoperational Stage

Jean Piaget has had a profound influence on our conceptualization of the cognitive development of children and on the education of the preschool child. Piaget's scientific background was in biology. A gifted child, he published a paper on an albino sparrow at age 10 and completed his doctorate (his dissertation was on mollusks) at age 21 (Beatty, 2009). He studied for a time at the Sorbonne in Paris, where he worked at the Alfred Binet laboratory helping to standardize intelligence tests. Piaget became intrigued by the wrong answers the children gave, and this inspired him to study the cognitive development of children. In the 1920s, Piaget observed and interviewed children at Maison des Petits laboratory school at the Jean-Jacques Rousseau school in Geneva. Initially using only observation and interviews to study children, he later developed experiments to assess a child's level of cognitive development. Piaget is considered a constructivist theorist. Piaget's cognitive constructivism is based on the premise that learning and meaning are constructed through personal experience and process (Powell & Kalina, 2008).

Piaget's preoperational stage encompasses ages 2 through 7 years. The **preoperational stage** is comprised of two substages: (1) preconceptual, ages 2 through 4, is characterized by exploration and imagination; and (2) the intuitive stage, ages 4 through 7, is characterized by intuitive thought rather than logic. As a biologist, Piaget was familiar with how organisms adapt to their environment, and perhaps this biological perspective shaped how he viewed cognitive development and adaptation. Infants enter the world with schemes or organized patterns of behavior through which they interact with the world (Ginsburg & Opper, 1987). Assimilation and accommodation are the mechanisms by which new schemas are developed and are thus intellectual adaptations. When a child encounters a new situation, the child initially applies an existing schema to the new situation. If the child discovers that an existing schema can be adapted to that situation, the child has **assimilated** the new information. However, when a child encounters a new situation that cannot be readily adapted into existing schemas, the child must **accommodate** the new information and modify the current schema; thus, the child has learned and expanded his or her understanding of the world and accommodated the new information.

As children encounter new experiences that they can readily assimilate into their schemas, they feel a sense of equilibrium or balance. Conversely, a sense of **disequilibrium** or unbalance signals the need to accommodate something new into existing schemas. This feeling of disequilibrium motivates the child to incorporate the new information and return to equilibrium (Ginsburg & Opper, 1987). Thus, the quest for equilibrium is the driving force behind increasing cognitive development as the child accommodates new experiences and information.

For example, consider 3-year-old Sally and her mother, who frequently visit the park near their home. The park has a pond with ducks, and Sally loves to bring bread to feed the ducks. One day, Sally is visiting at her aunt's farm and she points to a chicken and says "Duck!" Her aunt corrects her saying, "No, that's a chicken." Sally frowns and then tentatively says, "Chicken." Here, Sally had assimilated the concept of duck and applied this schema to her aunt's chicken. When her aunt introduces the word "chicken," Sally briefly experiences disequilibrium but then accommodates the new information and learns a new concept: chicken. Ducks and chickens are somewhat similar, but she is now able to distinguish the differences. The mental structure of "duck" has been modified, new information about the concept of "chicken" has been added, and her view of the world has expanded.

During the preoperational stage, children are egocentric, meaning they believe everyone else knows and experiences the world as they do. They are unable to realize the perspective of another. Another facet of egocentrism is **animism**, or the tendency of children to believe that inanimate objects have the characteristics and feelings of living things, as in a child saying "our house is sad when we aren't home." **Artificialism** is the belief that natural phenomena such as rain or sunrise are caused by people.

REFLECTION 7.2 EGOCENTRISM

When my son Daniel was a preschooler, he loved to have me scratch his back, but he would get very frustrated with me and say "No, Mom, scratch where it itches." He couldn't understand that I wasn't experiencing his itchy back, and he assumed I was pretty dense because I wasn't scratching where it itched. [~CD]

AN IMAGINATIVE INTERPRETATION OF LIFE EVENTS

My son John was 4 years old when my grandmother passed away. He was close to "Mama Lil" because I was her primary family caregiver/advocate once she relocated to Birmingham for assisted living and then nursing care. Anyhow, when she died we explained to John Sawyer that Mama Lil had died. He asked what that meant. I told him it meant that she was in heaven with God. He asked, "How is she going to get there? Does Santa take her there in his sleigh?" Later at the funeral home, we did allow John to enter the funeral home for visitation. He ran up to the casket and pulled on my arm while I was chatting with some guests and said, very excitedly, "Mommy, Mommy, Santa doesn't need to come get Mama Lil! She has her VERY OWN SLEIGH!" And that was his happy literal interpretation of how to get to our afterlife. And it made saying goodbye so much easier for all the adults. [~EB]

The preoperational stage is characterized by symbolic thought, wherein children think in terms of images and symbols; this leads to the creative imaginative play that is a hallmark of the preschool child. The later part of this stage is also typified by intuitive thought, which is the reason behind all those "why" questions children ask during early childhood. These questions are fueled by innate curiosity and simplistic reasoning.

During the intuitive substage of preoperational thought, children master the concept of **conservation**, the understanding that an object maintains its basic properties even if some attribute of the object changes. The classic Piaget experiment for conservation involves showing a child two identical beakers with the same amount of liquid in them. The contents of one beaker are poured into a taller, skinnier beaker and the child is asked which beaker has more liquid. A child who has not mastered conservation will state that the taller beaker has more liquid, whereas a child who has attained conservation will note that the amount of liquid is the same even though the beakers are different shapes (Ginsburg & Opper, 1987).

Another egocentric factor that occurs toward the end of the preoperational stage and into the concrete operations stage is the concept of **immanent justice**. Piaget postulated that children have an innate belief in a just world and would make causal connections between their own misdeeds and later adversity (Jose, 1990). The belief in immanent justice is the reason children tend to blame themselves for parental divorce: "Daddy moved out of the house tonight because I didn't clean my room." Piaget believed immanent justice was based in egocentric thought and that it declined as children aged; however, aspects of this type of reasoning can be found in older children, adolescents, and even some adults.

Concepts

Size, shape, and spatial ability are cognitive concepts acquired during early childhood. Shutts, Örnkloo, van Hofsten, Keen, and Spelke (2009) note that around 2 to 3 years of age, children begin to build simple stacks of blocks and start to gain spatial perception. Young children also develop spatial ability through play that involves tasks such as object fitting or placing a shape into the appropriate hole. The special skills needed for object fitting involve being able to understand how a three-dimensional object will fit into a two-dimensional silhouette. Practice during play with manipulative toys such as blocks and simple puzzles encourages the development of spatial abilities. Also, the attainment of language including words such as "build" allows children to cognitively think about and thereby map the properties of objects, thus improving their spatial abilities. Likewise, manipulative toys enhance a child's understanding of size and geometric shapes, particularly when these concepts are reinforced by adults interacting with children during play.

REFLECTION 7.4 ANOTHERDAY!

When my daughter Breann was 4 years old, her concept of time was limited to today and "anotherday." When we would reminisce over something we had done in the past, she would say, "We did that anotherday." When I would share with her our plans for tomorrow or next week, she would say, "We are going to do that anotherday." Quickly over the next year or so, she mastered the terminology of temporal ordering and was able to use tomorrow, next week, and next year, as well as yesterday, last week, and last year, with great accuracy. But to most 3- and 4-year-olds, there is just today ... and anotherday! [~BTE]

How do children acquire the ability to understand the concept of time? Interestingly, Piaget actually consulted with Einstein on the nature of time and how the mental representation of time is created by children (Actis-Grosso & Zavagno, 2008). Piaget theorized that there are three stages to the development of time perception. Prior to the development of language, the child does not have time perception; actions simply take place in the present. Therefore, the first stage of time perception, what Piaget referred to as intuitive time, occurs after language acquisition at about age 4. At this stage, children can understand order and sequencing of events. By age 8, children can link events to the past or the future; finally, after age 10, children have a fully organized concept of time.

Numeracy involves the understanding of numbers and the ability to do mathematical operations; essentially, it is number sense (Skwarchak, 2009). During the early childhood years, children learn to recognize numbers, count, add, subtract, and estimate. Practice in numerical skills and conceptualization both at home and in preschool will form the foundation for successful math achievement throughout life. While numeracy is typically included in a preschool curriculum, it is less likely to be intentionally included in home activities. Just as reading and language activities are vital parental activities, it is also important for parents to include exposure to numbers and numerical functions in the home.

Vygotsky's Sociocultural Theory

Lev Vygotsky was a Soviet psychologist whose work was relatively unknown in the West until the 1980s, after the dissolution of the Soviet Union. Vygotsky's theory is considered a social constructivist theory, wherein knowledge and meaning are constructed through interaction with others (Powell & Kalina, 2008). For Vygotsky, cognitive development was contextual and relational, and his theory is often referred to as a sociocultural theory due to the importance of cultural-social context and relational interaction in the cognitive development of the child (Couchenour & Chrisman, 2011). For Vygotksy, thought, language, and social context were all intertwined in the cognitive development of the child.

Vygotsky viewed language as particularly important in cognitive development. He noted that young children use private speech, talking to oneself, or thinking out loud to self-regulate and guide action (Yang, 2000). Through private speech, children develop strategies, make decisions, and evaluate results. The language process not only regulates the child's behavior; it also develops mental processes and increases cognitive functioning.

Vygotsky is probably best known for his concept of the **zone of proximal development (ZPD)**. The ZPD is the method by which development unfolds; it is basically the difference between what one can do independently and what one can do with assistance from a more experienced person, such as a parent, teacher, or peer (Powell & Kalina, 2008). **Scaffolding** is the process whereby a more experienced person helps or coaches a less experienced person to go beyond a current level of understanding and attain a new level of knowledge. Scaffolding provides a support system for the learner while a difficult task is performed and until new knowledge is internalized. Vygotsky believed education should be collaborative and that both teachers and peers should be actively involved in the scaffolding of the ZPD.

This social constructivist classroom emphasizes cooperative active learning, scaffolding, and language (both private speech and conversations) to increase knowledge, problem solving, and self-regulation. It is a classroom emphasizing relationships and cooperation.

As a clinical consideration, while Vygotsky's theory is prominent in educational contexts, its application in counseling is less well defined. Vygotsky's ZPD could be used by school counselors in the realm of personal and social interventions and could also be a beneficial systemic perspective for family counselors. Vygotsky's emphasis on the relationship of language and cognitive functioning and mental processes may be very useful for counselors. Language systems that differ from standard English speak to social worlds with distinct features or characteristics. If the therapeutic process proceeds from understanding the world of the child, accepting the child's linguistic system and the social world reflected by it enhances the potential of the therapeutic enterprise.

Information Processing

Information processing is a model that illustrates the cognitive processes of how information is attained, stored, and used (Bergin & Bergin, 2012). The basic components of the model include the sensory register, short-term or working memory, and long-term memory. Information processing involves the process whereby the **sensory register** takes in a tremendous amount of data through the senses, essentially all the environmental stimuli that the senses pick up. This information is held in the sensory register anywhere from 1 to 3 seconds. For the most part, one is not aware of the vast amount of sensory information racing through the sensory register.

In order to move sensory information into the working memory, a person must pay attention to it. According to Downing (2000), people pay attention to something if it is new, pertinent to what is being processed, or emotionally significant. St. Clair-Thompson, Overton, and Botton (2010) note the importance of a perception filter during the attention stage of information processing. People filter new information through their previous experiences and then select what is important and what to focus on in working memory. This perception filter also influences which information gets stored into long-term memory and how that information is elaborated and coded for storage. The concept of a perception filter certainly has implications for educational settings and the understanding of individual differences in learning.

Attention moves the information into working memory. **Working memory** is where we reason, comprehend, and problem solve; it has a limited capacity and a short duration, about 20 seconds. Adults can hold approximately seven (plus or minus two) items or chunks of information in working memory, usually through processes such as rehearsal (repetition) or visual imagery (St. Clair-Thompson et al., 2010). A good illustration of working memory is the process of remembering a phone number. If someone gives you a phone number, you repeat it over and over until you are able to dial the number. If you are distracted before dialing, the new phone number is gone from working memory and you have to ask for it again. It is possible to hold more information in working memory by **chunking** associated items, thereby making one item out of several. For instance, if the last four digits of a phone number are the same as the year you were born, you would be able to reduce those four items, the four digits, into one item, the year of your birth. While adults can hold about seven items or chunks of information in working memory, preschool children can only hold up to four items (Alvarez & Cavanagh, 2004). After age 5, working memory capacity and processing speed increase. Working memory is a component of intelligence testing, and there are several options for testing preschool children (Erford, 2013), including the Slosson Intelligence Test–Primary (SIT-P), the Wechsler Preschool and Primary Scale of Intelligence—Third Edition (WPPSI-III), Stanford–Binet Intelligence Scales—Fifth Edition (SB-5), Kaufman Assessment Battery for Children—Second Edition, and the Woodcock–Johnson Test of Cognitive Ability—Third Edition (WJ-III-COG).

I grew up on a farm but have lived many years in the city. Needless to say, nowadays I rarely encounter the smells of a farm. One fall I happened upon an "autumn display" at the supermarket; pumpkins and leaves were exhibited upon several stacked hay bales. As I smelled the hay, I was instantly taken back to a happy childhood memory in the hayloft of our barn, a childhood event I had probably not thought of since it happened. The scent took me there immediately. [~CD]

Long-term memory has a large capacity and long, perhaps unlimited, duration. Once information is stored in long-term memory, it can be accessed through retrieval pathways. Forgetting is likely the result of not being able to access retrieval pathways rather than actually losing the information from long-term memory. Just as a hiking trail or path becomes overgrown and disappears if not used, retrieval pathways in long-term memory become difficult to find if they are not used, or if they were not initially encoded in an elaborate manner during the long-term memory storage process. Our brain has the capacity to cross-reference memory, and the more ways we use and enrich information during the learning process, the more pathways we have to access this information. Our senses are a particularly strong memory prompt, as beautifully illustrated by Marcel Proust in *In Search of Lost Time*, or *Remembrance of Things Past*, where the narrator is flooded with childhood memories upon tasting a madeleine, a small cake he associated with childhood. Such involuntary memories are commonly known as **Proustian memories** or moments. This episode illustrates the power of our senses in retrieval of memories.

There are many ways to store information in long-term memory, the most common, and least effective, being rote memorization. Learning that has taken place via rote memorization does not create elaborate cross-referenced retrieval pathways in the brain; therefore, recalling rote-memorized information can be challenging. This is why cramming for a test is not an effective learning tool. The student might remember some of the information for a brief time but weeks later can recall little of the information. The pathway to retrieve the information learned by rote or through cramming is simplistic and quickly lost to the learner. To create easily accessed retrieval pathways, one must enrich or elaborate information. Elaboration strategies for long-term memory retrieval include concept or mind mapping, organized presentation of material, self-regulation, and self-explanation (St. Clair-Thompson et al., 2010). As mentioned previously, encoding information using the senses is very powerful. This is especially true for young children. And teachers and parents should strive to provide learning opportunities where children can use their senses when encountering new information.

Preschoolers are able to remember events, especially if these are repeated events such as going to preschool or dinner with family, using scripts, which are broad generalizations of repeated events (Rathus, 2012). Specific autobiographical memory emerges during the preschool years as children begin to remember their own noteworthy life events: birthday parties, the first day of preschool. These become part of the child's story. As self-awareness and increasing language ability develop during early childhood, children's capacity for remembering incidents and constructing their life stories is augmented. Adults can assist children in memory development. Asking young children to remember specific occasions and providing cues about these experiences will help them create enriched retrieval pathways, thus increasing their ability to remember these life events. Encouraging children to use their senses will boost memory attainment as well.

Language Development

If language is considered as a symbolic system that allows the organization and transmission of thought, a case can be made that language is what most distinguishes humans from all other species. The human odyssey is defined by the human species' ability to use language to communicate with others and to make meaning of our experiences. There are five major components of language acquisition: phonemes, morphemes, semantics, syntax, and pragmatics. A **phoneme** is a speech sound and is the smallest unit of language. There are about 50 phonemes in the English language, and phonological awareness is the ability to distinguish phonemes. A preschool child's capacity to recognize phonemes is not only important for verbal language development; it is also essential for providing the foundation for reading (Braten & Hulme, 2009). A **morpheme** is the smallest unit that has meaning. Schiller and Costa (2006) note that morphemes can be divided into two categories: open class, which include nouns, verbs, adjectives, and adverbs; and closed class, which include conjunctions, pronouns, and prepositions. **Semantics** refers to the use of words to express meaning and thought. **Syntax** refers to the manner in which words are arranged in a language—essentially, the rules within a language that govern the order and organization of a phrase or sentence (Society for Research in Child Development, 2009). **Pragmatics** involves the use of language within social context, such as asking a question, giving a command, or using a nonverbal cue. All of these factors must come together in order for a child to understand language and to construct meaningful verbal expression. In addition to the five components of language, Tamis-LeMonda, Bornstein, and Baumwell (2001) noted that there are five language milestones in children's development of language: "... first imitations, first spontaneous words, achievement of 50 words, combinational speech and the use of language to talk about the past" (p. 749). Preschool children learn roughly nine new words each day, and by age 6 they have attained a vocabulary of approximately 14,000 words.

As they acquire language, children begin to pick up grammar rules and apply these rules, but at first they seem to make up their own rules. Two- and 3-year-old children can sometimes come up with interesting grammatical constructions. For example, one time my thirsty 3-year-old son Jake returned from a family hike and proclaimed, "Soda of grape to me." This was an unconventional and interesting way to phrase it, but his meaning was clear. Jacobson and Schwartz (2005) note that preschool children, upon learning basic language rules, tend to over-generalize and stringently apply grammatical rules. Most commonly, this results in errors of past tense and irregular verbs and nouns such as "We goed to school." Over time, children learn the nuances of grammar and the tendency to over-generalize grammar rules diminishes.

Young children are capable of learning and speaking more than one language at a time (Couchenour & Chrisman, 2011). Upon entering preschool, English language learners (ELL) may be silent as they adjust to the new environment and concentrate on listening. But after this slight delay, ELL preschoolers begin to learn English at a rapid rate (Bergin & Bergin, 2012). A major problem facing bilingual children is the lack of access to preschool programs. Zehr (2011) noted that there are effective bilingual programs available for preschool ELL students; however, Latino children comprise the vast majority of ELL students and are less likely to be enrolled in preschool programs. This lack of access to ELL services at a young age puts these children at a disadvantage upon entering kindergarten. The major barriers to preschool education for ELL children are lack of funds to pay for school and lack of transportation. Another barrier for ELL preschoolers is the shortage of early childhood bilingual teachers (Gillanders, 2007); therefore, most ELL preschool children are in settings without bilingual instruction. In the preschool classroom with a non-bilingual teacher, it is important that the school day have a predictable routine so that the children can feel secure as they begin to acquire English. Teachers should also use stories and songs to augment acquisition of English.

One of the best ways for children to learn a second language is within a social context; however, not knowing the language is a considerable barrier for social interaction. Teachers can encourage social interaction by using games and activities that are not language dependent. This will encourage connection and give ELL students an opportunity to learn within communal interaction. Oral interaction is the best way for ELL students to acquire vocabulary, and it is important for teachers to engage ELL students in conversation (Lenters, 2004).

Emergent literacy skills, antecedents to reading and writing, are usually evident by age 3 (Bergin & Bergin, 2012). As children approach age 5 and kindergarten, the literacy skills developed during the preschool years will provide the foundation for reading, writing, and ultimate academic success. Failure to develop literacy skills can hinder a child's academic achievement. Dooley (2010) stressed that comprehension comes before decoding, describing the following progression of preschool literacy skills. Prior to age 2, books serve mainly as a prop during play; however, infants and toddlers who have been read to are aware of how to hold a book. By age 3, children recognize images and are aware of content and may recognize some words. By age 4 they may echo or mimic reading and use pictures as cues to comprehend content. By age 5 they understand content by images and words and may be able to read print with scaffolding. A vital scaffolding technique to boost literacy is for children to follow along with the print as an adult reads the story. Saccardi (1996) stressed the importance of predictable books for emergent literacy. Predictable books have repetitive language patterns and story lines, usually coupled with pictures illustrating the story. Preschool children quickly pick up on the pattern and experience success and confidence in "reading" the book. This confidence coupled with encouragement of literacy skills will establish a solid foundation for success in reading.

ELL students face special challenges in learning to read (Lenters, 2004). These include interference due to dissimilar sounds, the constraints of their vocabulary, lack of background cultural knowledge, and dissimilar grammar structure. It is essential that ELL students engage in oral communication to build their basic vocabulary and grasp of grammar. It is also important for teachers to forge good relationships with families and to encourage first-language reading, especially when matched with second-language texts.

Education

As children age, they develop unique interests and require multifaceted experiences to advance cognitively, emotionally, and socially. Levine (2005) stated that the early years are a time of cognitive growth trajectory; interfering with this course of growth or failing to support it can result in the need for remediation later. It is crucial for young children to have the advantage of appropriate educational opportunities. To ignore the importance of preschool education is to risk the academic achievement of children later, since early childhood education forms the foundation for subsequent success in school. Young children need a stimulating and motivating educational environment to best use the rapid brain development that occurs at this stage of life (Neuman, 2005).

Young children experience numerous child care and educational situations. According to the National Center for Education Statistics (2011), in 2005–2006 approximately 20% of 4-year-olds were cared for in the home by one or both parents. Other in-home child care arrangements included relative care, which accounted for about 13%, and non-relative in-home care, which accounted for about 8% of 4-year-olds. Center-based care constituted 57% of child care; 13% of the children enrolled in center-based care attended Head Start, and 44% of children were enrolled in other types of day care centers. Various child care settings are described in more detail in the Social Development section of Chapter 8.

Over the years, there has been an ongoing debate about the effect of day care on children. What we now know is that high-quality child care has beneficial outcomes for children, whereas low-quality child can be unhelpful or even harmful (Couchenour & Chrisman, 2011). Longitudinal studies indicate that individuals who had quality preschool education were more likely to graduate from high school and be more successful in their careers and relationships (National Education Association, 2011). Conversely, children who lack quality preschool education start out at a deficit when entering formal schooling at age 5, suffer academic impediments, and are at risk for negative life outcomes.

REFLECTION 7.6 GETTING A HEAD START

My first job out of college was at a Head Start in rural Indiana. I was a combination teacher/ bus driver/social worker. The fact that I drove the bus helped me develop relationships with the families, which in turn facilitated the monthly home visits that I made to each child's home. As the only staff member with a degree in early childhood education, I worked closely with the parent curriculum committee in planning curriculum and events for the children. I came to value the input of the parents and their commitment to their children's success. The inclusion of parents in Head Start programs is empowering and advantageous to both the preschool and the families. [~CD]

What constitutes high-quality child care? Burchinal, Roberts, Riggins, and Zeisal (2000) stated that high-quality child care involves a low student/teacher ratio, educational and social opportunities, well-trained and educated staff, as well as good communication between the family and school. Couchenour and Chrisman (2011) stated that high-quality child care also includes responsive interactions between children and adults, a developmentally appropriate curriculum, and assessment. High-quality education for children before they enter kindergarten provides the underpinning for long-term academic success. Unfortunately, the benefits of quality early education are often out of reach for low-income families. Children living in poverty, who are at great risk academically, are most likely to receive child care from family members and therefore miss out on stimulating educational experiences and opportunities.

Created in 1965, during the Johnson administration as part of the War on Poverty, Head Start began as a summer preschool program to help close the achievement gap for low-income children. The following year it was expanded to a year-round preschool program. Head Start was developed to provide education, health services, and good nutrition to children. A hallmark of the program is the involvement of parents in their children's education and in the program. Through hands-on involvement in the Head Start center, parents are given a voice and cooperative relationships between school and home are fostered. Head Start parents are involved in many ways, including classroom volunteers, policy committees, and fundraising.

Longitudinal studies indicate that Head Start children have gains in cognitive and social development over low-SES children who did not attend Head Start; however, these gains are likely to diminish in the elementary school years unless they are supported by additional intervention programs to scaffold achievement and development for low-income children (Ludwig & Phillips, 2007). The lack of long-term effects for Head Start has led some to question the program's value in combating the achievement gap for low-income children; however, Ludwig and Phillips noted that a cost-benefit analysis of Head Start indicates that it is a worthwhile intervention.

Think About It **7.3**

With budget cuts, many low-SES families are losing access to preschool education for their children. Do you believe this is an advocacy issue for counselors? Why or why not? If yes, how would you begin to advocate for access to preschool education?

One of the main benefits of Head Start is the program's emphasis on education of families as well as the child. Parenting programs are beneficial for most families and are frequently offered through child care centers and programs. There are numerous parenting program packages. One of the best-known parenting programs is the Systematic Training for Effective Parenting (STEP) series. Based on Adlerian theory, STEP teaches concepts of family relationships and basic communication (Dinkmeyer & McKay, 1989). STEP helps parents understand the goals of misbehavior and how to set up a system of natural and logical consequences that will lead to children learning responsibility for their choices. Another Adlerian-based program is Active Parenting (Popkin, 1989). Both of these programs urge the use of encouragement instead of praise. **Praise** focuses on the outcome or completion of a task, whereas **encouragement** provides feedback during the activity and stays focused on the child's effort and ingenuity. Encouragement highlights the child's effort rather than merely providing a critique of a final product.

Adlerian approaches to parenting also espouse the use of natural and **logical consequences** instead of punishment. Allowing children to experience the consequences of their behavioral choices teaches responsibility and helps children make the connection between their decisions and outcomes. A natural consequence occurs when a child's behavior results in unpleasant effects. For instance, a child who chooses to not put on a jacket on a chilly morning will become cold and will learn that wearing a jacket is a better choice. Logical consequences are developed by parents and teachers and are logically connected to the behavioral choices made by the child. Hence, a child who refuses to pick up his toys will lose the privilege of playing with those toys for a set amount of time. The adult stresses that the child chose to not pick up toys and therefore he chose to lose access to the toys. The key is to calmly emphasize the connection between the child's behavioral choice and the consequences.

▶ CASE EXAMPLE **7.2** JASON.

Your client, Jason, has just been awarded sole custody of his three children (ages 5, 9, and 12). He feels very overwhelmed by all the responsibilities of being a single parent. The children have been acting out, and Jason is ashamed that he often loses his cool and yells at the kids. He wants to create a home that runs more smoothly and is calmer. In working with Jason, what do you need to assess? What resources could be integrated into an intervention with Jason and his children? How would you go about choosing a parenting approach with Jason that fits with this family?

Jennings, Hooker, and Linebarger (2009) reported that preschool educational television can facilitate literacy in children. The quality of the programming is the key to enhancement of emerging literacy skills through television. Preschool programs that use puppets, stories, and songs to familiarize children with letters and letter sounds can have a significant impact on literacy development. Interestingly, the most well-known children's television program, Sesame Street, was originally funded by Head Start. While there are benefits associated with watching educational programs, care must be taken that children are not watching violent and low-quality programs. Parents should monitor and limit television viewing.

While preschool education is universally regarded as vital to child development and success, there are diverse approaches to early childhood education around the world. In Europe, the education of young children is viewed as essential, with particular emphasis being paid to school readiness and transitions from home to preschool and then on to primary school (Neuman, 2005). European preschool teachers are well trained and well compensated and the curriculum tends to be standardized. Pang and Richey (2007) noted that while in the United States early childhood education is child-centered and tends to focus on individualism, self-expression, and free creative play, in China preschools are more structured, teacher-centered, and focused on academic success. Preschools in Japan are likely to follow a compensatory model, in which cognitive deficits are identified and instruction is tailored to help each child reach his or her full potential. While early childhood education is generally viewed as essential in the industrialized world, in emerging nations it is a new concept. As emerging nations develop, the need for preschool education will become more important, since early childhood education is the key to long-term success of a populace (Neuman, 2005). According to Levine (2005), by 2015 the world's most populous nations (i.e., China, Brazil, India, and Indonesia) will each educate more children than will be educated in the United States. While currently these nations lag behind in early childhood education, there is a great deal of interest in emerging nations in adopting best practices for the health, well-being, and education of their children.

Summary

During the preschool years, children continue to grow, but in spurts rather than a continuous growth trajectory. Normal weight and height ranges are broad to accommodate the considerable variability of individual growth rates found among preschool children. The brain grows rapidly during the early childhood years, and it has plasticity that can allow for adaptation and adjustment following brain injury.

The development of large and small motor skills is very important during the preschool years, and lack of appropriate development can hinder cognitive and social growth. Children should be encouraged to play and engage in large motor activities. This is particularly important due to the tendency toward sedentary activity in U.S. society. Small motor skills include using scissors, buttoning, drawing, and writing. The development of small motor skills is vital to the long-term academic success of the young child.

Minor illnesses are common in preschool children. It is very important for children to adhere to an immunization schedule for their own health and to avoid the emergence of more dangerous diseases. Children from lower SES strata have a lower rate of immunization due to lack of access to health care and lack of funds; they are also more likely to have dental decay or caries, which is a preventable disease. Again, lack of funds and access to dental care are major contributing factors. The most alarming health problem among young children is the rising rate of obesity. Better education for families on health and exercise is suggested to counteract the obesity trend. The most common cause of death in early childhood is unintentional injury; education about home safety can provide injury prevention.

Vision and hearing impairment create academic and social problems for children, and screening to identify these impairments is crucial. Preschool children may also experience sleep problems. Having a routine and security items can help children form good sleep habits. It is not uncommon for young children to experience nightmares and night terrors, especially during times of stress. In many families, co-sleeping is practiced. While there are people who argue against co-sleeping, there is little evidence that it is emotionally harmful, and it is a norm for many cultures.

Both Piaget and Vygotsky had an immense impact on preschool education. Most preschool aged children are in Piaget's preoperational stage, which includes two substages: preconceptual and intuitive. Piaget viewed learning as occurring thorough a process of assimilation and accommodation whereby new information is either aligned with an existing schema or adapted into a new schema. Preoperational children are egocentric in their worldview. Vygotsky's contribution to the field of cognitive development was relatively unheard of in the West until the dissolution of the Soviet Union. Vygotsky's concepts of the zone of proximal development and scaffolding are widely used in preschools.

Information processing is the mechanism by which we attain and store knowledge. The information processing model includes the sensory register, working memory, and long-term memory. Another aspect of cognitive development is language. Children must master the components of language and the rules of grammar during the preschool years. Language and literacy skills are crucial for education, and early childhood education forms the foundation for future academic success and is vital for long-term achievement.

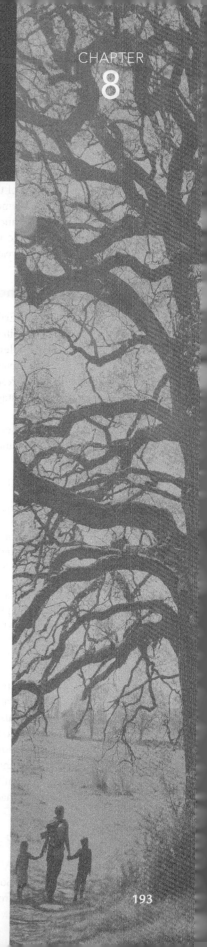

The Preschool Years: Early Childhood Emotional and Social Development

By Stephen Parker and Charlotte Daughhetee

L ife is not a solitary journey. We traverse our lifespan in relationship with others. The formation of a sense of self and the extent of one's ability to form bonds and connections with others is a crucial aspect of development during the preschool years. Through multifaceted familial and societal influences, individuals form a basis of emotional and social competence that will guide their personal odyssey across the lifespan.

SECTION I: Emotional Development

One cannot overemphasize the importance of secure, nurturing relationships to the overall emotional well-being of young children (Shonkoff, 2010). Through these relationships, children learn the basics of emotional and social interactions and establish the foundation of their relational framework. By early childhood, children have not only developed basic emotions such as happiness and anger, but also more complex emotions such as jealousy and guilt (Kail & Cavanaugh, 2010). It is also during the preschool years that children learn to regulate themselves and their emotions (Boyer, 2009). Consequently, these are critical years in the development of emotional understanding of the self and of others.

Erik Erikson's Psychosocial Theory

Erik Erikson's stage theory of psychosocial development epitomizes the concept of the lifespan odyssey and adroitly illustrates the perilous journey individuals undertake as they develop psychologically within a social context. Erikson's eight-stage theory spans the lifespan, and each stage consists of tasks or crises that must be completed for the successful resolution of that stage. Failure to resolve a stage crisis will inhibit resolution of the future stages, thereby resulting in a psychosocial deficit (Erikson, 1982).

Erikson studied with Freud, and while his stage model theory parallels Freud's theory somewhat, Erikson departed from Freud's view of instinct, psychosexual stages, and the unconscious as the defining elements of ego development. In contrast to Freud, Erikson put forth the concept that the psychosocial factors occurring within a group context were the major forces behind personality development. Freud viewed child development as progressing through psychosexual stages in which, at each stage, the libido is focused upon a particular erogenous zone. Freud's **phallic stage** occurs during early childhood (ages 3 to 6 years), when children become aware of their genitals and of the difference between males and females. For males, this stage includes the oedipal complex, wherein boys focus their libido on their mothers and want to replace their father. For girls, Freud suggested the Electra complex, wherein girls focus their libido on their fathers and want to replace their mother.

Erikson's **initiative vs. guilt stage** occurs during the preschool years and is characterized by the child pursuing interests and independent activities (Erikson, 1982). Children at this stage engage in exploration of the environment and imaginative play. They learn to cooperate with others and also learn how to lead. Encouragement of this exploration will result in the child learning to take on new challenges, plan activities, and acquire a sense of purpose. Conversely, when adults discourage or impede initiative, children become ashamed and develop guilt about their interests and exploration. During this stage, it is important for teachers and parents to allow children to choose activities they are interested in and to provide materials for imaginative play (Goodnough, Perusse, & Erford, 2015).

> ### REFLECTION 8.1 JAKE AND OEDIPUS
>
> As I was washing dishes one evening, my 5-year-old son Jake was visiting with me in the kitchen. He sat at the kitchen table looking out the window at our herb garden, which was decorated with a ceramic angel. His little voice piped up: "Mom, when I grow up I'm going to marry you," to which I responded, "That's nice." He pointed out the window at the angel and said "That would be a great place to bury Dad." Wow! I thought, maybe Freud was right after all.[~CD]

Adler's Individual Psychology

Alfred Adler was a contemporary of Freud and a member of the Vienna Psychoanalytic Society; however, he began to diverge from Freud's theory and was eventually ousted from Freud's inner circle in what was to become the first split from Freud's central group.

The division was acrimonious and became a motivating factor for Adler to prove the superiority of his theory. Adler differed from Freud primarily in that Adler saw people as social beings, best understood when viewed within a social context. His approach was more holistic; he did not divide the self into concepts such as the id or superego. Adler was more interested in people's conscious rather than their unconscious, and his approach was ultimately more pragmatic and purposeful. This more practical and goal-directed approach has proved to be very beneficial in counseling, and the Adlerian approach is a commonplace theory in use today by counselors in a variety of settings, especially counselors working with families and children.

After the break with Freud, Adler went on to form the Society for Individual Psychology in 1912 and became a major influence on psychology and counseling. Adler believed that people could be understood by the patterns of their personalities, or what he called the "lifestyle" of the person (Dinkmeyer & Carlson, 2001). Additionally, he believed that people endeavored to belong, a concept known as **social interest**. Social interest can be observed in young children when they want to help and be a contributing part of the group. Adler's concept of **lifestyle** is the way in which the person interfaces with social context. If a person has a healthy lifestyle, that individual will experience mental health and positive social interactions. A person's lifestyle is profoundly influenced by childhood experiences and can be thought of as the self, the personality, or the uniqueness of the individual.

Adler viewed behavior as being goal directed and having social significance. The phrase "Nobody ever throws away a behavior that works" (Dinkmeyer & Carlson, 2001, p. 42) sums up the Adlerian stance on how behavior reveals inner choices and rationales. When someone's behavior is puzzling, consider how that behavior might be paying off for that individual. Though Adler focused on the conscious, he also recognized that behavioral goals could be unconsciously driven.

One of the most valuable ideas to come from Adlerian theory is the concept of the four **goals of misbehavior** developed by Rudolph Dreikurs (Dreikurs & Soltz, 1991). Dreikurs believed that children want to belong and feel that they matter. If a child is not able to belong in a positive way, he will try to find significance and belonging in what society considers a negative manner, or through mistaken goals that fuel negative recurring interactions between parents and children (Bitter, 2009). These mistaken goals arise out of the child's sense of discouragement. Adlerians believe that a misbehaving child is a discouraged child. The four goals are: attention seeking, power, revenge, and inadequacy. One of the most interesting and useful aspects of Dreikurs' four goals of misbehavior is the manner in which a parent or teacher can ascertain which goal the child is engaged in. When a child is misbehaving, the adult examines his or her internal emotional reaction to the child's misconduct; thus, the child's goal of misbehavior can be uncovered by the adult's internal response. It should be noted that of the four goals of misbehavior, attention seeking and power are the most common, especially among preschool children. The goals of revenge and inadequacy present more difficulties for intervention and may require counseling interventions.

The **attention-seeking** child believes she matters only if she is being noticed, and therefore, she engages in behavior that will draw the attention of the adult. For instance, she might intentionally make noise when an adult is trying to talk on the phone. The adult pauses in conversation and shushes the child, who is quiet for a brief moment and then once again engages in noisy behavior. Dreikurs (Dreikurs & Stoltz, 1991) referred to this type of interaction as shooing a fly. Just as a shooed fly comes back around, the shooed child will once again engage in attention-seeking behavior. Dreikurs suggested that parents ignore the behavior rather than feed the attention seeking by punishing or coaxing the child to behave. Parents are advised to pay attention to children when they are behaving appropriately, a concept commonly known as "catching them being good."

A child with a goal of power is trying to achieve significance by being in control and by proving no one can have **power** over them (Dreikurs & Stoltz, 1991). When encountering a power-seeking child, an adult feels angry and may be tempted to engage in a power struggle with the child. It is important for the adult to remain calm and not fight with the child. If the adult "wins" the power struggle and forces the child to defiantly acquiesce, the child has simply learned a lesson in the influence of dominance and control. Alternatively, if the parents give in to the child, they also underscore the importance of power. Allowing children to have choices within parameters set by the parent can help children learn responsibility and initiative without resorting to power struggles. An example would be dressing for school. Rather than engaging in a power struggle with a preschooler over what he will wear, the parent can provide the child with a range of appropriate clothes and allow him to choose his outfit for school. The child's need for power can be redirected into a sense of empowerment when parents elicit the child's help and collaboration and facilitate the child's experience of power in a constructive manner (Dinkmeyer & Carlson, 2001).

The third goal of misbehavior is **revenge** (Dreikurs & Stoltz, 1991). The revenge-seeking child has been hurt in some way and is lashing out at those around her. Her sense of belonging comes from making others hurt as much as she has been hurt. The parent or teacher experiences feelings of hurt and may be tempted to lash back. It is important to rebuild the relationship with the child and use natural and logical consequences for behavior management. The use of punishment with such children will only exacerbate the feelings of revenge and behaviors of retaliation.

The final goal of misbehavior is **inadequacy** (Dreikurs & Stoltz, 1991). The child displaying inadequacy has given up and displays hopelessness. Parents and teachers will experience feelings of giving up on the child, but they must not throw in the towel or exhibit pity for the child. The child with a goal of inadequacy is the most discouraged child of all, and he will not benefit from praise. In fact, the use of praise or gold stars and awards will feel hollow and fake and will have little or no effect. This child is in great need of encouragement, and the adult should look for ways to authentically encourage small attempts. Above all the adult must not criticize the child (Dinkmeyer & Carlson, 2001). Parents and teachers should find ways for the child to experience success and work to build the child's confidence.

Because of Adler's focus on the importance of the social and belonging needs of humans, he was the first to clearly recognize the importance of the family; he can thus be regarded as the first family therapist (Bitter, 2009). Adler put forth the concept of the **family atmosphere**, the climate that exists within and between people in a family system. He used the term **family constellation** to describe the structure of the family system and how each person defines his or her place within the family system. Adler's concepts of belonging and social interest reflect the significant relationships within a family system, the most powerful influence in a child's life.

A major facet of the family constellation is the effect of **birth order**. Adler was the first theorist to emphasize the significance of birth order, and Adlerians have written extensively on the topic over the years. Eckstein et al. (2010) reported that an extensive review of birth order research reveals support for the existence of distinctive birth order characteristics. It should be noted that Adler emphasized that birth order should be considered within context and that factors such as gender and the years between siblings were important elements. A daughter born more than five years after a son should not automatically be assumed to possess the characteristics of a second-born; each case must be considered individually. Also, Adler was more interested in the psychological birth order, the role the child assumes, than the simple ranking of oldest to youngest. With those caveats in place, let's examine the concept of birth order.

The oldest child has the luxury of parental attention; if this child is an only child, the attention continues and the child is never dethroned by the birth of a sibling (Bitter, 2009). Oldest and only children tend to be high achievers, responsible, organized, traditional, and more anxious than subsequent children (Eckstein et al., 2010). With parental attention firmly focused on them, oldest and only children are the center of attention and may prefer the company of adults over peers. The parents of first-born children can be anxious,

REFLECTION 8.2 LEARNING TO SHARE MOM

My oldest son Daniel was 3½ years old when my second son, Jake, was born. We brought Jake home from the hospital and Daniel wasn't exactly thrilled about his baby brother. Daniel brought over a toy telephone to show Jake and I said, "That's nice, you're showing him your toys," to which Daniel replied, "He can call him mom." I said, "But I'm baby Jake's mom just like I'm your mom." Daniel's response: "No, he can call his real mom to come get him." It took a few weeks, but Daniel eventually accepted the reality of baby Jake. [~CD]

overprotective, and very focused on the child. If another child is born, the firstborn is dethroned and is no longer the center of the parental universe. This dethronement may lead the firstborn to act out in an attempt to recapture parental attention; however, it should be noted that the dethronement effect may be more pronounced within competitive family systems.

The second child, particularly if this is the second of only two, is very focused on competing with the firstborn and may seek to be very different from the firstborn in an attempt to capture parental attention (Bitter, 2009). The second child may avoid direct competition in arenas where the firstborn excels, and will seek to carve out a unique role for him or herself. In a sense, the second child is playing catch-up. If another child is born, the second child becomes a middle child and feels competition from both the eldest and the youngest children. It is easy for a middle child to feel somewhat lost and insignificant; a middle child may believe the parents favor the older or younger sibling. Middle children are often excellent negotiators and tend to be very loyal to peers.

The youngest or baby of the family is never dethroned (Bitter, 2009). Youngest children tend to be charming and affectionate. Skilled at getting what they want and at being the center of attention, youngest children can seem to be manipulative and spoiled. Parents tend to be more lenient with youngest children. The parents are no longer anxious about child rearing, are busy with the other children, and are more lenient with discipline; as a result, youngest children may at times feel overlooked and unattended. "Once the baby always the baby" is another issue for youngest children, and as youngest children age, they may struggle with not being taken seriously within the family. Youngest children tend to be very social and are usually viewed as entertaining and humorous; however, they may also be more rebellious and tend to be risk takers.

Family Systems Theory

Families are the most important influence on a child's development (Venetsanou & Kambas, 2010), and since all members of the family are interconnected, changes in one person within the family system will impact the entire family. That concept of interconnectedness is at the core of the family systems perspective. It is important to remember that no one person or family exists or develops outside of systemic influence. Individuals and families do not develop in isolation but develop within the context of multiple systems, and they are simultaneously acting upon and influenced by multiple systems. A child is an individual who dwells within the multiple contexts of his or her family of origin, extended family, community (school, neighborhood), and larger societal and cultural context (Couchenour & Chrisman, 2011). Hence, the most effective interventions for children are those that involve multiple systems working together collaboratively.

Just as children are influenced by multiple systems, they are also affected by developmental progressions across time as well as traditions passed down through time. McGoldrick and Carter (1999) postulated that families are influenced by **horizontal stressors**, the expected and unexpected developmental events that occur across time. Examples of horizontal stressors include the expected family stress of a child becoming an adolescent or the stress from the unexpected death of a young person. Horizontal stressors also include events that occur within historical context such as economic downturns or war. McGoldrick and Carter also noted the influence of vertical stressors on family systems. **Vertical stressors** include patterns such as familial behavioral and communication styles passed down through generations, as well as the influence of long-term poverty and oppression on generations of a family. When working with young children, teachers and mental health professionals should remain cognizant of the influence of both multiple systems and stressors.

➤ CASE EXAMPLE **8.1** THE CLARKS.

The Clark family has come for counseling. The Clarks (Brent and Sandra) have been married for 15 years and they have a 14-year-old son and a 3-year-old daughter. Brent comes from a poor family and has worked hard to achieve a middle-class lifestyle. Sandra grew up in an upper-middle-class household and works part-time as an industrial design consultant. They had only planned on having two children, but Sandra just found out that she is unexpectedly expecting. Brent just started a new job that isn't working out well, but with a new baby coming and very few jobs in his line of work, he feels he has to tough it out. Brent tries to not worry Sandra with his problems because she has enough to worry about with the kids and her consulting business. Brent has been drinking more at night, and Sandra expresses concern about this because alcoholism runs in both of their families. What types of stressors can you identify in this family? What systemic issues should you explore when working with the family? What strengths might this family possess that could be accessed as part of the treatment plan?

Gladding (2011) provided a broad definition of family that is inclusive of the myriad family configurations in our society: "those persons who are biologically and/or psychologically related, whom historical, emotional or economic bonds connect, and who perceive themselves as part of a household" (p. 6). Gladding noted that there are many types of family structures with the most prevalent being nuclear, single-parent, and blended families.

Just as individuals develop across the lifespan, so do families. Carter and McGoldrick (2005) developed a family lifecycle model that highlights typical developmental trends that occur across specific life stages. Their changing family lifecycle stage model begins with single young adults and covers the lifespan to the elderly. Early childhood falls within the families with young children phase. This is a very stressful stage. Parents with young children become exhausted simply trying to meet the physical and psychological demands of preschoolers (Gladding, 2011). Adding to the stress of rearing young children is the fact that most couples in the United States are dual-career couples. Managing young children, a home, and a job means that parents are spread very thin, and the emotional and psychological strain during this phase can take its toll on parents. Couple satisfaction decreases during this stage as the parents put all their energy into child-rearing and may put their relationship and their own self-care on the back burner. For single parents, this is a particularly difficult stage as they shoulder the burdens of child care, home, and work by themselves. An additional stressor that emerges during this stage is the stress of interfacing with new systems as young children enter preschool. Beginning preschool is a happy event, but it does bring with it new concerns and challenges, which are addressed later in this chapter.

Families that are too inflexible or disordered struggle with the developmental changes and stressors that occur across the family lifecycle. There must be a healthy balance of bonding and constancy in order to cope with the constant systemic modifications that must be made as children grow and develop. Olsen's circumplex model illustrates the various types of systemic connectedness and stability that can be found in families (Olson & Gorall, 2003). The model shows the interaction between **cohesion**, how close or distant family members feel themselves to be, and **flexibility**, the amount of structure in a family. On the extreme ends of the cohesion scale, families are either enmeshed (over-involved) or disengaged (distant), with midpoint scale descriptors of connected and separated. The flexibility scale includes rigid families on one extreme and chaotic families on the other. Midpoint scale descriptors of flexibility include flexible and structured. Families that are extreme (e.g., enmeshed and chaotic or rigid and disengaged families) have the most stress and difficulty dealing with life events and development. The more balanced or centered a family is on the circumplex model, the better able the family is to deal with life and the expected changes encountered across the lifespan. There is no perfect definition of a family in this model, but the model does illustrate how various family systems can be organized in ways that are more conducive to healthy navigation through family development and life stressors across the lifespan.

Emotional Competence

As preschoolers develop cognitively, their ability to name and discuss their own emotional states increases. Hansen and Zambo (2006) indicated that "Emotions or affect are both physiological and psychological feelings that children have in response to their world" (p. 274). The development of language allows children to express emotional states and find clarity in discussing emotions, thereby developing emotional competence. **Emotional competence** is extraordinarily important to the overall well-being of preschool children. Emotionally competent children have awareness of their own and others' emotions and can regulate their emotional responses. This development of emotional competence is critically important, as it is linked to later social and academic success (Denham et al., 2003). Children who exhibited emotional competence by ages 3 or 4 were more likely to experience success in kindergarten. Conversely, a lack of emotional competence was found to hinder social and academic achievement.

An important factor in emotional development is the capacity of the child to experience empathy. Empathy is a congruent affective response to the emotional condition of another person (Hinnant & O'Brien, 2007). By age 4, children have the ability to understand the feelings of others and can exhibit caring behaviors to a friend who is hurt or upset. Empathy skills are associated with cognitive and language development (Moreno & Klute, 2008). The development of empathy is crucial to friendship skills and the understanding of social context. It is the cornerstone of emotional competence.

> **Think About It   8.1**
>
> Can empathy be taught? If so, how could preschools and families encourage the development of empathy and other pro-social behaviors?

A major component of emotional competence is the ability of the child to regulate his or her emotions and responses to emotion. Self-regulated children are able to respond to social and emotional situations appropriately. They can obey directives, begin or halt behaviors according to contextual cues, modulate the intensity of their responses, and delay gratification (Boyer, 2009). Essentially, self-regulated children have learned to think before they act. Hansen and Zambo (2006) suggested that parents and teachers model emotional regulation and encourage children to name and clarify feelings. Hansen and Zambo emphasized the power of

---

REFLECTION   8.3   KATIE AND ANNIE

Many years ago I did a student teaching internship at a preschool in Bloomington, Indiana. I've always remembered one particular incident. It was a chilly day and the children were getting their coats and mittens on for the playground. In all the excitement, Annie wet her pants. The teacher took the children outside and I stayed with Annie to help her change into clean dry clothes. Annie was very embarrassed and teary-eyed. As we walked down the hall toward the playground, I noticed that Annie's friend Katie was waiting outside. When we exited the building, Katie, with a very concerned look on her face, walked up to Annie, hugged her, took her hand and said "It's OK, Annie, last week I peed in my snowsuit." Katie and Annie laughed and ran off to play. At the time I was struck by the kindness, but it wasn't until I was working on my master's degree in counseling 10 years later that I realized what I had witnessed was a delightful display of early childhood empathy skills. Not only did Katie understand Annie's emotions, she displayed concern, compassion, and even threw in some appropriate self-disclosure. Maybe Katie has grown up to become a counselor; she certainly exhibited some excellent empathy skills at age 4. [~CD]

children's literature to enhance emotional development. They point out that children's books are an easy way for adults to help children recognize and interpret the increasingly complex emotions they are experiencing as they develop. These authors listed books that address a wide range of emotions including anger, anxiety, disgust, fear, guilt, shame, and pride.

A basic emotional concern for young children is fear. Robinson and Rotter (1991) pointed out that children's fears are usually short-lived and that children learn to cope with fears; however, about 10% of children may develop phobias. Fears can be protective, such as fear of strangers, or they may be incapacitating, as when a child cannot go to sleep due to fear of the dark. Children's fears are for the most part normative and an expected facet of early childhood development.

Meltzer et al. (2008) stated that while the strength and ranking of children's fears differ across cultures, some fears are common among children, including fear of animals, the dark, blood, doctors/shots, thunder, and imaginary beings. Younger children tend to be more frightened of imaginary beings and natural phenomena such as storms, whereas older children have fears more grounded in typical life experiences, such as fear of doctors. Girls tend to exhibit fears more often than boys, which might be accounted for by gender socialization. In fact, preschool children classified adults as less afraid than children and boys as less afraid than girls (Sayfan & Lagattuta, 2009). The ability to regulate fear grows as children develop cognitively. Children aged 7 and older are able to reason with themselves that "monsters aren't real, so there can't be one in my closet," while younger children ages 3 or 4 might cope with fear through imaginary means: "I'll fight that witch with my toy gun." Fears are very common for preschool children and are only problematic if the fear becomes a phobia that inhibits the child's daily functioning (Meltzer et al., 2008).

Separation anxiety is common among preschool children, especially as children begin attending preschool. For the most part, children adjust and the anxiety passes; however, as the following story from a colleague illustrates, fear of separation can be a long-standing problem for some children.

Robinson and Rotter (1991) recommended several strategies for helping children cope with fear. These include reading stories related to conquering fear, helping children understand the natural world to soothe fears about storms and the dark, and helping children to

---

REFLECTION 8.4 THE PERFECT PARENT

Despite my knowledge of child development, gleaned from graduate work in counseling and guidance, I discovered that I was not completely prepared, as I had erroneously assumed, to be "The Perfect Parent"—especially to two children with distinctly different personalities. I learned all too soon that I had much "on-the-job training" ahead of me.

My son arrived in the world equipped with an impressive case of separation anxiety that persisted, to some degree, into middle school. This condition began with nightly struggles to get him to sleep, followed by my (usually unsuccessful) attempts to tiptoe out of his bedroom without his waking up and shrieking at the shocking realization that I was leaving him alone in his crib. In desperation, I attempted to implement the "Ferber Method," which involves allowing your child to "cry it out" and learn to self-comfort; however, after he cried for four hours straight and began banging his head on the crib, I accepted my defeat—and total failure as a Ferber-approved mom—and picked him up. After many weeks of nightly struggles, I finally lost the battle altogether and began putting him in bed between my husband and me in order to get any uninterrupted sleep at all.

Engaging the services of babysitters, other than his grandmothers, was out of the question as well, we learned; he would make himself physically ill (and the babysitter, as well), crying until we returned. Mom's Day Out was possible only because of the infinite patience of two kind and caring women who bravely endured his crying nearly the entire morning of his attendance there each week. (I'm nominating them for Methodist sainthood.) When the elementary school years arrived, the teacher reported teary episodes daily for weeks on end. My accompanying the class on all field trips was a mandatory condition in order for my son to agree to go on the trip himself.

In stark contrast, my daughter, born six years later, never displayed the slightest indication that parting from me presented a problem for her. She slept soundly through the night early on, happily occupied herself when left with a babysitter, and, as a toddler, engaged immediately with her peers at Mom's Day Out. Even on the dreaded (by most children and their parents) First Day of Kindergarten, she stepped out of the car and went straight into the school, never looking back even to wave goodbye. Unlike her brother, my daughter actually complained when I went along with her class on elementary school field trips. She approached virtually all new situations with a level of independence that I found extraordinary, particularly in contrast to my experience with her brother.

Interestingly, the chasm between the levels of independence they exhibited as children has closed completely as they have become young adults. Both are friendly, gregarious (to a fault)—and far too rarely call their mother! [~MH]

develop an overall sense of self-efficacy and confidence. Children who feel self-assured are more able to overcome fearful circumstances.

Angry outbursts and temper tantrums are normal occurrences with preschool age children; however, early childhood is also the time when children learn to understand and manage their emotions. For most children, as they develop emotional competence, they will learn to manage strong emotions such as anger in a pro-social manner. Sometimes preschoolers "melt down" or have a temper tantrum. A **temper tantrum** is an explosive external presentation of an inner emotional state, usually a mixture of both anger and distress (Potegal & Davidson, 2003). Giesbrecht, Miller, and Muller (2010) explored the impact of emotional reactivity on the ability of children to manage anger. Emotional reactivity can be viewed as a manner in which humans adapt to the environment. Essentially, people are going to have emotional reactions to environmental stimuli, but how people cope with the emotional reactivity determines one's level of emotional competence. Giesbrecht et al. found that whether or not a child had a temper tantrum was associated with their level of emotional reactivity and their emotional competence ability; high emotional reactivity and low emotional competence were associated with temper tantrums. Obviously, a child with higher levels of emotional competence is able to perceive his or her emotions and also able to recognize emotions in others. Additionally, emotionally competent children can make decisions about appropriate behavior within a particular circumstance. Parents and teachers can model appropriate behavior. The use of Adlerian or behavioral techniques to help children learn emotional management is also helpful at home and in preschool settings.

Mental Disorders in Early Childhood

According to the Surgeon General (2011) of the United States, good mental health in children is indicated by successful attainment of developmental milestones, secure attachments, healthy social relationships, and good coping skills. There is little research on the frequency of mental disorders in early childhood. The Centers for Disease Control and Prevention (2008) reported on the rate of mental health services provided to children in 2005–2006. In this report, 14.5% of children aged 4–11 years had a parent who talked with school staff or a health care provider about emotional or behavioral problems during that year. This data does not give us specific information about early childhood, and is more indicative of the mental health concerns of elementary-aged children.

Though little research has been conducted on mental disorders in preschool children, the prevalence of early childhood psychopharmacological treatment is rising each year as more young children are prescribed psychotropic medications (Egger & Angold, 2006). While there has been a rise in the treatment of young children with medication, there are still many mental health professionals who are reluctant to diagnose young children with mental disorders.

The early childhood years involve rapid development, particularly of emotional competence and regulation; therefore, it is wise to exercise caution before labeling a child as having a disorder. That said, children diagnosed later in childhood were found to have exhibited symptoms of their disorders in early childhood, so there may be a benefit to early diagnosis and intervention. When diagnosing preschool children, one must consider whether the observed behaviors are chronic and outside the norm, or fall within the expected range of developmental behavior.

The most common diagnosis found in preschoolers is attention-deficit/hyperactivity disorder (ADHD), with about three times as many boys diagnosed as girls (Egger & Angold, 2006). This disorder is characterized by inattention, hyperactivity, and impulsivity, and these symptoms must be chronic, severe, and cause impairment to warrant a diagnosis. Since preschoolers are just developing the ability to pay attention and regulate themselves, one can see how challenging it would be to recognize ADHD and distinguish it from naturally occurring behaviors.

Other disorders that can be recognized in young children are oppositional defiant disorder (ODD) and conduct disorder (CD) (Egger & Angold, 2006). Once again, young boys are more likely to be diagnosed with these disorders. These disorders are characterized by anger, aggression, opposition, and negative affect that are persistent, pervasive, and severe. Since young children are learning how to regulate and control their emotions, care must be taken in determining a diagnosis. The use of structured assessment for ODD and CD is encouraged.

While major depressive disorder is rarely diagnosed in early childhood, depressive symptoms do occur in young children, with approximately the same rate of occurrence in boys and girls (Egger & Angold, 2006). Depressed children exhibit sadness and low energy; they may be irritable and have altered eating and sleeping habits. Due to their age, preschool children do not have the cognitive ability to express their inner feelings of sadness. With adult clients, a counselor can ask questions about suicidal thoughts and assess the level of suicidal ideation; however, this is not possible with preschoolers. Luby et al. (2002) suggested that by observing children's play, themes of suicide and death can be detected and suicidal ideation assessed. In addition, a family history of mood disorders should be taken into account when assessing for depression in young children. As for the rate of mania and bipolar disorders in early childhood, there is not enough research or data to determine how prevalent these conditions are in the preschool population. There is also very little research on anxiety disorders in preschoolers, but young children who have been diagnosed with anxiety disorders were found to be significantly impaired socially and academically (Egger & Angold, 2006).

Egger and Emde (2011) examined the need for a mental health diagnostic method that would be reliable for infants, toddlers, and preschool aged children. While diagnostic research regarding adolescent and school-aged children has grown in the past few decades, little research has been done to address the mental health needs and diagnosis of infants and young children. As it pertains to mental health, Egger and Emde define infancy as the period from birth to 5 years of age. They espouse a relational approach that examines the multiple systems and environmental circumstances that affect the child, rather than relying on classification of symptoms. They note, "The challenge of applying the DSM criteria to very young children is greater than in later childhood because of the rapid developmental changes, the limitations of language, and the interdependence of the child with his or her caregivers that characterize early childhood" (p. 98).

Think About It 8.2

Does diagnosing preschool aged children provide early intervention and help, or does it label them? Are behaviors within the normal range of preschool development being pathologized?

Child Maltreatment

There is a connection between child maltreatment and the development of subsequent mental disorders in childhood and adulthood; this is particularly true when chronic maltreatment occurs during the preschool years (Manly, Kim, Rogosch, & Cicchetti, 2001). Additionally, Kim and Chicchetti (2010) found that child maltreatment interfered with the development of emotional regulation and appropriate peer relationships. According to the Centers for Disease Control and Prevention, in 2008 state and local child protective agencies received approximately 3.3 million reports of child abuse and neglect in the United States (CDC, 2010b). For preschool children, the child maltreatment victim rate is about 11 per 1000. Of these, 71% were victims of neglect, 16% physical abuse, 9% sexual abuse, and 7% emotional abuse. Children with multiple forms of abuse are counted more than once in these statistics. Of these children, 1740 died from abuse and neglect, with about 80% of cases occurring with children 4 years old and younger. The majority of perpetrators in child abuse cases are parents. It is important to note that these data are from cases actually reported to child protective agencies, so the rate of child maltreatment is actually thought to be much higher due to unreported child abuse incidents.

Educators, medical providers, mental health professionals, and members of law enforcement agencies are considered mandated reporters and are required by law in all 50 states to report suspected child abuse (Remley & Herlihy, 2010). A mandated reporter is not supposed to investigate the abuse, but must report when abuse is suspected. Fear of being sued is not a reason for failing to report abuse since most states include a "good faith" provision in laws to protect reporters (Sperry, 2007). Mandated reporters should become familiar with state laws and know the appropriate reporting agencies and protocol. It is also important to leave the investigative interviewing to forensic interviewers who are trained in investigative techniques and proper procedures (National Child Advocacy Center, 2012). An individual without appropriate forensic interviewing training could re-traumatize the child during an interview, and the fact that an untrained interviewer questioned the child could be used by a perpetrator's defense attorney to nullify a charge. The National Child Advocacy Center has information about the forensic interviewing process and training. Table 8.1 lists the signs and symptoms of abuse and neglect as specified by the Child Welfare Identification Gateway (2007).

The National Child Advocacy Center was created in 1985 with a mission to provide child abuse response and prevention (National Child Advocacy Center, 2012). There are more than 800 Child Advocacy Centers in all 50 states and 10 foreign countries. The centers use a multidisciplinary approach, coordinating treatment and intervention among law enforcement, criminal justice, medical and mental health professionals, and child protective services. Many Child Advocacy Centers use trauma-focused cognitive behavioral therapy as a treatment model. Ongoing outcome research on this approach will provide useful information for mental health professionals and families. Regardless of which therapeutic model is used in the treatment of child abuse and neglect, the importance of building a strong, trusting, therapeutic alliance and providing a safe environment for the children is paramount (Capuzzi & Gross, 2004).

Another issue that affects children is parental substance abuse. According to the Children of Alcoholic Families organization, one in four children will be exposed to alcohol/substance abuse or dependence in the family before the age of 18 (Children of Alcoholic Families, 2011). Substance abuse in the family has a detrimental effect upon children. Couchenour and Chrisman (2011) stated that children in families with members who abuse alcohol and other substances sometimes reverse roles with the parent and become the caretaker, often taking on responsibilities well beyond what would be expected given their age, although some of these children may become more irresponsible. They are often fearful, angry, mistrustful, or sad, sometimes displaying chronic depression. It is not uncommon for these children to struggle academically and socially. Early mental health intervention with both the child and the family is vital for successful developmental progress. Jaffee and Maikovich-Fong (2011) found that providing mental health intervention with the families and caregivers of abused children led to significant lessening of psychopathological symptoms in the children. Early intervention and increased access to counseling services for maltreated children and their caregivers are essential elements for appropriate lifespan development.

TABLE 8.1 ✦ SIGNS AND SYMPTOMS OF ABUSE AND NEGLECT

Physical abuse:
- Unexplained burns, bites, bruises, broken bones, or black eyes
- Fading bruises or other marks noticeable after an absence from school
- Fear of parents, protests or crying when it is time to go home
- Shrinking at the approach of adults
- Reports of injury by a parent or other adult caregiver

Neglect:
- Frequently absent from school
- Begs or steals food or money
- Lacks medical or dental care, immunizations, or glasses
- Is consistently dirty and has severe body odor
- Lacks sufficient clothing for the weather
- Abuses alcohol or other drugs
- States that there is no one at home to provide care

Sexual abuse:
- Difficulty walking or sitting
- Refuses to change for gym or participate in physical activities
- Nightmares or bed wetting
- Sudden change in appetite
- Has unusual or advanced sexual knowledge or behavior
- Pregnancy or venereal disease
- Runs away
- Reports sexual abuse by parent or other adult caregiver

Emotional abuse:
- Exhibits extremes in behavior; overly compliant, demanding, extremely passive or aggressive
- Either inappropriately adult-like or infantile
- Has attempted suicide
- Reports lack of attachment to parent

SECTION II: Social Development

Sex Role and Gender Role Development

When a child is born the typical announcement is not "It's a person" or "It's a human." Indeed, those pronouncements seem rather silly. Rather, we loudly and proudly shout, "It's a girl" or "It's a boy." It is not a stretch to use this simple observation to suggest that the sex of a child is the single most important characteristic that can be communicated. Thus, it is important to take a step back and ask the basic question, "Why?"

Why is the future reproductive capacity of the infant so very important? Why are infants dressed in coded colors? Why, in the extreme, do female babies with little or no hair end up with bows taped to their heads? Why are we so deeply apologetic if we ever mistake the sex of a child and compliment a parent on what a cute little girl she is, only to be corrected by the maligned parent with "His name is Mike." Information about a person's identity is provided to others only if there is an expectation that this information is important with respect to how interaction should take place. We work diligently to make sure others know the sex of a child because we expect interactions to be affected by whether the person (the child) is male or female. We expect boys and girls to be different. These expectations are called **gender stereotypes**.

Explaining and legitimizing these differences has been the subject of theoretical debates for centuries. These explanations vary widely and have important implications for how children are raised. This is true interpersonally as well as with respect to social policy. Thus, it is worth reviewing and offering a critique of some of the major theories addressing gender.

Biological Approaches

Biological approaches to understanding gender tend to see male and female differences as normal, natural, and necessary. Many theorists suggest evolutionary advantages to early humans in the type of gender expectations that exist in contemporary society. In the **"Man as Hunter" hypothesis** (Ardrey, 1976) men have always been hunters. As a result, characteristics such as aggression, ambition, leadership, and interest in technological innovation have long been traits associated with being male. Because men were providing the basic sustenance for the group, men were of a higher status than women. And thus the seeds for patriarchy and male dominance were established.

Perhaps even more basic has been a focus on the differential reproductive capacities of men and women as they relate to early evolution. It was in men's best interest to have as many children with as many women as possible in order to ensure the continuation of their genetic line. At the same time, because women could have only a limited number of children, they had to be much more selective with respect to whom they would allow to be the father of their children. Women therefore sought out the most highly successful and high-status men with whom to produce a child. This then provided another motive for men to be aggressive, ambitious, competitive, and successful. Doing so increased the probability of having sexual mates and thus continuing one's genetic legacy (Fischer, 1994). However, these hypotheses are contradicted by the accepted archeological and anthropological evidence (Sussman & Hart, 2008). Humans were much lower on the food chain than the hunting hypothesis assumes. Humans operated much more like scavengers than noble hunters. Additionally, it seems clear that women contributed much more to the sustenance of early human groups than is traditionally assumed.

Psychoanalytic Theory

Psychoanalytic theory is most directly associated with Sigmund Freud (1856–1939). According to Freud, children pass through a series of psychosexual stages as part of their personality development. Gender is not a major issue in either of the first two stages (oral and anal). It is during the third stage, at around the age of 4, that gender becomes a major focus. It is during this "phallic stage" that children become aware of their own genitals and the fact that the genitals of boys and girls are different. In addition, in the traditional nuclear family, children understand that their genitals are similar to those of one, but not both, of their parents. This establishes the basis for the identification of the child with the same-gendered parent. Much of Freud's work then concerns the tensions, competitions, and dynamics of child–parent relationships that arise out of these biological differences. Because so much of this occurs unconsciously, it has been difficult to investigate empirically. In addition, Freud seems to overstate the stability of these early experiences and leaves little room for growth or change on the part of individuals. Finally, it is difficult to deny a fundamental anti-female bias in Freud's work. Women are defined as inadequate, insecure, and even masochistic. Perhaps the only positive outcome of the misogynistic ideas of Freud is that it established a framework within which the feminist criticisms of individuals such as DeBeauvoir (1972) arose.

Others have remained more in the psychoanalytical tradition of Freud while attempting to address the inherent difficulties of his original propositions. Chodorow (1978, 1994) has used some of the basic precepts of Freud to address the question of how "mothering," caregiving responsibilities, and the emphasis on affective interpersonal relationship skills are learned by females. She suggests that boys need to separate from their mothers as part of their gender identification. Their identification is with an individual largely absent, physically and emotionally. Continuing an intimate relationship with one's mother is a direct threat to their gender-based identification. Put succinctly, intimacy is a threat to being a man. In contrast, young girls identify with their primary caregivers. They are able to maintain an intensely intimate relationship and in doing so learn the skills of intimacy and desire for such relationships. Chodorow's work is thought provoking and challenging. It continues, however, to be culturally bound. Studies from around the world demonstrate a lack of universality with respect to the relationship of intimacy and gender, and indeed for the assumed relationship between caregiving responsibilities (and skills) and gender.

Behavioral Theory

Behavioral theories (including social learning theory) suggest that boys and girls learn gender-appropriate behavior as a consequence of observing adult models of the same gender. Sometime during the second and third years of life children develop a **gender identity**; that is, they recognize their own gender and are able to identify others of the same gender. Gender is one substantive area among many that can be explained using models of conditioning (classical and operant) and reinforcement (reward and punishments) (Bandura, 1986). Children who behave in gender-appropriate ways are rewarded, while non-appropriate gender behaviors are punished. In addition to experiencing rewards and punishment directly, children may learn simply by observing the consequences experienced by others (Bronstein, 1988).

There are understandably appealing aspects to behavioral approaches. We have all witnessed and experienced reinforcement in practice and are aware that children regularly imitate the behavior of others. In addition, this perspective is characteristic of our general cultural beliefs regarding socialization. It is, however, important to distinguish between cultural beliefs and academic theory. As an explanation of how individuals learn appropriate gender behaviors, this perspective can be challenged in a number of important ways. First, if individuals learn by modeling the behavior of others, how do we explain changes in gender expectations? Overemphasizing modeling would seem to point toward a cultural inertia with respect to gender that does not hold in the face of changes with respect to gender expectations in the last half century. Second, behaviorism seems to overstate, or over-assume, societal consensus with respect to gender expectations. There is tremendous disagreement with respect to what is appropriate for males and females today. How do individuals (or perhaps groups) disentangle all of the mixed messages as to what it means to be male or female in our society? Put another way, behaviorism tends to look at the individual as overly passive in the socialization process. There is a need for some sort of cognitive model that explains how received information is interpreted, evaluated, and given meaning. Various theories under the banner of "cognitive development" represent attempts to address some of these remaining questions.

Cognitive Development Theory

Cognitive development approaches to gender are grounded in the theories of Piaget and Kohlberg. In some ways, these approaches stand in contrast to behaviorism. The outcomes of gender socialization are the same in both models; what differs is the temporal relationship of behavior and thought. For behaviorists, children learn appropriate behaviors and then construct a general understanding of what it is to be male or female. For cognitive development theorists, a cognitive understanding of gender is established, and as a result children learn to behave in gender-appropriate manners.

The passivity that characterizes behaviorism is challenged by cognitive developmental theorists. In this approach children actively seek patterns in their physical and social worlds. "Once they discover those categories or regularities, they spontaneously construct a self and a set of social rules consistent with them" (Bem, 1993). Sandra Bem has taken the basic framework of the cognitive development approach and made significant contributions to its application to gender formation. According to Bem and her gender-schema theory, cultures consist of a set of hidden assumptions, or "taken-for-granted" knowledge about how individuals should think, feel, and look. These assumptions are communicated both explicitly and tacitly. They are embedded in every aspect of cultural discourse, social institutions, and the behavior of individuals. Bem calls these assumptions "lenses." She identifies three distinct lenses that characterize the United States and other Western cultures.

First, **gender polarization** describes our tendency to dichotomize the world of gender. Things are either male or female and there is no room for ambiguity. While this may seem natural and normal, it is important to note that this is a product of particular cultures. Many, perhaps even most, cultures accept that gender is more complex than just male/female designations (Fausto-Sterling, 1985). Second, **androcentrism** refers to the tendency to view things masculine as superior to those things associated with femininity. Finally, **biological essentialism** is a concept used by Bem to describe the tendency to ground gender differences in biology, thus becoming natural, normal, and necessary.

While Bem's approach is appropriately viewed as an extension of cognitive development theory, it is also accurate to view her model as an integration of cognitive learning and a behaviorist approach. It extends behaviorism in that she recognizes that the messages children receive from others are not limited to simple and isolated behaviors. Children actively look for themes and overarching principles to understand why others act as they do. And then, based on those themes, or lenses, intentionally and actively choose courses of behavior for themselves. Recognizing that children are actively involved in their own socialization is an important contribution. However, Bem's theory is individualistic, and therefore may not accurately describe the socialization of children with respect to gender and more generally.

Interpretivist Theory

Interpretivist approaches differ from cognitive development and other theoretical models in their emphasis on the collectivist (vs. individualistic) nature of socialization. These approaches have been influenced by developments in a number of disciplines. Researchers investigating issues of socialization and gender have drawn upon work in anthropology (Geertz, 1973a, 1973b), psychology (Vygotsky, 1978), sociology (Cicourel, 1974), and philosophy (Schutz, 1970). In the interpretivist approach, as opposed to most of the more traditional theoretical perspectives already described, the world of children must be recognized as creative, collective, and autonomous. Creativity implies that children are not passive recipients of the messages provided to them by adults. These messages must be interpreted, contextualized, and generalized. In this regard, interpretivist theory builds upon some of the work described in the section on cognitive development. A focus on the collective is where interpretivist and cognitive development approaches differ. Cognitive development approaches continue to focus on individuals as the unit of analysis. As opposed to the individual processing information on one's own, interpretivists look at friendship, play groups, and peer cultures as sites within which understanding and meaning are constructed. It is during peer interactions that notions of what is appropriate for boys and girls are negotiated. Peer groups are safe arenas within which behaviors and identities are constructed and evaluated (Fine, 1987). Autonomy is the tendency, often tacit, of most theories of socialization to assume that adulthood is an end point. Children are typically studied with an eye to how, more or less, they have acquired the characteristics of adults. From an interpretivist perspective, 3-year-olds are not incomplete adults; nor are they better adults than 2-year-olds. Rather, they are participants in the culture of 3-year-olds, and what needs to be understood is this age-specific culture.

There are particular methodological implications of this approach. Interpretivists call for more ethnographic and

Think About It   **8.3**

As a child, how were messages about what it means to be a boy or a girl communicated to you through your family and culture? What were some of those messages?

participant observation research. The assertion is that understandings are created within and require context. Therefore, what needs to be studied are the settings within which these processes take place (Corsaro & Eder, 1990; Gaskins, Miller, & Corsaro, 1992).

Diversity

When sociologists discuss diversity, gender, ethnicity, and social class are considered the trinity of concepts. Each of these concepts is important in its own right. However, it is increasingly understood that these variables are interconnected and should be studied, analyzed, and understood as an intersection of characteristics. What this means is that the meanings and implications of being female are different depending on whether the individual is rich or poor, Black or White. The consequences of being poor are textured by one's gender and ethnicity (Foley, 2010).

Focusing on the preschool years adds a twist to more typical and general analyses of social diversity. Preschool children are more aware and self-conscious of their gender than of their ethnic identity or social class. This is largely explained by again referencing a central principle of family and socialization. That is, children experience their family not as their family, but rather as "The World." In the cases of both ethnicity and social class, recognition of one's own identity is possible only with extended experiences with individuals and groups with distinct identities. Given the rather segregated nature of American society with respect to ethnicity and social class, these trans-ethnic and trans-class experiences are largely limited for many, if not for most, American preschoolers. With these caveats, it is still possible to discuss some aspects of the relationship of ethnicity, social class, and the worlds of preschoolers.

Ethnicity

Let's start with a basic assertion. Ethnic categories are cultural constructs. As adults we largely accept these categories as a given, as representing some sort of objective reality. But this does not change the fact that these categories must be learned. And individuals must learn what factors are to be used in classifying individuals.

Social Class

Preschool children's experiences with diverse social classes are even more limited than their experiences with diverse ethnic groups. Extended family, residential neighborhoods, and the composition of preschool populations are largely class specific. This does not mean that preschoolers are not affected by social class; rather, it means only that they remain largely unaware that their life experiences are tied so closely to the economic conditions of their families. The most basic material conditions of their lives (e.g., food, clothing, access to health care, quality of physical environment) are directly determined by their families' social classes.

REFLECTION 8.5 NO WHITE KIDS IN MY CLASS

When my son was 3 or 4 years old, I attended some sort of preschool program. Afterward I wanted to know the name of one of the other children in his class. He asked me what he looked like and I said, "He's sort of tall and was wearing a red shirt." This did not ring a bell for my son. I added, "He's White." (The class was approximately 50/50 White and Black.) My son responded, "We don't have any White kids in my class." I was, of course, surprised by this. I asked what color he was and he stated, "I'm Brown." as he held out his arm. I asked if there were any Black kids in his class. After reflecting for a moment he confidently said, "No. We're all just Brown." Please understand that I am not suggesting that somehow my wife and I raised our children to be color blind. Rather, he had not yet learned the ethnic classification system of central Alabama (or the United States). He was still thinking of colors in the context of, well, actual colors. [~SP]

Unfortunately, across academic disciplines there has been a history of assuming that only in the case of the poor do economic conditions have cultural consequences. The concept "culture of poverty," a term first coined by Lewis (1961), speaks to this tendency. As typically interpreted, the implication is that individuals and families living in poverty develop cultural practices that operate to keep these people in poverty. A tacit assumption is that while living in poverty can result in a specific and (mal)adaptive culture, middle-class people have no class-based culture: they are just normal. Confusing middle-class culture with "normal" is incorrect, inconsistent with a theoretical understanding of the culture, and serves as the basis of yet another barrier for individuals attempting to achieve greater economic stability.

Coles' (1977) work with children of affluence is a wonderful example illustrating the fundamental link between culture and social class throughout the entire spectrum of stratification in our society. Coles asserts that children of affluent families develop a worldview characterized by such features as a greater attachment to the future, an assumption of competence, and the existence of options. In the case of attachment to the future, perhaps the most telling contrast might lie in the work of Kotlowitz (1991), in which he tells of children in the Cabrini Green housing project of south Chicago responding to his question of what they want to be when they grow up with, "IF I grow up, I want to. ..." In this case, these children have developed a worldview in which a future as an adult is not a given, and this worldview is tellingly expressed linguistically.

Social classes have cultures that represent adaptations to material conditions. And institutions have cultures, including educational institutions. Here is another example where the tendency to see middle-class culture as something "normal" has tremendous implications for poor and modest income families. Heath's (1983) research on the relationship of diverse cultures (largely grounded in ethnicity and social class) and the early educational experiences of children is especially provocative. Schools' assumptions about basic constructs such as time and space differentially affect children based on the relative similarities of the schools' constructs and the children's home-based cultures. Middle-class families are more likely to have schedules organized around specific times for specific activities (e.g., piano lessons, soccer practices, aerobics, committee meetings) than more economically limited families. The cliché "a place for everything and everything in its place" is more likely to be a working principle for families with enough space to assign specific tasks to specific territories. These constructs of time and space are consistent with how schools operate. As a result, school is more of an extension of the home environment for middle-class children than for children from homes where time is less structured and space more characterized as serving multiple purposes. Adding to this the tendency to mistake culture for "normalcy," and children's difficulties adjusting to the expectations of the school, lead to negative evaluations of individual students instead of a recognition that what is going on has to do with their relative inexperience with new and novel cultural (tacit) expectations.

The point is not to somehow think we can, or should, rid educational institutions of particular cultural elements. Rather, the chances of children from modest economic backgrounds adapting to middle-class culture are improved when the cultural assumptions of our schools are acknowledged. This is true for professionals working with preschoolers as well as professionals in K–12 educational environments.

School/Day Care Influences on Socialization

As the percentage of women in the labor market continues to increase, a greater number of young children are spending more and more time outside of family settings. The tremendous variation with respect to the types of day care settings makes it difficult to make many statements regarding the impact of day care on children's development. Clarke-Stewart and Allhusen (2005) have offered a typology of day care.

Care in the Child's Home

In this case, a member of the extended family is usually the caregiver. Because this arrangement is negotiated and structured within the family, less is known about it than any other type of day care. Advantages include that the child is familiar with the physical environment and the caregiver. In addition, there is a greater probability of scheduling flexibility. Some suggest that disadvantages include the lack of formal training on the part of the caregiver and the fact that the child does not have the opportunity to participate in the peer activities provided by child care centers.

Family Day Care

In this case, caregivers provide child care in their own homes. States vary with respect to licensing requirements for these services. The number of children cared for may range from one to 15. Surveys indicate this is the most common type of day care and may be the least expensive option for families needing to look for services outside of their extended family. Many parents appreciate the home-based, neighborhood setting that may characterize these sites, as well as the opportunities for group play. The lack of accountability and stability is the major drawback.

Child Care Centers

This is the type of child care most people have in mind when using the term **day care**. Within this general category there are a number of distinct types of centers.

- *Private day care centers* are available to anyone with the ability to pay the fees. These local, independent businesses are typically limited in size (e.g., 10–20 children).
- *Commercial day care centers* are of a larger size and often part of a national or regional chain. Facilities, staff training, educational activities, and general offerings tend to be more standardized.
- *Community church centers* rely on the facilities of local religious congregations. They are often viewed as part of the social ministry of the church. Their size, the professional training of the staff, and their physical facilities vary greatly depending on characteristics of the church.
- *Company centers* are typically offered as a part of employees' fringe benefits. They are most often characterized by good facilities and a professionally trained staff.
- *Public service centers* are state sponsored and funded. Their primary charge is to provide services for low-income families. It is unfortunate that their availability is so limited.
- *Research centers* are typically associated with institutions of higher education and often are a part of undergraduate programs in child development and elementary education. More research has been done in these settings than in any of the other types of day care centers. The distinctive elements of this setting prevent many of the findings from being generalized to non-research centers.

In addition to all of the above settings, the most affluent American families have the additional options of au pairs and nannies. The issue of economic inequality and stratification is far too often ignored in discussions of child care in the United States. In 2014 the average cost for one child in a child care center was $500–$800 a month. Thus, modest and low-income families are particularly limited with respect to child care options. These families are most likely to rely on family members and family-based day care arrangements. As a result, these children face greater difficulties when it is time to transition into elementary school.

Even with the caveats concerning the difficulties of generalizing research on the effects of day care on children, it is possible to identify a few important factors for parents to consider when deciding about day care.

1. Site characteristics should include a good staff-to-child ratio, high-quality staff training and education, high wages for staff, and a safe, clean physical environment.

<table>
<tr><td>

REFLECTION 8.6 FLEXIBLE CHILD CARE
DECISIONS

As I was looking over the typology of child care alternatives I just described, I realized my two children attended six of the eight settings listed. In talking with other parents, I have found this amount of variation is not particularly unusual. Whether it be the age of the child, changing employment conditions, instability of care centers, geographic relocations, or any number of other factors, parents do not typically make a single decision with regard to child care. Rather, parenting a preschool child involves a series of decisions as to how the child will be cared for. [~SP]

</td></tr>
</table>

2. Curriculum or program characteristics should include active encouragement of creativity, supervised motor activities, particular attention to language development, and opportunities for peer-based play.
3. Specific characteristics of the child and family assumes there is no "one size fits all" when evaluating the appropriateness of any day care situation. Each child has unique qualities and needs. Each family has a distinct combination of resources, needs, and challenges. This is an important consideration not only for families deciding on how to handle issues of day care, but also for professionals working with families. It is important to reserve judgment (especially of the negative variety) and recognize the difficulties families face as they attempt to make decisions about child care.

Parenting Styles

There are a number of different models and typologies used in discussing various parenting styles. A significant percent of these models make use of Baumrind's (1971, 1980, 1996) research on the relationship of parental child-rearing styles and the social competencies of their children.

Authoritarian Parenting

Authoritarian parents are demanding, actively attempting to shape and control a child's behavior. In the extreme form, these parents are sometimes referred to as autocratic. The standards used to evaluate behaviors are grounded in what may be considered traditional and absolute values and standards of conduct. There is little room for discussion, and indeed the perspectives of the child are not legitimized. These parents see little need to provide explanations for their demands. They express less affection and tend to restrict emotional expressions on the part of the child. Children growing up with this parenting style are at risk of being discontented, rebellious, withdrawn, and distrustful (Weiss & Schwarz, 1996).

Authoritative Parenting

Authoritative parents provide structure and direction to the child while still allowing a significant amount of freedom and room for exploration and self-expression. These parents promote autonomy and individuality while clearly communicating consistent standards and expectations of mature behavior. These families are characterized by high levels of two-way communication. The authoritative parenting style is associated with self-reliant, explorative, and contented children, yielding the best outcomes among all of the parental styles. Baumrind's later research (1996) found this style was particularly effective during adolescence. Sometimes authoritative parents may be referred to as using a democratic parental style.

Permissive Parenting

Permissive parents are accepting, affirmative, and tolerant of their children's behavior. Their goal is to create an environment in which the child exercises significant amounts of discretion with respect to their own behaviors. There are few demands placed on the child, and punishment of any type is seldom employed. Children raised in this manner are less self-reliant, explorative, and self-controlled than children raised by parents with other styles.

Uninvolved Parental Style

Maccoby and Martin (1983) distinguish between a permissive parenting style and the **neglecting-uninvolved style**. In making this distinction they maintain that permissive parents remain in communication with the child and continue to express affection. Neither of these characteristics is true for neglecting-uninvolved parents. From these brief descriptions of parenting styles based on Baumrind's model, it seems rather clear that one style, authoritative, is superior to the others. Baumrind's original sample was limited to White, middle-class families. It is legitimate to question whether her findings are applicable across ethnicities, cultures, and/or social classes. For example, Chao's (1994, 2001) studies of Chinese-American family relationships found that broader cultural values that emphasize respect for elders and stress parental responsibilities for teaching children socially appropriate behaviors acted as a lens, or filter, whereby parental styles that Baumrind might describe as authoritarian were interpreted very differently by both Chinese-American parents and children.

Play

What is it that children do? Well, they eat, they sleep, and they play. In fact, eating often involves a significant dose of playing. Play allows children to actively encounter and engage with their environments. Children manipulate physical objects, amuse themselves, make and sustain relationships, make sense of the world, and develop skills allowing them to understand how others are making sense of the world.

A number of different models portraying the stages of play have been offered by theorists going back at least to George Herbert Mead (1934). What all of these models have in common is a recognition of the increasing complexity of play activities as children age and the greater emphasis on coordination of behaviors between play participants. Before children are even 1 year old, we can observe them being aware of one another. Young children will look, smile, and point to one another (Rubin, Bukowski, & Parker, 2006). By their first birthday we see what may be termed **parallel play**. These play activities remain solitary in that there is no coordination of activity among children. Rather, there is a noticeable interest in, and awareness of, the activities of others.

A 1-year-old child is no longer content to merely observe others. Instead, the child makes active attempts to mimic the behaviors of others. Children are also more active at responding to others as well as encouraging responses from others to themselves (Howes & Matheson, 1993). This represents a move from parallel play to what may legitimately be considered **simple social play**. By the beginning of the third year the "simple" modifier can be dropped. There are open, active, and intentional efforts to cooperate in order to create play activities. And, it is important to note, these efforts are often successful. Children are now creatively constructing interactional frames within which social performances and relationships can be fostered, developed, and sustained.

Cultural differences can affect play in numerous ways. Efforts to sustain imaginative play require a sharing of assumptions concerning what behaviors are called for and how those behaviors are to be interpreted. Imagine the different assumptions children might have about something as simple as "playing house." Does "the mom" prepare dinner? Does "the dad"? Or is dinner prepared cooperatively? Do parents express affection or do they ignore each other? Are "the children" comforted or told to "Stop bothering me"? Young children do not experience their families as unique families with particular quirks, routines, and/or practices. Rather, they initially experience their particular families as "the way families are." Any differences between the dynamics of families are potential hindrances to accomplishing cooperative play. On the other hand, it can be the case that the challenges presented by these differences provide children the opportunity to understand and appreciate family diversities as well as recognize the distinctiveness of their own worlds. To the degree cultural groups based on ethnicity, social class, and religious values have particular family dynamics, children from these groups will experience the challenges and opportunities described above.

More cross-cultural research on children's play is needed, and students interested in child development would be well served by paying greater attention to the research that has been done. Opie and Opie's (1959, 1969) now classic compilation of children's folklore spurred interest in the social worlds of European children, but remains less than an integrated part of the literature on child development in the United States. Identifying similarities in children's activities across cultures can contribute to a more universal model of child development. On the other hand, research pointing to culturally specific play routines among children aids in making sure theories of child development are not based on assumptions of the normalcy of White, middle-class American culture (Gaskins et al., 1992).

Childhood Friendships

It is hard to separate information on friendships from that focusing on play. As children grow older, more and more of their play activities involve others. These activities form the basis of friendships. By the age of 3, children are interested in and able to sustain play with peers. Simply gaining access to play groups as well as sustaining play activities are significant and formidable accomplishments that should not be dismissed. Children's skills at sustaining play are in their earlier stages of development, and at some level they seem to recognize the fragility of their interactional frames. They tend, therefore, to be very protective of their ongoing activities (Corsaro, 1985). Joining others already playing usually is not as simple as asking, "Can I play?" Children as young as 3 years old develop an elaborate repertoire of "access rituals" in order to overcome peer resistance to allowing new (and potentially threatening) play partners (Corsaro, 1979; Dodge, 1983).

One particularly common access ritual includes a reference to friendship status: "We're friends, right?" (Corsaro, 1981). It should be noted that this strategy is not always successful, although its rate of success increases over time. The explanation for the change in the effectiveness of this strategy lies in children's changing ideas as to what being a "friend" means. Younger children tend to define friendship in terms of who they are immediately playing with, whereas over time they begin to develop more abstract yet permanent notions of the implications of friendship. Apart from the substance of this finding, it is illustrative of the importance of not imposing adult conceptualizations of concepts such as friendship upon young children. Children's understandings of friendship (as well as other concepts) are developed within the context of their own peer cultures and need to be understood in their own right (Corsaro & Eder, 1990; Willis, 1977).

Corsaro and Eder (1990) identified three major themes that characterize the play activities of children. First, children learn how to share and get along in a group. Children spend a significant amount of time creating and sustaining activities that they find enjoyable and exciting. These activities provide children with emotional security and a sense of accomplishment. Second, many of the activities constructed by preschool-aged children allow them to deal with common fears and conflict. Children are made aware that the world is a dangerous place from interactions and communications with parents, other adult caregivers, fairy tales, and various popular media. Much of the shared fantasy play of children is directed toward making sense of the sources of these threats, and children often find comfort in the security of their friends. The final theme involves children's need to challenge adult authority and rules. This is a theme adults might prefer to ignore, but doing so does not serve the goal of understanding the lives of children. Dunn (1988) and Miller (1986) have pointed out that children challenge the rules of parents from the very first years of life. By age 3, children have begun to develop an awareness of common interests of children (vs. adults) and coordinate efforts to both mock and evade authority (Corsaro, 1985).

Play Therapy

The Association for Play Therapy (2013) defines play therapy as "the systematic use of a theoretical model to establish an interpersonal process wherein trained play therapists use the therapeutic powers of play to help clients prevent or resolve psychosocial difficulties and achieve optimal growth and development." While play therapy can be used with individuals of all ages, including adults, children ages 3–12 are the main recipients of this type of counseling intervention (Schaefer, 2011). Play therapy is especially beneficial when counseling preschool-aged children, as they are usually not developmentally able to fully express their thoughts and feelings verbally. Play therapy can be based on many different counseling theories, and while the overall configuration of a play therapy room might differ according to the theoretical perspective of the counselor, the essential function of play therapy is the use of symbolic play for therapeutic purposes. Since play functions as a mechanism for children to work through fears and make sense and meaning of their lives, the use of play in counseling interventions is highly effective and is the primary mode of therapy for young children.

Summary

Erikson is pivotal to our understanding of children's psychosocial development. Erikson's stage theory spans the lifespan and is composed of eight stages that have specific tasks or crises that must be resolved. Preschool children fall into the initiative versus guilt stage, wherein children begin to develop interests and independent activities. Failure to successfully resolve this stage will result in guilt.

Alfred Adler's individual psychology theory has contributed a great deal to our understanding of children and families. Adler viewed behavior as goal directed and purposeful and believed that people wanted to belong. Adler's four goals of misbehavior (i.e., attention, power, revenge, and inadequacy) provide a helpful conceptualization for understanding why children misbehave. Adler's concept of birth order provides insight into child behavior; however, Adler cautioned that perceived psychological order matters most, not just the order of birth.

Family systems theory postulates that children should be viewed within the context of multiple systems, including family of birth, extended family, community, and the larger society. Families should be defined in a broad manner, and it should be understood that there are many different types of family configurations. Within these various types of families, there is a progression across the lifespan with special challenges at each stage. Families with young children face challenges related to the time and energy put forth in caring for children. The degree to which a family has cohesion and flexibility can indicate the overall health of the family system and the family's ability to cope with stress and developmental change.

Emotional development begins to occur during early childhood as children develop more advanced language skills. Identifying and understanding emotions leads to emotional competence and self-regulation. A significant emotional competency is the development of empathy. Self-regulation is important as growing children learn how to manage anger in a pro-social manner and deal with fear.

Very little research has been conducted regarding mental disorders in early childhood, but the rate of psychotropic medication use in preschoolers is on the rise. Common diagnoses in preschoolers include ADHD, ODD, CD, depression, and anxiety. Diagnostic criteria should be adapted to fit this unique population. Another issue facing young children is abuse and neglect. Mandated reporters should be aware of signs of abuse and neglect and should report suspected abuse to child protective services.

The social development of a child occurs in many ways. When a child is born, the most important characteristic that is communicated by parents is the child's sex. There are various theoretical approaches to understanding sex and gender role socialization, including biological, psychoanalytic, behavioral, cognitive, and interpretivist approaches. It is important to realize the impact of the complex intersection between gender, race, and SES when exploring the socialization of the preschool child.

School and day care settings are major aspects of child socialization. These settings include child care in the home, family child care, and child care centers. How a child is parented is also a critical aspect of their social development. Parenting styles include authoritarian, authoritative, and permissive. Children socialize through play and friendships. Play is their work, and social skills aimed at accessing play groups and making friends are critical to child development.

Middle Childhood: Physical and Cognitive Development

By Stephanie Puleo

The lifespan odyssey proceeds through middle childhood beginning around age 6 with the adventure of entering elementary school, and continues until about age 11. In this chapter, changes in physical and cognitive functioning that occur during middle childhood will be discussed. As attention is focused on these domains, it is important to keep in mind that each develops in conjunction with emotional and social development (see Chapter 10) and is influenced by environmental factors. The development of each child is unique and contingent on the interaction of a variety of factors, so a range of phenomena that occur during middle childhood is presented in this chapter.

SECTION I: Physical Development

Despite Freud's contention that middle childhood is an interlude of relative quiescence (Hunt & Kraus, 2009; Jacobs, 2004), anyone who observes the population of an elementary school can see that there is much activity and quite a difference between kindergartners and fifth graders. As children navigate middle childhood, they experience physical and cognitive changes that allow them to think differently about themselves and to interact differently with the world.

Middle childhood seems to be a healthy time for developing individuals. In the United States, mortality rates for individuals in this age group are lower than for any other age group, including early childhood and adolescence (Kochanek, Xu, Murphy, Minino, & Kung, 2011). In 2010, 82% of children in this age bracket enjoyed very good to excellent health, while only 2% of children were in fair or poor health (U.S. Department of Health and Human Services, 2011). Only 5.2 % of elementary school children missed more than 10 days of school due to illness or injury.

Growth and Physical Development

Growth and Physical Changes

During middle childhood, children continue to grow steadily, but at a slower rate than when younger. Between the ages of 6 and 11, children grow an average of 2–3 inches per year and nearly double their weight, gaining 5–7 pounds per year. The average 6-year-old girl is 46.9 inches tall and weighs 51.5 pounds. The average 6-year-old boy is 47.5 inches tall and weighs 53.3 pounds. By age 11, girls have grown to 59.6 inches and 108.4 pounds, and boys have grown to 59.1 inches and 103.2 pounds, on average (McDowell, Fryar, Ogden, & Flegal, 2008). In addition to increases in height and weight, there are changes in body proportion, dentition, muscle development, and brain structure.

Among the noticeable changes in the appearance of children in middle childhood are changes in body proportion. Whereas the head size of younger children makes up about one-fourth of total body size, this proportional relationship decreases during middle childhood. Arms and legs extend, and the torso becomes more elongated, giving children a slimmer, thinner appearance. In addition to the head becoming proportionally smaller compared to the total body size, the shape of the face and lower jaw change as "baby teeth" are lost and replaced by permanent ones. Although girls tend to retain a bit more fatty tissue than boys, muscle mass for both boys and girls gradually increases, and bones become more ossified.

Brain Development

During middle childhood, most neurological development occurs in the brain's cortex, that part of the brain responsible for executive processes. Various centers within the cortex have specific functions, and each develops and differentiates at a different rate. As this part of the brain develops, children become better able to reason, plan, and communicate. In contrast to younger children who may be inattentive or prone to emotional outbursts, children in middle childhood pay attention to their environment, analyze consequences, and demonstrate self-control. As the brain and its cortex develop, children become better able to attend to and process multiple sources of sensory information simultaneously. In the classroom setting, this allows children to write and listen to their teachers at the same time. During play, they are able to know and follow rules, focus on the ball, and keep track of their own and opposing team members.

Brain development is a dynamic process that involves billions of interactions and component parts (Perry, 2009). The component parts include nerve cells (neurons), glia, and synapses. Healthy development is dependent upon interactions among and between these components as well as interactions with the environment. There are four anatomically distinct regions of the brain: the brain stem, the diencephalon, the limbic system, and the cortex. These regions develop somewhat in order of complexity (Perry, 2009). While each region is distinct in its functioning, all are interconnected. Systems that develop and become organized in lower brain areas project to and impact systems developing and organizing in other brain areas. This process is guided by use and dependent on cues that come from biological factors such as neurotransmitters, neurohormones, and amino acids, as well as environmental factors and experience (Perry, 2009).

Two important processes that occur during brain and central nervous system development are myelination and pruning (Wenar & Kerig, 2006). **Myelination** is a process whereby glial cells grow around the axons of nerve cells, encasing them in a sheath known as myelin. This sheath, which gives "white matter" its color, serves to increase the speed and efficiency with which information is carried through nerve cells. Myelination occurs throughout brain development; however, there is a sharp increase that begins to take place around puberty and continues into adulthood. During middle childhood, much growth in myelination seems to occur in connections between the brain's temporal lobe, which is important for memory and auditory perception, and the parietal lobe, which is important for spatial understanding and sensory perception (Giedd, 2003).

Pruning is the process by which the brain rids itself of unnecessary or redundant cells or cell connections. A significant amount of pruning occurs prior to birth, subsequent to a period of rapid neural growth. However, a second critical pruning stage begins during middle childhood and concludes later in adolescence (Giedd, 2003). This pruning follows a period in early childhood when an abundance of new synapses appear and gray matter seems to be at its largest volume. This excessive development of synapses allows children to be prepared for a multitude of physical and cultural environments. As children adapt to their unique environments, neural connections that are not used wither away.

In addition to increasing the amount of information to which they are able to attend, children in middle childhood gain the ability to engage in some cognitive activities automatically, without much conscious thought. As patterns of thought and behavior are repeated, the neural connections involved are strengthened and less effort is required. This process is known as **automatization**.

The way in which neural structures develop and become organized depends on the child's experience. The child's sensory experience affects the timing, frequency, and pattern of activation of neural factors necessary for brain development. Thus it is important to note that neglect or trauma may alter the normal or healthy course of brain development (Perry, 2009).

Motor Development

Gross Motor Development

Motor development is supported by maturation of the cerebral cortex, the cerebellum, connections between the two, and automatization. During middle childhood, motor skills become smoother and more coordinated. With gains in muscle mass and an overall slower rate of growth, children in middle childhood have more time to become comfortable with their bodies and practice motor behavior (Crandell, Crandell, & VanderZanden, 2009). Children become adept at controlling their own bodies and gain mastery of most basic skills that do not require strength or instant judgment. As neural connections are made, myelination occurs, and automatization takes place, reaction time as well as hand-eye coordination improves. These advances allow children to progress from T-ball to baseball, and to begin enjoying competitive and team sports.

Fine Motor Development

As their coordination improves, children make gains in fine motor skills as well. Upon entering middle childhood, children progress from crayons to pencils. Printing makes way for cursive writing, although an increasing number of school systems no longer provide instruction in or require cursive handwriting. Toward the end of middle childhood, children can manipulate both hands independently and engage in tasks requiring complex movements. Using their developing fine motor skills to engage in crafts or learn to play musical instruments allows children to experience productivity.

Children whose motor skills develop more slowly or more poorly tend to be less accepted by their peers (Livesey, Lum Mow, Toshack, & Zheng, 2011). This phenomenon may lead to repercussions in the development of social relationships and self-esteem.

Physical Activity, Play, and Sports

Physical Activity

To support their growth and developing motor skills, elementary age children need to be physically active. During middle childhood, children need at least 60 minutes of physical exercise each day (U.S. Department of Health and Human Services, 2008). Much of this time should be devoted to aerobic activity of moderate to vigorous intensity, but muscle- and bone-strengthening activities should also be included. Bone-strengthening activities are particularly important because the greatest gains in bone mass occur during middle childhood. In addition to the benefits provided for muscle and bone development, physical activity leads to better cardiorespiratory fitness and a lower risk of being overweight or obese (Physical Activity Guidelines Advisory Committee, 2008). Research also shows that aerobic fitness may contribute positively to the development of cognitive skills and executive functioning in children (Hillman, Buck, Themanson, Pontifex, & Castelli, 2009).

Play

When entering middle childhood, much of children's physical activity is in the form of rough-and-tumble play, which peaks at about 8 to 10 years of age, especially for boys (Friedman & Downey, 2008). Rough-and-tumble play involves running, chasing, wrestling, and a variety of other actions using large muscle groups and gross motor skills. To many, it appears to mimic aggression; however, children's facial expressions and laughter suggest otherwise. Rough-and-tumble play is a pro-social activity, and through it children gain experience being in relationships, practicing assertiveness, burning energy, and having fun. For both boys and girls, rough-and-tumble play leads to cooperative games with rules such as tag and jump-rope, which in turn have a role in the development of social competence (Frye, 2005).

Sports

Rough-and-tumble play and games with rules provide skills that allow children to begin to participate in organized sports. Organized sports require children not only to refine their motor skills, but also to follow rules and cooperate with team members. Participation in organized sports is associated with enhanced communication, cooperation, connection, self-confidence, empathy, and leadership (Gano-Overway et al., 2009; Zarrett et al., 2009), all aspects of social development. In addition, children who participate in sports and physical activities are more likely to be active adults (Schmalz, Kerstetter, & Anderson, 2008).

Diet, Nutrition, and Weight

Diet

Although physical growth slows during middle childhood, children in this age group are more active and use more energy than in early childhood; thus, they need to consume more calories per day. Depending on their age, gender, and level of activity, children between the ages of 6 and 11 need to take in between 1200 and 2200 calories per day. According to the 2010 Dietary Recommendations for Americans, a balanced diet for 6-year-old girls who are sedentary should include around 1200 calories per day, while a balanced diet for active 11-year-old boys might include around 2200 calories per day (U.S. Department of Agriculture & U.S. Department of Health and Human Services, 2010). To help Americans conceptualize a balanced, healthy diet, the U.S. Department of Agriculture and U.S. Department of Health and Human Services have launched a campaign called "My Plate" to replace the food pyramid icon originally released in 1992 (see Figure 9.1). Similar to previous guidelines, it is recommended that a healthy diet include foods from five groups—fruits, vegetables, grains, protein, and dairy—and that fruits and vegetables should make up about half of each day's calories.

Body Weight

Using the body mass index (BMI) as a measure, body weight status can be classified into four categories: underweight, healthy weight, overweight, and obese. The BMI is derived by comparing a person's weight and height; it is computed using the formula kilograms of body weight per meter of height squared ($kg \div m^2$) in the metric system, or pounds of body weight per height in inches squared, multiplied by 703 in the English system ($lbs \div in^2 \times 703$). For example, if an 11-year-old child weighs 103 pounds (46.8 kg) and is 59 inches tall (1.50 m), then, in the metric system, BMI = $46.8 \div (1.5)^2$ = 20.8, which is normal at just below the 85th percentile; in the English system the child's BMI would be the same: BMI = $103 \div (59)^2 \times 703$ = 20.8. Children whose BMI falls at or above the 85th percentile when compared to others the same age and gender are considered overweight, and those with a BMI that falls at or above the 95th percentile are considered obese. In the United States, the prevalence of obesity in children ages 6 to 11 has risen from approximately 4% in the 1970s to over 20% in 2008 (U.S. Department of Agriculture & U.S. Department of Health and Human Services, 2010). These children are at risk for a number of health problems such as type 2 diabetes, hypertension, high cholesterol, and cardiovascular disease, conditions once diagnosed primarily in adults. Many of these children are also at risk for social and emotional consequences.

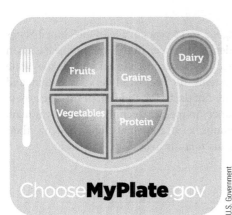

Figure 9.1 Choosemyplate.gov nutritional graphic from the U.S. Department of Agriculture and U.S. Department of Health and Human Services.

Retrieved from http://www.choosemyplate.gov/

U.S. Government

Think About It **9.1**

In the last 30 years, rates of childhood obesity have tripled. In 1980, there were approximately three children out of every 50 in the 6–11-year-old age group who were obese. Think about it: In the average elementary school classroom in 1980, there might have been one child who was obese. Thirty or more years later, there are approximately 10 children out of every 50 who are obese. These children are at risk for numerous health-related problems including type II diabetes, hypertension, and cardiovascular disease. In addition to health risks, what other risks might children who are obese face? What factors have contributed to the increased rate of obesity in elementary school children? What might be done to turn these statistics around?

Accidents and Illness

Accidents

Although relatively few elementary children miss school because of unintentional injuries, when accidents happen, they can be quite serious. While the death rate for school-age children is the lowest of any age group, the leading cause of death in this age group is accidents. In the United States in 2009, almost 1000 children died as a result of motor vehicle accidents, and over 700 more died of injuries from other types of accidents (Kochanek et al., 2011). For every child who died as a result of an accident or injury, scores of others received medical treatment for falls, bicycle accidents, sports injuries, and injuries sustained in automobile accidents. Many of these injuries might be avoidable through education and prevention measures such as bicycle helmets and automobile safety belts.

Chronic Illnesses/Conditions

Most children get sick once in a while, but some experience illnesses that persist for longer periods of time. In 2010, there were more than 10 million children (14%) in the United States who took prescription medications regularly for health problems lasting more than three months (U.S. Department of Health and Human Services, 2011). Some of the chronic conditions that have become common are asthma, allergies, and attention-deficit/hyperactivity disorder.

Cancer

The second leading cause of death of children ages 5 to 14 years of age in the United States is cancer (Kochanek et al., 2011), and the incidence of cancer in this age group has risen slightly in recent years. Areas most often affected by cancer in children include the white blood cells (leukemia), endocrine and lymph systems, the brain and nervous system, and bones. Although cancer is the second leading cause of death for children in this age group, the survival rate continues to improve with advances in medical technology and treatment. Children undergoing cancer treatment face a number of stresses that could challenge their development. One such story is told by Wes, a leukemia survivor.

REFLECTION 9.1 WES' STORY

On a warm September evening when I was 6 years old, my world changed forever. This was the day I was diagnosed with a form of cancer known as acute lymphoblastic leukemia (ALL). When I stepped into the lobby of the emergency room in my hometown, I was surprised to find my grandparents, my extended family, and even my kindergarten teacher, and they were all tearful. I had no idea what was going on.

But children are resilient, and I am living proof of this. I underwent an aggressive chemotherapy regimen for the next month, went into remission, and then continued maintenance chemotherapy for the next three years. The poisonous chemotherapy was tolerable and I took it in stride despite the nausea, weight loss, and difficulty in general occupational functioning.

There was one side effect, however, that was utterly devastating and made the task of adjusting to elementary school all the more difficult: I was bald. Not surprisingly, I was embarrassed and extremely self-conscious. Some classmates were very sympathetic to my predicament and made special efforts to try and include me. Sometimes I was unable to participate in games and physical activities because I was physically too ill. In these cases I was content to just stand and observe while my classmates actively learned to socialize and resolve conflict. On the other hand, some classmates didn't help much; frankly, they were cruel. They bullied me in order to agitate me. I felt tortured. I was insulted verbally and had my hat taken. I was picked on for the remainder of elementary school by these children.

In response, toward the end of elementary school I became reactively aggressive. Some of this aggression was channeled appropriately through karate lessons and sports teams. However, I also on occasion picked fights (usually with children I perceived as weaker). I was merciless toward these children, and unfortunately this behavior carried on into middle school.

Academically, I was generally superior to my peers. I attribute this to the special attention given to me by teachers who were acutely aware of my predicament. In other words, adults babied me. This special treatment by adults was not unique to teachers and other school staff; this was true also of my parents, extended family, adults within my spiritual community, and hospital staff.

In the summer after first grade I was introduced to a wonderful program designed specifically for children who have cancer. This program was an immense help to me socially during my elementary school years. Camp, in contrast to school, home, and church, held me accountable for my behavior while nurturing my social development. It was at camp that I made my earliest friends, was encouraged to set goals for myself, and even got my first kiss!

SECTION II: Cognitive Development

> CASE EXAMPLE **9.1** REBECCA'S STORY.

Rebecca, at age 7, was referred to counseling shortly after the war in Afghanistan began. Rebecca was displaying signs of anxiety and depression, and although she could verbalize that she was feeling "a little scared," she could not articulate much else about how she was feeling or why. According to her parents, Rebecca did not know anyone who had been deployed to Afghanistan for military service, media coverage, or any other reason; however, she became visibly upset whenever the television in her home was tuned to the news of the war.

Tim, a counselor experienced in working with children, listened to the concerns expressed by Rebecca's parents, and then led the child to the play therapy room. The room was a standard play therapy room complete with a sand tray, art media, and a variety of toys including toy soldiers, tanks, and helicopters. Because her parents indicated that her troublesome behavior seemed to be triggered by the television news coverage of the war, Tim expected Rebecca to gravitate toward the military toys. Instead, Rebecca pulled out two baskets and placed them on opposite sides of the room. Into each basket she placed two medium-sized stuffed animals. Next, she found a car, and placed a smaller stuffed animal in it, along with two she had removed from one of the baskets. She proceeded to drive the car with the three stuffed animals over to the other basket. "They're visiting Grandma and Grandpa," she declared.

"Tell me about Grandma and Grandpa," Tim probed.
Rebecca responded by bursting into tears. "They live far away."
Following Rebecca's lead, Tim asked, "Where is far away?"
"It's where the war is."

And then it made sense. To Rebecca, far away is far away. The difference between 70 miles, 700 miles, or 7000 miles is imperceptible.

Once he learned that Rebecca's grandparents lived in a U.S. city about 200 miles away, Tim began by going to his computer and pulling up two maps; one showed the two U.S. cities where Rebecca and her grandparents lived, and the other showed Afghanistan and western Asia. These screen shots did little to allay Rebecca's fears about her grandparents' vulnerability to war-inflicted harm. Next, Tim found an old, two-dimensional world map depicting all of the continents. Tim put a pin in the map to mark the city where they were, and another a few millimeters away to mark where Rebecca's grandparents were. A third pin was placed on Afghanistan. Rebecca looked at all three pins and still was worried.

Finally, Tim found a globe. He spun the globe until North America showed, and stuck two pins side by side in the approximate location of the cities where Rebecca and her grandparents lived.

He spun the globe again and placed a pin in Afghanistan. "Now," he said to Rebecca as he turned the globe back to North America. "Here you see where you live, and you also can see where Grandma and Grandpa live." Rebecca looked at the two pins. "But you cannot see where the war is." Tim continued to rotate the globe to demonstrate that North America could not be seen from Asia, and that Asia could not be seen from North America until Rebecca seemed satisfied that far away could be many places and that her grandparents were safe.

Piaget's Concrete Operations

Rebecca's is a story illustrating a child's odyssey from preoperational to concrete operational thought. The stage of development described by Piaget as **concrete operations** spans approximately ages 7 through 11, or most of middle childhood. In this stage, children become able to reason and to use logic to solve problems about the concrete elements of the world around them. Concrete operations, which include reversibility, grouping, and conservation, are made possible because children's perceptions expand and they are able to entertain more than one dimension, category, or piece of information at a time. In middle childhood, children are less egocentric, understand spatial concepts better, and can appreciate cause-and-effect relationships.

Reversibility

Reversibility of thought, in its simplest form, is the child's ability to mentally undo or reverse an action. In order to do this, the child must be able to observe an action and then hold and manipulate a mental representation of that action. For example, children with reversibility of thought are able to note that clay they have seen transformed from a ball to a rope can be transformed back to a ball.

Grouping

Grouping, also often called categorization, involves the child's ability to sort objects by various dimensions such as color or shape. Initially, they are able to attend to only one dimension at a time, but as they gain concrete operational thinking capabilities, they can consider multiple dimensions simultaneously. Asked to sort red and blue, round and cube-shaped beads, younger children most often will attend to only color or only shape. Children with concrete operations can attend to both dimensions and have little difficulty developing four categories: red round, red cubes, blue round, and blue cubes. The ability to focus on more than one dimension at a time is sometimes referred to as **decentration**.

Seriation

Children in the concrete operational stage of thinking also have mastered the concepts of seriation and transivity. **Seriation** is the ability to arrange items in order along some quantitative dimension such as height. For younger children it is often necessary to physically compare each item to the others in order to complete this task; however, by about age 7 or 8, children no longer need the physical comparison and are able to accomplish this task more quickly.

Transivity

Transivity is a more sophisticated variation of seriation. To master **transivity**, children must understand the relationship between items in a series and be able to draw conclusions based on their understanding of these relationships. For example, if asked to consider three blocks—a red one, a yellow one, and a blue one—and told that the blue block is the heaviest and the yellow block is the lightest, the concrete operational child will understand that the red block is heavier than the yellow and lighter than the blue one.

An additional concept related to grouping is **class inclusion**. Mastery of this concept involves the ability to perceive part-to-whole relationships and to distinguish categories and subcategories. While waiting for an amusement park ride in a line consisting of three girls and six boys, and asked whether there are more boys or more children on the line, a preoperational child is likely to say that there are more boys. This conclusion is influenced by the younger child's consideration of only one dimension, rather than the relationship of the part to the whole. By about age 8 years of age, children are able to reason that both boys and girls are subclasses of the category of children.

➤ CASE EXAMPLE **9.2**   GRACE.

Shortly after her seventh birthday, Grace went on vacation with her extended family, including her aunts and older cousins. Some of the adults on the trip filled their quiet time with crossword puzzles and Sudoku (a puzzle in which numbers are to be filled into a 9 × 9 grid of squares so that every row, column, and 3 × 3 box contains the numerals 1 through 9). Grace had little interest in the crossword puzzles, but was intrigued by Sudoku and wanted to learn. Her aunt explained the rules and found an easy puzzle they could work on together. Grace began by determining which numerals were needed to complete some of the rows. As she entered numbers in the boxes, her aunt reminded her that the columns needed to be completed as well. Grace shifted her attention to columns. Overall, Grace was successful in placing numbers in boxes and being certain that each row and each column to which she attended contained each numeral only once; however, the completed puzzle contained many "boo-boos," as Grace did not yet have the cognitive ability to consider rows, columns, and boxes simultaneously. Grace was not yet fully able to decenter.

Conservation

At the concrete operational stage of thinking, children are able to acknowledge that quantities do not change regardless of appearances. Over time, as mental operations such as reversibility of thought, decentration, and seriation and transitivity develop, children become able to solve more complex conservation tasks. Conservation skills seem to develop in a particular sequence, beginning with conservation of number. By about age 7 or 8, children are able to solve problems involving conservation of substance and length. A bit later they acquire conservation of area skills, followed by conservation of weight and finally, by about age 12 or 14, conservation of volume (Crandell et al., 2009).

Time

Being able to tell time comes after children gain the concept of seriation. Most children in elementary school can look at a clock and announce what time it is. However, some internal concepts related to telling time develop a little later. When given an instruction to complete a task at a point later in time, younger children very often fail to follow through. When they agree to clean their rooms or take out the trash "later," but do not succeed in getting the job done, it is likely because they have not yet mastered strategies for time monitoring. Research on "prospective memory," being able to remember to carry out an action at some point in the future, shows that older elementary age children are strategic and consistent in monitoring time, and therefore more successful in completing tasks assigned to be completed in the future than their younger schoolmates (Voigt, Aberle, Schonfeld, & Kliegel, 2011).

Information Processing

Information processing refers to the way in which individuals receive, think about, mentally modify, and remember information (McDevitt & Ormrod, 2012). Often, information processing in humans is compared to that of computers, in that humans can receive and store vast amounts of data and employ a variety of applications to use those data.

Several mental structures and processes are involved, including sensation and perception, attention, and memory. As each of these mechanisms matures, so does the child's efficiency in learning, performing mental activities, and using knowledge and information.

Structures

Information processing begins with the sensation and perception of information from the environment. Raw material is received through the senses (the sensation) and is immediately interpreted as perception. The mechanism that receives raw material from the senses often is called the **sensory register** or **sensory memory**. Experience plays some role in the development of perception; however, there seems to be very little difference between the sensory memory of school-age children and that of adults. Many pieces of information that enter the sensory memory are lost or discarded, but significant information passes along to the working memory.

Information that is selected for attention flows from the sensory memory to the **working memory**. According to information processing theory, working memory, often called **short-term memory**, is that part of the memory system where conscious mental activity occurs. Information enters the working memory in limited quantities, and remains there for a brief period of time while it is processed and then either dismissed or moved into long-term memory for storage. It is in the working memory that thinking, problem solving, and other cognitive activities occur. The capacity of working memory increases during middle childhood. Although it is not clear what processes account for the change, recent studies examining visual working memory performance have shown that sixth- and seventh-grade children can handle a higher working memory load than first- and second-grade children (Cowan, Morey, AuBuchon, Zwilling, & Gilchrist, 2010).

Because new information from sensory memory is constantly available, material in the working memory stays only for a very short period of time. After about 15 to 30 seconds, meaningful information is transferred from the working memory to the **long-term memory**. Whereas the working memory is that part of the cognitive system where mental activity occurs, long-term memory is the part of the system where information is stored. In contrast to short-term memory, which is limited in capacity and duration, long-term memory is thought to have unlimited storage capacity over an indefinite period of time. As children mature, the amount of knowledge stored in long-term memory increases dramatically. To manage the vast amount of knowledge stored in long-term memory, a variety of organizational strategies and techniques develop. These strategies allow new material to be integrated into long-term memory with greater efficiency.

Processes

While the structures involved in information processing seem to change little during middle childhood, the processes involved change quite a bit. Eleven-year-old children are better thinkers than six-year-olds, in part because they have more knowledge, but mainly because they can use their minds more strategically and efficiently (Berger, 2008). During middle childhood, advances are particularly notable in attention and in processing speed.

Whether information moves through the parts of the memory system or is discarded depends on whether attention is paid to it. Attention is the primary process through which information moves from the sensory memory to the working memory (McDevitt & Ormrod, 2012) and through which information is retained and manipulated in the working memory. Attention changes along several dimensions as children mature. Younger children are distractible. As various stimuli catch their attention, they shift focus quickly. Over time, children gain the ability to control their attention. They become less susceptible to distraction and better able to deliberately focus on selected stimuli. Furthermore, older children are more purposeful in choosing the focus of their attention.

The ability to focus on relevant information and screen out irrelevant information is known as **selective attention**, a skill essential to learning. It appears that older children are more proficient at selectively attending than younger children. The ability of younger children to selectively attend seems to be influenced by the capacity of the working memory. In comparisons of first and second graders with older children and adults, Cowan et al. (2010) showed that the younger children pay attention in a manner similar to that of older children and adults. Like older children and adults, to complete short-term memory tasks, they are able to focus on relevant information and filter out irrelevant information. This ability is compromised, however, when the amount of information added to the capacity of the working memory is increased.

Another cognitive development that distinguishes older and younger children is **processing speed**. With time and practice throughout middle childhood, children become quicker at responding and performing mental activities, sometimes with very little conscious effort at all. As mental activities are repeated, the neural pathways used become myelinated and automatization occurs. With faster and more automatic processing taking place, the working memory has more capacity available to take in information and perform more complex tasks.

Strategies are more deliberate, less automatic mental activities that are involved in learning and moving information to long-term memory. Several strategies that seem to gain sophistication during the school years are rehearsal, organization, and elaboration. **Rehearsal** is simply the conscious repetition of one or more pieces of information as a way of holding the information in the working memory temporarily. In general, younger children do not begin to use this strategy spontaneously until about age 7 or 8, but 6-year-olds can be taught the strategy. By about age 9 or 10, children use rehearsal with more complexity, often using association to combine things to be remembered into groups or categories.

By looking for associations and combining information into groups or categories to make it easier to recall, children are beginning to use the strategy of **organization**. While younger children may be observed organizing information in order to be able to remember it, the organization seems to lack logic and doesn't have much effect on recall. By the later elementary years, children are more intentional about learning, organizing information into patterns that are more intricate and sophisticated.

Another strategy that children seem to use intentionally to help them learn and remember is elaboration. The process of **elaboration** involves reasoning, logic, and sometimes imagination. To elaborate, information to be remembered is linked with information that is already known. For example, a child might find it easier to remember that the new soccer coach's last name is Cleatus if the coach can be visualized putting on cleats in preparation for a game. As the strategy of elaboration becomes more complex, it allows the possibility of assumption. When new information is encountered, it is broadened by the addition of information that is already known. This strategy begins to emerge during the later years of middle childhood.

When children deliberately employ strategies to help them remember or learn, they are demonstrating that they have the ability to think about thinking. Knowledge about cognitive states or processes, known as **metacognition** begins to emerge at around 8 years of age (Veenman, Van Hout-Walters, & Afflerbach, 2006) and expands across the middle childhood years. Metacognition can be divided into two categories: self-appraisal of knowledge and self-monitoring of cognitive processes (Vasile, 2010). Cognitive self-appraisal generally involves awareness of three types of knowledge: declarative, knowing about oneself as a learner and about factors that influence learning and performance; procedural, knowing how to execute skills; and conditional, knowing when and why to employ various cognitive operations (Broderick & Blewitt, 2014). Self-monitoring of cognition involves the use of executive processes such as planning, evaluation, and monitoring or regulation.

Language Development

As children enter elementary school along their odyssey, their use of language is similar to that of adults in many respects (McDevitt & Ormrod, 2012), including their use of grammar, questions, negative statements, and complex sentences. They know and apply basic rules of syntax and continue to learn more complex and "exceptions to" rules as they mature. Beginning with about 8000 words at the beginning of middle childhood, children's vocabulary grows to about 50,000 words by the end of middle childhood. As words are added to children's vocabularies, their meanings, at first, are not fully understood, and these words may be used incorrectly. In particular, elementary-aged children have difficulty mastering "function" words such as prepositions and conjunctions, which are used to represent relationships among words and phrases in sentences. As they develop, children increase their understanding of temporal and comparative words.

Because children in middle childhood think concretely, their understanding of abstract words emerges later than their understanding of more concrete words. Thinking concretely also affects the way they make meaning of what they hear; thus, younger children are likely to interpret verbal messages literally. As their cognitive abilities mature, however, they become better able to understand and use figurative language. Increasing cognitive maturity also allows children to consider the perspectives of their listeners and adjust their conversation accordingly. This development plays a role in social development as well.

Intelligence

Changes in cognitive development are reflected in measures of intelligence. Numerous theories of intelligence have been proposed, and each is tied to its own definition. In general, intelligence may be thought of as mental capacities or functions such as learning, problem solving, and reasoning that are required for survival and advancement in a particular culture [American Association on Intellectual and Developmental Disabilities (AAIDD, 2010)]. An intelligence quotient (IQ), the measure of intellectual functioning, is an expression of an individual's mental capacity at any given point in time compared to others the same age. Although mental abilities are gained throughout middle childhood, IQ remains relatively stable since it is a measure of the developing child's ability in reference to other developing children. Variations in IQ may be attributed to the influence of environmental and biological factors as well as differences in the rate at which individual children develop.

Measures of intelligence currently in use in the United States correlate highly with measures of academic achievement. Thus, it stands to reason that intelligence has an important role in children's learning and academic performance. On the other hand, it is important to note that the content of intelligence tests resembles what is taught in school. Factors such as poverty, parental involvement, changes in the family structure or home conditions, and severe or prolonged illness are related to measured intelligence in much the same way that they are related to scholastic achievement.

Mindsets

The way children think about their own intelligence contributes to their academic achievement and resilience (Yeager & Dweck, 2012). Resilience may be thought of as a positive outcome or adaptation to challenges and stress, and indeed, many children are challenged by the way they and others around them think of intelligence. Frequently, intelligence is thought of as a "fixed entity," that is, something of which there is a fixed amount that cannot be changed. When children receive and internalize this message, they may attribute difficult academic experiences to not being smart or to limited intelligence. Such thinking may compromise resilience and conclude with giving up, cheating, learned helplessness, or other negative outcomes (Dweck, 2006; Yeager & Dweck, 2012). In contrast, intelligence may be thought of as a malleable construct that develops incrementally. Individuals who hold an "incremental" or growth mindset about intelligence see themselves as able to grow, learn, and develop their intelligence. These individuals tend to demonstrate more academic resilience.

Research has shown that children can be taught to think about intelligence as incremental rather than a fixed entity, and when they adopt this mindset, its benefits are seen in academic achievement and resilience (Dweck, 2006; Yeager & Dweck, 2012). Helping children to view intelligence as malleable or incremental may be accomplished by being intentional and attentive to the words used in praise. Two types of praise that have been studied for their effects are person-praise and process-praise. Feedback that includes statements about stable, global traits is considered **person-praise**. Examples of this type of praise are, "You're so smart," and "You're really good at math." These statements suggest that ability is static and unchanging and contribute to a fixed-entity mindset. While on the surface this type of praise seems positive, it may be detrimental as it links success to ability as a fixed entity. The assumption that intelligence or ability is a fixed entity leads children to avoid challenges and limits their performance. **Process-praise**, on the other hand, focuses on effort rather than a fixed ability. Children who are given feedback such as "You tried really hard" learn to link success to task engagement. Process-praise fosters the view that intelligence may be developed incrementally, leads children to prefer challenges, and enhances their performance (Pomerantz & Kempner, 2013).

Exceptionalities

Precursors of the intelligence tests most widely used today were developed in the early part of the 20th century as a way to identify children who were unlikely to succeed in traditional academic settings and might require modified instruction. Today, tests such as the Wechsler Intelligence Scale for Children—Fifth Edition (WISC-V) and the Stanford–Binet Intelligence Scales—Fifth Edition (SB-5) serve a similar purpose. These tests help in diagnosing developmental disabilities and exceptionalities, and often the specific information gained from them assists in the construction of individualized educational plans for children with special needs.

Intellectual Disability

Some children learn and acquire mental capacities at a rate much slower than others. Compared to other children the same age, they may have significant limitations in intellectual functioning and adaptive behavior. Once called mental retardation, this impairment is now known as **intellectual disability** (AAIDD, 2010). On standardized assessments of IQ, these children score below 70 and make up the bottom 2% of their age group. They have difficulty with conceptual skills and with everyday social and practical skills, and seem to function similarly to children who are much younger.

Learning Disability

Many children score within the normal or above normal range of measured intelligence but still have difficulty with scholastic performance, and are identified as having a **learning disability**. These children may have difficulties in specific cognitive processes involving perception, memory, language, or metacognition. Their cognitive difficulty interferes with their ability to succeed in specific academic areas such as mathematics, reading, or written expression. About 5% of children enrolled in school receive education services for specific learning disabilities, making this the largest single category of special education services provided in the United States (U.S. Department of Education, 2011). By the middle elementary years, children with such difficulties often have fallen behind their peers in achievement in one or more academic areas. When the discrepancy between their actual achievement in a specific academic area and the level of achievement predicted by their IQ scores is fairly great and cannot be attributed to other behavioral or emotional problems, they may be diagnosed with a specific learning disability.

Attention-Deficit/Hyperactivity Disorder (ADHD)

Another problem that may contribute to difficulty in school performance is attention-deficit/hyperactivity disorder (ADHD). Two qualities that characterize children with ADHD are inattention (i.e., difficulty focusing and maintaining attention) and/or hyperactive or impulsive behavior. Many children with ADHD exhibit only one of these qualities; many exhibit both [American Psychiatric Association (APA), 2013]. It is generally thought that the attention problems of ADHD reflect deficits in working memory and selective attention (Barkley, 2006). Research suggests that it may be more realistic to consider ADHD a disorder of self-regulation (Barkley, 2011), which will be discussed in the Chapter 10 along with other disruptive behavior disorders.

Summary

Children begin middle childhood with many of the characteristics of younger children. Their body proportions and motor skills resemble those of younger children, and their thinking is preoperational and often magical. As children mature through middle childhood, they become more adult-like. Their body proportions are more similar to adults, as is their use of language. They are able to carry out complex mental activities, to think about themselves and others, and to participate in a wide range of socially interactive activities.

Children grow steadily during middle childhood. As they mature from early childhood to adolescence, their weight doubles, their body proportions change, and their baby teeth are replaced by permanent dentition. Much brain development occurs in the cortex, and neural pathways are created and strengthened that allow for increased executive functioning. Neural pathways strengthened through myelination and automatization also allow children more control of their bodies and motor behaviors. Physical development is supported by play as well as good nutrition.

Physical and brain changes that occur during middle childhood support a tremendous amount of cognitive growth. Conversely, the repetition of newly acquired cognitive skills strengthens neural connections. Cognitively, children during middle childhood develop competencies and strategies that allow them to reason and

use logic. They learn to read, write, and do basic arithmetic through their use of concrete operations. Among the cognitive functions that Piaget described as concrete operations are reversibility, grouping, seriation, and conservation. Together, these emerging abilities allow children to better appreciate cause-and-effect relationships and to interact with their environments with more intention.

Another way to conceptualize children's cognitive development is to consider it in terms of the way information is processed. During middle childhood, children develop structures that allow them to attend to new information and store it for later retrieval. New information is acquired through sensory memory, processed through short-term memory, and stored in long-term memory. Improved information processing allows children to selectively attend, and to improve the efficiency with which they gain new knowledge and skills. In addition, they gain the ability to think about the way they think, a phenomenon known as metacognition.

Children begin elementary school with language skills that are similar to those of adults. They know grammar and syntax and use complex sentences. As they mature, their vocabularies expand and they begin to comprehend words that have abstract meanings. With abstract reasoning comes the ability to see other perspectives and to develop socially and emotionally.

Middle Childhood: Emotional and Social Development

By Stephanie Puleo

While family influences remain important, the school environment plays an increasingly greater role in the child's cognitive, emotional, and social development during middle childhood (Maldonado-Carreno & Votruba-Drzal, 2011; McDevitt & Ormrod, 2012). Before they can learn to read, write, and compute, children must be able to function in the absence of their primary caretakers for extended periods of time. As their attention shifts from home to school and from fantasy to reality, children in middle childhood acquire skills and concepts necessary for daily living. Their attention spans increase, their motor abilities grow more complex, they gain better understanding of right and wrong, they begin to think logically, they become integrated into social networks, and their developing self-awareness permits them to compare themselves to others and to refine their self-concepts.

Freud and Erikson

According to Freudian (psychoanalytic) theory, middle childhood is a period of relative calm known as the latency stage of psychosexual development. In previous stages of development, Freud noted, psychological energy (libido) shifted through different parts of the body, thereby calling attention to different sources of pleasure and changing the nature of relationships with others. By middle childhood, the three components of the psyche—the id, the ego, and the superego—are complete and the child has learned to cope with conflict and tension through a complex system of defense mechanisms. During latency, then, the focus of attention turns to mastery of nonsexual developmental tasks (Hunt & Kraus, 2009; Jacobs, 2004).

Erikson, schooled in psychoanalytic theory, agreed with Freud's basic concepts regarding stages of development. Similar to Freud, Erikson postulated that at each stage of development there is a conflict or crisis to be resolved. For Erikson, however, the nature of the developmental crises was more social than sexual. Thus, according to Erikson, middle childhood is a period filled with much developmental activity as the child's social focus expands to include the aspects of school, peers, and the community. The acquisition of skills necessary to confront the tasks of school and socialization contribute to a sense of either competency or inferiority. This developmental crisis is known as **industry versus inferiority**.

Walk into the home of any elementary school child, and there likely will be a refrigerator door covered with school work, art work, and a variety of other crudely manufactured items attributed to that child. These items are all examples of the child's growing desire to make things and to be recognized for these efforts and accomplishments. Children at this stage of development are beginning to see themselves as capable of being productive and industrious. They are learning new skills that will help them to function and be accepted in society. During middle childhood, school is a major context in which the emergence of a sense of industry may be observed, but it is important to notice other accomplishments as well. Children's sense of industry also grows through activities such as organized sports, music, online and video games, clubs, and extracurricular programs. Adults play an important part in the development of industry in two ways. Adults have a role in providing opportunities for children to experience making things and being productive; they also have a responsibility to noncritically recognize effort and accomplishments.

Children who are allowed to participate in productive activities, who gain skill mastery, and whose efforts and accomplishments are recognized resolve this stage of development with a sense of competence. For some children, successful resolution of this stage of development is difficult. If they are denied opportunities, if they are criticized, or if they view their emerging skills as inadequate compared to those of their peers, they may develop a sense of inferiority.

Developing Self

Self-Concept

The way in which children view themselves as either industrious or inferior contributes to their emerging self-concept. **Self-concept** entails the content of what one thinks about oneself as well as how one assesses that content (Wenar & Kerig, 2006). Younger children, who are limited by concrete, all-or-nothing thinking, tend to view themselves in absolute (and mostly positive) terms. During middle childhood, children acquire the ability to consider two or more concepts and dimensions simultaneously and therefore begin to develop self-concepts that are more complex and multifaceted (Steinberg, Bornstein, Vandell, & Rook, 2011). Prior to entering the cognitive development stage of concrete operations, younger children (ages 5 to 7) may still hold onto unrealistically positive self-perceptions, or self-descriptions that are compartmentalized and absolute. As children develop more versatile cognitive abilities (by about ages 8 to 11), their self-concepts become more complex and integrated. They are able to describe themselves in terms of overall self-worth or self-esteem, as well as in terms of specific domains such as academic competency, physical appearance and ability, and social acceptance (Harter, 2006; Manning, Bear, & Minke, 2006).

Self-Esteem

Self-esteem refers to the evaluative component of self-concept, and it appears to be driven by both cognitive development and socialization (Harter, 2006). Some research suggests that children may experience a drop in self-esteem as they enter elementary school and are faced with new academic and social challenges and begin to compare themselves to their peers. At about age 8, children are able to comprehend that they are individual people, and they can reflect on whether they are happy or unhappy with themselves. As they become less egocentric in their thinking, their feelings about themselves are influenced by how they compare with others and how they sense others reacting to them. These self-judgments may be related to children's mindsets about their abilities, that is, whether they think of their abilities as fluid and developing or as fixed entities (Dweck, 2006). Self-esteem influences children's behavior and achievement. Children who judge themselves positively are likely to engage in behaviors that lead to further accomplishment, whereas children who judge themselves negatively are less likely to continue to engage in success-promoting behaviors. While it is generally thought that self-esteem is related to perceived competence, it also is dependent upon the personal importance of the specific areas being evaluated (Harter, 2006). For example, if physical ability has more personal importance than academic performance, the child who is an accomplished athlete but a weak student might be expected to experience positive self-esteem. Overall, the more an individual perceives personal competence in areas of high importance, the more likely that person's self-esteem will be positive. Disturbances in self-esteem place children at risk for a number of psychological disorders.

Emotions

As children grow older and acquire more complex cognitive abilities, they also acquire a broader range of emotions. They become increasingly aware of the feelings of others and aware of the connection between thoughts and feelings. By middle childhood, children realize that situations may be perceived and interpreted differently by different people, leading to different emotional reactions. By the later years of middle childhood, they also recognize that it is possible to have ambivalent or conflicting feelings, and that some feelings may be hidden.

Emotional Intelligence

Emotional intelligence is a set of interrelated abilities that allow individuals to process information about their own and others' emotions and to use that information to guide their thinking and behavior (Mayer, Salovey, & Caruso, 2008). Central to the concept of emotional intelligence is the ability to empathize. Young children understand the feelings of others only superficially, but as they progress through middle childhood, they gain appreciation for the needs, feelings, and perspectives of others. During middle childhood, emotional intelligence is refined and tested as children's cognitive abilities and self-concepts become more complex.

Emotional Regulation

Implied in the concept of emotional intelligence is the notion of **emotional regulation**. During middle childhood, children increase their capacity to manage their emotions, thoughts, and behavior. Whereas in early childhood much responsibility for the control of behavior was assumed by parents and caretakers, in middle childhood children take more responsibility for themselves. As new stressful situations are encountered, new coping skills are learned. Throughout middle childhood, children become better able to assess the situations in which they find themselves and to evaluate the benefits and disadvantages of using particular coping strategies. Ultimately, they learn when it is safe and appropriate to express emotions publicly and when they would be better served by concealing or curbing their emotional responses (McDevitt & Ormrod, 2012).

Emotional Problems in Middle Childhood

Disruptive Behavior Disorders

The executive skills that are required for self-regulation appear to be the same skills required for attention and behavior inhibition. Deficits in these skills often are associated with **attention-deficit/hyperactivity disorder** (ADHD) (Barkley, 2006, 2011). The executive functioning deficits associated with ADHD appear to affect inhibition, paying attention, rule following, self-directed speech, motivation, and self-awareness, all abilities required for self-regulation. In the United States, it is estimated that more than 7% of children ages 6 to 11 have been diagnosed with ADHD (Pastor & Reuben, 2008). ADHD is generally recognized as a neuropsychological disorder that results in significant problems in attention, often accompanied with impulsivity and excessive activity (Barkley, 2006). Children who have ADHD have a great deal of difficulty concentrating for long periods of time, particularly if they find no motivation in the task at hand. Lacking in some self-regulatory skills, many of these children are also easily distracted by other, irrelevant, stimuli. Distraction often leads to impulsive behavior and the appearance of being overly active. Children with ADHD typically have difficulty attending to details, following through on instructions, being organized, and completing tasks. In addition, many children fidget, squirm, and are often out of their seats without permission from the teacher. According to the American Psychiatric Association's (2013) *Diagnostic and Statistical Manual of Mental Disorders* (DSM-5), there are three types of ADHD: predominantly inattentive presentation, predominantly hyperactive/impulsive presentation, and combined presentation. To be diagnosed, symptoms that cause distress must appear before the age of 7, be present for at least six months, and be observable in more than one setting. Most individuals who receive a diagnosis of ADHD are considered to have the combined type (Barkley, 2011).

Without intervention, children with ADHD may be at risk for poor school performance. Their inability to attend and concentrate may lead to gaps in information processing and the acquisition of new knowledge. Approximately 3% of all children in the United States have both ADHD and a learning disability (Pastor & Reuben, 2008). In addition to learning problems, many children with ADHD may experience anxiety and depression and may have problems with social functioning. They often are perceived as troublesome by adults, and are rejected by their peers. It is not uncommon to see some aggressive behavior in children with ADHD who become frustrated. Aggressive and impulsive behaviors also put children with ADHD at higher risk for accident and injury.

ADHD is considered one of three disorders characterized by "disruptive behavior" (APA, 2013). Two other disorders that are characterized by disruptive behavior are oppositional defiant disorder (ODD) and conduct disorder (CD), and children with ADHD have an increased risk of developing one of these problems as well. **Oppositional defiant disorder** is characterized by hostile, negative behavior, particularly directed toward adults. Behaviors associated with ODD typically emerge prior to age 8. Children with ODD are viewed by others as being deliberately annoying, uncooperative, disobedient, disrespectful, blaming, and vindictive (APA, 2013). While many children fail to comply with parental commands, or engage in temper tantrums, it is the frequency and intensity of such behavior that suggests a problematic pattern. About half of the children in the United States who

---

Think About It   10.1

In a controversial book, Dr. Richard Saul claims that ADHD does not exist (Saul, 2014). Using DSM-5 (APA, 2013) criteria, a diagnosis of ADHD may be assigned if an individual exhibits six of nine possible symptoms in either of two categories. Among the symptoms are difficulties in attending to details, organizing activities, following through on instructions, and waiting one's turn. Some individuals would argue that these are traits that define elementary school children! Dr. Saul, a researcher and clinician who specializes in pediatrics and behavioral neurology, contends that the traits, behaviors, and difficulties that are grouped together to describe ADHD are just that—a group of symptoms, not a condition or disorder. He maintains that there may be as many as 20 conditions that could lead to these symptoms including hearing or vision problems, nutrition or metabolic issues, sleep deprivation, mood disorders, and anxiety. Rather than diagnosing so many children with ADHD and prescribing stimulant medications for them, Dr. Saul would prefer to see underlying conditions identified and treated, and healthy lifestyle habits promoted. What do you think?

---

are identified with ODD have also been diagnosed with ADHD (Hinshaw & Lee, 2003). In addition, ODD seems to be more prevalent in children with depression and anxiety.

Conduct disorder tends to be more problematic than ODD. Whereas the hostility of children with ODD tends to be aimed at authority figures and people they know, the hostility of children with CD tends to be more diffused and directed at others in society. Children with CD seem to have a general disregard for the rights of others and a tendency to violate basic rules and norms of society. The behaviors of children with CD are grouped into four categories: aggression against people and animals, destruction of property, deceitfulness and theft, and serious violations of rules. Without intervention, children with CD may develop into adults with antisocial personality disorder. In addition to being associated with ADHD, CD in children is associated with mood, anxiety, and learning disorders. Both ODD and CD are more prevalent in boys than in girls (APA, 2013).

The Counselor in the Child's Journey through Disruptive Behavior Disorders

Many children with disruptive behavior disorders are positively influenced by the counselors they meet during their odyssey. A number of promising evidence-based psychosocial intervention strategies for disruptive behavior have been identified in the literature (Eyberg, Nelson, & Boggs, 2008), including anger control training, assertiveness training, and problem-solving skills training for both individuals and groups. Intervention strategies that involve parents and families are also associated with positive outcomes for children with disruptive behaviors. Additional evidence suggests that counselors can expand their impact by teaching or training parents and peers to have a role in helping children with disruptive behaviors.

Compared to other disruptive behavior disorders, much more research has been conducted on counseling strategies for children with ADHD. Many of these studies suggest that children with ADHD are most successful when a strengths-based behavioral approach is taken (Jarrett & Ollendick, 2012; Portrie-Bethke, Hill, & Bethke, 2009; Schultz, Storer, Watabe, Sadler, & Evans, 2011). Behavioral strategies that record, reward, and reinforce appropriate attentive behaviors help many children. These strategies might include daily report cards or token economies, and their effectiveness is increased when counselors enlist and guide teachers and parents as allies (Jarrett & Ollendick, 2012; Levine & Anshel, 2011; Schultz et al., 2011). Research suggests that cognitive counseling strategies offer limited assistance to elementary school children with ADHD (Schultz et al., 2011); however, the cognitive strategies may be helpful when used to challenge negative self-attributions such as laziness or incompetence (Levine & Anshel, 2011).

Several studies suggest that experiential counseling strategies may be beneficial for children with disruptive behavior disorders. Children with ADHD and those with aggressive behavior have shown improvement when given opportunities to participate in experiential forms of counseling such as play therapy or adventure-based counseling (Levine & Anshel, 2011; Ray, Schottelkorb, & Tsai, 2007; Ray, Sullivan, Blanco, & Holliman, 2009).

Anxiety, Depression, and Grief

Sometimes children in the United States are inattentive, have trouble concentrating, or exhibit problematic behavior, yet their difficulties are not related to one of the disruptive behavior disorders. Because young children do not have the cognitive and emotional maturity to recognize and articulate how they are feeling, their behavior and school performance may be the first signs that they are experiencing depression or anxiety. It is often the case that these experiences and symptoms are related to stressors and events in children's lives. Many times, children exhibit changes in behavior, anxiety, or depressed moods when they are having difficulty adjusting to new or different circumstances, for example, a new brother or sister, a different housing arrangement, or an altered routine. When children's reactions to change are more than might be expected, an **adjustment disorder** (APA, 2013) might be present. Changes in behavior, anxiety, and depressed mood also may signify grief and **bereavement** if the altered life circumstance involves loss.

Children who experience the death of a loved one wrestle with their emotions and with finding ways to express their emotions. A predominant feeling identified by children who are grieving is sadness, but many are not aware that it is appropriate for them to cry or verbalize this feeling (McClatchey & Wimmer, 2014). Bereaved children also tend to worry; they worry about their own safety, security, and care, and tend to focus their worry on fears about the health and commitment of their surviving parents. Younger children, whose thinking is still somewhat egocentric, may feel guilty and worry that their own actions or thoughts caused the death (Worden, 1996). In addition to these feelings, older children whose cognitive abilities are more advanced, often report feelings of anger toward the person who has died. Children's grief reactions may be further complicated if their loved one's death was traumatic (McClatchey & Wimmer, 2014).

About 2% of children experience depressive disorders including **major depressive disorder** and **dysthymic disorder** (APA, 2013). Children with depression may seem sad, lonely, irritable, negative, hypersensitive, and overreactive. Often, children who are depressed express self-criticism and low self-esteem. Their low energy and loss of motivation may prevent them from fully participating in school or social activities. If they engage in disruptive or aggressive behavior, their social relationships and academic performance may be further affected (Wenar & Kerig, 2006).

It is generally thought that depression is the result of a complicated interaction of environmental and biological factors. When working with children, it is especially important to pay attention to environmental factors. Stressful, chaotic, and abusive family environments may be breeding grounds for depression. Having parents who are depressed increases a child's risk for depression (APA, 2013). In addition, children who are depressed often have poor peer relationships, but it is not clear which is the causal factor. Finally, perhaps because of their limited cognitive and emotional development, depressed children may see suicide as a viable coping strategy.

All children (and adults, for that matter) have some fears, but as they mature they are able to use concrete operations and their emerging emotional regulation to calm themselves (Wenar & Kerig, 2006). Some children, however, are not as successful in applying coping mechanisms and are at risk for anxiety disorders. Anxiety disorders are distinguished from normal fears by their intensity, persistence, and involuntary nature. In children, many symptoms of anxiety look similar to symptoms of depression. Anxious children may be withdrawn, have physical complaints, and may cry. In contrast to children with depression, anxious children worry; they worry a lot. Worries about specific situations or objects generally suggest phobias, and it is not uncommon for children to have school or social phobias. Some children, however, carry their worry with them wherever they go. Many of these children, who seem to find things to worry about, may be diagnosed with generalized anxiety disorder.

Children with **school phobia** experience irrational dread related to going to school. As the thought or reality of school attendance becomes more imminent, they experience physiological symptoms of anxiety. School phobia should not be confused with school refusal, which may be attributed to other causes such as conduct disorder, depression, separation anxiety, or social phobia. School phobia sometimes is mistaken for **separation anxiety**, but the two can be distinguished by observing when and where the child appears anxious. Children with school phobia are generally comfortable in any setting that is not school, with or without their caretakers present. Children with separation anxiety are anxious and uncomfortable in any setting where the caretaker to whom they are attached is not present. School phobia is more prevalent in older boys from higher socioeconomic strata, and separation anxiety is more prevalent in girls from lower socioeconomic strata (Wenar & Kerig, 2006).

Social phobia is characterized by anxiety symptoms that are similar to those of school phobia and separation anxiety. Children with this disorder seem to experience anxiety in most social situations in and out of school. What they seem to fear most is being embarrassed or humiliated; as a result, they avoid situations where they feel they would be judged or evaluated. Avoiding social situations often means avoiding school. If it is not possible to avoid school, school is endured with a great deal of distress and anxiety, limiting learning. Lack of participation in social activities further interferes with their social development, possibly leading to low self-esteem and additional rejection by peers.

As is the case when children are exhibiting symptoms of depression, it is important to examine environmental factors when children develop symptoms of anxiety. While some anxiety may be related to school and social worries, some may be triggered by traumatic events. **Traumatic stress disorders** are characterized by symptoms of anxiety and arousal, avoidance, and psychological reexperiencing of trauma (e.g., nightmares, intrusive thoughts, flashbacks). Anxiety reactions may be triggered by anything that remotely reminds the child of the traumatic event. Often, the traumatic event responsible for this type of anxiety is something that is obvious, such as a disaster or crisis event, but all too often acute stress disorder and post-traumatic stress disorder are the consequences of abuse and victimization.

The Counselor in the Child's Journey through Anxiety, Depression, and Grief

Similar to children with disruptive behavioral disorders, children with mood and anxiety disturbances may be positively influenced by the counselors they meet during their odyssey. Many counselors are called upon to work with children whose anxiety, depressed mood, and altered behavior are related to grief. According to a model proposed by Worden (1996, 2002; Worden & Winokuer, 2010), a foremost researcher and author on the subject of grief and grief counseling, there are four tasks to be accomplished during periods of mourning: (1) accept the reality of the death; (2) experience pain and other feelings associated with the death; (3) adjust to an environment without the deceased; and (4) find ways to "relocate" and memorialize the deceased. While these tasks are difficult enough for adults, for children they are complicated by cognitive development. To accept the reality of death, children must learn what death means, namely that all life functions end at the time of death and that death is irreversible. Conversations aimed at helping children understand death should include language that is simple and concrete, as children may be confused by euphemisms and abstract concepts. Children should not be shielded from others' expressions of emotions; seeing other people appropriately express emotions sends a message of permission and validation for their own feelings. Expressing and talking about their feelings is easier for children if they believe they have permission and that someone is genuinely interested and listening. Conversations that include religious beliefs that have been introduced by the child's family may facilitate the child's understanding of death and how to relocate the deceased; however, it should be noted that religious concepts may also be confusing for children who are not yet capable of abstract thinking (see Case Example 10.1). Overall, any number of techniques and activities may be employed to help a child accomplish the tasks of mourning, but it is important for them to be simple, concrete, and consistent with the child's level of cognitive development and individual needs.

While cognitive counseling strategies seem to be of limited benefit to children with ADHD, research suggests that they may be very beneficial to children with anxiety, depression, and grief (Erford, Lee, Newsome, & Rock, 2011; Jarrett & Ollendick, 2012; Rolfsnes & Idsoe, 2011; Silverman, Pina, & Viswesvaran, 2008). Studies examining the effects of cognitive and cognitive-behavioral counseling strategies applied to individual children, to children in groups, and to families all have shown positive results.

As alternatives to cognitive counseling strategies, there are additional counseling approaches that may benefit children with anxiety, depression, and grief. Some studies have shown that social effectiveness training as well as play therapy may be helpful for children who are socially anxious, shy, or withdrawn (Silverman, Pina, & Viswesvaran, 2008; Wettig, Coleman, & Geider, 2011). Play therapy also is a treatment of choice for children who may be experiencing trauma-related anxiety (Fitzgerald, Henriksen, & Garza, 2012; Rolfsnes & Idsoe, 2011).

Play therapy may be a particularly beneficial adventure for children during the middle childhood years, for a number of reasons. During this time of their developmental odyssey, children are operating in the concrete stage of cognitive development. Their ability to express complicated emotions is limited by their lack of abstract thought. In contrast to cognitive therapy, in which children are asked to discuss their experiences and emotions but are restricted by the limitations in their cognitive development, play therapy allows children to communicate their emotions and experiences through toys and other play media (Landreth, Ray, & Bratton, 2009).

➤ CASE EXAMPLE **10.1** WHERE IS HEAVEN?

Antoine is the 6-year-old great-nephew of Sophia. (He is the son of Sophia's niece.) One day while Sophia was caring for Antoine in her home, she put him to work with a feather duster. As he dusted around books and objects on the shelves he was cleaning, a particular object caught his attention. "What's that?" he asked as he pointed to a memorial urn. Sophia's mother, Antoine's great-grandmother, had recently died and been cremated. The urn contained her remains. Sophia had a moment of panic as she wondered about this child's awareness of death and spirituality, what his parents already had attempted to teach him, and what to say.

Sophia took a deep breath and asked Antoine to sit beside her on the couch. "Do you remember Grandma Rosa?"

"Yes," Antoine said. "She was a nice lady. She used to give me jars of pennies when I would visit her."

"And do you remember that she died last month? And after she died we all went to her funeral?"

"Yes."

Sophia took another deep breath. "Well, after the funeral, Grandma Rosa was cremated." Antoine sat silently and stared at the urn.

Sophia followed his stare, pointed to the urn, and in a quiet voice said, "She's in there."

Antoine jumped off the couch and ran to the urn, "You mean, THAT'S heaven?!"

REFLECTION 10.1 UNCLE MALCOLM

The year that Antoine's great-grandmother died was a rough year for the family. I am Antoine's other great-aunt, and I have another nephew, Jerome, who is about three years older than Antoine. About a month before Antoine's great-grandmother died, my own husband, Malcolm, died. Malcolm had a relationship with each of these boys and it was interesting to me to watch their developmental differences as they grappled with understanding death and relocating their deceased relatives. Antoine had been told that his great-grandmother and his great-uncle both were in heaven. As a 6-year-old with very concrete thinking, he concluded that heaven must be a memorial urn.

Jerome's story was a bit different. Jerome was 9 years old when his Uncle Malcolm died. Several months later, Jerome and his parents were visiting a park where it happened that helium-inflated balloons were being sold. Jerome pleaded and insisted that his parents buy a balloon. Once the balloon was paid for and handed to Jerome, he intentionally let go of the string. Caught by surprise and confusion, his parents asked him why he would do such a thing. His response was, "I wanted to send it to Uncle Malcolm in heaven." It was clear that five or six months after his uncle's death, Jerome was still thinking about him and grieving. It seemed to me that in some way he was longing for him and wishing to connect.

Antoine and Jerome both had been taught that their deceased family members were now in heaven. They both seemed to understand the concept of death and that neither Antoine's great-grandmother nor Uncle Malcolm would be returning to life. As I juxtaposed their two stories, it was interesting to me to observe the developmental differences between Antoine and Jerome as they struggled with understanding death, "relocating" their deceased family members, and making sense of an abstract concept such as heaven. [~SP]

SECTION II: Social Development

One of the most significant areas to change during the odyssey through the middle childhood years is the area of social understanding. As children enter elementary school they are developing the cognitive capacity to be less egocentric. At the same time, they begin to see their peers as frames of reference against which to measure their own competencies. While recognizing that they are separate from their peers, they also recognize the importance of cooperation, collaboration, and relationships. Advances in cognitive and emotional development pave the way for friendships and group membership.

Moral Development

In order to interact with others and function in groups, people must develop a common set of values and standards to govern their conduct. The standards provide a framework for protecting individual and group rights while promoting interdependent functioning. **Moral development** refers to the process through which children adopt principles and guidelines that allow them to judge whether behavior is right or wrong so that they might interact with others, join groups, and contribute to society. Children acquire morals through socialization, emotional maturation, and cognitive development.

Initially, children begin to learn about right and wrong from their parents and others around them. As they see appropriate behavior modeled and are themselves rewarded for acceptable behavior and punished for behaviors that are harmful, they begin to internalize basic values and guidelines for conduct. Upon entering middle childhood, the number of models around them increases to include siblings, friends, schoolmates, teachers, and other authority figures. With a widening array of social contacts, new rules, different from those imposed by parents, are encountered. Children continue to learn right and wrong as they practice the rules they know, construct new ones, and observe the consequences of rules being broken.

In addition to being contingent upon socialization, moral reasoning seems to be affected by emotional maturation. During middle childhood, children become more **empathic**; that is, they are more able to understand and appreciate the feelings and needs of others. They are better able to read the emotional cues of others and to understand the feelings and thought processes that are associated with them. At the same time, as they become better able to self-regulate, they are less likely to be overwhelmed by their own emotions. These emotional developments contribute to children's increasing demonstration of pro-social behavior.

To some extent, the ability to judge whether behavior is right or wrong requires reasoning, a cognitive ability. Prior to middle childhood, children tend to consider rules as external and fairly absolute. Their level of cognitive development prevents them from considering the intentions of those who may deviate from the rules, or recognizing that rules are implemented by social consensus and are changeable.

➤ CASE EXAMPLE **10.2** CROSSING THE STREET.

A rule in the Lyons family was that young children should cross busy streets only while holding the hand of an adult. This rule especially applied to Main Street, a thoroughfare about two blocks from the Lyons' house. Stacy Lyons had internalized this rule and lived by it without question. By about age 8, as Stacy was becoming more independent, her parents would permit her to walk or ride her bicycle to Main Street. Stacy adhered to the rule about not crossing Main Street alone, however, so she visited only the stores on her side of the street. One Saturday, Stacy had an appointment with the pediatric dentist whose office was on Main Street. Busy with other family responsibilities, the Lyons told Stacy to go on ahead so as not to be late. Without any trepidation, Stacy walked the familiar two blocks to Main Street. When she got there, however, she suddenly realized that the dentist's office was on the other side of the street, and there was no adult to hold her hand as she crossed. Stacy stood at the corner for quite some time, trying to figure out what to do. There are rules about honoring commitments and not being late, but there are also rules about not crossing busy streets unassisted. Finally, she noticed an older neighbor walking by. Problem solved. "Hey, Mrs. Glenn! Would you cross me?"

By middle childhood, children are better able to think about rules and their purpose. They are able to see perspectives other than their own and understand concepts such as caring, fairness, and justice. With advanced cognitive skills, they recognize that rules are constructed by social agreement to promote cooperation, equality, and reciprocity. They also recognize that it is as important to judge behavior by intent as it is to judge it by outcome.

Gains in cognitive abilities in middle childhood allow children to demonstrate more mature moral reasoning. Kohlberg (1963) posited that there are six patterns of thought that are used to solve moral dilemmas. The patterns, or modes, of thought are grouped into three levels of moral reasoning which have become known as preconventional morality, conventional morality, and postconventional morality. Engaging their egocentric, preoperational thought, children in early childhood tend to make moral decisions based on obedience and the avoidance of punishment. As they mature a bit, their moral decisions reflect some consideration of the needs of others, but are still guided by the possibility of external consequences. Most elementary school children choose behavior based on these types of preconventional moral reasoning. Kohlberg observed that the use of these less mature thought patterns decreases with age, and that mature patterns of moral reasoning emerge as the child interacts with the social environment.

By the end of the middle childhood years, some children begin to make decisions based on relationships and social considerations, and are able to take intention into account when evaluating behavior. They are interested in pleasing others, keeping promises, establishing trust, and following the Golden Rule. Stacy's story (Case Example 10.2) is a demonstration of a child about to make this transition. Similar to a child engaging in the first stage of conventional moral reasoning, she knows she must keep her promise and commitment to her dentist; however, she is still motivated by preconventional reasoning in that she does not wish to be disobedient by crossing the street unaccompanied. Most conventional moral reasoning is dependent on being able to think about abstract ideas. Since children in the middle childhood years have not yet acquired formal operational thought, their moral reasoning continues to be predominantly preconventional.

The story of a dad's dilemma (see Reflection 10.2) describes a father's attempt to influence the moral reasoning of a child who has not quite entered the conventional level of moral development. From a conventional reasoning perspective, Dave explained how shared needs and social order are more important than self-interest. Ultimately, the choice he made violated his own reasoning. Knowing that his behavior was incongruent with the moral values he was espousing caused some anxiety for Dave. Jessica, on the other hand, seemed unaffected. It is likely that her cognitive and moral development prevented her from comprehending lofty concepts such as social order, but allowed her to see that her father had the adventurous good intention of getting her to the top of the Empire State Building.

Moral development is influenced by and influences children's ability to interact socially. By middle childhood, children become increasingly likely to engage in behaviors that are helpful and that benefit others. They cooperate, share, help, and comfort others as they perceive the need for these interactive behaviors. At younger ages, the moral reasoning behind such behavior may be based on self-interest (e.g., gaining approval for being helpful), but as they mature, children become more able to focus on serving a common cause. With maturity, children are better able to use cognitive reasoning along with emotions such as empathy and sympathy to guide their pro-social behavior.

REFLECTION 10.2 A DAD'S DILEMMA (DAVE'S STORY)

Jessica and I were in New York City when she was about 11 years old. I believe it was the first time we were visiting Manhattan and I was showing her "the sights." For the past month or two, I had taken every opportunity I could to talk to her about honesty and ethical behavior.

One afternoon, I decided to show her the Empire State Building and take her to the top for the view. We walked to the building and were confronted with a line of tourists that wrapped around the block. Discouraged, we strolled around, looking up at the building only from street level. We ended up in a drug store at the base of the skyscraper with the intention of buying a snack or something like that. While walking around the drug store, I noticed a door that led directly into the lobby of the Empire State Building and to the line for the elevator. The honest and ethical thing would have been to acknowledge it as well as my temptation and then not cut in front of the line. That is not the choice I made. We walked out of the drug store and into the Empire State Building lobby, waited on line for only 10 or 15 minutes and ascended to the top of the tower, where we looked out over New York City as best we could through clouds, wind, and rain. On the way up, and for the rest of the afternoon, I tried to tell Jessica that I knew what we did was wrong and dishonest and there was no real way I could make it otherwise. I made it clear that I consciously chose to do "wrong" and did not try to justify it or make it any other way. It was a tough one and I am not sure what the actual lesson was that was learned. I can only hope that the act of consciously recognizing a moral dilemma was modeled as best it could be. [~SP]

Social Awareness

Social awareness consists primarily of social cognition and social perspective taking.

Social Cognition

Social cognition refers to the way that children think about people and relationships. Social cognition allows children to think about themselves and other people and thus plays an important role in the formation of self-image as well as social relationships. In many ways, children learn about themselves and others by watching. They take notice of the consequences of various actions, and construct personal rules and guidelines for behavior based on what they have noticed. Observing others also gives children a frame of reference for evaluating their own talents and competencies, an important component in the development of their self-concept.

Social Perspective Taking

To further the development of self-concept, people must understand how they and their actions are viewed by others. This mental operation, which becomes possible as children decenter, is known as **perspective taking**. Without being able to understand that there are perspectives other than their own, children would not be able to experience emotions such as empathy, recognize a need to refine their communication skills, or develop meaningful relationships.

Peer Relationships

Social perspective taking plays an important role in the development of peer relationships and friendships. When children enter elementary school their circle of peers increases dramatically. While peers may serve as sources of amusement, entertainment, and fun, they also serve several important developmental functions (McDevitt & Ormrod, 2012). Since peers are their equals, children can practice new and existing social skills with them. In this way, they learn about the perspectives of others, negotiating, and regulating their own emotions and behaviors. Peers serve as role models and help each other learn what is acceptable. Peers teach each other what is "cool" or admirable. They learn from each other what is acceptable to wear, to play, and even to be interested in. By associating with particular groups of peers, children's identities begin to take shape. Finally, peers are a source of emotional and social support, offering comfort in times of anxiety and clarity in times of confusion.

When children are asked about which of their peers they like and which they dislike, four categories of acceptance emerge: accepted, rejected, neglected, and controversial. Children who are accepted by their peers seem to be psychologically better adjusted. They have higher self-esteem, fewer behavioral problems, are happier, and perform better in school (Harter, 2006; Wenar & Kerig, 2006). In relating to other people, they are dependable, cooperative, and sensitive to the feelings of others (Wenar & Kerig, 2006). Children who are rejected, on the other hand, have poor social skills and tend to be distractible and impulsive. In addition, many children who are rejected are aggressive. Neglected children are another group of children who seem to be deficient in social skills. These children are identified as neither liked nor disliked by their peers. They tend to be quiet, sometimes anxious, and associate with only one or two close friends, if any. In contrast to neglected children, controversial children are strongly liked or disliked by their peers. These children do possess social skills and the ability to impress and attract. They are perceived both positively and negatively because of their charisma and their tendency to be identified as troublemakers and class clowns.

Social Exclusion

Much research on social exclusion in childhood has focused on interpersonal rejection, and has examined individual traits possessed by children who are not accepted by their peers.

Often, children who are not accepted have deficits in their ability to read the social cues and intentions of others, as well as deficits in temperament, attachment, and confidence. In general, there are two profiles described for children who are rejected or excluded. One group tends to be subject to victimization by virtue of their extreme shyness, fearfulness, and anxiety. Beyond not being accepted, these children may also be perceived as nonthreatening prey. By contrast, a second group is characterized by uninhibited, externalizing behaviors. These children may become aggressive and predatory (i.e., bullies), and are perceived as troublesome. Neither predators nor prey experience optimum social acceptance (Killen, Mulvey, & Hitti, 2013).

In addition to interpersonal factors that contribute to peer rejection and exclusion, by middle childhood, intergroup factors begin to influence peer relations as well. During middle childhood, awareness of group identity and societal structures begins to emerge, along with inherent attitudes, judgments, biases, and stereotypes. Consistent with their cognitive development, which supports categorical thinking, children form "in-group" and "out-group" classifications which inform their decisions about whom to include and whom to exclude in their friendship groups (Killen, Mulvey, & Hitti, 2013). The disadvantages (particularly within the context of power and social status) of belonging to multiple categories of social group membership, a construct known as **intersectionality** (Crenshaw, 1989), may increase children's risk for exclusion.

Friendships

Friendships are distinct from other forms of peer relationships and serve a number of functions for children. Through friendships, children have companionship, stimulation, support, a reference for social comparison, and intimacy and affection.

Taking cognitive development into consideration, Selman (1980) proposed a stage theory of friendship development based on maturing social perspective taking. Prior to middle childhood, most children are egocentric. They have little awareness or appreciation of the thoughts and feelings of others (or of themselves), and, while they might name people whom they call "friends," their understanding of the concept of friendship is very limited. Once they begin elementary school, children begin to understand that other people have points of view different from their own. Again, their limited cognitive development prevents them from being able to see their own and another perspective simultaneously. While they may acknowledge the perspective of the other person, they continue to make decisions based on their own. With some encouragement, they might reflect on the thoughts and feelings of another person, but for the most part their friendships are defined by personal benefit. During these early elementary years, friendships appear to be unilateral, and there appears to be little understanding that choices can be made and problems can be solved by mutual consensus.

Toward the later elementary years, children are able to think about other perspectives more consistently. They can psychologically put themselves in the position of others and understand motivation and intention. They also understand the possibility of conflicting feelings, motivations, and behaviors. By this stage, the friendships of children in middle childhood are more reciprocal, and decisions are based on mutual desire and emotional investment (Selman, 1980).

Friends are usually chosen because of their similarity in age, gender, and race. By middle childhood, children are able to identify their friends as "best friends," "good friends," or "casual friends" depending on their level of intimacy and the amount of time they spend together (Poulin & Chan, 2010; Vitaro, Boivin, & Bukowski, 2009). Girls in this age group tend to have narrower friendship networks than boys. More than other peer relationships, friendships are important to social and emotional development. Children who reported having best friends during both the fall and the spring of their fifth-grade years had better social adjustment, were more popular, and engaged in more pro-social behaviors than children who lost or did not have best friends (Bowker, Rubin, Burgess, Booth-LaForce, & Rose-Krasnor, 2006).

To honor their relationships, friends put effort into seeing one another's points of view and resolving disputes. This, in turn, leads to further development of social perspective taking and conflict resolution skills as well as trust and loyalty.

> CASE EXAMPLE **10.3**   PATRICIA.

Patricia is 9 years old and the youngest of six sisters. During the summer before the start of fourth grade, Patricia and her family moved to a small village on Long Island, New York. The population of the village is predominantly White middle class, and most people work locally in the fishing, boating, and coastal industries, while a small percentage commute to jobs in New York City, about 90 minutes away.

Patricia's father works for the United Nations as a diplomat representing Mexico. Upon receiving his assignment to the United Nations Headquarters in New York City, he moved his family from Mexico to New York State. He felt strongly about not having his wife and daughters live in New York City itself and chose to buy a house in the small village on Long Island instead, knowing it would mean commuting a total of three hours each day.

The school system that serves the village where Patricia lives has a large central high school, a large central middle school, and eight small elementary schools. Reflective of the community's demographics, the majority of children zoned to attend the same elementary school as Patricia are White. Many of these children are first- or second-generation descendants of European immigrants. In addition, there is one African-American family and one family from Puerto Rico with several children attending the elementary school.

Several days before the start of school, Patricia's father was transferred once again, this time to Cyprus. Accepting this one-year assignment, Patricia's father made the difficult decision to travel to Cyprus alone and leave his wife and daughters at their new house in the United States.

Given Patricia's situation, what might she expect on the first day of fourth grade? How will the school year unfold for her? How might she be accepted socially? How and with whom will she make friends? What factors might influence whether she is included or excluded? What emotions will she likely experience? What will counselors who are available to her need to consider and need to do?

Pro-Social and Antisocial Behavior

As children become less egocentric and more fluent in social perspective taking, they engage in more pro-social behaviors. Pro-social behaviors are those that are intended to be of benefit to others. Children who are accepted by their peers are likely to engage in helpful behaviors and to assume the best about others. Even if there has been a slight transgression, well-liked, well-adjusted children prefer to assume that there has been an accident or an oversight rather than that another person intended harm. When problems arise, these children do not react with fear or anger. Instead, they attempt to understand the other person's side and to use that understanding to try to solve the problem.

Compared to children who are well accepted, children who are rejected seem to be less likely to engage in pro-social behaviors. They are less likely to acknowledge the thoughts and feelings of others and less likely to engage in helpful behaviors. They are poor listeners and often misinterpret the words and actions of others. Many children who are not well accepted react to others with fear or anxiety and withdraw from social situations. Many others react with anger and may engage in hostile and aggressive behavior.

Aggression may be physical or verbal, and is related to the way some children process social information (Ostrov & Godleski, 2010). There are two types of aggressive children: those whose aggression is proactive, and those whose aggression is reactive.

Children who engage in **proactive aggression** do so deliberately. Their behavior is an attempt to obtain a desired goal through coercion. Obtaining the goal reinforces the belief that aggressive behavior is effective. In contrast, **reactive aggression** may not be so deliberate. Children who react aggressively may be reacting to their own misinterpretations of the intentions of others. Though the action of another person may have been accidental, children who are prone to reactive aggression may see the action as purposeful. This type of social information processing suggests a hostile attribution bias. Assuming that others are out to hurt them, these children view their own responses as retaliation or self-defense.

Bullying

Bullying generally is regarded as a subcategory of aggressive behavior. It is defined as deliberate, repeated attempts to harm, offend, or embarrass another person, usually a peer (Schoen & Schoen, 2010; Solberg, Olweus, & Endresen, 2007). In describing his experiences with childhood cancer in Reflection 9.1, Wes remembered feeling tortured by peers, who deliberately attempted to agitate him by taking the hat he wore to cover his bald head. Bullying behavior may be physical (e.g., hitting, kicking, shoving) or non-physical (relational aggression; e.g., gossip, name-calling, insulting, avoiding), direct or indirect. Boys typically use bullying tactics that are physical, whereas girls are more likely to use verbal assaults and ridicule. In Wes's case, the bullying was both physical and verbal. Whether direct or indirect, this pattern of interaction is based on and reinforces an imbalance of power between the bully and the victim. Both bullies and victims tend to be children who lack social skills and are rejected by their peers. Most often, victims are rejected children who are anxious, withdrawn, and have few friends. They are prone to loneliness, depression, self-esteem issues, and underachievement in school (Dempsey & Storch, 2010). Some victims of aggression are bullies themselves (Solberg et al., 2007), and indeed, Wes recalled the emergence of his own bullying behavior. In contrast to their victims, middle childhood bullies do have friends, but the friendships are not without some problems. Bullies often are admired by their friends for their strength and unapologetic attitudes. They also are feared, however, and over time, their popularity decreases as their peers increasingly judge their behavior more negatively. In reaction to negative judgments of peers and adults, bullies become more hostile and aggressive, qualities that tend to continue into adulthood (Bender, 2011; Kim, Catalano, Haggerty, & Abbott, 2011).

Empathy, which has both cognitive and affective aspects, is a key feature of pro-social and antisocial behavior. Children who engage in pro-social behaviors are able to sense the perspectives and feelings of others. On the other hand, children who are involved in bullying relationships often have some deficits in social skills and in their ability to sense the perspectives of others. Numerous intervention programs have been implemented based on the premise that bullying tendencies may be decreased if the development of empathy could be fostered in children who engage in these behaviors (van Noorden, Haselager, Cillessen, & Bukowski, 2014). A program developed in Canada called Roots of Empathy has shown success in ameliorating aggression and bullying among elementary-aged children. In this program, children periodically are visited in their classrooms by a mother and infant who live in the community. Roots of Empathy instructors coach the students to attend to the infant's development and to label the infant's feelings while reflecting on their own and those of others (Schonert-Reichl, Smith, Zaidman-Zait, & Hertzman, 2012). Studies examining the relationship between empathy training and bullying have had mixed results. Although a number of studies failed to show a relationship between bullying and empathy, in general, aggressive bullying behaviors seem to decrease as empathy increases, particularly when dimensions of affective empathy are fostered (van Noorden et al., 2014).

Social Influences

A variety of factors have been studied to determine the degree to which they influence social development in middle childhood. Peer relationships provide a context through which children refine their interpersonal skills and self-concepts, but a number of other variables influence social development as well. The influence of family begins at birth and continues throughout childhood. Extracurricular and leisure activities such as sports, gaming, and television watching are influential as well.

Sports

A number of studies have examined the relationship between participation in organized sports and children's social development. Most show that participation in sports has a positive effect on areas such as communication, cooperation, connection, self-confidence, empathy, and leadership (Gano-Overway et al., 2009; Zarrett et al., 2009). Participation in team sports has been associated with self-esteem and self-concept. Compared to children who participate in individual sports or no sports at all, team players have higher self-esteem, regardless of gender, ability, attitude, or peer acceptance (Slutsky & Simpkins, 2009). Attitude and peer acceptance do seem to have an effect on which sports children choose to pursue, however. By middle childhood, children have begun to identify many sports and recreational activities as either masculine or feminine, although the number of activities once described as exclusively masculine has decreased in recent years. Sports classified as masculine typically involve face-to-face competition and bodily contact, such as football and wrestling, whereas sports classified as feminine are more likely to involve grace and aesthetics, such as gymnastics and dance. Recent research examining sports participation and gender attitudes suggests that elementary-age boys participating in masculine athletic activities are more sensitive to gender stereotypes and stigmas than are girls participating in feminine athletic activities (Schmalz, Kerstetter, & Anderson, 2008). Additional research suggests that there is a positive association between aggressive or antisocial behavior and power sports. An examination of boys in the later years of middle childhood who participated in power sports such as wrestling, boxing, weightlifting, and martial arts found them to have higher levels of aggression and antisocial behaviors outside the sports arena than their nonparticipatory peers (Endresen & Olweus, 2005).

Screen Time

School-age children in the United States often spend countless hours per week in front of video screens watching television or videos, playing video games, or engaging in other computer-assisted activities. Given the power of observational learning, many questions arise about the impact of screen time on children's social and cognitive development. In particular, questions have been asked about whether screen time displaces other activities such as reading, studying, sports, physical activity, meals, and sleep. In addition, questions are asked about the impact of these media on achievement and social behavior. The answers to these questions suggest that while children may organize their time differently than they did when television, computer technology, and video games were less available, the use of these media is not necessarily bad (Hofferth, 2010; McDevitt & Ormrod, 2012).

Nearly all elementary-age children watch at least some television (Hofferth, 2010; National Survey of Children's Health, 2007). Almost half of all children over the age of 6 in the United States have televisions in their bedrooms (National Survey of Children's Health, 2007; Sisson, Broyles, Newton, Baker, & Chernausek, 2011). On average, children between the ages of 6 and 12 watch about 14 hours of television per week (Hofferth, 2010). Boys in this age group tend to watch a little more television on average than do girls, and children from lower-income families tend to watch more than children from higher-income families (National Survey of Children's Health, 2007; Sisson et al., 2011).

Not surprisingly, the more hours children in middle childhood spend watching television, the less likely they are to get enough sleep or engage in outdoor activities or non-video play (Hofferth, 2010). Furthermore, if they have televisions in their bedrooms, they are less likely to eat meals with their families, and more likely to be overweight (Sisson et al., 2011). Television viewing time also seems to displace some time that children might otherwise be studying, reading for pleasure, or participating in organized sports. Although increased television viewing is associated with decreased reading and studying, it does not appear to be associated with overall academic achievement when other variables such as socioeconomic status and family background are controlled. Similarly, when content is disregarded, the amount of time children spend watching television appears to have a minimal effect on behavioral problems (Hofferth, 2010); however, those problems do seem to increase somewhat when a television is present in the bedroom (Sisson et al., 2011). For the most part, negative associations between television viewing and aggressive or problematic behaviors are associated with the content that children are viewing. Over the last few decades, there have been several thousand studies examining the relationship between media violence and aggressive behavior, and almost all have shown that there is indeed a relationship (American Academy of Pediatrics, 2009a). In addition, what children watch has an effect on their assumptions about the world around them, as biases and stereotypes depicted in the media often constitute children's perceptions of reality.

While television viewing time is associated with decreases in many behaviors, it does not seem to be related to the amount of time children spend playing video games. Almost 57% of boys ages 6 to 12 play video games. In contrast, only about 16.5% of girls seem to be interested in video games, spending an average of about 48 minutes per week playing them. Boys, on the other hand, spend an average of four hours per week playing video games (Hofferth, 2010). Similar to watching television, playing video games is related to decreased sleep, studying, reading for pleasure, non-screen play, and outdoor activities. There appears to be no relationship between time spent video gaming and participation in organized sports. For boys, video game time does not appear to affect academic achievement, but it does seem to be related to behavior problems. For girls who play video games, there is some mixed news. Some girls show gains in scores on tests measuring problem solving, while others show lower scores on tests measuring specific reading skills. Unlike boys, girls' problematic behavior does not seem to be associated with video game time.

Compared to usage in the latter part of the 20th century, computer usage among children in the 6- to 12-year age group has been increasing dramatically during the first part of the 21st century. During non-school hours, computers are used by at least 29% of children in this age group for play, study, and communication, and it is estimated that children in this age group (including those who do not use computers at all) spend an average of 80 minutes per day in front of computer screens for these purposes (Hofferth, 2010). The majority of time outside of school that children spend on the computer is spent on play, and boys spend more time playing on the computer than do girls. Girls, on the other hand, are more likely than boys to use the computer for communication or Internet surfing. Neither boys nor girls in middle childhood spend very much time using the computer for study.

Computer screen time seems to affect elementary children differently than television or video game time. Neither reading nor studying decreases with computer use, and reading for pleasure actually increases in children who use the computer for studying. Children who use computers outside of school tend to spend less time watching television or playing video games, and to gain in academic achievement (Hofferth, 2010).

Social awareness and behavior seem to be affected by the content of video media. Children are influenced by what they see and through video media, including television; they have opportunities to learn basic skills, problem solving, history, and culture. Unfortunately, most programming does not attend to or even consider the influence it might have on the social development of school-age children.

Family

In addition to helping children obtain basic physical necessities (e.g., food, clothing, shelter) families help children in middle childhood to feel safe, secure, and supported. Families play an important role in nurturing peer relationships, academic achievement, and self-esteem.

Once children enter elementary school, they spend much less time with parents than they did when they were younger. While parents continue to play an important role in discipline, children take on more of a co-regulatory role in their own behavior as they become more independent. With advances in cognitive and moral development, parents have more freedom to incorporate reasoning into their disciplinary techniques. Parenting styles begin to have an effect on children's social development very early on. In middle childhood, it appears that the children who are the most happy, self-confident, successful, and liked are those whose parents practiced authoritative parenting styles. Conversely, children from authoritarian homes tend to be unhappy, less confident, anxious, and less successful in social relationships. The most disobedient, unmotivated, and demanding children seem to be those whose parents are permissive or uninvolved (McDevitt & Ormrod, 2012).

Unlike a few generations ago when most children grew up in families with two married parents, fewer than two-thirds of elementary-age children in the United States now live in such families. Today, about a quarter of children in the United States live with single mothers, about 4% live with single fathers, and many live with grandparents, other relatives, or foster parents (Kreider & Elliott, 2009). In general, children from two-parent homes benefit from financial, emotional, social, and community resources that are more available to them. Two-parent households tend to have higher incomes and more time for parent–child interaction. When everything is working well, children from these families perform better in school and have fewer behavioral problems, but these outcomes seem to be more related to resources, stability, emotional well-being, and parenting styles than to the number of parents in the home.

Divorce

When parents divorce, children react in a variety of ways, and their reactions tend to change over time. According to the divorce variability and fluidity model (DVFM) (Demo & Fine, 2010), there is substantial variability in the way children (as well as adults) experience, cope with, and adjust to divorce. Furthermore, adjustment is subject to change over time. While many studies suggest that children who experience divorce have significantly less positive adjustment than those who have not experienced divorce, the differences between these two groups tend to be relatively small (Demo & Fine, 2010; Harvey & Fine, 2010). Compared to children from intact families, children of divorced parents are somewhat more likely to have emotional problems such as anxiety and depression, behavioral problems, health problems, and poor school performance (Amato, 2010; Demo & Fine, 2010; Harvey & Fine, 2010). Many children do well during parental separation and continue to do well after divorce; many children have difficulty at first, but adjust well later; and many others have difficulty in both the short and long term. Strong evidence supporting the notion that divorce is linked to long-term harmful effects exists for only a minority of children of divorced parents (Harvey & Fine, 2010). Coping and adjustment seem to be contingent upon a number of risk as well as protective factors (Demo & Fine, 2010). Risk factors include family conflict before and after divorce, financial hardship, and diminished parenting. Protective factors, on the other hand, include coping skills, self-esteem, social support, and competent parenting. How well children adapt and adjust to divorce seems to be determined by the balance of risk and protective factors.

Many children who were in middle childhood when their parents separated later regard their parents' divorce as a major influence in their lives. Children who are in middle childhood when their parents divorce tend to feel hurt, afraid, powerless, and disillusioned at first (Harvey & Fine, 2010). Many children report losses and missed opportunities. Some children are prevented from participating in extracurricular activities such as sports, music, or summer camp, in part because financial resources decrease with divorce, and also because parents may not be available to transport them to lessons and activities, or because custody arrangements and visitation schedules are prohibitive (Wallerstein & Lewis, 2004).

While divorce may lead to stressful life circumstances, it may also provide relief and new opportunities for personal growth. There is evidence indicating that some children experience gains in self-esteem, maturity, and empathy following the divorce of their parents. These positive outcomes suggest successful acceptance of responsibility (Demo & Fine, 2010; Harvey & Fine, 2010; Hetherington, 2006) and demonstrate the children's resilience.

In the past several decades, there has been considerable attention devoted to research on the effects of divorce of children, with seemingly conflicting conclusions depending on the investigator's point of view and methodology. Overall, several themes seem to be consistent: (1) Divorce is a stressor for children and increases their risk for psychological or adjustment problems; (2) even with the added stress and risk, most children of divorced parents function as well as children from intact families; (3) divorce is associated with pain and unpleasant memories; (4) the nature of post-divorce family and contextual variables plays a role in determining how well children cope and adjust; and (5) most children are resilient in coping with divorce (Harvey & Fine, 2010).

Summary

The context of children's lives changes during middle childhood. Children are more independent, less reliant on parents, and more involved in school and community. Their social development reflects gains they have made physically, cognitively, and emotionally, and is influenced by a variety of factors. Physical and brain changes, cognitive advances, emotional regulation, and social awareness work together to promote the child's developing competencies and self-concept.

Improved cognitive abilities pave the way for emotional development. Children can use their cognitive abilities to calm themselves in uncomfortable situations and to add complexity to their self-concepts. In middle childhood, children become more aware of others and how others feel. Emotional intelligence develops as children process information about their own and others' emotions and use that information to guide their thoughts and actions. Being aware of others also allows children to make comparisons. Children compare their emerging skills to those of their peers and judge themselves to be competent or inferior. These judgments form the basis of self-esteem and contribute to children's self-concepts. Emotional development and cognitive development together influence social development. An important component of social development is moral development, which would not be possible without concurrent gains in cognition. As children mature, they acquire a more complex set of guidelines and principles to help them distinguish between right and wrong. These morals are attained through social interaction and observation and become ensconced through practice. Central to moral development is emotional development, and in particular the ability to be empathic. In middle childhood, as children come to appreciate others, they become able to sense how others feel. Having a sense of how others feel further guides social interaction.

Being able to think about people and relationships is known as social cognition. Through social cognition, children learn about themselves. They gain understanding of how they are viewed by others and thus modify their self-concepts. Social cognition, along with emotional intelligence, social perspective taking, and moral development also makes friendships, healthy peer relationships, and pro-social behavior possible. Being accepted by peers seems to be associated with happiness, higher self-esteem, fewer behavioral problems, and better school performance.

Friendships are a unique form of peer relationship. The ability to make friends develops in stages that parallel cognitive development. Through friendships children gain companionship, support, intimacy, and affection. Not having friends puts children at risk. Those who do not have friends or who are rejected by peers are less likely to engage in pro-social behaviors, and more likely to be hostile or aggressive.

Aggression may be reactive or proactive. Reactive aggression often is seen in children who misinterpret the intentions of others. Children who demonstrate proactive aggression, on the other hand, are deliberate about their behavior. Proactively aggressive behaviors are intended to harm, and the perpetrators may be considered bullies. Bullies, as well as victims, tend to be children who have gaps in their social skills and are rejected by peers. It is often the case that victims turn to bullying behaviors themselves.

In addition to peers and friendships, there are a number of other social influences on development during middle childhood. Participation in sports provides opportunities to enhance communication, cooperation, empathy, and connection. Team sports in particular seem to be associated with higher self-esteem; however, children who participate in certain sports such as wrestling and martial arts also tend to exhibit aggression.

During the elementary years, children spend many hours in front of video screens, watching television, playing games, or interacting with digital technology. The more hours they spend in front of video screens,

however, the less time they have to spend sleeping, engaging in outdoor activities, studying, or interacting with family and friends. Spending many hours in front of video screens is also associated with being overweight.

With or without television, video games, and computers, elementary-aged children spend less time with parents than they did when they were younger. Parents and families have an important role in helping children feel safe, secure, and supported. Although a slightly decreasing trend from decades past has been observed, many elementary children experience the divorce of their parents. One in three children in middle childhood is likely to live with a single parent, foster parents, grandparents, or other relatives. These types of living situations often place stressors on children and decrease the availability of tangible and intangible resources from which they could benefit. Increased stress and decreased resources often contributes to negative outcomes; however, the right balance of protective factors such as appropriate parenting and support mediate these outcomes. Development in middle childhood is impacted by an ever-expanding social context. The interactive influences of school, peers, media, and family all contribute to the developing child's readiness for adolescence.

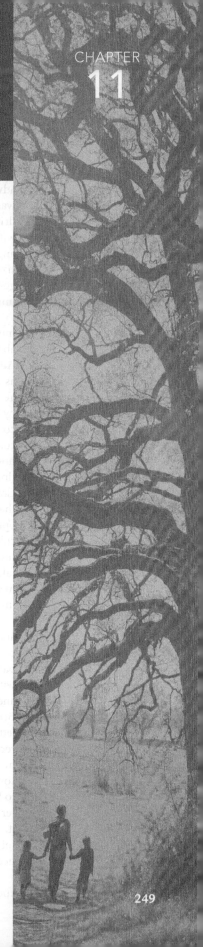

The Adolescent Years: Physical and Cognitive Development

By Ann Vernon

The purpose of this chapter is to revisit adolescence, a unique and important stage of development that connotes the passage from childhood to adulthood, by looking at what occurs with regard to physical and cognitive development. It is important to note that there are some significant dynamics in early adolescence (about ages 11–14 years) that are different from middle adolescence (about ages 15–18). Parents, teachers, and adolescents welcome this change, although, depending on the rate at which they reach formal operational thinking, some older adolescents still appear much like young adolescents.

Adolescent Development

Imagine that you are in a time capsule, zooming through the years. Instead of moving forward, however, you are going backward. When the time capsule comes to a halt, imagine that you are once again an adolescent. Depending on how you experienced this period of your life, you may be elated or devastated. Some may remember adolescence as an adventure: that first date which may have been sealed with a kiss, a driver's license which was synonymous with independence, or trying out more "adult" behaviors such as smoking, drinking, or being sexually active. But some may look back on this period of development with less than fond memories, recalling conflicts with parents when freedom was restricted, angst as a gaze into the mirror reflected a pimple on the nose that at the time seemed the size of an orange, or anxiety about being rejected by peers. Whether the memories were good or bad, the reality is that adolescence is a period of development characterized by immense changes which are accompanied by rather major challenges.

There is a certain amount of fascination with adolescence, characterized by the metamorphosis from childhood to adulthood. Biological, psychological, and social transitions abound, and it is a time of life when young people become more sophisticated and wiser. **Adolescence** is a concept that actually did not even exist until the middle of the 19th century as a result of the industrial revolution (Steinberg, Bornstein, Vandell, & Rook, 2011). Years ago adolescence was often described as a period of "storm and stress," a term used by G. Stanley Hall to describe the moody, rebellious nature of adolescents (Jaffe, 1998). In contrast to this typical view of adolescence as turbulent, Martin (2003) noted that the more contemporary view maintains that this is not a uniquely stressful period, but rather part of a normal, healthy developmental process. In fact, most adolescents mature in a gradual, continuous manner and navigate through adolescence without major disturbance (Crandell, Crandell, & VanderZanden, 2009; Kaplan, 2000; Santrock, 2011, 2012). That is not to say that young adolescents do not struggle during this developmental period, but the current opinion is that this is not an extremely difficult phase of development. And as Crandell and colleagues (2009) noted, "In the United States, adolescence is depicted mainly as a carefree time of physical attentiveness and attraction, vitality, robust fun, love, enthusiasm, and risk taking activities" (p. 351). It is also reassuring to know that most adolescents do not engage in self-destructive behaviors such as delinquency, acting out, drug dependence, school failure, eating disorders, or sexual promiscuity (Berk, 2008).

Readers of this chapter and the next are encouraged to reflect on their own adolescence and ask whether teens' experiences today are similar or dissimilar to others' journeys from past decades through this period of development. This question was answered for me in part several years ago when I was counseling a 17-year-old who was in constant combat with her mother because she wanted more freedom. As she shared her frustration, anger, and confusion, it reminded me so much of what I struggled with when I was that age. Because my mother and I found it difficult to discuss things in a rational manner, we wrote letters to each other, which I think helped us both deal with issues more effectively. I had recently come across a few of these letters as I was sorting through some of my childhood memorabilia and had taken them to my office, thinking that I would incorporate them into something I was writing at the time. So when my client talked about her repeated attempts to help her mother "see the light," I thought it might be appropriate to share one of my letters with her. I didn't mention that I had written it, but just asked her if she could relate to it. As soon as she finished reading the letter she said, "That is exactly how I feel." And then I told her that I had written it many years ago when I wanted my mother to understand that I needed to be more independent in order to prepare myself for leaving home to go to college.

So in some respects, it seems as if adolescents throughout the generations have experienced similar things. On the other hand, there are some new challenges that adolescents in

Think About It   11.1

The following questions may stimulate your thinking as you read this chapter about the changes that occur during the adolescent years:

- What is one of your most significant positive memories associated with early or mid-adolescence?
- What is one of your most significant negative memories associated with early or mid-adolescence?
- If you could go back and change one thing about your relationship with your peers during this time in your life, what would it be?
- If you could go back and change one thing about your relationship with your parents during this time in your life, what would it be?
- Do you agree with the experts who contend that adolescence is not a period of "storm and stress"? What was it like for you?
- What advice would you give adolescents today based on your experiences growing up?
- Do you agree with developmental experts who contend that adolescence is not an exceptionally difficult phase of life? What was it like for you?

a contemporary society are forced to deal with that weren't prevalent years ago, such as the drug culture, social networking via the Internet, the impact of the media exposing them to things they might not be mature enough to handle, and the complexity of lifestyle options. However, too many adolescents do not have sufficient support or opportunities to develop into competent adults.

It is also important to recognize that adolescence takes place within a cultural context, which means that while there are similarities, there are also unique differences. Papalia, Olds, and Feldman (2009) concurred that adolescence is not the same throughout the world, pointing out that adolescents in the United States experience and desire more separation from parents than do adolescents in India or Latin American countries, for example, who maintain closer family ties. Culture also has gender implications. In Africa, Asia, Latin America, and parts of the Middle East, males have more freedom and sexual experiences are judged less severely. Puberty is more restrictive for females, who must remain virgins in order to uphold family status and enhance their marriage eligibility. Furthermore, young girls from Middle Eastern, African, or Asian countries are at risk for serious health problems or death because genital mutilation is practiced in these countries as a way of guaranteeing chastity, which makes them a more valuable commodity when they marry (Crandell et al., 2009). Also, adolescents in developed countries such as the United States or in Europe reach sexual maturity earlier than youth in developing countries. As Papalia and colleagues noted, globalization and modernization have had an effect on adolescents throughout the world. Traditional patterns are changing and long-standing cultural values are being challenged.

SECTION I: Physical Development

As Crandell et al. (2009) noted, the physical changes that adolescents experience are quite dramatic, as well as confusing, exciting, and variable. In *The Diary of a Young Girl* (Frank, 1963), Anne Frank aptly captured the essence of early adolescence as she wrote:

> Yesterday I read an article . . . it might have been addressed to me personally . . . about a girl in the years of puberty who becomes quiet within and begins to think about the wonders that are happening to her body. I experience that, too, and that is why I get the feeling lately

of being embarrassed about Margot, Mummy, and Daddy. … I think what is happening to me is so wonderful, and not only what can be seen on my body, but all that is taking place inside. (p. 115)

Not everyone would take as positive a stance on puberty as Anne Frank did, but like it or not, going through puberty is a certainty. In fact, Steinberg et al. (2011, p. 331) suggested that "without puberty there would be no adolescence." And although one typically thinks of adolescence as being synonymous with puberty, Atwater (1996, p. 5) pointed out that "adolescence also includes psychological and social changes that may begin earlier and last longer than the biological changes of puberty," which result in the ability to reproduce (Papalia et al., 2009; Steinberg et al., 2011).

Think About It   11.2

Reflect on your own experiences with puberty. Do you recall at least one "first," such as getting your first bra, discovering that your penis had grown, or noticing facial or pubic hair? How did you feel? Were you proud? Embarrassed? Confused?

Puberty is a phase, as opposed to a single event, and can last as long as six years in girls and five years in boys—or it can be much shorter, ranging from a year and a half in girls and two years in boys (Crandell et al., 2009; Steinberg et al., 2011). The differences in the rate and nature of puberty can be confusing, agonizing, or exhilarating; some adolescents develop the "ugly duckling" syndrome, feeling self-conscious and embarrassed about their appearance, whereas others feel attractive and self-confident.

Changes Resulting from Puberty

Puberty begins when the pituitary gland is stimulated by the hypothalamus to produce hormones (Broderick & Blewitt, 2014), resulting in the development of testes and ovaries, as well as a rapid acceleration in growth, in terms of both height and weight. These changes are accompanied by the development of primary and secondary sex characteristics, changes in body composition, and increased strength and endurance resulting from changes in the respiratory and circulatory systems (Steinberg et al., 2011). Females generally begin puberty two years earlier than males, and there is a wide age variation for various changes. The onset of puberty may begin as early as age 7 in girls and 9.5 in boys, or it may not start until age 13 in girls and 13.5 in boys (Steinberg et al., 2011). Papalia et al. (2009) suggested that it typically begins at age 8 in girls and age 9 in boys. Regardless of when it begins, the ensuing changes in growth and development are profound.

Research suggests that boys who mature early have more self-confidence and experience more popularity than those who mature later. They are also less moody, and because they are larger and stronger, they tend to excel at sports and are more likely to be leaders. On the other hand, early-maturing boys are more prone to deviant behaviors, including school problems and experimentation with drugs and alcohol (Steinberg et al., 2011).

Quite the opposite is true for early-maturing females, who are more vulnerable emotionally, have a lower self-concept, and experience more depression, anxiety, and eating disorders (Santrock, 2011). Despite these problems, early-maturing females are more popular, particularly with boys. And like their male counterparts, they too are more likely to experiment with drugs, alcohol, and sexual intercourse, have problems in school, and are less likely to graduate. Early-maturing girls also tend to marry earlier.

It is interesting to note that there appears to be some correlation between the onset of puberty and family stress. Broderick and Blewitt (2014) cited several studies conducted in various parts of the world that supported the notion that stress affects hormone production. Thus, boys and girls living in stressful conditions are more likely to enter puberty sooner than those who experience a more stable environment. Sigelman and Rider (2012) noted that, particularly for females, family situations can affect the timing of puberty. Thus, physical and sexual maturation are influenced by the interaction between heredity and environment.

The onset of puberty appears to be occurring at an earlier age on average today than in previous generations. According to developmental research spanning several generations beginning about 100 years ago, this pattern has been described as the **secular trend**. This secular trend involves increases in weight and height, as well as earlier onset of puberty (Dacey, Travers, & Fiore, 2009; Papalia et al., 2009). Possible explanations for this trend include a higher standard of living, resulting in children who are better nourished and cared for, and who consequently mature earlier. This trend would not be as evident in underdeveloped countries.

Hormonal Changes

During puberty, young males and females experience visible physical changes called **secondary sex characteristics** that include signs of maturation not associated with the sex organs: breast development and pubic hair in girls; facial, pubic, and body hair in boys. **Testosterone** in males also increases their muscle size and bone structure and contributes to changes in vocal cords, which results in a deeper voice later in adolescence (Crandell et al., 2009). Boys have greater heart and lung increases than girls, as well as thicker bones and more muscle tissue, resulting in greater physical strength and endurance (Crandell et al., 2009). Girls have a bigger pelvic spread and breast size (Broderick & Blewitt, 2014). Both sexes experience increases in height and weight. Initially, since girls mature earlier than boys, they tend to be taller and heavier than boys the same age, but after the growth spurt, boys are taller and heavier than girls.

Primary sex characteristics also emerge during puberty. These are the organs needed for reproduction: the prostate gland, seminal vesicles, testes, scrotum, and penis for males; ovaries, fallopian tubes, uterus, clitoris, and vagina for females. These organs mature during puberty (Papalia et al., 2009).

The tremendous growth spurts that occur during puberty, which are as significant as those during infancy, are regulated by the central nervous system and the endocrine system. Initially, both males and females will notice changes in height and weight, generally at about age 12 in girls and 14 in boys (Crandell et al., 2009). According to Papalia et al. (2009), this growth spurt usually lasts about 2–4 years, and during this period the rate of growth almost doubles. Broderick and Blewitt (2014) noted that on average during the pubertal growth spurt, boys gain 42 pounds and grow 10 inches, while girls also grow 10 inches and gain 38 pounds. Not all parts of the body grow at the same time. Typically, hands, feet, and limbs grow before the torso, so many adolescents feel awkward and gangly until their body catches up with their extremities. By the end of mid-adolescence, most have reached their final height.

Female Development

As previously noted, the growth spurt begins approximately two years earlier for girls than for boys (Crandell et al., 2009; Santrock, 2011, 2012). Girls gradually develop breasts, beginning at about age 9 or 10, with breast buds which eventually increase in size over the next 3–4 years (Crandell et al., 2009). In addition, pubic and underarm hair appear, as well as oil- and sweat-producing glands that can result in acne. Females also experience an increase in fatty tissue in their hips and buttocks, their pelvis widens, and their vagina, uterus, and ovaries grow. As a result of the hormonal changes during this period, girls begin the process of shedding the lining of the uterus, otherwise known as menstruation (Sigelman & Rider, 2012). There is considerable variation as to the onset of menarche, or the first menstrual period, but the average is between ages 12 and 13 for Western populations, and earlier for African-American and Hispanic girls (Balter & Tamis-LeMonda, 2006). Age of onset is affected by nutrition and birth weight in conjunction with the amount of weight gained during childhood (Sigelman & Rider, 2012). Initially, menstrual periods are irregular, so it isn't until about a year or two after their first period that ovulation takes place. According to Steinberg et al. (2011), it takes several years after the first period for a girl to be fertile and capable of reproduction.

Male Development

Around age 11 to 11.5 years, boys begin the sexual maturation process (Sigelman & Rider, 2012). Initially, the testes and scrotum enlarge, followed by the appearance of pubic hair. Approximately six months later, the penis starts to grow rapidly. Around age 13, boys have their first ejaculation, emitting seminal fluid either during masturbation or in a wet dream. This first ejaculation is called semenarche and signifies sexual maturation. However, they do not produce viable sperm until sometime after this first ejaculation.

Later in the puberty cycle for males, facial and body hair emerge, along with a deepening of the voice, which usually does not occur until mid-adolescence. In addition, the sweat glands increase in development, often resulting in acne and oily skin (Steinberg et al., 2011). Increased amounts of testosterone appear to be linked to acne, which is more common in boys than in girls (Papalia et al., 2009).

Adolescent Health

During this period of rapid development, it is critical to encourage teens to develop healthy behavior patterns related to eating and exercising. Many adolescents live on junk food and foods high in fat and sodium. Obesity is a major concern (Kail & Cavanaugh, 2010), and the number of overweight adolescents has tripled in the past 25–30 years. "U.S. teens are about twice as likely to be overweight as their age-mates in 14 other industrialized countries" (Papalia et al., 2009, p. 363). In fact, Papalia and colleagues reported that 34% of U.S. teens have a body mass index at or above the 85th percentile for sex and age. Overweight adolescents are at risk for diabetes and high blood pressure and are usually less popular and have low self-esteem. Furthermore, because of unhealthy eating habits, overweight adolescents may not get enough calcium, which negatively affects healthy bone development. In addition, spending long hours on the Internet or in front of televisions or video games affects the amount of exercise one gets.

Sleep is also important, particularly because sleep patterns change during adolescence, and most teens do not get adequate sleep (Santrock, 2011), which affects mood as well as school performance. During adolescence, biological clocks change, and teens do better if they can sleep later in the morning because they are more wakeful at night. As a result, high schools would most likely see a decrease in tardiness or absenteeism if they started school later in the morning.

Other health issues emerge for adolescents, including drinking and smoking. Although it appears to be slightly on the decline, adolescent drug use remains high, particularly in the United States (Santrock, 2012). Substance abuse leads to academic problems and is also related to car accidents, one of the leading causes of death among adolescents. Because of adolescents' tendency to think that they are invulnerable, substance abuse programs are not as successful in preventing abuse as one would hope. In fact, adolescents fail to understand the consequences of their behavior, as Case Example 11.1 illustrates.

➤ CASE EXAMPLE **11.1** AMAYA.

Amaya, a 9th grader, was approached by a high school student who asked her if she wanted to buy some drugs. She said she didn't have any money, but later that day her friend repaid her money that she had borrowed, so Amaya found Adam and gave him $7.00 for some drugs. Although Amaya had only smoked pot in the past, her boyfriend was a pretty regular user, so she felt safe being with him while she experimented with something more powerful than marijuana. As Amaya shared with me at her next counseling session, she was scared to death by what happened to her. She remembered hallucinating and thinking that she was dying. She was shaking so hard that her boyfriend was frightened and called his dad, who suggested taking her to the hospital. But Amaya didn't want her parents to know, so she just "hung in" and eventually she felt better. She was convinced that what she had taken was laced with something bad. "I know this sounds stupid," she said, "but I would like to do it again to see if it could be as good as all my friends describe. None of them has had a bad experience like mine, so I want to see what it could be like." How would you handle this issue with Amaya? What resiliencies, resources, and supports does she have in place, or need to have in place?

Numerous similar cases involving illogical thinking and lack of awareness of the consequences of behavior almost result in the death of adolescents. Many clients are lucky, but not all adolescents live to tell their story. Educational success and involvement in sports and other extracurricular activities can reduce the likelihood of drug and alcohol abuse.

Body Image and Eating Disorders

Many readers can readily recall being preoccupied with their bodies, which is very typical during adolescence, especially during puberty. I recently attended a reunion where eight of my high school girlfriends were together for a weekend. One of the topics that came up as we were looking through an old yearbook was how we felt about our bodies as we began to develop. One of my friends who developed very early talked about how self-conscious she felt, while others who matured later also felt the same way. We all reminisced about being "sick" on physical education (gym class) days so that we didn't have to undress and expose our bodies. I was a bit surprised that we all had such clear memories associated with body image and development.

According to Santrock (2011), there is a gender difference associated with body image. Girls have a more negative image than do boys, and in contrast to boys, whose satisfaction with their body image increases through puberty as their muscle mass increases, girls become more dissatisfied because their body fat increases. Some teens resort to eating disorders, hoping that being thin will help them feel better about their bodies (see Case Example 11.2).

➤ CASE EXAMPLE **11.2** CASSIE.

Early in my career as a mental health counselor I worked with several adolescents with severe anorexia nervosa. In fact, one of the times I was "duped" by a client was when I was doing after care for a 14-year-old who had recently been released from an inpatient treatment program. As part of her program, she was required to weigh in each week, and because she didn't want to miss school to see me as well as the doctor for a weigh-in, I agreed to do this for her. I was so pleased that each week she gained about a pound and stayed very close to her target weight. Her food charts indicated that she was eating well-balanced, healthy meals, and emotionally she appeared to be doing well. Of course, I was aware that she could cheat on her food charts, but the fact that she was steadily gaining weight seemed like proof that she was finally on the road to recovery. Imagine my dismay a few weeks later when I discovered the reason for the weight gain—ankle weights, not increased food consumption!

Anorexia Nervosa

Case Example 11.2 shows how desperate clients with anorexia can become. They resort to all sorts of ways to control what they eat and how much they exercise because they become obsessed with being thin. One of my former clients only permitted herself to eat a bowl of rice and drink a glass of water for supper after she had re-washed all the dishes in the dishwasher and had cleaned the house. Others carried heavy backpacks wherever they went in order to burn more calories during the day, and one girl sneaked out of the house each morning before her parents were awake in order to run several miles and be back in bed before they woke her up for school. They had no idea she was doing this until months later when she wasn't in bed when they went to her room. Then the pieces began to fall into place regarding how she was still so thin even though she appeared to be eating fairly well.

Anorexia nervosa is self-starvation and can be life threatening. It is more prevalent in girls than in boys, but is increasing in males (Papalia et al., 2009). According to Santrock (2012), this disorder typically begins in the early to mid-adolescent years, although some clients start becoming obsessed about their weight when at age 8 or 9. Individuals with anorexia are in relentless pursuit of thinness and limit their food intake to almost nothing. They have a very distorted body image, weigh themselves obsessively, and weigh less than 85% of what should be their normal body weight, which is basically a body mass index of less than 18 (Santrock, 2012). They have an intense fear of gaining weight and see themselves as fat even if they are only "skin and bones." Oftentimes individuals with anorexia nervosa are perfectionists and hold themselves to high standards. When they can't live up to these self-imposed standards they need to find something that they can control: their weight. Depression, anxiety, obsessive compulsive disorder, and low self-esteem are common co-morbid conditions with this disorder. Treatment is imperative and difficult, in part because society is obsessed with "thin as beautiful." But cognitive behavior therapy targeting the adolescent as well as the family can be effective.

Bulimia Nervosa

Quite the opposite of self-starvation, bulimia nervosa is a disorder characterized by binge eating (consumption of excessive calories over a short time period, usually minutes to hours), followed by purging of the calories by using laxatives, diuretics, over-exercising, or inducing vomiting. Like clients with anorexia, individuals with bulimia nervosa are obsessed with food, and although most are not substantially overweight, they see themselves as overweight. Bulimia is more difficult to detect because these individuals generally maintain a fairly normal weight range (Erford et al., 2013; Santrock, 2012).

Bulimia nervosa typically begins in late adolescence or early adulthood and is more prevalent among women, although it is a frequently used method of weight control among wrestlers. People with bulimia have low self-esteem and feel ashamed of their behavior, which is often difficult to hide because of the need to purge. As with clients with anorexia, people with bulimia lie about what they eat, avoid eating in public, and in general experience anxiety related to food. The most successful treatment for bulimia nervosa is cognitive behavioral therapy, although many counseling approaches are effective in treating the symptoms of bulimia (Erford et al., 2013).

Think About It 11.3

After reading about the physical changes that take place during early and mid-adolescence, you may have wandered down your own memory lane, recalling what it was like for you as you matured. Did you know what was happening to your body, and if so, how did you get this information? What feelings do you recall experiencing? Did you talk with parents, siblings, or peers about what you were going through or did you keep it to yourself? Do you think teens today are better informed than you were about growth and development during adolescence? If you could share one piece of advice with them about the metamorphosis occurring within their bodies, what would it be? Ponder these questions and then read further to learn more about cognitive development during adolescence.

CASE EXAMPLE **11.3** CARRIE.

I worked with a young adolescent and her father, who was very upset with his daughter for not being more responsible. He shared with me that his daughter had a paper route and she needed to get the newspapers delivered by 5:00 pm each evening. One day last week she didn't get home from basketball practice until 6:00 pm. Her irate father said, "Why didn't you just call home to let us know you had to stay for practice so that your brother could have delivered the newspapers? Don't you know how important it is for people to get their papers on time?" Carrie looked him in the eye and said, "Dad, I honestly didn't think about that. The coach just said that if we didn't stay we wouldn't get to play in the game on Saturday, so I didn't have a choice." Dad looked a bit incredulous as he asked me how a smart kid like Carrie couldn't have figured out something as simple as a phone call home. My mini-lesson on cognitive development ultimately helped Dad understand that abstract reasoning develops gradually in the adolescent world; one day it seems like they are using good mature judgment and the next day they may be total space cadets who seem incapable of simple problem solving. What are some additional ways you can help parents and adolescents understand the cognitive changes being experienced.

Brain Development

During adolescence, the synaptic connections that are used are strengthened. The unused ones are "pruned," which means that they are replaced by other pathways or they disappear (Santrock, 2012). Consequently, adolescents have fewer but more effective neuronal connections than they did when they were children.

There are also structural changes in the brain during adolescence. The corpus callosum, which affects how adolescents process information, thickens, and the amygdala, which is where emotions are stored, matures (Santrock, 2011). Just as there are physical growth spurts stimulated by hormones during puberty, hormonal changes also trigger growth changes, particularly in the prefrontal cortex (Steinberg et al., 2011), which doesn't actually reach full maturity until between 18 and 25 years of age (Santrock, 2011). These changes, in addition to the growth of the subcortical regions, have a tremendous impact on the teenager's cognitive abilities (Dacey et al., 2009). Broderick and Blewitt (2014) reported that new brain research supports the notion that puberty and other maturational processes act in accordance with growth in the brain, resulting in a significant increase in cognitive abilities and in the acquisition and processing of information.

There are actually two distinct growth periods, one in early adolescence around age 12 and 13 years, and the second during mid-adolescence (Dacey et al., 2009). The cognitive changes that occur during this period are not nearly as significant as those that take place in childhood, so adolescence is actually a transitional period that ultimately results in more mature cognitive thought processes. By the end of mid-adolescence (about age 18 years), most adolescents are capable of more abstract thinking and typically can reason and problem solve in a more sophisticated manner than can younger children. They can distinguish the real and concrete from the possible and abstract, and their thinking becomes more multidimensional and relativistic (Owens, 2002). Their thought processes are more flexible; they are less likely to think in either/or terms, which has a positive effect on how they problem solve (Vernon, 2009).

They are also better at planning and thinking ahead. However, because the changes in the brain are gradual and uneven, there is considerable variation in their ability to control impulses, weigh risks, and process social and emotional information. Steinberg et al. (2011) speculated that because the prefrontal cortex matures relatively late, especially within the limbic system, which processes emotions and social information, this may have implications for risk taking and behavioral problems during adolescence. Apparently, the brain changes result in a craving for stimulation and novelty, and it is not until the brain fully matures that adolescents are able to make better decisions and control their impulses.

Like other aspects of human development, thinking is highly individualized. Variation also occurs in the degree to which adolescents use formal operational thinking consistently, especially among younger adolescents. For example, it is not uncommon to find an early adolescent using formal operational thinking to solve math problems but not when dealing with problems with friends.

Piaget's Formal Operational Stage

Piaget (1970) developed the concept of formal operational thought, and indicated that it begins to develop at around age 11. This stage is characterized by an ability to think more abstractly, which allows adolescents to make logical inferences, hypothesize, and be more analytical. In addition, adolescents using formal operations develop the ability to think about things they have never previously experienced, such as what it would have been like to be held hostage during a war (Meece, 2002). The changes in cognition allow adolescents to think about possibilities, which improves their problem-solving abilities. They also are more likely to understand subtle humor, puns, and analogies. In addition, adolescents become better arguers: They often do not accept other's viewpoints without question.

Other characteristics of formal operational thought include the ability to "think about the thought itself" (Santrock, 2011, p. 242), called **meta-cognition**, and detect logical consistency or inconsistency in statements. Adolescents often engage in idealization and then compare themselves and others to these ideal standards. They are more speculative and reflective about themselves, peers, teachers, and parents (Crandell et al., 2009). They also have the ability to think about future changes, such as how their relationships with their parents or their peers will likely be different in 10 years, and are better able to predict the consequences of their actions. However, adolescents are not always consistent in their ability to do this. For example, it is not unusual for an adolescent to fail to see that if he repeatedly forgets to do his homework his grades will suffer.

Adolescents are also developing the ability to think about things in multiple dimensions (Papalia et al., 2009). They may describe themselves or others in more complex ways, such as stating that they are outgoing and also shy. They are better able to look at things from other points of view and consider other alternatives. They also see things are more relative, which is one of the reasons that they challenge others' opinions and don't readily accept the statements of others as absolute truths.

REFLECTION 11.1 THE LATE NIGHTS OF PARENTHOOD

On this topic of arguing, I am reminded of an exchange I had with my son during his junior year of high school. I was teaching summer school and needed to get to bed earlier than usual because I had early morning classes. For him to arrive home after 11:00 pm during the week just didn't allow me enough sleep. I tried to explain this logically to him, but his response was, "How is that my problem? I'm not the one that needs the sleep." Eventually we talked it through and agreed on a compromise. [~AV]

Evaluation of Piaget's Theory

There is little doubt that Piaget's stage theory (1970) has had a major impact on our understanding of cognitive development, but there have been criticisms. Specifically, there is considerable debate about the specific age when adolescents think more abstractly; the current view now is that many American adults never become formal operational thinkers as Piaget defined it. Critics also point to the fact that Piaget did not take individual differences into consideration. For example, some adolescents are very intelligent and can think abstractly sooner than Piaget proposed. Piaget also did not acknowledge that cognitive development is uneven, so adolescents do not necessarily think abstractly or logically in all areas; that is, an adolescent may be able to solve complex algebra problems very logically but fail to see the consequences of not doing homework. Another concern relates to culture; adolescents in rural parts of the world may never reach formal operational thinking. In fact, Dacey et al. (2009) emphasized that formal operational thinking might not be useful in some cultures, and so never develops.

There has also been criticism of Piaget's stage theory with regard to gender, because according to Gilligan (1982), most developmental theories focus on male-centric focal points and overlook female-oriented alternatives. Often, using the male model of development emphasizes independence and separation as ultimate goals, while ignoring the interdependence that often defines female interactions and thinking.

Despite the criticism, Piaget contributed a great deal to our knowledge about young people's thinking. His legacy will live on as current researchers continue to learn more about cognitive development and the changes that occur specifically during adolescence.

Hypothetical-Deductive Reasoning

As the brain matures, adolescents become capable of **hypothetical-deductive reasoning**, which means that they can develop a hypothesis and test it out, reasoning from general ideas to specific implications. This reasoning ability provides them with problem-solving tools that they can apply to an infinite number of situations (Papalia et al., 2009). Essentially, this is the approach that scientists use, and as adolescents develop the capacity for formal operational reasoning, they can form hypotheses and test them through experimental methods (Sigelman & Rider, 2012).

Piaget associated this ability with the formal operational stage of development, but culture and education also play a part. For example, Papalia et al. (2009) shared the example of a reasoning problem that adolescents in Rwanda and New Guinea were unable to do, but teens in Europe, the United States, and Chinese youth who had been educated in British schools were able to solve. Thus, formal operational reasoning is probably learned or facilitated in some cultures but less so in others.

Information Processing

As the frontal lobes in the brain mature, there are changes in how adolescents process information, although these changes vary significantly within the adolescent population depending on the rate of maturity. There are two main categories of cognitive change: structural and functional.

Structural Change

Though adults often refer to adolescents as being scatterbrained and forgetful, the reality is that their learning and memory improve considerably during adolescence (Sigelman & Rider, 2012). As they expand their working memory they become better able to tackle difficult problems. Papalia et al. (2009) identified three types of information that are stored in long-term memory: declarative, procedural, and conceptual. **Declarative knowledge** is factual knowledge that the individual has learned, such as when the Civil War ended. **Procedural knowledge** relates to skills that have been learned, such as how to play a musical instrument. **Conceptual knowledge** refers to knowing why—understanding why something is the way it is.

Functional Change

As their brain develops, so do adolescents' abilities to learn, remember, and reason, which comprise the functional aspects of cognition. They can process information more rapidly and become more skilled in the areas of selective attention and decision making, as well as controlling impulses. Adolescents are also better able to ignore irrelevant information which has a positive impact on their ability to concentrate on specific tasks. Because their attention spans are longer, adolescents can study for longer periods of time and stay focused during longer class periods (Sigelman & Rider, 2012).

Language Development

As formal operational thinking develops, adolescents usually become better at discussing abstract concepts such as love or freedom. Many enjoy engaging in debates about these concepts and are eager to engage in more philosophical discussions. They are more conscious of puns and irony and can "get" the humor in comedy programs. Although there is considerable variation, the average 16–18-year-old knows about 80,000 vocabulary words (Papalia et al., 2009).

Moral Reasoning

During adolescence there are significant "leaps" in moral development. However, because moral reasoning develops in varying degrees along with the ability to think abstractly, it is important to give young adolescents the opportunity to discuss moral issues and make choices that facilitate development of more complex moral decision making. Adolescents are very concerned with morality as they transition from childhood innocence to an awareness of adult morality, which is often disillusioning. Nevertheless, adolescents champion the cause for high moral principles and often try to reform their parents, teachers, and others. Adolescents also look up to parents, teachers, and popular classmates for guidance about what is right or wrong (Meece, 2002). They place a high priority on trust and loyalty in relationships, as well as on keeping promises and commitments (McDevitt & Ormrod, 2012). Motivation for good behavior comes from the approval of friends and relatives (Berk, 2008). Although they are idealistic and lack life experience, they still have a tendency to judge a person as "good or bad," as opposed to someone who makes mistakes and has limitations but is still a good person.

There are minor gender differences in the area of care-related moral reasoning (Papalia et al., 2009), with girls in the United States valuing care-related concerns more than boys. This is not surprising given that girls are more relational than boys, who, on average, think more in terms of justice.

Typically during mid-adolescence, there is some "existential examination" as teens struggle to figure out who they are and what they will do with their lives. They become more concerned with philosophical, political, and religious issues. As their thinking becomes more flexible, adolescents can understand different points of view about issues and form their own opinions. They learn more about their beliefs through philosophical arguments and questioning societal and family values.

REFLECTION 11.2 AGATHA'S FUNERAL
_____

I remember going through the questioning stage as a high school senior. One of my friends received a baby chicken from his girlfriend at Easter time, and sad to say, the little chick didn't live very long. Several of us decided that it was only appropriate to have a funeral for "Agatha," so we put her in a box which we placed in the back of the "hearse," which happened to be my father's station wagon. We started the funeral procession at one end of our small town, slowly moving toward the other end with our headlights on. Believe it or not, we must have had 30 cars following the hearse on our way to the cemetery, which was a farm outside of town where another friend assumed the role of the minister and laid Agatha to rest. News of the funeral spread throughout town and our parents weren't pleased to hear that we had been mocking our religious upbringing and societal rituals. As I look back on this event now, I think it was a pretty "safe" way to explore our beliefs and probably something today's more "sophisticated" teens wouldn't be caught dead doing! [~AV]

Stages of Moral Development

The person most famous for a theory of moral development is Kohlberg, who believed that people evolve through a sequence of six stages of moral development, divided into three levels: preconventional, conventional, and postconventional. At the **preconventional level**, children conceptualize things as good or bad as related to the consequences of their behavior, which could result in punishment or rewards. At the **conventional level**, children see rules and expectations as good. At this level, there is a focus on social relationships as well as compliance with social norms. At the **postconventional level**, which is often not attained on a consistent level, morality would be defined by self-chosen principles that they see as having validity. Moral development is closely related to more sophisticated thinking, which evolves as adolescents transition into the formal operational stage as described by Piaget.

There appears to be considerable variation regarding when adolescents reach the conventional level. In fact, some younger adolescents remain at the preconventional level, where their moral judgments are influenced by rewards and consequences, as opposed to what is right or wrong (Meece, 2002). They will also make moral decisions based on their own best interests as opposed to considering the needs of others. They will obey people in authority, but at the same time, they will also disobey them if they think they can get away with it (McDevitt & Ormrod, 2012). By mid-adolescence, more teens are functioning at the conventional stage of moral development. Although they may know what is right and wrong, we all know that there are adolescents who illegally drink alcohol or use drugs, drive above the speed limit, cheat in school, or engage in unsafe sex even though they know better morally. As they progress through the teen years, they will increasingly be confronted with moral dilemmas. Clearly peers, parents, and cultural norms will affect adolescents' moral decisions. Providing opportunities to discuss moral issues and make choices can enhance the development of more complex moral decision making.

> **Think About It   11.4**
>
> Think back to when you started middle or junior high school. Was this a difficult transition for you? What was more important to you: learning or socializing with your friends? What was the transition to high school like for you? What significant memories, positive or negative, stand out for you as you reflect on your middle school and high school years?

The School Experience

Like it or not, adolescents spend a great deal of time in school. For many, school is where they socialize with peers, while learning is a secondary outcome. The transition from elementary to middle school and then again to high school can be somewhat disruptive with regard to school performance, behavior, or self-image. In particular, the transition from elementary to middle school is more difficult because class sizes are typically larger, there is not as much nurturing as in primary grades, and the environment may be less supportive. There is often more emphasis on discipline, which sometimes puts students and teachers at odds with each other. At this age, adolescents want more independence and teachers want control of an orderly environment. Schulz and Rubel (2011) noted that authoritarian teachers are not well accepted by students. Furthermore, many middle schools and high schools are not as developmentally "sensitive" as they could be. For example, peer relationships are perhaps the most important aspect of a teen's life. Yet within the school day there is very little time for socializing—only a few minutes between classes and very short lunch breaks. Increasing lunch time and time between classes might cut down on some of the talking, note passing, and texting that distract students in classes because they want to communicate with their peers. Using a small group learning format where students work on tasks with peers but are held accountable for high-quality end products as well as efficient group behavior is an effective practice for this age group.

It is also important to build a "sense of community" in the school in order to increase attendance and class participation and decrease cliques, which are especially common in middle school. Schultz and Rubel (2011) stressed the importance of building an inclusive climate, noting that "adolescent alienation is particularly relevant in the school environment" (p. 286). Schultz and Rubel described how alienation negatively affects adolescents' academic performance as well as social interactions. Students who feel alienated are often hostile, passive, disinterested, and uninvolved. At the extreme, alienation can result in violence. There appear to be several factors that contribute to this sense of alienation, including harsh discipline policies, low teacher expectations, irrelevant curriculum, discriminatory practices, and a perceived lack of control in the school environment.

Also, school schedules are often at odds with adolescents' biological clocks. Adolescents stay up later and are tired if they have to go to school early. Starting school later could have a positive impact on both performance and attendance. In addition, educators should take into account the young adolescents' preoccupation with appearance and bodily changes as it affects school performance.

CASE EXAMPLE **11.4** STAGE FRIGHT.

I remember working with three seventh graders from the same middle school. All three had been good students throughout elementary school but suddenly they were skipping school, which had never been a problem. I learned that they were all taking the same language arts class and the teacher required them to stand in front of the room to deliver their speech. Imagine being 13 years old, feeling self-conscious about the pimples on your face or worrying about getting a spontaneous erection. What would you do? The answer for these students was to skip school because then they could give the speech just to the teacher and they wouldn't have to embarrass themselves in front of their peers. Of course, they didn't consider the negative consequences of skipping the whole day, but they achieved their goal, which was to avoid standing in front of the class by themselves. My suggestion to the teacher was to let them give their speeches to a small group initially and gradually move the presentation to the entire group. This appeared to be an acceptable solution and the students did not skip school again. What are some other ways to address such emotional reactions and school truancy, whether due to anxiety, substance abuse, or other conduct issues?

In terms of the school experience, adolescents are more satisfied with school if they think their classes are interesting and meaningful and if learning goals can be co-constructed. There is probably still too much emphasis on rote memorization and routine class experiences in secondary schools, which has a negative impact on students' desire to put effort into learning. Some school systems have established smaller schools within high schools to form a closer learning community, which can have a positive impact on involvement in school (Papalia et al., 2009). Another way of engaging students that is becoming more common is **service learning**, where adolescents volunteer in various community agencies. **Mentoring programs** can also enhance the school experience by giving adolescents access to relationships with successful community members who provide additional career and educational support, advice, and encouragement. Participation in extracurricular activities such as debate, music, drama, or sports provides an opportunity to explore potential career choices and assume leadership roles in clubs and organizations; such opportunities enhance skills in a non-academic arena and usually make school a more appealing experience.

> **Think About It** **11.5**
>
> Think about adolescents you know. Do they want to perform well in school, or don't they care. Or are they somewhere in between? Why do they put effort into some classes and not others?

Academic Achievement

Students achieve better when they are in schools with reasonable structure, a safe environment, an emotionally supportive academic atmosphere, high-quality teachers, high standards, and where students and teachers feel as if they have some say in rules

MOTIVATION, ADOLESCENT STYLE!

When I asked one of my clients the question "Why do you put effort into some classes and not others?" he looked at me like I was stupid. His reply was, "I don't like the math teacher, so why should I work hard for her?" It made sense to him, but not to me! [~AV]

and procedures. They learn best if teachers provide clear feedback about expectations and performance, moderate structure, and high levels of academic support (Steinberg et al., 2011). In contrast, student achievement and motivation decline when teachers are unsupportive and critical.

As they enter middle school, students often experience a decline in both academic motivation and academic achievement (Papalia et al., 2009; Steinberg et al., 2011). In part, this is because elementary schools are generally smaller and teachers are more nurturing. Adolescence can be a very difficult period and students at this age need nurturance and support, which lead to increased academic motivation to learn. It is thought that the desire to achieve is closely tied to parents who set high expectations, encourage their children to learn, reward school success, and become involved in the educational process by attending school functions. These parents show interest in student assignments, monitor homework, and provide assistance as needed (Steinberg et al., 2011). Unfortunately, during middle school and high school, many parents are not as involved in many aspects of schooling, including attending conferences, monitoring homework, or going to school performances.

While parents and teachers obviously have some influence on adolescents' achievement, friends actually influence achievement more, especially with regard to doing homework and putting effort into their classroom performance (Schulz & Rubel, 2011). However, this influence can be negative as well as positive. Adolescents worry about how their friends will react to their success in school and may not want their friends to know how much they study or desire good grades because that may not be the "cool" thing to do. Academic self-efficacy is key: If adolescents believe they are good at something, they are more motivated to learn and put more effort into it, which has a positive effect on their performance. Differences in achievement due to ethnicity, gender, and the intersection of the two are explored next.

Ethnic Differences

There are ethnic differences related to educational achievement, with Asian-American students achieving more than Caucasian students and Caucasian students achieving more than African-American and Hispanic students. Several explanations have been offered to explain this gap. It is possible that Hispanic and African-American students do not see as many positive outcomes of educational achievement because they think they will be discriminated against in the job market regardless of their level of education (Steinberg et al., 2011). It could also be that more of these students are raised in single-parent families where it is less likely for parents to be as involved in their child's school activities. Schools must address the issue of ethnic differences in achievement by providing viable role models as proof that educational achievement is important and pays off.

Gender Differences

Who are smarter, girls or boys? In general, and on average, adolescent girls are better in verbal activities that involve language and writing, whereas boys perform better on visual and spatial tasks (Papalia et al., 2009). On average, adolescent girls are better readers than boys, while boys tend to be better at math. And while there is still a gender gap, with boys performing higher on standardized math and science tests, girls are catching up because in recent years girls have been taking more challenging math and science courses. The differences in the way their brains are structured accounts for these differences. Simply stated, girls have more gray matter and boys have more connective white matter, the latter having a direct link to visual and spatial performance that is needed in math and science. Also, the corpus callosum is larger in girls than in boys, and this affects language processing. Because the corpus callosum connects the two brain hemispheres, girls have a broader range of cognitive abilities, which allows them to integrate left-brain (verbal and analytical) and right-brain tasks (spatial and holistic), whereas boys tend to operate within each hemisphere (Papalia et al., 2009).

It is interesting to note that on the whole, girls like school more and get better grades. On the other hand, boys are expelled and assigned to remedial classes more frequently. There has been controversy over the years about how sexist practices affect both boys and girls in school; because girls are often more compliant than boys, teachers tend to favor girls.

The Dropout Problem

A major concern related to the quality of education and academic achievement is the dropout rate, which traditionally has been higher for African-American and Hispanic-American students, and those from low socioeconomic groups. The dropout rate among Hispanics is far greater than that for African Americans, probably because they are more likely to be less proficient in English (Steinberg et al., 2011). High school dropouts are more likely to come from low-income or single-parent families. Because of their disadvantaged socioeconomic background, these students may not have good role models who value school attendance and achievement. Parents may be too busy to supervise or monitor homework or support them in school. Teachers may not hold these students to high expectations or may not provide the support and encouragement they need to stay in school. Students who drop out are usually underachievers and have a poor record of academic performance, which becomes a self-fulfilling prophecy and reinforces their self-perception as failures.

An important factor to consider regarding the dropout problem is that students who drop out feel disconnected (Schulz & Rubel, 2011). Students who feel alienated and disengaged are more likely to give up before they graduate, with males having a higher rate of noncompletion than females (Greene & Winters, 2005). As a result of dropping out, these students will most likely live in poverty, be unemployed or have low-paying menial jobs, and be involved in criminal behavior. Fortunately, the number of students who drop out of high school has been declining, from 14.1% in 1980 to 8.1% in 2010 (National Center for Education Statistics, 2013), but given the importance of education on future success, it is important to continue to address this problem by making sure that high-quality educational experiences are available for all students.

Adolescent Egocentrism

David Elkind (1984) is credited with developing the concept of the invincibility fable, as well as the personal fable and the imaginary audience. If you subscribe to the **invincibility fable**, you believe that bad things might happen to others who take risks, but not to you.

Think About It **11.6**

As an adolescent, do you remember feeling like you were under a microscope, with everyone seeing all your imperfections? Do you remember thinking that you were invincible—that nothing bad could happen to you, even if you were engaging in some behaviors that had significant negative or dangerous consequences? If so, you were not alone ... most adolescents have an "imaginary audience" and subscribe to the "invincibility fable."

REFLECTION 11.4 RISKY BEHAVIOR

Recently at a reunion with some of my high school girlfriends we were talking about some of the risky things we did as teenagers. One incident that came to mind was walking on the railroad tracks over a lengthy viaduct that ran across the major highway running through our town. I remember being excited about this, but I don't recall being aware of the potential danger—that a train could come around the corner and if we happened to be walking across the track on the viaduct, the only thing we could have done was jump onto the highway and most likely be killed by the impact. Looking back, I can't imagine myself taking chances like this, but back then it seemed pretty exciting. [~AV]

That is why it is sometimes difficult to reason with adolescents, because even if they are aware of the consequences, they nevertheless engage in the risky behavior because those consequences only apply to others, as least in their minds. Often, adolescents think they are unique and immune from negative consequences. Closely tied to this is the personal fable. This occurs when adolescents believe they will be world-famous, heroic, or special in some way at something when they grew up. Adolescents who adhere to the **personal fable** think that they are unlike everyone else—that no one experiences things in the same way as they do. Consequently, they believe that nobody will understand what they are going through if, for example, they get rejected by their girlfriend, even though it happens to many teens. Statements such as "My parents will never understand how I feel" typify this type of thinking.

The **imaginary audience** is related to self-consciousness and the idea that an adolescent is the focus of everyone's attention. As a result of the imaginary audience, adolescents become supersensitive and overly concerned about their appearance or their performance. Girls in particular are self-critical about how they look, and can become obsessive about their physical appearance. This is more prevalent during early adolescence, and lessens during mid-adolescence as teens develop more self-confidence and are less focused on what everyone else thinks about them.

Think About It **11.7**

As you read about cognitive development during adolescence, what did you identify with in relation to your own journey? Do you remember "arguing your case," engaging in philosophical arguments as a way of exploring your values and beliefs? How about your school experience—was it positive or negative? Looking back, what would you change about that experience if it were possible? Evaluate your level of abstract thinking that developed over the course of early and mid-adolescence. Do you recall becoming more flexible in your thinking, better able to hypothesize and identify consequences? Ponder these questions as you read Chapter 12 about emotional and identity development during adolescence.

Summary

This chapter focused on adolescent physical and cognitive development, including during early adolescence (ages 11–14) and mid-adolescence (ages 15–18). The chapter began with a brief discussion about how adolescence is a distinctively different period that is often associated with a certain degree of fascination captured through various forms of media. Adolescence used to be characterized as a period of "storm and stress," but the current view is that most adolescents mature in a gradual, mostly continuous manner and navigate through adolescence without major disturbances. The impact of culture on adolescence was addressed, as well as some new challenges that adolescents in contemporary society are forced to deal with that weren't prevalent years ago.

The first section of the chapter dealt with physical development and the many significant changes that affect the adolescent in various ways. In separate sections, male and female development was addressed, including physical growth, primary and secondary sex characteristics, and differing rates of development. A general discussion of what is associated with puberty was covered, as well as information about adolescent health and eating disorders.

The second section described the cognitive changes that occur during adolescence, including a discussion about brain development and the contributions of Piaget, who developed the concept of formal operational thinking. The chapter included information about the structural and functional changes that occur relative to informational processing and then addressed the stages of moral development. This section included a discussion of how adolescents experience school, describing gender and ethnic differences in achievement and the dropout problem. Finally, David Elkind's concepts of the invincibility fable, the personal fable, and the imaginary audience were presented.

The Adolescent Years: Emotional, Identity, and Social Development

By Ann Vernon

The purpose of this chapter is to explore the emotional, identity, and social development that occurs during adolescence. Early adolescence is generally considered to be a more emotionally volatile time, while mid-adolescence is a more emotionally stable period, where the "yo-yo" nature of early adolescence is replaced by greater stability, less dependence on peers, greater self-reliance, and more flexible and rational thought patterns. In addition to the challenges associated with "mood management," adolescents also are faced with the very major task of developing an independent identity and navigating more complex social relationships. Parents, teachers, and adolescents welcome these changes, although depending on the rate at which they reach formal operational thinking, some older adolescents may still appear much like young adolescents.

SECTION I: Emotional and Identity Development

As people reflect on their own experiences as adolescents, they may recall feeling more emotionally vulnerable, volatile, and confused about mood swings that could vacillate from anger to sadness in the blink of an eye. Of course, not all adolescents experience this emotional upheaval.

Emotional Development

Who would like to re-experience adolescence?! When asked, most counselors in training say that they definitely would not like to be 13 or 14 years old again, but many agree that being an older adolescent wasn't nearly as full of drama as those earlier years. What's the difference? In terms of emotions, there is considerable difference between early and mid-adolescence. Most current research suggests it is actually not the hormonal fluctuation that affects emotions as much as other changes during this period that may be occurring in conjunction with puberty that causes the mood fluctuations and heightened emotionality (Steinberg, Bornstein, Vandell, & Rook, 2011). However, because of the significant brain changes that also affect how emotions are processed, as well as rapid increases in many hormones (especially during early adolescence), there is some connection between mood fluctuations and hormonal changes during puberty.

> **REFLECTION 12.1** RIDING THE EMOTIONAL ROLLER COASTER
>
> In addition to negative emotions, mood swings are not uncommon. I worked with so many young adolescents who characterized their moods as being like a yo-yo: high one minute, low the next. These mood swings are confusing, and it was not at all uncommon for my clients to share that they felt like they were going crazy—that they didn't understand why this was happening to them. They actually sighed with relief when I explained that their mood swings had nothing to do with being crazy; it's just that they were going through a phase of life associated with lots of changes—and that in time they would be off the emotional roller coaster. [~AV]

It is true that negative and painful emotional states are experienced more frequently in early adolescence (Cobb, 2001; Siegler, DeLoache, & Eisenberg, 2003), along with troublesome emotions: anxiety, shame, depression, embarrassment, guilt, shyness, and loneliness (Vernon, 2009). Conflicts with parents and teachers may increase as adolescents search for autonomy, resulting in frustration and anger (Meece, 2002).

Because younger adolescents are becoming more aware of how others think and feel, they are more sensitive to the ups and downs associated with social interactions, often overreacting to who said what about whom. Some people will remember sitting at the lunchroom table and watching some whispering. Some people may even recall thinking that their peers were saying negative things about them. It is not unusual for such events to lower mood and ruin the rest of an adolescent's day. What power is given to others to control our moods!

Thankfully, adolescents gradually wean their way out of this intense emotionality, and in contrast to the upheaval characteristic of early adolescence, more emotional stability comes in mid-adolescence. This is a relief to parents as well as adolescents themselves, who are now better able to deal with emotionally charged issues because they are less likely to be overwhelmed by their emotions. As a general rule, during mid-adolescence, teenagers are not as vulnerable or volatile and are more amenable to receiving help if they need it. However, professional counselors need to be knowledgeable about anxiety, depression, and anger, in particular, as these emotional difficulties are prevalent during adolescence.

Adolescent Anxiety

The imaginary audience can contribute to significant anxiety during adolescence. Teenagers worry about how they look, what others will think about them if they perform poorly, or how peers would react if the teenager committed some type of social *faux pas*. Because there are so many changes associated with adolescence, anxiety is prevalent as teens struggle with decisions about whether or not to give in to their sexual urges, how to handle peer pressure concerning drugs and alcohol, or what to do after high school graduation. In addition, peer relationships and romantic liaisons create stress. Although for the most part they aren't as dependent on their peers for approval and support by mid-adolescence, younger adolescents are more vulnerable and worry about peer acceptance and rejection. Because they don't want to be "different," and think that they are the only human beings experiencing anxiety, adolescents struggle to hide their anxiety and depression.

Adolescent Depression

➤ CASE EXAMPLE **12.1** LIVING DEPRESSION.

> It comes out of the blue, this insidious feeling that envelops me, scares me, and changes me from an outgoing, upbeat teenager to a sullen, withdrawn stranger whose fleeting thoughts of suicide as a way to deal with the hopelessness accompany apathy and confusion. Why me? Why do I have to struggle like this? It's so hard, but I try my best to hide the pain because I'm ashamed . . . and afraid that people will think I'm crazy. Am I? I don't know; I just don't understand what's going on with me. (Vernon, 2006, p. 212)

Imagine being this client's counselor, which I was, and reading this explicit description of how depression was affecting her. I was so grateful that she shared her journal with me because she hadn't been able to articulate her degree of pain this profoundly. This 15-year-old continued to use writing as a way of charting her journey through depression. (If you are interested in reading several poems that she wrote about her experiences, see Vernon, 1998.) For her, it was a long road to recovery. I remember getting a phone call from her in between our sessions, in which she described what she was experiencing. She said, "This week has been pretty good so far. It felt like I was just about at the top of the brick wall, ready to climb down the other side, when all of a sudden I lost my grip and slipped back into my depression." Conversations like this are ones you don't forget.

Prevalence and Symptoms

Unfortunately, adolescent **depression** is all too prevalent; it is the most common psychological disturbance that occurs during this developmental period (Steinberg et al., 2011), and the most overlooked and undertreated. Depression is complex. In its simplest form, it can be described as intense sadness. But it also includes multiple cognitive, emotive, and behavioral symptoms including pessimism, hopelessness, loss of interest in usual activities (which often results in social withdrawal), lack of motivation and drop in grades, loss of concentration, difficulty making decisions, apathy, changes in eating and sleeping patterns, lethargy or listlessness, diminished self-esteem, and feelings of worthlessness (Koplewicz, 2002; Paterson, 2011). In addition, depressed adolescents may be irritable, angry, or act out, which often results in some sort of punishment. These additional affective expressions just compound the problem, as these symptoms often overshadow the signs of depression; that is, it is easier to identify anger than depression. Depression may begin with a situation that seems too difficult to control, or an important interpersonal loss, such as breaking up with a significant other or being rejected by peers. Adolescents who are prone to depression assume self-blame, and are less resilient. Counseling is an effective intervention for depression in adolescents (Erford, Erford, et al., 2011). Although there is some controversy regarding prescribing antidepressant medication for adolescents, medication may be necessary as an adjunctive treatment.

Factors Contributing to Depression

While there is a sharp increase in the prevalence of depression corresponding with puberty, depression can be difficult to diagnose because many of the symptoms (e.g., changes in eating and sleeping patterns, irritability, apathy) are also typically experienced during adolescence.

Other changes contribute to depression. For example, because they are better able to think hypothetically, adolescents may have a more pessimistic outlook on life. Changing schools, relationship issues with peers, increased preoccupation with body image, and uncertainty about the future can also cause stress and depression. Compounding matters, even though they are experiencing cognitive changes that ultimately result in more flexible and abstract thinking, adolescents are still quite concrete in their development. As such, they may over-generalize, blow things out of proportion, engage in dichotomous thinking, and have a tendency to personalize. Sometimes, adolescents can be like sponges, soaking up negative comments and putting themselves down.

There is also an environmental influence on depression (Steinberg et al., 2011). Depression is more common in families where there is high conflict, and in families whose birth parents have divorced. Depression is also more common among socially unpopular students and gay and lesbian youth (McFarland & Tollerud, 2009).

Who Is Most Vulnerable?

Who is more vulnerable to depression: boys or girls? Although prior to puberty the rate of depression is about equal for the two sexes, that changes by about age 12 years and on into adulthood, with about twice as many girls as boys experiencing significant depressive symptoms (Friedberg & McClure, 2002; Paterson, 2011; Shaffer & Waslick, 2002). Why do you think this is so? For one thing, girls are more social and therefore more vulnerable when peer relationships are strained. In addition, girls have lower self-esteem than boys, which puts them at higher risk for depression. They also engage in more self-blame, which increases their vulnerability to depression. Biological factors also play a role. Remember that prior to puberty, the rate of depression among boys and girls is about the same, but the female sex hormones that kick in at puberty may have a special effect on the mood regulators in the brain (Paterson, 2011).

Other factors that may predispose girls to depression more than males can be attributed to the observation that boys are generally more independent, which increases their sense of competence. Another sad reality is that girls are more often the victims of sexual abuse, which affects their sense of self-worth and contributes to depression. Furthermore, girls are more self-conscious about their physical appearance, which results in anxiety and can make them more susceptible to depression (Paterson, 2011; Steinberg et al., 2011). Girls who reach puberty early are more susceptible to depression if they feel pressured to engage in activities they may not be developmentally ready to handle. Finally, girls are less likely to express their feelings, reacting to stress by turning their feelings inward. Adolescent girls tend to ruminate about their problems and feel helpless, which results in depression.

Suicide

REFLECTION 12.2 HANDLING TEEN SUICIDAL IDEATION

If you asked a group of practicing counselors what keeps them awake at night, I would venture to guess that many would say that they worry about whether their client will follow through with their suicidal ideation. Indeed, I went through this worry with a significant number of adolescents when I worked in private practice. Suicide is on the radar for many depressed adolescents. Part of this can be attributed to lack of formal operational thinking in many adolescents, which in turn predisposes them to over-generalizing (things will never get better), awfulizing (everything is terrible), blowing things out of proportion (this is the worst thing that could ever happen to me). Couple this with a sense of time that is still quite immediate. As one of my clients said, "I just took an overdose because I wanted my pain to stop now. I didn't think about tomorrow." Unfortunately, some don't live to tell that tale. [~AV]

> CASE EXAMPLE **12.2** LOSS.

The following case study is a good illustration of how an adolescent's thinking contributed to his contemplation of suicide. Jess was a senior in high school when he found out that his parents were moving to a community that was about 50 miles away from where they were currently living. To Jess, it was like they were moving to the end of the Earth. He told me how depressed he was about this, thinking that he wouldn't make any friends (over-generalizing), that he would hate the school ("awfulizing"). Most important, he would have to break up with his girlfriend and he would never find anyone to love as much as he loved her.

After talking about all of these issues for some time, I asked him how depressed he was on a 1–10 scale, and he said he was a 9. He said that everything in his life seemed horrible and he couldn't imagine that anything could be worse. He was angry with his parents for ruining his life. He said he could never forgive them and that he might as well be dead. I empathized with how difficult this transition might be, but I said, "Jess, let's think about this. Suicide is a permanent thing . . . are you sure that *everything* is so terrible that you just can't go on living?"

He thought about it and admitted that it was mainly having to break up with his girlfriend. I pointed out that he might not even have to break up with her since 50 miles wasn't too far away and he could maybe still see her sometimes since he did have a car. He immediately said that his parents would never allow that, but admitted upon questioning that he hadn't asked them about it.

Then I asked him if he had had a girlfriend in 9th grade, and he said yes. "Is it the same one that you have now?" "No," he replied. I proceeded to ask if he had had a girlfriend in his sophomore and junior years, and it turned out that he had had three! "So Jess, even though you really love Megan now, you have had four girlfriends, not counting her, in three years, who at the time you thought were the loves of your life, right? Based on your track record, you might even have another girlfriend before the year is over . . . but if you kill yourself, you'll never know. Maybe it's something to think about?"

After a few sessions, Jess was able to look at the situation more realistically and decided that even though this would be difficult, he could get through it. It would be nice if all cases were as easy as this one, but the reality is that they are usually very complicated, coupled with intense depression and distorted cognitions. Medication is often needed in addition to counseling.

Suicide is a serious problem in the United States. It is the third leading cause of death for 10–19-year-olds, with the greatest risk being during early adolescence (Santrock, 2011). According to Steinberg et al. (2011), close to 20% of adolescents have suicidal ideation—they think about killing themselves, and the majority of them have a plan. Females are more likely to attempt suicide than males, and in any given year more than 10% of female high school students and more than 6% of males attempt suicide. Males are more likely to complete their attempts, but in reality, many more adolescents contemplate or attempt it than actually complete the act (Santrock, 2011). Females typically use more passive methods such as pills, while males are more likely to use more lethal methods such as guns or hanging (McWhirter, McWhirter, McWhirter, & McWhirter, 2007).

Depression and alcohol use are closely linked with suicide, as well as impulsivity, risk taking, low self-esteem (sense of worthlessness), irrational thinking, and loneliness, which is often associated with peer rejection (McWhirter et al., 2007). Adolescents contemplating suicide may make statements such as "I have nothing to live for," or "I wish I were dead," or communicate suicide ideation through journals, artwork, or poems. They may seem preoccupied with death, show a loss of interest in usual activities, or give away valued possessions. It is important to take into account any family history of suicide, as well as any current family problems or other stressors. Above all, suicide ideation needs to be taken seriously, and a multifaceted approach to assessment and treatment is necessary.

SECTION II: Identity Development

"Who am I?" and "What will I become?" are central to the gradual process of identity development that begins at birth and solidifies during adolescence or early adulthood as adolescents integrate childhood identities, their own desires, and cultural and societal expectations (Meece, 2002). As they develop a stronger sense of self and begin to appreciate their uniqueness, adolescents are less dependent on others' opinions and are generally better able to maintain personal boundaries.

Holcomb-McCoy (2005) characterized the task of self-definition as the time when adolescents begin to think about their own identity and where they fit in the world, stressing that they need to achieve a coherent identity. In some ways, it is like putting together a puzzle, trying out various roles and responsibilities to see which ones fit. Papalia, Olds, and Feldman (2009) noted that a large part of identity development is tied to social interaction; as they relate to their peers, adolescents either identify with certain characteristics of others or reject them, eventually figuring out how to come to terms with themselves.

During the identity development process, adolescents will speculate about the future and engage in a good deal of self-questioning and experimenting. Cultural values, as well as family, peers, the school and community, and one's personality all influence identity development.

Erikson's Theory of Development

Erik Erikson is credited with significant contributions in the area of identity development. According to his theory, a critical task of adolescence is to address the issue of identity versus identity (role) confusion, the goal being to achieve a coherent sense of self and a valued role in society (Papalia et al., 2009). Naturally, some degree of role confusion is normal and is characterized by varying levels of self-consciousness, intolerance of differences, and more chaotic behavior, which Erikson believed served as a defense against identity confusion.

Erikson maintained that identity develops as adolescents choose an occupation, adopt values that guide their lives, and develop a sexual identity. Adolescence provides a type of "time out" period, which he called the psychosocial moratorium, in which to develop a stable view of self. In many ways, developing a stable view of self may be more difficult for young people today, who have access to more adult information through media, information that they may not be prepared to assimilate. Couple this with the pressures that American culture has placed on adolescents to grow up fast and to excel in many arenas. David Elkind, who wrote *The Hurried Child* (1988), argued that identity formation cannot be delayed until late adolescence because of the pressures to act like adults.

Because Erikson's theory is based on a male identity model that emphasizes individuality and autonomy, it has been criticized. Specifically, Erikson maintained that women achieve their identity through the intimacy that comes with marriage and parenting, whereas men develop identity before this intimacy. Regardless, his theory has prompted research in the area of identity development.

Marcia's Identity Theory

Another person who has contributed to the research in identity development is James Marcia, who identified four types of identity status: identity achievement, foreclosure, moratorium, and identity diffusion (Papalia et al., 2009). Starting at the lower end of the continuum is **identity diffusion**, where adolescents are unsure of themselves and have not actively explored many options relative to what they want to do with their lives. These adolescents have difficulty making firm commitments about their beliefs, relationships, or occupational choices. They may struggle to make friends, complete schoolwork, and make decisions about their future. These adolescents in identity diffusion tend to be dependent, isolated, and experience anxiety as well as apathy. During the **moratorium period**, adolescents struggle with decisions, but it is a crisis period. They may appear to be self-confident on the one hand, but anxious on the other. During this period, adolescents are actively exploring relationships and career options, and they experiment with different identities. They may have a vague idea of what they want but cannot make a commitment and achieve identity. In **foreclosure**, adolescents may have committed themselves to certain choices, but they haven't explored all alternatives. Instead, they may adopt their parents' values and choose something that others want for them as opposed to exploring options and making a personal commitment. In this stage, adolescents can be very dependent and are easily influenced by others. **Identity achievement** is the desired goal; it occurs when adolescents have explored options and thought about what they want in life. They may adopt some of their parents' values and reject others. Self-control, high self-esteem, and self-directedness characterize this phase. A logical conclusion would be that adolescents in the identity achievement category are more mature. It is important to note that these are not stages per se; they change in one direction or the other as the adolescent continues to explore and develop.

> ### Think About It   12.1
>
> Think back to your own identity development. How did you decide "who" you were going to be? Do you recall going through the process identified by Marcia? At what age do you think you reached the identity achievement stage?

Gender Considerations

Identity development cannot be discussed without considering gender. As noted previously, Erikson's research has been criticized for being a male-oriented model that emphasizes the development of a separate identity. In contrast, Carol Gilligan (1993) maintained that female identity is achieved through establishing relationships as opposed to developing a separate identity. Researchers have questioned Gilligan's approach and seem to veer in the direction of suggesting that individual differences may be more significant than gender differences. In fact, Marcia's research on identity revealed very few gender differences with regard to identity development (Kroger, 2003).

Gurian and Stevens (2005), however, contended that there are brain and hormonal differences that influence how males and females operate. During puberty, young males have more dopamine in their brain, which increases their impulsivity and aggressiveness. Consequently, they have more difficulty attending to school tasks and experience more behavioral problems than girls. Gurian and Stevens cautioned that adolescent males need strong role models or mentors to facilitate healthy identity development.

Gender does play a role with respect to self-esteem. As girls transition from childhood to adolescence, their self-confidence and sense of mastery decline and they experience a rather dramatic decline in self-esteem, according to Vernon and Clemente (2005). The fact that they enter puberty earlier than boys, when they do not have adequate coping skills to help them deal with their physical changes may account for the decline in self-esteem.

It is interesting to note that in general, girls achieve better in school than boys and do not have as many behavioral problems, yet they still experience this decrease in self-esteem. Although the gender gap is not nearly as prominent as it once was, inequities still exist. Adolescents need strong female role models and opportunities to make their own decisions. Parents tend to allow their teenage sons to be more independent and autonomous than their daughters, which has a negative impact on the daughters' self-confidence.

If mental health practitioners were surveyed to determine whether they see more adolescent girls than boys in their practices, it should come as no surprise that young females seem to have more problems than males with regard to identity and self-esteem.

As Crandell, Crandell, and VanderZanden (2009) noted, young adolescent girls model their appearance and behavior after famous celebrities, often sex symbols who have multiple legal, ethical, and substance abuse issues.

Ethnic Considerations

Obviously, race and ethnicity are intertwined with identity development, and the process of forming an identity may be more complicated for adolescents from ethnicities other than White, who may experience conflict between their own culture and the values of the larger society. Meece (2002) pointed out that some ethnic minority adolescents may develop negative attitudes toward their own culture as a result of their desire to fit in, even to the point of rejecting their own cultural values.

Phinney (1990) identified the following ethnic identity statuses: diffuse, foreclosed, moratorium, and achieved, similar to Marcia's model. In the **diffuse** status, the adolescent has not explored his or her ethnic identity. In the **foreclosed** status, the adolescent has clear feelings about his or her ethnicity even if there has been very little exploration of ethnicity. During **moratorium**, there has been some exploration but the adolescent is confused about what it means to him or her personally. In the **achieved** status, the adolescent has explored his or her identity and accepts his or her ethnicity.

Papalia et al. (2009) noted that "perceived discrimination during the transition to adolescence can interfere with positive identity formation and lead to conduct problems or depression" (p. 395). They pointed out that parents should teach their children about their ethnic heritage and expose them to cultural values and traditions in order to increase their sense of pride. This practice, cultural socialization, promotes more positive ethnic identity.

The Transition to Adulthood

Adolescence is a developmental transition, typically beginning around age 11 and lasting until 19 or 20 years of age. It isn't altogether clear when adolescents transition to adulthood. In general, adulthood is associated with being financially independent, securing full-time employment, or assuming adult roles such as marriage or parenthood (Crandell et al., 2009). Several factors can impede this process. One is that adolescents who attend college postpone their full "adult" status until they have graduated. Another factor is that, for economic reasons, young people may live at home longer and be financially dependent on their parents because they are unable to get a well-paying full-time job. Furthermore, many young people postpone marriage and parenthood, so they don't assume adult roles as early as in previous generations.

It appears that the transition to adulthood has become more complicated, especially in Western cultures, because adolescents receive conflicting messages about growing up. On the one hand, adolescents are told to grow up, but on the other hand, they are still dependent. Those living in materialistic cultures may appear to have everything they need, but they still are confused about who they are and what they want in life. Crandell et al. (2009) noted that the United States and other Western countries actually promote an extended adolescence that can become problematic because adolescents develop their own youth culture that may interfere with their transition to adulthood.

Western cultures also do not have as many obvious rites of passage to adulthood that many non-Western cultures have. Getting a driver's license, voting, graduating from high school and college are examples of rites of passage, but they are not as significant or ceremonial as in many other cultures. For example, in many cultures there are ceremonies that include music, food, extensive time with elders, physical and spiritual cleansing, prayers and blessings, and other rituals to mark the transition from adolescence to adulthood. In Latin American countries, 15-year-old girls celebrate their transition from girlhood to

As you read about emotional and identity development during adolescence, what did you identify with in relation to your own journey? Did your moods fluctuate, or did you maintain your emotional equilibrium during this period? How would you characterize your self-esteem and your search for an independent identity? Did you "try on" various roles and responsibilities as you attempted to define yourself? At what age do you think you transitioned from adolescence to adulthood? Ponder these questions and then read on to learn more about social development during adolescence.

womanhood with the *quinceañera*, which involves a mass and a celebration consisting of elaborate rituals and a meal for relatives and guests (Crandell et al., 2009). Suffice it to say that in Western cultures, the line between adolescence and adulthood is not very well defined.

SECTION III: Social Development

In this section family and peer relationships will be explored, as well as the influence of sexuality, religious affiliation, social identity, and school on social development.

The Family

As children transition into adolescence, time spent with parents generally decreases as time with peers increases. And although the parent–child relationship changes, parents still play a major role in adolescent development. Because there may be increased conflict, it can seem as if adolescents don't need their parents, but in fact parents need to set limits, provide structure, and be emotionally available and supportive during this period of development.

Although teens, particularly in Western cultures, strive to be more autonomous and independent, parents still must monitor and supervise. Crandell et al. (2009) noted that among African-American adolescents, higher parental monitoring resulted in less substance abuse, delinquency, and aggression. These authors also pointed out that as a rule, boys receive less monitoring by parents and consequently are more likely to engage in criminal or delinquent activity, as well as drug and alcohol abuse. Their conclusion was that parents need to encourage adolescents to make their own decisions, while at the same time offering support and encouragement. I often used the analogy with parents that even though their adolescent might appear to be rejecting boundaries and advice, parents actually provided a

Think back to your own adolescent years and reflect on your relationships with your peers, parents, and siblings. What stands out most for you? As mentioned earlier in the chapter, my mother and I handled our conflicts, which actually weren't very major, by writing letters to each other. How I wish I had more of them today—it would be interesting to see what the issues really were. I do remember thinking that my parents were stricter than some of my friends' parents, and at least at the time I believed there was some validity for that when I had my first boy–girl party at age 16. Imagine my embarrassment when my mother came to the top of the steps leading to our family room and flicked the lights at 10:00 pm. I was upstairs in a flash demanding to know what she was doing. "It's time for everyone to go home," she announced in a loud voice. I still remember walking back down those steps and telling my friends that they had to go home. I felt like I was 6, not 16. [~AV]

type of "safety net" for their adolescent, being there to redirect them or help them pick up the pieces when things didn't go well.

As they move through adolescence, adolescents become less dependent on parents. The relationship is more balanced, which allows the adolescent to develop his or her individuality and begin to assume more adult roles. Most parents, and adolescents as well, would probably agree that as teens engage in the process of individuation, there may be some conflict over curfews, chores, appearance, choice of friends, performance in school, or behaviors such as drinking, smoking, or being sexually active. In reality, Broderick and Blewitt (2014) reported that these conflicts are quite minor and that many teens and parents don't experience much conflict at all. They also noted that conflict is more frequent during early adolescence but decreases by mid-adolescence, and that it was more prevalent when parents imposed rules related to personal issues such as what music to listen to, how to dress, whom to associate with, and so forth. Regardless, even these minor conflicts can create stress in the family. Parenting style has a big impact on how these conflicts play out.

Parenting Styles

Recall the four different parenting styles from previous chapters: authoritarian, authoritative, permissive, and ignoring. Each yields different results when applied to adolescents. **Authoritarian** parents are demanding and rigid, using harsh punishment and anger to try to change behavior. They do not let their adolescents argue or question them, they assume they (the parents) are always right, and they frequently behave in a very dictatorial manner. With this type of parenting, the relationship is usually tense, and there is little warmth or evidence of mutual caring. Adolescents raised with this type of parenting are often fearful or rebellious and may succumb to peer pressure. They have poor self-esteem and often do not do well in school.

In contrast, **authoritative** parents maintain a reasonable amount of control, clear expectations, and reasonable rules and consequences that are often developed collaboratively. They are supportive of their adolescent, displaying warmth and caring. They encourage their adolescent to be independent and invite discussion about concerns or areas of disagreement. Without a doubt, adolescents raised with this type of parenting fare best. These adolescents are confident, competent, responsible, and self-reliant. They have good self-esteem and are less likely to be rebellious or engage in self-destructive behaviors.

Permissive parents think they can't stand conflict, so they give in because it is easier. These parents generally have very few rules, and they might be uninvolved in their adolescents' lives. They may display warmth, but they are very low in control. Adolescents with permissive parents are often anxious because rules aren't clear or consistent and they don't know what to expect. Interestingly, many parents believe that adolescents want permissive parents, but younger adolescents in particular need structure, though they might not admit it.

Adolescents of **ignoring** parents are generally left to their own devices and receive very little parental guidance because the parents put their own needs first. Adolescents with ignoring parents may go to extremes to get their parents to pay attention to them—acting out, abusing drugs and alcohol, failing at school, or becoming sexually active. Unfortunately, these behaviors create other problems with negative consequences. Adolescents raised by ignoring parents lack social competence and have low self-esteem.

▶ CASE EXAMPLE **12.3** ALLISON.

I remember working with a family whose 15-year-old daughter was running all over them. Although Mom tried to impose rules, Allison knew she just had to go to her dad when she wanted anything and he would give in because it was easier than having her throw a fit. This pattern had been going on for quite some time, with Allison getting more and more out of control by the week. When they finally decided that things had gone too far, they made an appointment with me. As you might guess, Allison was not willing to come and she made that very evident in the first session, claiming that her parents had the problem and she didn't need help. I agreed with her that her parents might need help and asked if we could include them in the next session. She reluctantly agreed, and during that meeting, she accused her parents of being overprotective and worrying too much, basically taking no responsibility for any misbehavior. Although Mom protested, insisting that Allison's behavior was concerning because she was staying out late and she was quite sure she had been drinking each time she came home. Allison denied it, and Dad capitulated, making Allison "promise" to do better.

Allison reluctantly agreed to a next meeting, but prior to the appointment, Dad called, saying that they had a "little problem," which was that his daughter had stayed out all night. "That's probably more than a little problem, since you are responsible for your minor daughter's whereabouts," I said. He said that he and his wife were now on the same page and that they wanted to work on some reasonable rules and consequences in the next session. During that meeting I thought we might be making some progress, but in the final analysis, Allison promised things she couldn't deliver. Just a few days later Dad called again . . . this time saying that not only had she stayed out all night, but she came home at 6:00 am and was still very drunk. He said they needed an appointment as soon as possible and that they wanted her admitted to an inpatient treatment program at the end of the visit.

At this session, both parents were in agreement that Allison had crossed the line. Despite her protests, they left my office and drove to the treatment center. What might have been a happier ending, however, didn't turn out that way. As soon as they got there to check her in, Mom decided that if they followed through Allison might never speak to them again. When she called me to talk about this, I reminded her that Allison really wasn't speaking to them now and that she needed treatment before something more serious happened. The parents didn't heed my advice because it was too uncomfortable for them to follow through. Several months later Allison turned 16 years old, was driving while intoxicated, and had a very serious car accident, injuring herself and a friend. That was the wake-up call for the parents, who then put her in treatment. As this case illustrates, permissive parents need to put aside their own discomfort and consider the consequences of doing it the "easy way."

Broderick and Blewitt (2014) described another dimension related to responsive and demanding parenting. Responsive parents encourage their adolescents to be self-accepting, assertive, and confident. They are warm and involved and impose reasonable limits. On the other hand, demanding parents make and enforce rules, monitor their adolescent's behavior, and are confrontive.

According to Karpowitz (2000), the preferred parenting style includes realistic limit-setting, clear explanations, consistency, warmth and communication, and consequences instead of physical punishment. In return, adolescents will have higher self-esteem, better school performance, more positive social skills, and greater personal happiness. It is interesting to note that across cultures, there seems to be support for a more democratic family structure characterized by the authoritative parenting style (Broderick & Blewitt, 2014). However, in order for this parenting style to work, adolescents must be willing to share information about who they are with and what they are doing, which they are more likely to do if they see their parents as understanding, accepting, and reasonable.

Family Structure

As noted previously, the family remains an important source of influence on the adolescent, and even though adolescents may spend more time with peers, they still look to their parents for security. Some of the variables to consider include the quality of the parents' marital relationship, sibling relationships, and family reorganization due to divorce or remarriage. Crandell et al. (2009) maintained that adolescents who are more socially competent are raised in families where the marriage is strong, and that if the family atmosphere is positive, adolescents tend to have no serious problems. In contrast, if sibling relationships are distant or hostile and parents are inconsistent, coercive, or absent, there is greater likelihood that teens may become more antisocial or engage in more deviant behaviors. Adolescents from divorced or remarried families tend to be resilient, but may engage in more antisocial behaviors than adolescents from intact families.

As adolescents become more autonomous and spend more time with their peers, the sibling relationship also changes; they are not as close, nor are they likely to be influenced by them. There is some indication that the sibling relationship mirrors the parent–child relationship in that if there is parent–child conflict, sibling conflict is more common (Papalia et al., 2009). Not surprisingly, sisters are more intimate with each other than are brothers or mixed pairs, and although there may be more conflict during early adolescence, this decreases in mid-adolescence as a general rule. But parents are not the only source of influence on adolescents. Peer relationships and how they influence adolescent development are examined next.

Seltzer's Adolescent Social Identity

It is no secret that peers are very influential in the development of an adolescent's identity. Seltzer (1982) developed a model explaining how the changes that occur during puberty result in anxiety and instability. He labeled this **frameworklessness** because the adolescent flounders, caught between the familiarity of childhood and the unfamiliarity of adolescence. Just as toddlers gradually have to give up the security of their parents, adolescents also have to do this, becoming less dependent on parents and more autonomous. Broderick and Blewitt (2014) stressed that giving up this familiarity can result in a loss of security, which increases adolescent anxiety. As they seek independence from parents, adolescents gravitate to their peers and transfer emotional dependency, especially during early adolescence.

According to Seltzer's theory, peers are extremely important during this period because they all share this sense of frameworklessness. Since they are all about the same age, experiencing similar feelings, they naturally tend to associate with others who share these commonalities. They begin to compare themselves to others and also engage in a process called **attribute substitution** (Broderick & Blewitt, 2014), which means that they imitate behaviors and other characteristics they see in others. This reduces their anxiety because they now have a "model" of how to be. For example, shy adolescents might begin to imitate others who are more outgoing or they may develop an interest in photography, for example, because a classmate has expressed interest in it. All of this experimentation is an important part of adolescents coming to terms with who they are.

Peer Relationships

As you may recall from your own adolescence, peers can be a tremendous source of intimacy and support, as well as empathy and understanding. At the same time, peer relationships can also be quite stressful, particularly during early adolescence when teens are more vulnerable and sensitive, worried that they will be rejected or humiliated. Broderick and Blewitt (2010) reported that adolescents who have close, stable friendships are more sociable, have higher self-esteem, and do better in school.

Cobb (2001) described the importance of peers by stating that "in larger numbers, they are socialization agents, guiding adolescents into new, more adult roles. And one on one, they are mirrors into whom adolescents look to glimpse the future within" (p. 591). The peer group becomes a place for experimenting with new beliefs and behaviors, and without a doubt peers are a major influence on identity development.

Particularly during early adolescence, there is more conformity to peer norms because young adolescents have such a strong need to be accepted and to belong. They generally have a close relationship with one or two good friends, but they also become part of a **clique** (perhaps 6–10 peers), adopt the mannerisms of this group, and socialize with its members. In addition, they are part of a crowd, which is not necessarily characterized by friendship as much as by similar behaviors, interests, and attitudes (Broderick & Blewitt, 2014). Crowds can be very influential and may carry various labels, such as popular, jock, dirt head, or druggie. The **crowd** is based on image and reputation.

Peer pressure, or peer influence, becomes a significant factor that can be positive or negative. If it is negative, adolescents tend to conform to what others demand or what they think others want, often despite their better judgment. Peer influence is strongest during early adolescence when teens may try drinking or smoking or stealing to prove to their peers that they are independent and willing to take risks. However, although we typically attribute negative behavior to peer pressure, in reality, it is quite variable. Broderick and Blewitt (2014) suggested that teens more frequently engage in peer-sanctioned behavior voluntarily as opposed to being coerced. That is to say, adolescents did not feel pressure to conform; they conformed because they wanted to.

It is interesting to note that there are some brain changes that occur during adolescence that have some effect on the need to be accepted by one's peers. Broderick and Blewitt (2014) described how there is a proliferation and also a pruning of dopamine receptors that leads to reward seeking. There is also a link between the reward system and social processing that results in greater interest in peers after puberty.

> **Think About It   12.3**
>
> Do you remember your first date? Were you nervous or excited? Were you in a consistent relationship during your middle or high school years? Do you think adolescent dating has changed since the time you had your first dating experiences?

Romantic Relationships and Dating

Around age 11–13, adolescents become more interested in romance, though at this age they typically date in groups of young females and males. Some adolescents date at this age (Vernon, 2009), but more frequently these young adolescents just have a "crush" on someone and share this "secret" with a friend. In fact, having antagonistic feelings toward the opposite sex isn't uncommon at this age.

More serious dating generally begins after age 15. In the beginning it is more casual dating, which is often short lived, and adolescents still also date in groups (Santrock, 2011). Typically, girls start dating earlier than boys and are more interested in dating than boys. As they move through mid-adolescence, dating relationships become more intimate, usually around age 17, with some teens actually "falling in love," or at least thinking so. There are so many myths surrounding the notion of romantic love that it is hard for adolescents to know what love really is. Although not all romantic relationships are sexual, sexual experimentation generally increases during this period and teenagers are more likely to be sexually active (Cobb, 2001).

Romantic relationships can be a source of pleasure and contribute to identity development. At the same time, romantic relationships can be a source of heartache when terminated. A breakup of this nature can be a trigger for depression and, in rare cases, suicide.

Risky Behaviors

Risky behaviors can be conceptualized as points along a continuum, ranging from less risky to more severe. They escalate during adolescence, and although not all teens engage in risky or reckless behaviors, Broderick and Blewitt (2014) reported that a high percentage do. "Behaviors traditionally considered deviant are increasingly becoming part of the experimental repertoire of teens who are considered well adjusted" (p. 339). At present, drinking, smoking, and sexual activity appear to be things that you "just do" during adolescence.

Why do teens engage in risky behaviors that may lead to delinquency? The answer is multifaceted. In part, it is due to their egocentrism and their belief that they are invincible— bad things may happen to others but not to me. To these adolescents, risky behaviors are exciting and not potentially catastrophic. In addition, Broderick and Blewitt (2014) noted that adolescents are sensation seekers. They want new and varied experiences and are willing to take risks to get rewards. Brain changes that affect emotional and cognitive development play a key role, and because maturity is uneven, the connections between logical thinking and the emotional system develop more slowly, which affects the way adolescents evaluate the risks. Another factor that influences risky behaviors is the peer group, whose members may serve as role models for deviant behavior, and also a sort of collective egocentrism. An example of this is illustrated in Case Example 12.4.

➤ CASE EXAMPLE **12.4** JAMIE.

Jamie was 14 years old when she had her first bad experience with alcohol. In fact, she almost died. Throughout the summer she and her friends had been drinking, and because her friends didn't seem concerned about getting caught, she didn't worry either (collective egocentrism). One day Jamie and her best friend went to another friend's house in the afternoon just to hang out. It just so happened that neither parent was home, so the girls decided to raid the liquor cabinet. All three drank large amounts of vodka and gin, but Jamie apparently drank the most. They were all passed out when another friend happened to stop by. He was able to wake up two of the girls but not Jamie. They all were so scared that the boy decided to call his mother, a nurse, to ask for advice. She immediately called for an ambulance.

Just as the ambulance was arriving, so was Jamie's father, who had come to pick up his daughter. Imagine his shock when the paramedics came out with his daughter on the stretcher. The paramedics advised him to ride in the ambulance to the hospital because his daughter might not make it there alive. What transpired over the next few years was not a pretty picture. Jaime almost died from alcohol poisoning and became very depressed, anxious, and obsessive compulsive. She dropped out of school and was in and out of several different treatment programs, although none were very successful. And believe it or not, she still was binge drinking. During high school there were at least two other occasions similar to the first. It's a wonder she is still alive. What are some strategies or approaches to help Jamie and her family?

Drug and Alcohol Use

As Case Example 12.4 illustrates, Jamie put herself at risk because she wanted the short-term reward without considering the long-term consequences. Although experimentation with substances is quite common during adolescence, McWhirter and Burrow-Sanchez (2009) noted that some teens develop more significant substance abuse problems. Indeed, of industrialized nations, drug use places the United States near the top of the list despite some decline in the use of illicit drugs in recent years. In the United States, adolescents most frequently use alcohol, tobacco, and marijuana. It is also quite common for teens with a substance abuse disorder to have a conduct disorder, depression, ADHD, anxiety disorder, or Bipolar Disorder.

Risk factors for substance abuse include individual characteristics, peer factors, family factors, and school and community factors. Individual characteristics include aggressiveness, anger, and impulsivity. Those who associate with peers who use substances are more likely to use substances themselves. Family factors include harsh parenting, lack of parental supervision, low emotional support, high levels of family conflict, and parental or sibling substance abuse. School and community factors can also influence adolescents to turn to substances. School failure, an unsafe school environment, or unclear expectations increase dropout risk. Adolescents who drop out of school are more likely to abuse substances than peers who stay in school. Finally, the community plays a role.

Poor neighborhoods, easy access to drugs and alcohol, and lax laws about underage substance use contribute to the problem.

Delinquency

All are familiar with the term "juvenile delinquency." Delinquency is influenced by peers, family, and community. Papalia et al. (2009) distinguished between **early-onset antisocial behavior**, which begins by age 11 years, and **late-onset antisocial behavior**, which occurs after puberty and generally involves only minor offenses. Early onset is the most serious in that it generally leads to chronic delinquency resulting from inconsistent, harsh parenting practices, hostility toward parents, and deviant behavior by peers. Community and neighborhood structures may also be a factor, as well as socioeconomic status.

Fortunately, most adolescents who engage in delinquent behaviors do not get into serious trouble or become full-fledged criminals. The ones who engage in serious criminal activity most likely come from dysfunctional families and have poor school performance (Papalia et al., 2009). Harmful social conditions, racial discrimination, poverty, and alienation also contribute to this problem (Bemak, Chung, & Murphy, 2003). Prevention efforts need to address parenting practices with an emphasis on authoritative parenting, encouraging parents to monitor their adolescents' activities and discourage association with peers who engage in delinquent behaviors. It is also important to develop neighborhood and community support systems such as after-school programs, sports camps, church activities, and job skill programs to encourage adolescents to become involved in pro-social, constructive activities.

Violence and Gangs

The fact that there have been several school shootings in the past decade would seem to indicate that youth violence is increasing. McWhirter and Burrow-Sanchez (2009) stressed that youth violence is a growing concern that results in fear and intimidation, as well as more serious ramifications. Teen violence takes many forms: dating violence, rape, bullying that results in violent behavior, crime, shooting rampages, and so forth.

What causes youth violence? Modeling is a key factor. Teens growing up in violent homes learn to see violence as normal behavior. Additional factors include the immature adolescent brain, which affects impulse control, and a media that is replete with violent acts.

Closely tied to youth violence is involvement in gangs. Like a clique, a **gang** is a group of teens or young adults who spend time together. Unlike a clique, gang members engage in activities that typically involve violence. There are leaders and followers in the gang, and they differentiate themselves from other gangs by names, logos, tattoo symbols, clothing, or secret signs and signals. There are both male and female gangs. Initiation into the gang often involves the new member engaging in a violent or illegal act to prove themselves worthy of membership (Burnham & Arnold, 2000).

Fortunately, most teens are not in gangs because gang membership substantially increases one's chances of being killed or injured. Gang violence disrupts lives and creates a major problem for society. Gang violence, as well as youth violence in general, is a pervasive problem that needs to be addressed on many levels.

Adolescent Sexuality

Sexual exploration, sexual experimentation, and developing a sexual identity constitute an important part of adolescent development. As Santrock (2011) stated, "adolescence is a bridge between the asexual child and the sexual adult" (p. 233). Several challenges are associated with this transition: managing feelings, including anxiety about feeling aroused or engaging in sexual activity; learning how to avoid negative consequences of sexual experimentation

REFLECTION 12.4 TEENS AND STDS

I recall working with a 15-year-old who expressed concern about being tested for sexually transmitted diseases. When asked if there was good cause for her anxiety, she replied, "Probably not. I've only had two partners and most of my friends have had eight or ten. And now that I know what flavored condoms are for, I shouldn't be too worried!" I struggled to maintain my composure face as she casually discussed some of her sexual experiences, which were way beyond what I thought a 15-year-old would even know about, much less experience. [~AV]

such as pregnancy or sexually transmitted diseases; and knowing "what to do" and how to do it. In today's society, the Internet, movies, advertising, and television encourage sexual expression, and teens are becoming sexually active at earlier ages, when they may not be emotionally mature enough to deal with sexual experiences.

Think About It 12.4

Do you remember how you learned about sexuality? What do you remember about the progression of your sexual activity? Did you masturbate? How old were you when you first held hands or were kissed? Did you like it? At what age did you first have sexual intercourse and what was that like for you? Based on your experiences, what advice would you give to teens today about being sexually active?

Sexual activity often begins with masturbation, which is associated with erotic fantasies, and gradually transitions to sexual activity with a partner. Readers may remember their own stages of sexual activity: holding hands, kissing, and petting, which may or may not lead to orgasm. Gradually petting gets more involved—feeling breasts or a penis, first with clothes on and then off, and ultimately intercourse and oral sex.

Steinberg et al. (2011) noted that 40% of teenagers in America have had sexual intercourse by the end of their sophomore year in high school, and that by age 18 years, two-thirds have had intercourse. On average, African-American youth have their first sexual experiences earlier than White youth, purportedly because more African-American youth grow up in poverty and in single-parent families, both of which are risk factors for early sexual behavior. Sexually active adolescents aren't necessarily in romantic relationships, either. Many talk about having "friends with benefits" or "hooking up" with others just to have casual sex outside of a dating context. Their rationale for engaging in this type of relationship was that it wasn't as stressful as being in a more committed relationship and having sex.

The problem with sexual activity is that far too many adolescents still think they are invincible, fail to see the consequences of engaging in risky sexual behaviors, and consequently do not use contraception regularly. Some do not use contraception because their partners object to it, while others don't like to admit that they are sexually active and plan for it (Steinberg et al., 2011). Another factor is that some adolescents may lack information about conception and therefore not understand how important contraception is or how to obtain it. Alternatively, some adolescents may not use contraceptives because they want to get pregnant.

Early sexual activity is often associated with poor school performance, substance abuse, and other behavioral problems. Teen parents have many struggles, especially financial troubles, often raising children in poverty and single-parent families. As Santrock (2011) noted, programs to reduce teen pregnancy are critical, as is sex education. Unfortunately, sex education has been and continues to be a controversial subject. There are two basic types of sex education programs: (1) abstinence-only programs, which address the social, physiological, and health benefits of abstaining from sex; and (2) more comprehensive sex education programs that not only attempt to reduce the rate of early sexual activity and adolescent pregnancy, but also provide education about contraception and sexually transmitted diseases. According to Santrock, comprehensive sex education programs (as opposed to abstinence only) do not increase sexual intercourse, as critics believe, and can reduce the risk of adolescent pregnancy and sexually transmitted diseases. One factor to keep in mind about sex education is that adolescents mature at vastly differing rates, so it is very important to continue exposing them to information about puberty, sexuality, pregnancy, and so forth over a span of several years.

Teen Pregnancy

According to Santrock (2011), the United States ranks among the highest in teen pregnancy and childbearing among developed countries, even though the pregnancy rate seems to be on a bit of a downward trend. Still, Dacey, Travers, and Fiore (2009) noted that in the United States each year, about a million teens become pregnant. What is interesting is that although the U.S. pregnancy rate is eight times as high as in the Netherlands, teenagers in the Netherlands are as sexually active as those in this country. Although some U.S. teenagers opt for abortion and even fewer choose adoption, the vast majority of pregnant U.S. teens give birth to the babies and raise them as single parents, which generally creates a domino effect of problems ranging from poverty to dropping out of school. If sex education programs aren't successful in preventing pregnancy, the good news is that, increasingly, there are more teen parent programs that educate them about raising children, encourage them to pursue their education in order to better their lives, and help them plan for the future.

Sexually Transmitted Diseases

Teens who engage in sexual activity may not realize that there are risks in addition to becoming pregnant. **Sexually transmitted diseases (STDs)**, also known as sexually transmitted infections (STIs), are serious infections that primarily result from unprotected sexual contact. Santrock (2011) reported that a fourth of sexually active adolescents in the United States acquire a sexually transmitted disease such as genital herpes, gonorrhea, or chlamydia. They are also at higher risk for contracting AIDS than sexually inactive youth. In fact, according to Kail and Cavanaugh (2010), adolescents and adults age 24 and younger account for nearly half of new AIDS cases. Clearly, increased effort to educate teens about these risks is imperative because these diseases can have serious consequences.

Date Rape

Date rape, also known as **acquaintance rape**, is becoming more common among teens. Of significant concern are statistics from a recent study that revealed that 75% of men and 55% of the women who were raped had been drinking or were given the date rape drug Rohypnol (see www.incestabuse.about.com). Even more shocking is that 38% of the women who were raped were between ages 14 and 17 years of age. The problem is perpetuated because these attacks are often not reported. Date rape occurs more often if boys see violence modeled in their own homes and if girls have low self-esteem and think they "deserve" to be treated in this manner (Kail & Cavanaugh, 2010). Clearly this is a significant social problem that needs to be addressed and one that counselors will deal with if they treat adolescents and young adults.

Sexual Identity

Developing a sexual identity is one of the major tasks of adolescence, encompassing sexual behaviors, arousal, and interests, as well as sexual attraction. This can be particularly stressful for youth who are attracted to same-sex partners. Although the majority of adolescents are romantically involved with members of the opposite sex during early and mid-adolescence, approximately 15% question their sexuality (Carver, Egan, & Perry, 2004), but for most adolescents, this is just part of the identity experimentation. Same-sex attraction is somewhat different for boys than for girls. Usually, boys begin to feel different and become more interested in activities that are not typical for their gender, whereas girls first begin having a strong feeling toward another female (Kail & Cavanaugh, 2010). According to McFarland and Tollerud (2009), the average age of self-identification has been decreasing, and often by age 16 years these adolescents will self-identify as gay or lesbian. Santrock (2011) noted that most adolescents who are attracted to the same sex have also had some other-sex attractions.

Gay and lesbian youth face many challenges with immense social pressures. On average they experience more mental health and substance abuse problems, but the most critical fact is that the suicide rate among gay and lesbian youth is increasing, reportedly resulting from verbal and physical abuse, prejudice, and stress related to their sexual identity (McFarland & Tollerud, 2009). Many of these youth have social and academic problems at school and are at risk of dropping out because they are harassed if they have "come out" or if others suspect they are gay or lesbian. If they haven't come out, there is high anxiety about being discovered and subsequently rejected, threatened, and abused. They feel alone, inferior, and hopeless. Navigating through adolescence is difficult enough, but much more of a challenge for this population.

Fortunately, there are more school-based support groups for lesbian, gay, bisexual, and transgendered (LGBT) youth, which provide a network and a safe place for them to discuss issues pertaining to their sexual identity. Equally important are anti-harassment policies in schools.

Career Development

Throughout childhood and adolescence, career development is occurring as we engage in imaginary play, explore interests through organizations and recreational activities, and join clubs and participate in extracurricular activities during the secondary school years. Another source of career development often occurs through part-time employment during high school. In this section we will explore the concept of work and leisure, as well as occupational choices, and postsecondary opportunities, including college.

Leisure and Work

Adolescents often just "hang out" with their friends, siblings, or just by themselves in their rooms. Parents of adolescents are sometimes concerned that this is unproductive time, but in reality, there are positives as well as negatives regarding hanging out. On the positive side, hanging out in a social context is a time when adolescents explore interests and opportunities. On the negative side, if there is too little structure, adolescents may get into trouble. There is growing concern that today's adolescents may not have enough down time because some are overcommitted and overscheduled with extracurricular activities, community involvement and volunteer work, church activities, or with clubs and organizations. While all of these activities can promote skill mastery and help clarify interests, too much involvement can result in stress.

Advantages and Disadvantages of Working during High School

Working during high school can compound stress due to balancing work, leisure, studying, and extracurricular activities. On the other hand, work can be a very good experience in that it helps adolescents learn to manage time and money, be more responsible, and develop a work ethic. Adolescents can learn social skills as well as job-related skills that may be helpful in future employment. In addition, having a job helps adolescents clarify career goals and work values and gives them extra money to spend on clothes or entertainment. Broderick and Blewitt (2014) noted that adolescents from lower socioeconomic groups are not as likely to be employed as are middle-class teens. You might think it would be the opposite because youth from a lower SES group probably need the money more than middle-class youth do. However, that depends on how one defines "need."

Steinberg et al. (2011) noted that the advantages of working may be overstated, especially when it comes to learning money management. They reported that few adolescents actually save money; they just spend it on their own needs and activities, rather than saving it for college or contributing to family expenses. In fact, having disposable income that enables adolescents to buy what they want may establish bad habits regarding spending and impulse buying that could have negative future ramifications.

One might think that working would keep adolescents out of trouble, but there is some indication that working long hours (over 20 hours a week) can also lead to increased behavior problems, misconduct in school, and increased substance abuse (Broderick & Blewitt, 2014; Steinberg et al., 2011). Working long hours also affects school attendance; if adolescents are tired after working late the night before, skipping school to sleep may seem like a viable option. Furthermore, work can interfere with participation in extracurricular activities. Although Steinberg et al. reported that the impact of working on school achievement is not that significant, students who work long hours are less attentive in class, may take easier courses, or cheat in order to keep their grades up. It appears that working per se isn't the issue—it is how much students work. Working less than 20 hours a week seems to be more manageable, but anything over that can be problematic.

Vocational Choices

In reality, choosing a career isn't easy, and most people change careers several times throughout their working years. But there is a lot of pressure placed on adolescents to figure out what they want to do, resulting in varying degrees of anxiety. Kail and Cavanaugh (2010) described the three stages of career development according to Super's theory. Around age 13 or 14 adolescents engage in a process called **crystallization**, in which they begin to develop ideas about careers based on their ideas about their interests and talents. At this stage adolescents are just "trying on" ideas about what they might want to do when they grow up. Discussions with parents, teachers, and counselors can facilitate this process, as well as exposure to options and opportunities provided by attending career fairs and other school-sponsored career education activities. They may also take career inventories to generate awareness.

The second phase begins around age 18, when adolescents enter the **specification** phase, which is when they begin to limit their options by learning about specific jobs. It is at this point that adolescents may begin training and skill development for a future career by entering college or a vocational school or starting a job. There can still be considerable confusion and exploration at this stage.

The third phase, **implementation**, begins in the early 20s when young adults get a job and move into the workforce. This can be a reality check in that the job they had fantasized about and planned for may actually not be as glamorous or fulfilling as they thought it would be. Due to the nature of the job, the person may need more training. It is not uncommon at this point for adolescents to veer in another direction, perhaps because of the economy and its impact on the job market or because they don't think they are cut out for the job they trained for. Other factors affect career choices, such as stress in the workplace, compensation, and the working environment itself. As Akos, Niles, Miller, and Erford (2011) pointed out, this phase is about adapting to the work environment. Like any transition, beginning a job will affect individuals' roles, routines, responsibilities, and assessment of self (Schlossberg, 2009).

Career development and personal development are closely intertwined, and adolescents need skills not only for selecting and implementing a career, but also skills to help them adjust to various life roles (Akos et al., 2011). It is critical that school counselors implement sound educational and career planning and technical preparation programs that help prepare students for the future. Such programs need to be implemented systematically and be integrated as part of the total educational process. Programs also need to be comprehensive, not just informing students about various career options, but also helping them learn decision-making skills, clarify their values, and assess their strengths, weaknesses, and interests. It is also imperative to avoid stereotyping students who attend technical college rather than four-year programs or who get a job instead of going on for further training. Saginak (2003) noted that training in technical and two-year programs can be rigorous, and professionals need to dispel the myth that students who attend these programs are not strong academically.

Influences on Vocational Choices

Of course, young people dream about the ideal career, and during adolescence it is not uncommon for teens to fantasize about being a famous rock star or athlete, never taking into consideration the steps that it takes to reach the top. In reality, vocational choices are influenced by such factors as gender, ethnicity, socioeconomic status, cultural contexts, and other people, including parents, peers, teachers, coaches, and counselors.

Some adolescents make career decisions based on what others want for them, which may end up not being the right decision. Parents sometimes put pressure on their adolescents to become what they want them to be, or adolescents might assume that their parents expect them to follow in the footsteps of one or the other, even if this isn't what they want to do. This can create a great deal of stress and anxiety for both adolescents and their parents.

Culture also affects career decision making. My son is an ESL teacher, helping immigrant adolescents learn English. He spends considerable time working with his high school students to help them explore postsecondary options that they and their families might not have even considered. Because of equity gaps, efforts such as this are critical because there are simply more opportunities for bright, middle- and upper-class adolescents who come from homes where education is valued and college is a given, not an option. But for under-advantaged youth who might be the first individual in the family to go to college or technical school, the decision-making process is much more complex and there are more barriers to break through.

REFLECTION 12.6 THE FAST TRACK TO KINDERGARTEN?

How times have changed. I am retired now, but I remember going to my high school counselor during my senior year for some advice about college or careers. I still vividly recall him saying to me that my only choices were nursing or teaching—and he actually said that I should teach kindergarten because I was small and wouldn't be able to handle the discipline at the secondary level. Luckily I wanted to be a teacher and I never considered being a lawyer, a doctor, a veterinarian, or a dentist, for instance, because those careers weren't presented as options for young women at that time. Thankfully, this is not the case for today's adolescents—the doors have finally opened and young women have more choices. That is not to say that gender stereotyping doesn't still exist, but it is much more common now for young females to pursue careers traditionally limited to males. [~AV]

College Planning

It is important to help students who may not be able to, or choose not to, go to college to not feel inferior. College isn't for everybody, and there are many options available for young people. As Saginak (2003) noted, there are many people who have pursued meaningful careers and didn't have a four-year college education.

For those adolescents who intend to pursue college, planning is an important part of a process that can be confusing and overwhelming. Decisions about where to go, what is affordable, scholarship availability, and types of academic as well as extracurricular opportunities are all part of the decision-making process that involve adolescents and their parents. Beginning early in high school, adolescents need to begin taking courses that will prepare them to meet entrance requirements. As they progress through high school they may take college prep or AP courses, attend meetings with college representatives at school, and visit various campuses to find out more about them.

Transitions after High School

High school seniors display considerable ambiguity and anxiety about transitioning out of high school into another world, whether that will be attending college or technical school, or entering the workforce or the armed forces. As previously noted, transitions involve a change in roles, relationships, routines, and assessment of self. For some adolescents this can be overwhelming because they are going from the familiar to varying degrees of unfamiliarity. Adolescents may be moving away from home to a different city or part of the country. They will most likely be leaving old friends and gaining new ones. They may be living under a different set of rules and need to learn self-regulation skills. In many cases adolescents will be moving from familiar routines to unfamiliar ones that may necessitate more independence and present challenges greater than in the past. For example, some schools conduct brief tutorials during the senior year to teach students how to wash and iron clothes, change a car's oil, and other survival techniques needed when living independently. Another aspect of the transition involves a change in one's assessment of self. Maybe someone was the star of the high school basketball team but didn't make the cut in college. Maybe someone was the valedictorian of the high school class, but so are a lot of others in the new peer pool.

All of these factors can be difficult challenges depending in part on whether adolescents are looking at the transition from a loss perspective or as the beginning of a new stage of life. Other aspects that enter into these transitions have to do with comparisons. Adolescents from poor families usually don't have as many options open to them and may compare themselves negatively to those who appear on the surface to have privilege or a brighter future. There is often a degree of competition prior to the transition out of high school: competing for scholarships, acceptance into college or technical school, or jobs. Some adolescents may look down on their classmates who can't afford to go to college or move away from home. All of these factors can have an impact on this last year of high school. School counselors should encourage dialogue about these changes through a small group counseling format and introduce specific interventions designed to make this transition easier (Vernon, 2002).

Think About It **12.6**

What came to mind as you read this section about career development? Has your career path been similar to what was described? What influenced your career choices? As you reflect on career opportunities for young people today, do you think there is less stereotyping than in previous years? What are some things you consider important for today's youth in making informed decisions about their future?

Summary

This chapter included a discussion of emotional and identity development. A general discussion about how hormonal changes influence emotions was included, as well as specific information about anxiety and depression, two common emotional problems that affect many adolescents. Signs, symptoms, and who is most vulnerable to depression were described, as well as the connection between adolescent depression and suicide. In terms of identity development, both Erikson's and Marcia's theories were described, as well as gender and ethnic considerations relative to identity development.

The second section of the chapter was about social development, including the influence of both family and peers on adolescent development. With regard to family, the chapter discussed four parenting styles—authoritarian, authoritative, permissive, and ignoring—and how these styles affect the parent–adolescent relationship. Seltzer's social identity theory is described in this section, as well as peer relationships, peer pressure, and romantic relationships and dating. Other topics addressed included substance abuse, delinquent behaviors, violence and gang membership, adolescent sexuality, career development, and stages of vocational decision making.

With each generation it seems as if the challenges facing adolescents are more substantial. Consider the fact that all adolescents have the typical developmental tasks to deal with (which many do quite successfully), but in addition there are situational issues that affect more and more youth: living in divorced or blended families, growing up in abusive households, dealing with addicted parents, living in poverty, being victimized or bullied, and so on. As helping professionals we have an obligation to help adolescents living in a contemporary society to grow up without giving up.

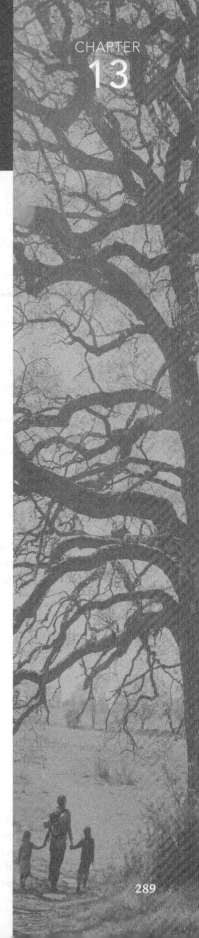

Young Adulthood: Physical and Cognitive Development

By Stephanie Crockett

I n Western cultures, the journey to adulthood is marked more by the achievement of certain developmental tasks than by a specific chronological age, although young adulthood is normative in the age range of 18 and throughout the 30s. Young adulthood is frequently associated with achieving the following tasks: accepting responsibility for oneself, making independent decisions, and becoming financially independent (Arnett & Tanner, 2006). This chapter provides an overview of the characteristics and developmental tasks that define young adulthood. The physical and cognitive changes that young adults experience are explored in detail.

Introduction to Young Adulthood

When do we become adults? In some cultures, the transition from adolescence to adulthood is abrupt and clearly marked by a rite of passage. For example, in the Jewish religion the transition to manhood is celebrated by a bar mitzvah ritual on a boy's 13th birthday. In Nigeria, the transition to womanhood is marked by a ritual that occurs over a span of several weeks. During this time young girls stay in fattening rooms with their legs bound by copper coils to restrict movement while they are pampered. Unlike many societies that have rite-of-passage rituals and celebrations to mark adulthood and the associated change in status, roles, and responsibilities, Western societies often have fuzzy boundaries between adolescence and adulthood.

While becoming an adult is one of the most important milestones in our journey through the lifespan, it is difficult to define exactly when one becomes an adult in the United States. Many adolescents believe adulthood commences with their 18th birthday and the right to vote. Still others may see adulthood as beginning on their 21st birthday with the right to legally drink alcohol in public. One's 18th and 21st birthdays are often important markers along the transition to adulthood, but they do not necessarily represent a clear transition to adult roles and responsibilities. Take, for instance, hung-over young adults the morning after their 21st birthday; they may call one of their parents to nurse their hangover symptoms or to ask for money after blowing a lot of cash at the bar the night before.

For many, the quest to become an adult does not end at a specific chronological age, but boils down to three fundamental accomplishments: (1) accepting responsibility for oneself, (2) making independent decisions, and (3) becoming financially independent (Arnett & Tanner, 2006). It also involves numerous role transitions that are marked by completing education, beginning full-time employment, establishing a household, getting married, and becoming a parent. Given that most individuals spread out these achievements over their 20s, the transition from adolescence to adulthood is a process that results in a development period called "emerging adulthood" (Arnett, 2004).

Developmental theorists have defined the period from late adolescence through the 20s as a distinctive developmental phase of the lifespan odyssey. This period is referred to as **emerging adulthood**, or **young adulthood**; it is characterized as a time when individuals have moved out of adolescence, but have not quite reached full adulthood (Arnett, 2004). Emerging adulthood is defined by five key features (Arnett & Tanner, 2006):

- *Identity exploration:* Young adults invest much time and energy into figuring out who they are as autonomous individuals and finding their niche in society.
- *Self-focused:* Young adulthood is also a time for self-focus and reflection. Young adults are free to make their own life decisions and have few commitments to other individuals or society.
- *Instability:* Young adulthood is characterized by instability and transition. Young adults often experience changes in residence, jobs, and relationships.
- *Feeling in-between:* Most young adults feel in transition, as they do not consider themselves either adolescents or adults.
- *Opportunity:* Young adults see their lives as full of opportunity and often have an optimistic view of the future.

These five key features capture a generalized experience of young adulthood, and can be a useful guide in deepening our understanding of young adult development. It is critical, however, that counselors understand how social structures, such as race, gender, class, and sexual orientation, interact with this developmental phase to create varied experiences of privilege and oppression for young adults. Such an understanding is often called **intersectionality** (Glenn, 1985). Intersectionality theory calls attention to the ways in which "identity categories intersect to produce distinctive social experiences that are not reducible to their component parts" (Meier, Hull, & Ortyl, 2009, p. 516). For example, a young Latina woman's experiences in dating is not simply the sum of her experiences as a Latina and as a woman, but the interaction of both cultural identities. The dating experiences of a Latina/o are different for men and women; likewise, the dating experiences of a woman vary across differing ethnic groups. In this chapter and the next, we will specifically attend to the ways in which multiple cultural identities and group memberships intersect to create inequities in the young adult experience.

SECTION I: Physical Development

Young adulthood, for most individuals, is characterized by a peak in physical functioning and minimal health concerns. Despite the experience of peak physical performance, young adults often engage in lifestyle behaviors (e.g., smoking, binge drinking, unhealthy eating habits) that negatively impact their current physical functioning and often have long-term consequences for their physical health. Counselors play an important role in helping young adults maintain physical health and wellness by helping their clients explore the effects of these detrimental lifestyle behaviors on their health, devise reasonable plans to reduce and/or eliminate unhealthy habits, and begin to engage in healthy lifestyle behaviors that promote physical, emotional, and spiritual wellness. In this section, we will further explore the physical functioning and health of young adults, and we will consider lifestyle factors that can adversely impact physical health in early adulthood.

Physical Functioning and Performance

Most individuals reach their peak physical performance between 19 and 26 years of age. By age 20, the majority of people have reached their full physical growth and are at their maximum height. Physical strength, coordination, dexterity, agility, and flexibility also peak around this time. Biological systems (e.g., cardiovascular, respiratory, neuroendocrine, digestive) are highly efficient, functioning at maximum capacity and effectiveness during young adulthood. The immune system is much more effective at defending against disease than in childhood. Women also reach their peak fertility during their early 20s and, if engaging in unprotected intercourse with a young adult male, encounter an 85% chance of becoming pregnant within a year (American Congress of Obstetricians and Gynecologists, 2011). Finally, the senses—touch, smell, vision, hearing, taste, and balance—tend to be most acute during young adulthood. Due to this peak in physical performance, many world-class athletes and professional sports players are between 20 and 30 years of age.

Not all individuals reach their physical peak at the same time. For instance, most women reach their full height by age 19 years, whereas men can continue to grow until their 30s. Research also shows that men reach their maximum potential in physical abilities such as running, jumping, and swimming approximately one year later than women (Schulz & Curnow, 1988). Substantial differences exist in the timing of peak performance for specific physical skills. Physical skills that involve muscle strength, flexibility, and speed of movement tend to peak early, whereas skills involving control, arm–hand steadiness, precision, and stamina peak later.

Early adulthood is also a time when our physical functioning starts to decrease and signs of aging gradually appear. Muscle tone and strength start to decrease by age 30, regardless of how many weights are lifted or laps run at the gym. Additionally, the body's fatty tissue increases around age 25. The added body fat and loss in muscle tone can lead some to have bellies that jut out and chins that sag; unfortunately, this is a drastic change from the effortlessly toned body of a 19-year-old. Lung tissues may also lose elasticity in young adulthood, causing respiratory muscles to weaken (Sharma & Goodwin, 2006). Finally, sensory acuity begins to decline toward the end of young adulthood. The lenses in the eyes of young adults become less elastic, making it more difficult to focus on near objects (Fozard & Gordon-Salant, 2001). Also, hearing sensitivity for high-pitched tones begins to decline somewhat, especially in men, by the late 20s (Gordon-Salant, 2005).

Physical Health in Young Adulthood

Individuals are often healthiest during young adulthood and are seemingly exempt from health issues caused by serious diseases (e.g., cancer) and senescence. In the United States, the majority of young adults rate their physical health as good to excellent, with fewer than 6% reporting health problems that interfere with daily functioning (Park, Paul, Adams, Brindis, & Irwin, 2006). Due to the general healthy status of most young adults, death from disease is very rare in early adulthood. For instance, the mortality rate for cancer in young adults, ages 15 to 29, is approximately four people per 100,000, as compared to 119 per 100,000 in adults age 29–44 years, and 1650 per 100,000 in adults over the age of 85 (Bleyer, O'Leary, Barr, & Ries, 2006). The leading cause of death in adults aged 25 to 44 is unintentional injury (26%), followed by cancer (14%), heart disease (12%), suicide (10%), homicide (6%), and HIV (4%) (see Figure 13.1) [National Center for Health Statistics (NCHS), 2010].

While the leading causes of death in emerging adults are parallel to those in adolescents, the mortality rates of young adults more than triple between adolescence and young adulthood as the incidence of injury, homicide, and substance use peak during this time. The experience of robust health during young adulthood is frequently taken for granted; emerging adults are typically not as concerned about their health and overall well-being as adults in their mid-30s. Additionally, young adults are more likely to live in poverty and have no access to health care. Indeed, young adults hold the lowest level of health insurance of any age group (Callahan & Cooper, 2005; Park et al., 2006). These self-imposed and environmental barriers can present challenges to health care professionals who seek to provide medical and mental health services to this population.

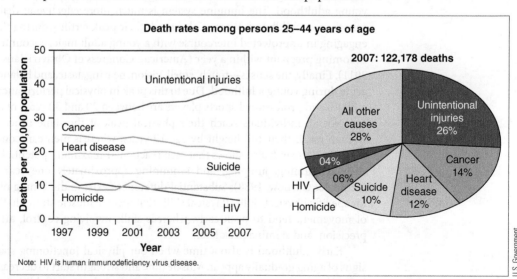

Figure 13.1 CDC mortality.

Lifestyle Factors Influencing the Physical Health of Young Adults

➤ CASE EXAMPLE **13.1** JASMINE.

Jasmine, an 18-year-old college freshman, was referred to the university counseling center by her academic advisor for poor academic performance. During the initial counseling session, Jasmine admitted that she was falling behind in her classes; she attributed her failing grades to feeling exhausted and lethargic during the day. As the counselor talked with Jasmine, she disclosed that she often stayed up late drinking at a sorority house. On average, she got less than five hours of sleep a night. Jasmine had also gained 20 pounds since starting college and started smoking in an effort to lose weight. When the counselor spoke to Jasmine about her lifestyle habits, Jasmine stated that these bad habits are probably affecting her health, but believes that drinking and staying up all night are just part of the college experience. She was unwilling to modify her habits, believing that it is important to have fun at this stage in life.

As Case Example 13.1 demonstrates, while Jasmine is supposed to be at peak physical health and performance, specific lifestyle choices are negatively affecting her health and well-being. Jasmine is not unlike most young adults in the United States. Poor lifestyle practices, which begin in childhood or adolescence, increase during adulthood. A longitudinal study that followed more than 14,000 adolescent individuals into their 20s found that diet, activity level, obesity, tobacco, alcohol, and illicit drug use, and the likelihood of contracting a sexually transmitted disease [STD; also known as a sexually-transmitted infection (STI)] increased as participants approached young adulthood (Harris, Gordon-Larson, Chantala, & Udry, 2006). Although most young adults are fully aware of the liabilities associated with their poor lifestyle choices and bad habits, they still engage in reckless behaviors that compromise their health and, in some instances, lead to untimely death. Professional counselors who strive to help individuals achieve health and wellness may wonder why young adults act in ways that are seemingly self-destructive. Broderick and Blewitt (2014) posit that the unhealthy habits and behaviors demonstrated by young adults are due to

> the poor application of problem-solving skills to practical problems, a continuing sense of invulnerability that began in the adolescent years, which may be exacerbated by the fact that young adults can bounce back from physical stress far more readily than they will in later years, and the stresses of leaving home and facing the social and academic demands of college and the workplace. (p. 358)

Not all of the factors that contribute to the health habits of young adults are known, but researchers have shown that poor physical and mental health choices affect adults in later life. A recent longitudinal study by Grant, Wardle, and Steptoe (2009) tracked participants for up to 50 years, showing that individuals who make unhealthy lifestyle choices as young adults have poorer health and lower levels of life satisfaction in later life, as compared to people who do not develop these habits in early adulthood. In particular, Grant et al. found that life satisfaction was positively related to not smoking, exercising regularly, limiting fat intake, and eating fruit. Clearly, adopting healthy habits during young adulthood can contribute to physical and emotional wellness in later life, but young adults may find it particularly challenging to initiate and maintain a healthy lifestyle. Counselors can play an important role in preventing young adults from developing destructive lifestyle habits and helping them to implement healthy behaviors. In the remainder of this section, we will further explore lifestyle habits that affect the health of young adults.

Tobacco Use

Smoking and the use of other tobacco products constitute the leading preventable cause of death in the United States. Smoking increases heart rate and blood pressure, as it reduces the heart's supply of oxygen. Consequently, cigarette smoking has been linked to increased risk for heart disease, stroke, and chronic lung disease (NCHS, 2004). The American Cancer Society further estimates that smoking is related to more than half of all cancers, including cancer of mouth, esophagus, larynx, and lung. It is estimated that one out of every five deaths in the United States is the result of tobacco use, and the Centers for Disease Control (http://www.cdc.gov/tobacco/global/#core1) estimates that more than 8 million people worldwide will die per year by 2030 from tobacco-related illnesses. In the United States, African-American men disproportionately bear the burden of tobacco-related deaths. For example, from 2005 to 2009 the average death rate from lung cancer was 26% higher in African-American men compared to White men (American Cancer Society, 2013). While nearly all deaths related to smoking occur after age 35 years, most individuals begin smoking during adolescence and young adulthood (Kandel & Chen, 2000; Mokdad, Marks, Stroup, & Gerberding, 2004). In fact, young adults are more likely to smoke than older adults, with more than 40% of 21- to 25-year-olds reporting the use of cigarettes (SAMHSA, 2007).

Given that the future is grim for tobacco users, one may question why young adults smoke. To start, the nicotine in cigarettes is highly addictive, with symptoms of dependence (e.g., irritability, anxiety, difficulty concentrating, increased appetite) occurring soon after the onset of smoking (DiFranza et al., 2007). Pressure from friends and acquaintances to smoke is another reason for tobacco use in early adulthood. Smoking may be perceived as fashionable, or make one appear to be more mature. Young adults, such as Jasmine, may also smoke to control their weight—a primary reason reported by many college females who smoke. Still others may believe that smoking improves their mental performance (Piper et al., 2004). Additional factors such as gender, ethnicity, education, and socioeconomic status (and the intersection of these characteristics) affect tobacco usage. The CDC (2010c) reported that more adult men (23.5%) smoke than do adult women (17.9%), and that Native Americans/Alaska Natives (23.2%) have a higher prevalence of tobacco use than do Whites (22.1%), Blacks (21.3%), or Hispanics (14.5%). Nearly half of all individuals with a GED and a third of adults living in poverty smoke, compared to 11.1% of individuals with a college degree. On a positive note, young adults who quit smoking show marked health improvement and significantly reduced their risk of developing heart disease and cancer (U.S. Department of Health and Human Services, 2010c).

Alcohol and Illicit Drug Use

Experimentation with alcohol and drugs typically begins during the adolescent years and increases during emerging adulthood when young adults leave home for college or a job, becoming free from the watchful eyes of their parents. In fact, SAMHSA (2006) reported that young adults have higher rates of alcohol and illicit drug use than any other age group. A major issue among youth is binge drinking. **Binge drinking** is defined as having five or more drinks in a row on at least one day in the past month. Binge drinking is more frequent among college students than their noncollegiate peers (SAMHSA, 2006), especially among students living in fraternity houses (McCabe et al., 2004; Wechsler & Nelson, 2008). It is also more widespread in men, although binge drinking in women aged 19 to 22 is increasing (Johnston, O'Malley, Bachman, & Schulenberg, 2012). Binge drinking peaks around age 21 and then slowly declines throughout the remainder of young adulthood. While often short-lived, binge drinking is associated with numerous health issues and can take a toll on the physical functioning of young adults. In particular, binge drinking has been found to inhibit the development of memory in young adults, and may cause cirrhosis of the liver, other gastrointestinal disorders (e.g., ulcers), pancreatic disease, certain cancers, heart failure, and stroke (American Heart Association, 2010). The use of alcohol is related to health risks such as traffic accidents, HIV infection, sexual risk taking (e.g., having sex without using a contraceptive, sexual assault), and illicit drug and tobacco use. Wechsler and Nelson (2008) found that college students who engaged in binge drinking were more likely to fall behind in their classes, drive under the influence of alcohol, and have unprotected sex than students who did not binge drink. Among young adults who were involved in fatal auto accidents in 2003, over a quarter had been drinking (NHTSA, 2010).

Young adults aged 18 to 25 also tend to have high rates of substance abuse (SAMHSA, 2006). Approximately 20% of young adults reported abusing one or more illicit drugs. Nearly 17% of young adults abused marijuana, making it the most widely used illicit substance among this age group. Other illicit drugs used by young adults included cocaine, crack, hallucinogens, inhalants, stimulants, and methamphetamines. Men are more likely than women to use illicit substances, and the nonmedical use of prescription drugs is more prevalent in Whites and Hispanics than in African-Americans and Asian-Americans (SAMHSA, 2006). Young adult women who are sexual minorities (i.e., lesbians and bisexuals) have also been found to have higher rates of alcohol abuse than their heterosexual counterparts (Dermody et al., 2013). Finally, full-time college students, in comparison to their nonstudent peers, are less likely to use cocaine, crack cocaine, and methamphetamines [National Survey on Drug Use and Health (NSDUH), 2005]. As with binge drinking, rates of illicit substance use typically decline after age 25. While the overall rates of drug use in early adulthood remain stable, abuse of cocaine and methamphetamines has significantly decreased in recent years (SAMHSA, 2007). Specifically, cocaine abuse dropped by 23% in young adults and methamphetamine abuse declined by a third.

The use of illicit substances has both short- and long-term effects on young adults' physical health (National Institute on Drug Abuse, 2012). For example, methamphetamine use can cause irregular heartbeat, anxiety, confusion, insomnia, mood disturbances, violent behavior, dental problems, and damage to the brain that mimics symptoms of Alzhelimer's disease. Likewise, cocaine use is associated with increased risk of heart attacks, strokes, seizures, gastrointestinal issues (e.g., abdominal pain, nausea), weight loss, malnourishment, irritability, panic attacks, and paranoia. Unexpected death may also occur any time one uses cocaine. While the health consequences associated with marijuana use have been the subject of much debate, one study indicated that heavy marijuana users reported that the drug interfered with their physical and mental health, negatively affecting their cognitive abilities, social life, and career (Gruber, Pope, Hudson, & Yurgelun-Todd, 2003). Withdrawal symptoms, such as irritability, insomnia, suppressed appetite, and anxiety, have also been reported by individuals who are trying to quit using the drug (Budney, Vandrey, Hughes, Thostenson, & Bursac, 2008).

Diet, Exercise, and Obesity

Diet and exercise are important components of maintaining physical health in early adulthood. To sustain a healthy lifestyle, the U.S. Department of Agriculture (USDA, 2010) recommends eating a variety of nutrient-rich foods from the basic food groups and limiting the intake of saturated fats, cholesterol, sugar, and salt. In addition to eating right, the American Heart Association (2007) advises individuals to engage in at least 30 minutes of aerobic exercise (e.g., jogging, swimming) a day. Young adults who eat nutritious meals and exercise regularly significantly reduce their risk of developing heart disease, diabetes, and high blood pressure in middle adulthood (Steffen et al., 2005). Exercise may even improve cognitive functioning in young adults. One study found that participants who jogged for 30 minutes two to three times a week improved their performance on memory tests (Cocke, 2002). Interestingly, their scores dropped when they stopped exercising due to decreased oxygen levels in the brain. So make sure to get plenty of exercise before your next exam!

REFLECTION 13.1 ADJUSTING TO COLLEGE

As counselors, we often do not think too much about providing information and counseling to clients regarding their eating habits. Reflecting back over my experiences as a young college student, it certainly would have been helpful to have a counselor discuss such issues. While I grew up in a health-conscious family and played team sports in high school, the academic rigor of college was particularly challenging during my freshman year, and I experienced a lot of stress trying to maintain good grades. To cope with the academic stress I began eating large amounts of junk food. To be honest, it never crossed my mind that I could develop health issues from lack of exercise and unhealthy eating. But I did. During my first year of college, I gained over 20 pounds and began to experience severe intestinal issues. By the end of my second year in college, my intestinal issues were so severe that they began affecting my daily functioning. While I did not seek out counseling or see a doctor, I often think about how helpful it would have been to have a professional help me to link the impact of stress and lifestyle habits on my physical health. A counselor could have played a key role in helping me to adopt adaptive ways of coping with the academic stress and referred me to a physician to change my eating habits. [~SC]

Despite the health benefits associated with diet and exercise, young adults often fail to eat nutritious meals and engage in regular physical exercise. Over a third of young adults aged 18–24 eat out four or more times a week and, by the time people reach age 20 years, half do not get the recommended amount of exercise. The excess fat consumption associated with restaurant food, coupled with the lack of physical activity, increases young adults' risk for heart disease and high cholesterol. Gender, race, and level of education (and the intersection of these characteristics) play a significant role in individuals' level of physical activity. Women are less likely than men to get the recommended amount of weekly exercise. African-Americans and Latinos/as are less likely to exercise than Whites, and individuals who did not graduate from high school get less exercise than college graduates (Kruger & Kohl, 2007).

A lack of healthy diet and exercise habits in adulthood has certainly contributed to the increase of obesity in the United States. The number of obese people in the United States, as well as internationally, has sharply risen in recent years, making obesity a worldwide problem [Ogden et al., 2006; World Health Organization (WHO), 2012]. **Obesity** is defined as having a body mass index (BMI; weight in kilograms divided by height in meters squared) above 30. Likewise, body fat percentages for obesity are generally cited as 30% for adult females and 25% for adult males. Adults between the ages of 20 and 40 are very likely to experience weight gain, with approximately 30% of men and women being classified as obese (Ogden, Carroll, Curtin, Lamb, & Flegal. 2010). African-American women have experienced the greatest increase in obesity over the last two decades, with nearly half of all African-American women being classified as obese (Ogden, Carroll, Kit, & Flegal, 2014). While an unhealthy diet and lack of exercise play a significant role in weight gain, it appears that minority status and oppression may also contribute to obesity. A recent study found that the frequent experience of racism was related to weight gain in African-American women (Cozier et al., 2014). Numerous health risks are associated with being overweight. Young adults with obesity increase their likelihood of developing serious chronic illnesses such as heart disease, type 2 diabetes, and cancer, as well as increasing their probability of dying in middle adulthood by as much as 40%. As a result, the current generation of young adults may actually have a shorter life expectancy than their parents (Olshansky et al., 2005).

Sleep

The National Sleep Foundation (2011) recommends that young adults get between seven and nine hours of sleep each night. Getting a good night's sleep can enhance complex motor skills (Walker et al., 2003), help to solidify and consolidate learning experiences (Stickgold &

Walker, 2007), and prevent the effects of sleep deprivation. Unfortunately, many young adults fail to get adequate amounts of sleep, and college students, with high levels of family and academic stressors, are likely to experience insomnia (Bernert, Merrill, Braithwaite, Van Orden, & Joiner, 2007). Sleep deprivation has a negative impact on physical and mental well-being. It can:

- cause increased feelings of irritability and aggravation;
- decrease attention levels and increase distractibility, having an impact on cognitive performance;
- impair verbal learning, memory, and high-level decision making; and
- cause drowsiness and fatigue, which can be dangerous if driving.

Sexually Risky Behaviors

Young adulthood is a period in which most people are sexually active, with 85% of 20–22-year-old males and 81% of females reporting they have engaged in sexual intercourse (Mosher, Chandra, & Jones, 2005). Casual sex is common during adulthood, and over half of young adults reported "hooking up" with a friend or acquaintance (McGinty, Knox, & Zusman, 2007). Monogamous relationships among college students tend to be short-lived and are subject to high rates of infidelity (Allen & Baucom, 2006). Condom use in emerging adulthood remains inconsistent (Lefkowitz & Gillen, 2006), with only 45% of males and 39% of females between the ages of 18 and 24 using condoms consistently (National Survey of Sexual Health and Behavior, 2010). Young adults may feel awkward asking their sexual partner to use protection, believing it implies they have an STD. Finally, young adults may believe that condoms are not needed in monogamous relationships even though these relationships may be short-term.

Having multiple sexual partners in combination with inconsistent use of condoms can place young adults at a high risk for contracting an STD/STI. Approximately half of all new STD cases in the United States occurs in individuals aged 15 to 24 (Weinstock, Berman, & Cates, 2004), and nearly a quarter of sexually active young adults (ages 15 to 24) will contract an STD each year (Kaiser Family Foundation, 2006). Chlamydia, a bacterial infection that may lead to infertility and causes few, if any, symptoms, is the most frequently reported STD in the United States. Young adults can also contract the following STDs: gonorrhea, syphilis, genital herpes, human papillomavirus (HPV), and genital warts. These infections can pose serious threats to individuals' physical health and may cause complications such as pelvic inflammatory disease, infertility, ectopic pregnancy, preterm birth, and fetal abnormalities. Given that several STD symptoms surface only many years after initially contracting the disease, young adults tend to have limited knowledge and poor understanding of STDs. Young people, on the other hand, are very familiar with HIV, the human immunodeficiency virus that leads to AIDS (autoimmune deficiency syndrome), and are aware of the risk associated with the disease. They perceive the health risks associated with HIV/AIDS to exceed those of other STDS. While the number of new HIV infections per year in the United States, about 50,000, has remained stable in recent years (CDC, 2012b), young adults remain at risk for contracting HIV. In 2009, 39% of all new HIV infections in the United States occurred in persons between the ages of 13 and 29 (CDC, 2011k). The risk for contracting HIV is especially high among younger gay, bisexual, and other men who have sex with men, with this population accounting for 69% of all new HIV infections among young persons (CDC, 2011k).

Alcohol and drug use can increase the likelihood that young adults will engage in sexually risky behaviors. A survey concerning the sexual attitudes and practices of young adults found that 88% of young adults reported using alcohol or drugs before engaging in sex at least some of the time (Kaiser Family Foundation, 2002). Most participants also reported that condoms were not frequently used when under the influence of drugs or alcohol, and nearly a third worried about contracting STDs or an unplanned pregnancy because of engaging in

Think About It   13.1

Given that most young adults are at peak physical functioning and relatively healthy, they often have difficulty understanding that poor lifestyle choices have a negative impact on well-being. How might a counselor assist a young adult who does not understand the consequences of his/her poor lifestyle choices? How might the cognitive development of a young adult affect the lifestyle decisions he/she makes? How might limited access to health care affect young adults who do seek out medical or counseling services?

unsafe sex while drinking or using drugs. More recent studies have shown that substance use increases the probability that young adults will initiate sexual activity, have unprotected sexual intercourse, engage in casual sex, and have multiple sex partners (e.g., Leigh, Ames, & Stacey, 2008; Roberts & Kennedy, 2006; Winters, Botzet, Fahnhorst, Baumel, & Lee, 2009).

The lifestyles of young adults can have a significant impact on their physical health and well-being. Engaging in bad habits such as smoking, drinking, using drugs, eating a high-fat diet, and practicing unsafe sex can prevent young adults from reaching peak physical performance and may negatively affect their health in middle adulthood, possibly contributing to premature death. Racial, gender, and sexual minorities (and the intersection of these characteristics) are particularly vulnerable to the negative consequences of poor lifestyle choices in young adulthood. Counselors can play a key role in helping all young adults to establish healthy lifestyles. Specifically, counselors can help young adult clients to understand the impact of their lifestyle habits on their current level of health and well-being. Counselors can provide information on healthy habits (e.g., diet, exercise, recommended sleep) and discuss the health consequences of unhealthy practices with their clients. It may also be helpful to provide the client with a referral to visit a general practitioner for further consultation and advice on maintaining a healthy lifestyle. Finally, counselors can empower minority clients who experience oppression and advocate for social justice in their broader communities.

SECTION II: Cognitive Development

Counselors working with young adults may notice dramatic shifts in their clients' thinking over a short span of time. For instance, a counselor may observe young adults who originally entered counseling searching for the "right" answers and demanding concrete solutions to their problems becoming more comfortable with the ambiguity that characterizes many of the problems experienced in life and starting to look within themselves for answers after just a few sessions. Cognitive development does not end with adolescence. Changes in the actual structure of the brain occur in early adulthood, giving rise to new perspectives and ways of thinking. As a result, counselors will notice that young adult clients experience advances in cognition, intelligence, and moral reasoning.

Brain Development

Advances in early adult cognition are, in large part, due to the continuing physical development of the brain. Several studies provide evidence that development in the human brain continues throughout early adulthood and may even extend into the third decade of life (e.g., Bennett & Baird, 2006; Grohol, 2006; Lebel & Beaulieu, 2011; Vaillant et al., 1998). The prefrontal cortex experiences a "growth spurt," causing gray matter in the brain to decrease and white matter to increase. During puberty gray matter is overproduced and must undergo a pruning process in early adulthood. **Synaptic pruning** involves the discarding of synaptic connections (i.e., gray matter) that are no longer used by the brain. The frontal lobes also undergo enhanced **myelination**, which refers to the development of fatty sheaths that provide insulation to the remaining synaptic connections. Enhanced myelination increases the brain's white matter and improves the efficiency of established neural connections (Ashtari et al., 2007; Lebel, Leemans, Phillips, & Beaulieu, 2008). Synaptic pruning and myelination ensure that young adults have fewer, but more selective and stronger, synaptic connections than they did as children. These stronger synaptic connections enhance the efficiency of cognitive processing (Kuhn, 2006; Steinberg, 2004) and contribute to increases in young adults' ability to understand and evaluate abstract material, and to assimilate emotion and cognition (Fischer & Pruyne, 2003; LaBouvie-Vief, 2006; Steinberg, 2004). While much attention has been paid to processes of synaptic pruning and myelination in young adults, Steinberg (2007) points out that the frontal regions of the brain also become more integrated in early adulthood. This process is likely to contribute to gradual enhancements in cognitive-emotional control. Specifically, Steinberg proposes that young adults are less susceptible than adolescents to acting on gut feelings without thinking through a situation, and less likely to over-attend to thoughts when feelings should also be given consideration.

Adult Cognition: Moving beyond Adolescent Formal Operations

Unlike Jean Piaget (1980), who believed the formal operational stage (characterized by logic, absolute truth, and correct solutions) was the final stage of cognitive development, contemporary theorists and researchers believe that adult cognition and thought processes are qualitatively different from adolescent formal operations (Kitchener, King, & DeLuca, 2006; Sinnott, 1998). Postformal thought emerges during early adulthood and may be fostered by experiences gained through exposure to higher education (Fischer & Pruyne, 2003; Labouvie-Vief, 2006). The term **postformal thought** is used to refer to the advances in adult cognition characterized by (1) relativistic thinking, (2) flexibility and pragmatics, (3) tolerance for ambiguity and contradictions, and (4) cognitive-affective complexity.

Adults who demonstrate postformal thought recognize that truth is not absolute, but is relative to context and varies from situation to situation. They also realize that solutions to problems in life must be realistic, and they are able to remain flexible in generating solutions to such problems. Adults accept that contradictions and ambiguity are the rule rather than the exception, as they are constantly confronted with contrary viewpoints and people in society. Finally, they are aware that emotion and other subjective circumstances play a large role in the way they think and make decisions. The transition from Piaget's formal operations to this proposed postformal stage of thinking is often difficult to navigate and requires individuals to exchange more assured ways of thinking about their world for worldviews that are often vague and uncertain. Such a change can cause young adults to experience discomfort, anxiety, and a sense of meaninglessness. Perhaps due to the discomfort associated with postformal thought, not all individuals reach the postformal stage of thinking, and those who do may expect to step in and out of this way of thinking (Sinnott, 1998). In order to better understand the transition to postformal thinking, consider Case Example 13.2.

➤ CASE EXAMPLE **13.2** ERICA.

Erica is a 20-year-old retail worker who attends the local community college part time. She recently sought out counseling for relationship issues. Erica has been dating her current boyfriend for the past three months. She enjoys his company and talks about how much fun they have together. She tells the counselor that her boyfriend recently asked her to move in with him. This request has made Erica very uneasy, and she believes that, even though she really likes her boyfriend, she needs to end the relationship before it becomes more serious. Upon further probing, Erica discloses that she is a devout Southern Baptist and her boyfriend, Chris, is an atheist. Her religious faith is very important to her and defines who she is as a person. Erica further states that her religious upbringing taught her that atheists are bad people who deny Christ and, as a result, do not go to heaven. However, she does not believe Chris to be a bad person at all. She describes how he is respectful of her, loves his family, and even volunteers his time at the local YMCA. He seems to embody several Christ-like characteristics, even though he is an atheist. Erica's relationship with Chris is beginning to cause her to question her own faith. She is experiencing anxiety because what she thought she knew does not seem to hold true with Chris in the picture. How can someone so loving and giving as Chris not be accepted into heaven? How can she, as a Christian, be in love with an atheist? Erica states that she is very confused; this cannot be God's plan for her life. She is supposed to fall in love with and marry a fellow Christian man. She cannot continue this relationship with an atheist and be a Christian at the same time.

Erica's relationship with Chris is forcing her to cope with new information that directly contradicts her current worldview and her religious beliefs. She is currently unable to reconcile her strong feelings for Chris with her religious beliefs, and this dissonance is causing her to experience anxiety. As Erica's counselor, how would you help her navigate the transition from formal operational to postformal thinking? This question will be considered throughout the remainder of this section as the theoretical observations of several well-known scholars help conceptualize the emergence of postformal thought in early adulthood.

Perry's Theory of Intellectual and Ethical Development in the College Years

William Perry (1970, 1999) was among the first to expand beyond Piaget's formal operational stage. Using hundreds of volunteer male students from Harvard, Perry developed a stage-based theory that outlined the intellectual and ethical development of students in higher education settings. From his research, nine stages of development emerged, indicating the transition from absolute adherence to authority and experts to the recognition that one must make personal commitments and decisions based on these commitments (see Table 13.1).

TABLE 13.1 ✦ TRANSITIONING TO POSTFORMAL THOUGHT: PERRY'S NINE STAGES OF DEVELOPMENT

Dualism
(Existence of absolute truth)

- *Position 1:* Characterized by dichotomous thought (e.g., good vs. bad, right vs. wrong), Authorities know the absolute truth.
- *Position 2:* Recognition that uncertainty can exist, but this lack of knowledge is attributed to unqualified authorities.

Multiplicity
(Acceptance of multiple viewpoints)

- *Position 3:* Accepts the fact that multiple viewpoints exist on some matters, but believes that the truth will eventually emerge from authorities.
- *Position 4a:* Recognition of diverse viewpoints as legitimate and that anyone has the right to an opinion.
- *Position 4b:* Authorities may not have the right answers and one must learn to think independently, supporting his/her conclusions with outside sources or data.

Relativism
(Truth is contextual)

- *Position 5:* All knowledge is contextual; there are rarely simple answers to defining right and wrong.
- *Position 6:* Recognize the importance of making personal commitments to certain worldviews rather than relying on an outside authority.

Commitment to Relativism
(Commitment to personal beliefs and values)

- *Position 7:* Initial commitments to specific worldviews and values are made.
- *Position 8:* Exploration of the implications of personal commitments and how they may conflict with societal responsibilities.
- *Position 9:* Personal identity is formed based on commitments, and individuals learn to balance these commitments with societal responsibilities.

Perry's nine stages can be divided among four broader categories: dualism, multiplicity, relativism, and commitment to relativism. **Dualism** refers to polaristic thinking (e.g., good or bad, right or wrong) and the existence of absolute truth. Much like Erica in Case Example 13.2, dualistic thinkers rely on authorities, such as teachers and religious leaders, to provide this absolute knowledge and truth. Dualistic thinkers often hold rigid worldviews that are dictated by black-and-white rules. For example, in Erica's worldview the Christian faith is seen as the one real truth and all other ways of thinking are seen as wrong. **Multiplicity** marks the transition from dualistic to more relativistic thinking. Individuals in this stage realize the legitimacy of multiple viewpoints and no longer believe authorities hold absolute truth. Erica can be seen as moving toward multiplicity. Her experience dating Chris is not congruent with her rigid religious beliefs, and the cognitive dissonance caused by this new experience is causing her to question the absoluteness of her own worldview. A counselor who can support Erica's current dualistic position while gently encouraging her to challenge her beliefs can help Erica move into multiplicity. **Relativism** refers to a significant cognitive shift in recognizing that whether something is right or wrong depends on the situation, and truth exists in a specific context. Individuals also begin to recognize the importance of making personal commitments in an ambiguous world as opposed to following authority. In the case of Erica, the relativistic thinker realizes the complexities of the situation and that no ultimate solution exists. The individual may realize that the religious authority does not account for the intricacies in this particular case, and may spend a great deal of time reflecting on the obligation to religious authority and family versus personal desires and viewpoints. A person may also wrestle over the consequences of both remaining in and leaving the relationship. Finally, **commitment to relativism** refers to the process of choosing and adhering to personal commitments; this is Perry's highest level of development. During this stage, individuals are able to commit to certain worldviews, while maintaining a sense of awareness and respect for divergent viewpoints. Those in this stage also attempt to balance their personal commitments with societal responsibilities.

REFLECTION 13.2 A PERSONAL JOURNEY THROUGH PERRY'S LENS

Every semester that I teach Perry's theory of development and inevitability, my students and I find ourselves discussing the complexities of why people move from dualistic to relativistic thinking and how this can be achieved with the assistance of a counselor. While I do not have exact answers to such complex questions, my own personal experiences do provide some insight into the movement from dualism to relativism. I grew up in a small, rural community with minimal exposure to diverse people and ways of thinking, which allowed me to view the world in very simplistic, black-and-white ways. While I was certain, in my late teens, that I knew what was "right" and "wrong," I did have a strong sense of curiosity and passion for learning. When I entered my freshman year of college, I was suddenly exposed to people and viewpoints that were starkly different than "my truth." This exposure to diversity was the impetus for my shift from dualistic to relativistic thinking. As the things I once believed to be ultimate truth became one perspective in a sea of multiple perspectives, I found myself questioning what I thought I knew and searching for answers. It was a particularly frightening and scary time for me as my ways of knowing were shifting. I had minimal support from my family and community, and felt like I was abandoning everything that was important to me. However, my passion for learning and innate sense of curiosity pushed me to challenge my thinking and ways of being in the world. I also sought support from professors and friends, and exposed myself to diverse viewpoints and people whenever I could. The support I received from those around me and the exposure to diversity were invaluable in my transition from dualistic to relativistic thinking, but I believe the driving force during this transition was my own curiosity and determination to keep pushing forward. It was important to me, at the time, to question my childhood ways of knowing and to search out my truth. I think it is important that counselors remember that not every client will be willing or have the desire to move from dualistic to relativistic thinking, and unless the client is motivated to move forward, the counselor's efforts may be futile. [~SC]

Women's Ways of Knowing

William Perry's theory of development provides important information regarding the process of cognitive maturity in adults, but he has been heavily criticized for basing the theory solely on male perspectives. Using Perry's theory as a framework, in addition to the work of Gilligan (1982), Belenky, Bond, and Weinstock (1997) conducted interviews with women from diverse socioeconomic backgrounds to determine whether women differ from men in their cognitive development. From the data collected during these interviews, Belenky and her associates developed a model that included five different knowledge perspectives through which women view themselves and the world. These five perspectives, which are outlined in Belenky et al.'s seminal work *Women's Ways of Knowing*, include:

1. *Silence.* This first stage is characterized by right versus wrong, similar to Perry's dualism stage. Women view themselves as "deaf and dumb," having no independent voice, being incapable of thinking, and being afraid of authorities.
2. *Received knowledge.* In the second stage, women learn by listening to authorities, believing that absolute truth comes from those in positions of power. They are also unable to tolerate ambiguity and discrepancies.
3. *Subjective knowledge.* During this stage, women begin to distrust outside sources of knowledge and start to recognize themselves as an authority. Consequently, women rely on their own subjective experiences for knowledge and truth.
4. *Procedural knowledge.* This stage is characterized by a recognition that multiple sources of knowledge exist and is coupled with the realization that both personal experiences and outside information are important for gaining knowledge. Procedural knowers, similar to Perry's position 4b, employ reflective reasoning and evaluate information within a given context.
5. *Constructed knowledge.* In this final stage of development, women acknowledge that all knowledge is constructed. These women have a high tolerance for ambiguity and even feel connected to other people when differences in worldviews exist. Finally, constructed knowers have the ability to listen, contribute, and work collaboratively without losing their own voice.

Kitchener's Model of Reflective Judgment

Young adults face a variety of complex dilemmas. These dilemmas may require making personal choices (e.g., choosing whether or not to pursue additional school and a high-powered career instead of starting a family and focusing on child-rearing) and/or societal decisions (e.g., how to reform U.S. health care). Kitchener (1983) referred to these dilemmas as ill-defined problems where no one acceptable solution or agreed-upon way to solve the issue exists. Kitchener further proposed that young adults develop reflective judgment to assist them in solving ill-defined problems. **Reflexive judgment** refers to the way in which adults analyze and reason through a dilemma, as well as justify the solutions they develop. Through research, Kitchener and her associates (King & Kitchener, 1994; Kitchener, King, & DeLuca, 2006) found that reflexive judgment develops through a series of seven predictable stages. Similar to Perry's findings, young adults move from believing in absolute truth to a position of relativism.

In the early stages (1 through 3) of reflective development, individuals demonstrate prereflective thought, believing in the existence of supreme knowledge and absolute certainties, relying on authorities or personal justification (e.g., that is just the way it is). Consequently, they fail to realize that problems do not always have a clear solution or absolute answer. A college student in the prereflective stages may push his professor to provide the "correct" answer to a subjective problem or elaborate on the "right" counseling theory to explain human behavior. The student may also unyieldingly adhere to a position when discussing controversial issues without showing respect or regard for other, viable positions.

The middle stages (4 and 5) of development, known as quasi-reflective thinking, are characterized by a recognition of the uncertainties inherent in knowledge and an over-reliance on personal opinion to justify reasoning (e.g., only reading books that support one's pre-established belief). Individuals in this stage of development realize that knowledge is subjective. A college student in these stages will remind the professor that nothing can be known for sure and is likely to change his/her viewpoints based on the context of the situation. When discussing controversial issues the student is less persuasive, insisting that everyone is entitled to their own opinion.

In the later stages (6 and 7), individuals begin to demonstrate true reflective judgment and have the ability to reflect on knowledge, understand the uncertainties inherent in knowledge, and recognize the importance of critically evaluating information. Students in these stages have given careful thought to their viewpoints, often considering several alternative perspectives, and hold firm to their beliefs. They realize, however, that these beliefs must be constantly reevaluated as new evidence emerges.

Kitchener and Fischer (1990; Kitchener, Lynch, Fischer, & Wood, 1993) indicated that progression through the seven stages is dependent on two factors: optimal level of development and skill acquisition. The term **optimal level of development** refers to the highest level of cognitive performance (i.e., information processing) that a person is capable of achieving. Kitchener and Fischer noted that people will fail at any task that is more complex than their optimal level. Individuals' optimal level of development increases as they age through "growth spurts" that mark significant changes in cognition. A period of stability will follow these growth spurts, providing individuals time to become adept at using their newly acquired cognitive skills. The term **skill acquisition** refers to the gradual process of learning new cognitive abilities. During the periods of stability, individuals slowly become proficient in using new cognitive skills through a series of small and often haphazard steps before they are ready to move to the next level of development. The presence of environmental supports may also affect an individual's level of development. King and Kitchener (1994) theorized that, on a daily basis, many people often operate at cognitive levels lower than their optimal level of development due to a lack of environmental supports. Kail and Cavanaugh (2010) illustrate this point by highlighting the nature of exams in a typical college course. For most, those dreaded exams ask students to choose the best answer, requiring that one correct answer be chosen when multiple correct answers to the problem exist. One must learn to master the dualism that characterizes the prereflective judgment instead of exercising high levels of reflective judgment that emphasize relativistic thinking. If college exams asked students to pick multiple answers to each question, thus encouraging higher levels of cognitive performance, then perhaps students would be able to demonstrate higher levels of cognitive complexity on a daily basis!

Schaie's Model of Adult Cognitive Development

Formal operational thought is characterized by the ability to (1) systematically apply logical reasoning to an abstract problem, and (2) consider the possibilities that may occur. In adolescent thinking, reality takes a back seat to idealism, leaving little room for realistic or pragmatic thought. Several researchers have proposed that as young adults face the constraints of reality, their idealism decreases and they rely less on logical analysis to solve problems (Labouvie-Vief, 1990). Instead, young adults focus on the practical integration of their knowledge and skills, and finding their place in the workplace and society (Labouvie-Vief, 1990; Schaie, 1993).

One well-known theory that addresses young adults' shift from acquiring knowledge and using logic reasoning to applying what they know in order to be successful in work and life tasks is derived from Schaie's (1993) work on adult cognitive development. Specifically, Shaie's theory addresses how adults adjust to the new roles, needs, and responsibilities that emerge throughout the lifespan. Through a series of seven sequential stages, Schaie describes how cognitive functioning shifts from the acquisition of information and skills (i.e., what I need to know about the world), to the practical integration of knowledge and skills (i.e., how to use what I know to be successful in the world), to searching for meaning and purpose (i.e., why it is important that I should know). Early in life children are sheltered from many of life's responsibilities, leaving time for them to focus on learning skills, such as problem solving and logical reasoning, that will assist them in being successful members of society. As young adults, individuals begin to face responsibilities and ill-defined problems (i.e., problems with no pre-established answers), such as whether to marry and have children, what career to pursue. At this stage individuals must make the cognitive shift from learning new skills and knowledge to practically applying the skills and knowledge they already know. Through the practical application of preexisting knowledge, individuals are able to effectively solve problems and pursue long-term goals. Table 13.2 outlines Schaie's seven life stages in detail.

Labouvie-Vief: Cognitive-Affective Complexity

In addition to the rise of relativistic, reflective, and pragmatic thought in early adulthood, Labouvie-Vief, Chiodo, Goguen, Diehl, and Orwoll (1995) also noted changes in the cognitive-affective complexity of young adults. **Cognitive-affective complexity** refers to the capacity to integrate one's emotions and pragmatic reasoning when solving problems and making decisions. Labouvie-Vief and DeVoe (1991) observed that the development of intellect and

TABLE 13.2 ✦ SCHAIE'S STAGES OF COGNITIVE DEVELOPMENT

Stage One: Acquisition	*Childhood and adolescence* Children are sheltered from most of life's responsibilities and can focus solely on learning the skills and knowledge needed to prepare for adulthood. In particular, children develop problem-solving skills and logical thinking.
Stage Two: Achieving	*Early Adulthood* (20s and early 30s) Young adults begin to take on life responsibilities and face ill-defined, complex problems. In order to effectively problem solve and work toward life goals, young adults must apply the knowledge and skills they learned in the acquisition stage. They no longer learn for the sake of learning, but focus on sharpening preexisting skills and knowledge.
Stage Three: Responsible	*Adulthood* (late 30s to 60s) Adults face the responsibility for caring for others in addition to themselves. They apply their knowledge and skills to caring for spouses, parents, children, coworkers, and community members.
Stage Four: Executive	*Middle Adulthood* (30s–50s) Adults in the middle stages of life may have executive responsibilities and be in charge of societal systems (e.g., local government, organizations). These individuals must learn to navigate complex relationships and demonstrate acceptance of diverse perspectives, commitment, and conflict resolution skills. This stage may overlap with the achieving and responsibility stages.
Stage Five: Reorganizational	*End of Middle Adulthood* This period may be marked by retirement and a decrease in responsibilities. Adults must reorganize their existing knowledge and skills to tasks associated with retirement (e.g., engagement in leisure tasks, budgeting and managing finances).
Stage Six: Reintegrative	*Late Adulthood* Older adults focus less on acquiring and applying new knowledge and skills. Instead they focus on creating a sense of purpose from meaningful tasks.
Stage Seven: Legacy-Creating	*Advanced Old Age* Adults who are nearing the end of their lives focus on providing a written or oral account of their lives to pass on to future generations. Given that the task of creating a legacy requires that cognitive energy be devoted to long-term memory recall, individuals rely less on problem-solving and decision-making skills at this point in life.

Think About It   13.2

Many of the theories related to cognitive development in young adulthood imply that higher stages of
cognitive development, such as relativism, are more
optimal than lower stages of cognitive development,
such as dualism. Do you believe it is imperative that
young adults must achieve the highest levels of cognitive development in order to be well adjusted, healthy
individuals? Explain. What are some scenarios where it
might be important for a counselor to assist a young
adult in moving from a more dualistic perspective to a
more relativistic perspective?

affect are parallel, believing that "the experience of emotions is qualitatively restructured as the growing individual
acquires more complex categories with which to think about
the world" (p. 172). In particular, Labouvie-Vief et al. (1995)
described the simultaneous development of emotions and
cognition throughout the lifespan through four sequential
stages: self-protective, dysregulated, complex, and integrated.
As individuals progress through these stages, they move from
an inability to fully understand their emotional experience
and emotions cloud their thoughts and problem-solving abilities to achieving high levels of cognitive-affective complexity. The capacity for cognitive-affective thinking originates in
early adulthood when the ability to think complexly about
affect emerges. Young adults, however, still have difficulty balancing their emotions with pragmatic reasoning, and their thoughts and decisions may be
easily swayed by emotions. Even though this age group demonstrates an improvement over
the emotionally driven stage of adolescents, Labouvie-Vief, Grühn, and Studer (2010) maintain that the highest levels of cognitive-affective complexity do not develop until midlife.

Intelligence

Intelligence in young adults is a highly complex and multifaceted concept. Most theories of intelligence are multidimensional, involving several aspects of cognitive ability
(e.g., abstract thought, creativity, emotional intelligence, problem solving, reasoning,
learning). One theory of intelligence, the Horn-Cattell-Carroll theory, has received a good
deal of attention in adult developmental research. This theory contends that intelligence
is comprised of several general factors, including fluid and crystallized intelligence. **Fluid
intelligence** refers to the ability to think logically, demonstrate mental flexibility, and solve
problems in new and unfamiliar situations. It allows you to understand and respond to
novel situations through identifying patterns, understanding relationships among concepts, and the use of inductive and deductive reasoning. Fluid intelligence does not rely on
acquired knowledge through educational experiences, but is largely determined by genetic
factors. Abstract reasoning problems, such as the one below, are considered an accurate
way to assess fluid intelligence.

Example: Which number should come next in this series? 45, 44, 42, 39, 35. . . ? A. 24; B. 25;
C. 30; or D. 34.

If you chose answer C, you are correct! For those who may need a helpful hint, the pattern decreases progressively: -1, -2, -3, etc. As you can see, no specific knowledge (e.g.,
algebraic formulas, vocabulary words) is required to complete this problem, which makes it
ideal for assessing fluid intelligence.

Crystallized intelligence refers to the breadth of knowledge acquired through formal
education and life experiences in a particular culture. It is the ability to use the specific
skills, knowledge, and experiences gained throughout a lifetime. For example, a child who
had just learned to read a simple sentence or to count to 10 has just expanded his/her
crystallized intelligence. One may demonstrate crystallized intelligence when spouting off
historical facts, sports trivia, or reciting the preamble to the Constitution memorized in
third grade. While crystallized intelligence involves acquiring knowledge specific to one's
culture, it relies heavily on the person's underlying fluid intelligence (Horn, 1982). For
example, the extent of knowledge regarding history is dependent to some degree on how
quickly one is capable of making connections between new historical facts read and the

historical information already known (a form of fluid intelligence). People with high fluid intelligence tend to acquire more crystallized knowledge at a faster pace.

Changes in Fluid and Crystallized Intelligence

Several longitudinal studies have shown that general intelligence (i.e., IQ) is highly stable throughout an individual's lifetime (e.g., Deary, Whiteman, Starr, Whalley, & Fox, 2004; Hoeksta, Bartels, & Boomsma, 2007). Fluid and crystallized intelligence, however, can undergo dramatic shifts over the lifespan. For instance, research has shown that mathematicians and theoretical physicists make their most important contributions to their respective fields by age 30 (Simonton, 1988). Likewise, chess players peak in their mid-30s, achieving their highest rankings during this period (Charness & Bosman, 1990). These "shooting stars" shine early, doing their best work in young adulthood, then fizzle out. You may wonder, what accounts for the fizzling out of some of the world's most promising young minds? Do theoretical physicists, mathematicians, and chess players become less intelligent as they age?

While there are no simple answers to this complex observation, one can logically speculate that changes in fluid and crystallized intelligence may partially account for this early intellectual peak. Fluid intelligence declines throughout adulthood, whereas crystallized intelligence improves (Schaie, 1993). The decline of fluid intelligences means that it becomes more difficult for adults to learn a new language or to employ higher-order problem solving needed in the mathematical and scientific fields. Although it is unclear as to why fluid intelligence declines as we age, Horn and Hofer (1992) attributed changes in this type of intelligence to structural and chemical changes that occur in the adult brain as a result of disease, injury, and growing older. As we age, very few adults devote time to solving abstract reasoning problems like the example on the previous page. Unfortunately, changes in fluid intelligence are fairly uniform throughout the lifespan, with all individuals experiencing a decline in their ability to employ logical reasoning and problem solving to novel situations. However, individual differences in crystallized intelligence as we age are dependent on our exposure to information and environments that facilitate learning. For example, as one reads through this text, one is working to improve one's crystallized intelligence of lifespan development. Other students in class may choose not to read the text and are missing an opportunity to expand their crystallized intelligence/knowledge.

As demonstrated in Figure 13.2, crystallized intelligence tends to peak in late adolescence and remains constant throughout the adult years and into old age. Conversely, fluid intelligence tends to peak in late adolescence and diminish throughout the adult years and into old age.

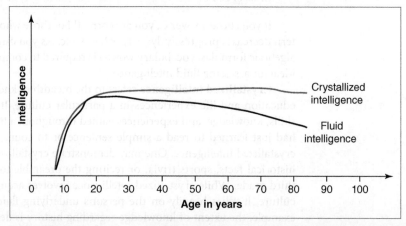

Figure 13.2 The longitudinal pattern of fluid and crystallized intelligences.

Changes in Divergent Thinking and Creativity

Additional answers as to why our mathematician and theoretical physicist "shooting stars" intellectually peak early may lie in our ability to engage in divergent thinking. Guilford (1967; Guilford & Hoepfner, 1971) developed one of the best-known general models of intelligence: structure of intellect. One of the most important contributions of the structure of intellect model is the distinction between convergent and divergent production. **Convergent production** refers to deriving a single, correct answer to an objective question. This type of thinking emphasizes speed, accuracy, and logic, and is most effective in situations where a correct answer needs to be recalled from memory. **Divergent production**, on the other hand, requires the ability to generate multiple solutions to a question or problem. Individuals who demonstrate divergent thinking are able to draw on ideas from multiple disciplines and sources of knowledge to create their own solutions to open-ended problems. According to Guilford (1975), divergent thinking is an important component of human creativity.

Several researchers have found that, similar to fluid intelligence, divergent thinking and creativity peak in early adulthood and slowly decline throughout adulthood (Alspaugh & Birren, 1977; McCrae, Arenberg, & Costa, 1987; Reese, Lee, Cohen, & Puckett, 2001; Ruth & Birren, 1985). Much like our physicists and mathematicians, Lehman (1960) found that people's most creative products were produced in their 30s, and 80% of the creative contributions were completed by age 50. Before all of us under that age of 50 seclude ourselves for months from our jobs and school work to develop an innovative contribution to society, it is worth noting that recent studies report that divergent thinking may not decline as rapidly as previous researchers suggested. Foos and Boone (2008), who studied adult age differences in divergent thinking, found that older adults had the capability to think as divergently as young adults, but did so at a much slower rate. The researchers concluded that divergent thinking remains intact throughout the lifespan, but slows as we grow older. Csikszentmihalyi (2000) also believes that everyone, regardless of age, is capable of achieving a creative flow (i.e., a heighted state of pleasure) when we take on mental and physical challenges that consume us. Consequently, all individuals should be encouraged to spend time in settings that stimulate creativity and to follow activities and ideas that spark personal interest.

Moral and Ethical Development

> A trolley is out of control, running rapidly down a track. Five people have been tied to the track by a crazy moral development researcher and are in the trolley's path. You have access to a switch that, should you choose to flip it, will divert the trolley down an alternate track and save the five people. Unfortunately, there is a single person tied to the alternate track. Should you flip the switch or do nothing?

As you mull this question over in your mind, it probably will not take long for you to realize that Foot's (1978) moral dilemma has no easy solution. Each possible decision leads to devastating consequences and raises moral issues about the value of human life. Such dilemmas force us to answer the question, "What is the ethical thing to do in this situation?"

Moral Reasoning

Young adults not only experience shifts in their information-processing and problem-solving skills; they also undergo changes in moral judgment. **Moral judgment** refers to the process of reasoning through and reaching a decision about moral issues. You may recall from earlier chapters that Lawrence Kohlberg (1969; Kohlberg & Hersh, 1977) believed moral judgment involved a process of rational deliberation, or reasoning, and developed through a series of six stages across the lifespan. Kohlberg's highest stage, postconventional moral reasoning, emerges in mid-adolescence to early adulthood and is thought to be facilitated by cognitive and environmental factors. The emergence of relativistic and reflective thinking, coupled with experiences that require one to encounter conflicting values (e.g., moving away from home to attend college) and be responsible for the well-being of others (e.g., parenthood), enhances young adults' ability to comprehend and evaluate moral dilemmas from new perspectives. Kohlberg argued that an individual's moral development could not exceed one's level of cognitive development; consequently, he expected that some adults would never achieve postconventional moral reasoning.

Young adults in Kohlberg's **postconventional stages of moral reasoning** come to rely less on external standards when making ethical decisions and more on a personal moral code rooted in universal ethical principles. Individuals in stage 5, Social Contract and Individual Rights, question the validity of societal laws/rules and begin to recognize that such laws/rules may not always promote justice or protect basic human rights. Also, people may work toward changing unfair laws/rules and improving society through a democratic process. Remember the classic "Heinz" dilemma Kohlberg posed to participants in his study? In case the reader is drawing a blank, here is a quick refresher: Heinz's wife is terminally ill with cancer, but he cannot afford the drug needed to save her life. The pharmacist is unwilling to bargain with him, so Heinz considers breaking into the drugstore to steal the drug. Kohlberg found that people at a stage 5 level of moral reasoning would reason in favor of Heinz stealing the drug to promote the universal value of saving human life.

At the highest level of moral reasoning, stage 6, Universal Principles, individuals operate by their own personal moral code and conscience, which are driven by respect for individual human rights and dignity. Persons are prepared to violate societal laws/rules that are in conflict with their ethical conscience. When presented with the Heinz dilemma, Kohlberg reported that people at a stage 6 level of moral reasoning would also approve of Heinz stealing the drug, arguing that they believed saving human life promoted universal rights and justice over breaking the law. Kohlberg posited that very few individuals reach the final stage of moral reasoning. He did believe that a handful of moral leaders (e.g., Martin Luther King, Jr., Mohandas Gandhi, Mother Teresa) successfully demonstrated this final stage of moral reasoning through their acts of civil disobedience, which served to advance universal principles of justice.

Carol Gilligan (1982) proposed that moral judgment consisted of more than principles of justice. Believing that Kolhberg's theory favored male moral development, Gilligan speculated that young women placed greater importance on social relationships and caring for others when making moral decisions. She further proposed that women defined morality as an obligation to exercise care and avoid hurting others. While research has failed to support the existence of gender differences in moral reasoning, it is important for counselors to consider that factors other than universal justice may be important in the process of developing moral judgment.

Moral Intuition

In contrast to Kolhberg, Haidt (2001, 2007) believed emotion, not reasoning, is fundamental to making moral judgments. Haidt proposed that it is individuals' immediate emotional reaction to the moral dilemma that drives their actions. Think back to the out-of-control trolley example that opened this section. What if the person tied to the alternative track was a close relative (e.g., partner, child, parent)? What are your immediate impressions of this new situation? Do you believe your emotions affected your thoughts on whether or not it was right to flip the switch? If so, moral intuition may be rendering a judgment about principles of morality.

Moral intuition refers to an instantaneous emotional reaction of approval or disapproval of a person's actions or behavior. Young adults using moral intuition make an immediate, intuitive judgment about a situation, and then employ cognitive reasoning to justify their initial "gut feelings" (Haidt, 2007). Your first instinct after reading that your mother was tied to the alternate track may have been not to flip the switch. To validate this decision, you may need to engage in some mental legwork, convincing yourself that your mother's life is certainly more valuable than the lives of five strangers. Anybody else in your position would certainly have reacted in the same manner, right? Moral intuition is supported by research; several brain imaging studies show that areas of the brain responsible for emotion are activated when people are asked to respond to a moral dilemma (Ciaramelli, Muccioli, Ladavas, & di Pellegrino, 2007; Greene, Sommerville, Nystrom, Darley, & Cohen, 2001). While moral intuition offers the benefits of immediacy and the use of emotion, it may lead to errors in moral judgment (Reyna & Farley, 2006). What if the "right" thing to do is to flip the switch and save five lives? We cannot overlook the importance of methodical deliberation and analysis to evaluate the complex nature of moral dilemmas.

Moral Relativism: The Impact of Technology on Moral Development

Laptops, iPads, e-readers, texting, Facebook®, tweeting, avatars, and Android phones are just a few of the technological advances of the past decade. These gadgets, along with the boom of the Internet, have exponentially increased our access to information and ability to communicate with one another. Never before has so much information been at one's finger tips. People have the ability to share information with a hundred of their "closest friends" at the click of a button. Emerging research suggests this increased exposure to information and people may affect the moral development of today's young adults. In particular, Stein and Dawson-Tunik (2004) have found that the Millennial generation, young adults born in the 1990s, exhibit moral relativism.

Moral relativism recognizes that differences in moral judgments (i.e., what is right vs. wrong) exist across diverse cultures. In other words, no universal moral standard can be applied to all individuals as people from different cultural backgrounds have different ways of interpreting right and wrong. Stein and Dawson-Tunik (2004) believe that Millennials' tendency toward moral relativism can be attributed to technological advances in the 21st century. Today's young adults, through advances like the Internet, have increased exposure to diverse people and ways of thinking, leading them to question whether "what is moral to me, is moral to you." As a result, they may not value universal codes of morality, but instead choose to define right and wrong from their own personal experiences and cultural norms.

Summary

Becoming an adult is a developmental process and is rarely associated with chronological age in Western cultures. Instead, adulthood is associated with achieving the following tasks: (1) accepting responsibility for oneself, (2) making independent decisions, and (3) becoming financially independent (Arnett & Tanner, 2006). The developmental phase of emerging adulthood, or young adulthood, marks this transitional period from adolescence to adulthood. Arnett (2004) proposed that this developmental phase of the lifespan is characterized by five key characteristics: identity exploration, self-focus, instability, feeling-in-between, and opportunity. In addition to these defining features, emerging adulthood ushers in a variety of physical and cognitive changes.

Young adults experience a peak in their physical performance. Biological systems are highly efficient and the senses are decidedly acute. Physical strength, coordination, dexterity, agility, and flexibility also peak. Most individuals are healthiest during young adulthood and are often exempt from health issues associated with serious illness. While young adults experience peak physical functioning and health, many engage in poor lifestyle practices that compromise their health and may lead to untimely death. The most common lifestyle habits that affect the health of young adults include tobacco use, alcohol and illicit drug use, poor diet and lack of exercise, sleep deprivation, and sexually risky behaviors. A particularly dangerous lifestyle behavior that increases in young adulthood is binge drinking. Binge drinking is defined as having five or more drinks in a row at least one day in the past month. Binge drinking peaks around age 21 years and declines throughout the remainder of young adulthood. While binge drinking behaviors are short-lived for most young adults, it is associated with numerous health issues and risky behaviors. As a professional counselor, it is important to help young adults understand the impact of lifestyle habits on their health and well-being, and to adopt healthy lifestyle practices.

It is now widely accepted that individuals experience gains in cognition during young adulthood. These gains are due in large part to the continuing maturation of the brain. Specifically, the brain of a young adult undergoes synaptic pruning and enhanced myelination. Synaptic pruning and myelination ensure that young adults have fewer, but more selective and stronger, synaptic connections, which enhance the efficiency of cognitive processing (Kuhn, 2006; Steinberg, 2004) and the ability to evaluate abstract material. Developmental theorists use the term postformal thought to characterize advances in adult cognition. Postformal thought is distinct from Piaget's formal operational stage of cognitive functioning and is defined by the following achievements:

(1) relativistic thinking, (2) flexibility and pragmatics, (3) tolerance for ambiguity and contradictions, and (4) cognitive-affective complexity.

William Perry (1970, 1999) was one of the first developmental theorists to delineate adult stages of cognitive development beyond Piaget's formal operational stage. According to Perry's nine-stage theory, individuals move from dualistic thought, an absolute adherence to authority and experts, to relativistic thinking, which recognizes the contextual nature of knowledge and involves committing to one's own worldviews rather than relying on outside authority. Kitchener (1983) also proposed that young adults move to a position of relativism and develop reflective judgment to help solve life's ill-defined problems. In addition to adopting relativistic thinking, young adults experience enhancements in cognitive-affective complexity. This increased capacity to integrate one's emotions and pragmatic reasoning when solving problems leads to decreased emotional reactivity. Young adults also demonstrate marked increases in divergent thinking and creativity. Specifically, they are able to draw on ideas from numerous disciplines and generate multiple solutions for a problem. Finally, individuals undergo changes in their moral judgment in young adulthood. Kohlberg's highest stage, postconventional moral reasoning, emerges in mid-adolescence to early adulthood due to the emergence of relativistic thinking and increasingly encountering life's ill-defined problems. As a result, young adults come to rely less on external standards when making ethical decisions and more on a personal moral code rooted in universal ethical principles. As the expansion of the Internet has increased our access to information and ability to share information globally, young adults today demonstrate moral relativism. They recognize that moral standards vary across cultures and that diverse individuals may have different ways of interpreting right and wrong (Stein & Dawson-Tunik, 2004).

Young Adulthood: Social, Emotional, and Career Development

By Stephanie Crockett

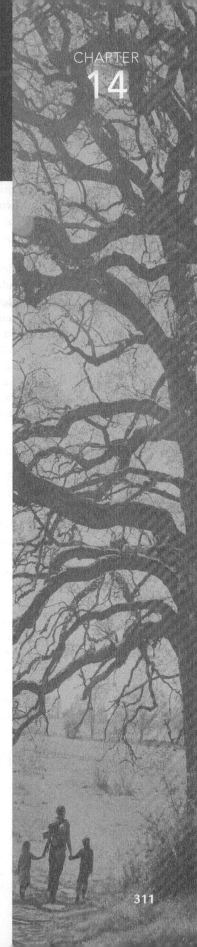

Young adulthood marks a transitional period full of social-emotional and career developmental changes. Most young adults have sufficiently resolved the identity issues associated with adolescence and can begin to focus on establishing intimate relationships and starting a career. Social development in young adulthood is characterized by the development and maintenance of close relationships with intimate partners, friends, and family. In addition to establishing relationships, young adults focus on becoming productive workers and achieving the tasks associated with finding and maintaining a career. This chapter will examine the ways in which young adults go about establishing and maintaining intimate relationships, and the vast variety in lifestyle choices made. Personality development and mental health in young adulthood are also discussed. The second half of the chapter focuses on career selection, vocational preparation, transitioning to the workforce, and balancing work and life roles.

SECTION I: Social/Emotional Development

Ben recently graduated with an associate's degree from a two-year community college. He has spent the past few years living at home, going to school, and working for his father's business. After graduating Ben suddenly finds that he is faced with several decisions to make about the next steps in his life. He received a job offer in a neighboring town that would give him an opportunity to use his new degree. And his partner, Marcus, has asked him to consider moving in with him. Ben wonders if he is ready to take a new job, leave home, and begin a life with his partner.

Like many young adults, Ben finds himself faced with several social and emotional developmental tasks that characterize early adulthood. Specifically, the transition to adulthood involves establishing independence, managing a household, starting a career, developing intimate relationships, and becoming a parent. Such tasks can present challenges to many young adults and require making tough decisions. If young adults are able to successfully complete these social and emotional developmental tasks, they are likely to achieve independence and lead well-adjusted lives. In this section, the developmental tasks specific to young adulthood and the impact of such tasks on the family lifecycle are discussed. In addition, how young adulthood affects personality development and the mental health of young adults will be considered. Finally, the formation of intimate relationships and lifestyle choices of young adults are explored.

Developmental Tasks of Early Adulthood

Robert Havighurst (1952), a developmental theorist, was among the first to introduce the idea of developmental tasks. **Developmental tasks** can be thought of as assignments that individuals are expected to complete during a specific period in their life. Havighurst believed people progress through a series of developmental stages during their lifespan and that each developmental stage consists of developmental tasks that need to be completed. Young adulthood involves the completion of seven developmental tasks: selection of a mate, learning to live with a partner, starting a family, raising children, managing a home, starting an occupation, and assuming civic responsibilities. These tasks of young adulthood arise from both social expectations and personal standards. For example, young adults often seek to move out of their parents' house and find a job after completing college, based on society's expectation that college graduates should support themselves. Those who are not able to support themselves after college are nicknamed "boomerang kids," because they are launched and then return home, and are sometimes perceived to be a burden to parents. The successful completion of developmental tasks in early adulthood reflects gains in intellectual, social, and emotional skills, and ordinarily leads to happiness and success as well as the opportunity to accomplish future developmental tasks. Failure to complete such tasks

---

Think About It   14.1

Consider a 20-year-old client who lives at home with his parents and attends a local technical school. As counselors, we would most likely consider this situation to be normal. However, what if the client was 30 years old and still living at home, where his mother cooks his meals and does his laundry? What would be your immediate reaction to this client? Most likely, some would pathologize the latter client, thinking that his circumstances were developmentally inappropriate. Some may also react negatively to an 18-year-old client who is pregnant and considering marriage, versus a 27-year-old client in the same situation. Bottom line: Both the task and the timing of completion play a role in early adult development.

REFLECTION 14.1 ON TIME? OFF TIME?

Reflecting back on my life, it is difficult to know with certainty what key events in my life have been "on time" and "off time." I got married in my early 20s and went back to school for my master's degree. I perceived these events to be very much "on time" as they conformed to societal and familial expectations regarding the timing when one should get married and pursue a career. I was never directly told that these events were expected to occur during my 20s, but I received several social cues that let me know my life was on track. Such cues included support for my decisions from family and friends, as well as financial resources. For example, my parents paid for my wedding, no questions asked. As I moved into my 30s, I feel like I fell behind on the social clock. My partner and I still rented; despite nearly 10 years of marriage, we did not have children; and I continued to pursue my education instead of beginning a career. Instead of feeling supported by family and friends, I began to feel pressure to achieve these developmental milestones. The messages I received were very subtle; for example, my dad would comment on how we were throwing away money by renting. I also started seeing friends post pictures of their children on Facebook and it reminded me of how isolated my life was becoming as my social clock became "off time." I internalized these messages and the societal pressure I felt; I started to doubt the educational choices I had made for myself and wondered if I was disappointing those around me. I went from feeling normal to feeling isolated and substandard. [~SC]

often leads to unhappiness, disapproval from others, social seclusion, and difficulty with later developmental tasks.

The Social Clock of Early Adulthood

While Havighurst (1956) focused on the specific tasks of early adulthood, it is important to also consider the timing of such events. The examples in Think About It 14.1 may elicit a negative reaction from counselors because they violate our social clock. The **social clock** refers to societal norms that dictate the age by which certain life events should occur (Neugarten, Moore, & Lowe, 1965). Young adults are considered to be "on time" if key life events are experienced at the normative age; "off time" adults experience key events at a nonnormative age.

Much like the experiences shared in Reflection 14.1, failure to conform to society's social clock can lead individuals to experience criticism from family and friends, societal disapproval, lowered self-esteem, isolation, lack of support, and access to fewer resources. The negative consequences associated with going against the social clock are many and, for this reason, most individuals find themselves conforming to society's expectations regarding the tasks of early adulthood. Two studies by Settersen and her associate (Settersen, 2003; Settersen & Hagestad, 1996) suggested, however, that the time of key life events is in fact becoming more flexible. Adults are beginning to wait until later in life to marry and have children. Also, many individuals are now pursuing a four-year college degree and starting a career in middle adulthood. While the social clock plays a key role in young adult development, it is important for counselors to remember that this is a socially constructed phenomenon. Whether a person considers oneself to be "on time" or "off time" depends on societal, cultural, and individual factors.

Family Life Development in Early Adulthood

Up to now the discussion of developmental tasks has involved only the individual (i.e., the young adult). Yet families, like individuals, change over the course of time, progressing through a series of developmental stages that parallel the individual tasks of adulthood. Evelyn Duvall (1967) developed the **family lifecycle** to explain the changes families are required to adapt to over time. The family life cycle consists of eight stages: married couples, childbearing families, families with preschool children, families with school children, families with teenagers, families as launching centers, middle-aged parents, and aging family members. Each stage in the family lifecycle involves a series of developmental tasks that must be accomplished in order to successfully move to the next stage. Failure to complete developmental tasks can lead to difficulty in later stages. Within the last decade, Monica McGoldrick and Betty Carter (1999) updated Duvall's family lifecycle stages and developmental tasks to apply to American middle-class families living in the 21st century (see Chapter 2 for more information specific to McGoldrick & Carter's family lifecycle).

According to the family lifecycle, early adulthood commences when single, young adults leave home. During this time, young adults take on both emotional and financial responsibility instead of relying on family members for such support. Individuals also begin to differentiate themselves from their family of origin, developing an identity that is separate from parental beliefs and expectations. Young adults are very much their own, independent persons, but they still benefit from parental acceptance and support. They must learn to navigate the ability to remain autonomous, while maintaining meaningful relationships with their parents. Early adulthood requires that one form adult relationships with parents and renegotiate the boundaries of the parent–child relationship established in childhood. The transition to adulthood and the negotiation of adult relationships with parents can be difficult for the family and inhibit the family's development if (1) the adult child's values and expectations are incompatible with parental values and expectations, and (2) the parents are unable to acknowledge and/or accept the changes that ensue when a child leaves home. Additionally, parents and their children may have a difficult time renegotiating their relationship when the young adult still lives at home and needs parental financial support.

Although most of the focus on family life development during young adulthood is on differentiating from one's family of origin and renegotiating childhood relationships with parents, it is important to note that young adults also begin to form deeper and more intimate peer relationships than in adolescence. The formation of intimate relationships with peers can lead to the development of a romantic relationship and the decision to marry or live with a partner. Marriage or cohabitation creates many new changes for young adults and their families. Young adults must adjust from being single and independent to living with a partner and forming a marital (or cohabitation) system that involves commitment and compromise. Relationships with extended families and friends must be adjusted to include one's partner. Most couples, for instance, initially struggle with deciding how to spend holidays with extended family members, or which set of friends to hang out with on the weekends.

As young adults adjust to living with a partner through marriage or cohabitation, they may have children. Welcoming children into the family gives rise to many new developmental challenges for the couple and their families. The marital system must adjust to make space for the children. The couple must take on parental roles in addition to their role as a partner. They may also have to renegotiate financial, household, and child care responsibilities. Finally, extended family members will assume new roles (e.g., grandparent, aunt, uncle) and may be asked to provide child care.

Personality Development in Early Adulthood

Do you believe that personality changes from adolescence to adulthood, or remains stable? Developmental theorists contend that changes in personality do indeed occur throughout the lifespan. In particular, these theorists propose that adults follow a prescribed, normative sequence of psychosocial and emotional stages as they age. Each stage of development is characterized by an emotional crisis that, if resolved, paves the way for continued personal growth. In this section, we will discuss five diverse theories of emotional-social development that provide insight into the formation of personality in young adulthood.

Erikson's Psychosocial Stages: Intimacy versus Isolation

Erik Erikson (1963) was the first developmental theorist to propose that personality continued to develop in adulthood. Erikson identified stages of psychosocial development that occur throughout a person's lifetime. The stage that emerges in early adulthood is **intimacy versus isolation**, and the principal developmental task facing young adults involves reaching out to other people to make connections and form intimate relationships. According to Erikson, young adults must resolve the previous psychosocial stage, identity verses role confusion, before they can develop intimate relationships with others. He believed it was imperative for individuals to have a strong sense of self before successfully merging their identity with another person. The ability to form intimate relationships requires having a genuine concern for another's needs, and a willingness to sacrifice one's own needs at certain times. If young adults fail to develop the ability to connect with others intimately, they risk becoming socially isolated. Isolation, contrary to intimacy, involves not being able to risk one's identity in order to form intimate relationships. Individuals may be fearful of becoming emotionally and physically close to another person and the consequences that ensue (e.g., being in a committed relationship, having children). Social isolation, for young adults, can lead to a life that is lonely and devoid of meaningful relationships.

Levinson's Seasons of a Man's Life

In an effort to construct a detailed account of male development over the lifespan, Daniel Levinson (1986) and his associates from Yale (Levinson, Darrow, Klein, Levinson, & McKee, 1978) conducted in-depth interviews with 40 middle-aged men. Like Erikson, Levinson's research revealed that men progress through a series of developmental stages, which Levinson called "seasons," throughout the lifespan. Personality development, according to Levinson, is contingent on the evolution of a **life structure**, which he defined as "the underlying pattern or design of a person's life at a given time." (Levinson, 1986, p. 6). Changes in a man's life structure occur as he progresses through six developmental seasons of life.

Levinson viewed early adulthood as a time of exploration, opportunity, and the accomplishment of several life events (e.g., financial independence, beginning a career, marriage, parenthood). Adulthood, the first developmental phase in a man's life structure, begins when he leaves his parents' home, perhaps to attend college, join the military, or take a job. During this developmental period a man achieves financial and emotional independence from his childhood family. While Levinson theorized that this period lasts approximately three to five years, today's young adults may choose to live at home longer, or may return home after finishing college, needing financial support from their parents due to the increasing costs of higher education and the unstable economy (Settersen, 2006). The next developmental stage in a man's life occurs when he enters the adult world and begins to commit to adult roles, responsibilities, and relationships. A man's initial identity and life structure are created as he forms adult relationships, engages in intimate sexual relationships, attains a professional degree(s), and/or takes on employment opportunities. During this period, men may begin to pursue a particular career path, become involved in a long-term committed relationship, and work toward achieving stability in their lives. Entrance into the adult world may be delayed for many of today's young adults as the workforce requires individuals to attain more and more education. Arnett and Tanner (2006) reported that this delay should not be seen as a barrier to young adult development, but should be viewed as a source of support for personal growth, as higher education offers the opportunity to establish a sense of identity, become competent, move toward self-sufficiency, and develop mature relationships with others. Unfortunately, researchers have provided very little information regarding the development of young adults who do not attend college.

Vaillant's Adaptation to Life Approach

George Vaillant (1977) also studied the development of personality in adult men. In 1938, Vaillant began a longitudinal study, following 268 male Harvard undergraduates throughout the course of their adulthood. When the study began, the participants were 18 years of age, and by the time they reached midlife, Vaillant noted that a typical developmental pattern seemed to emerge. Men in their 20s were still heavily influenced by their parents, but were concerned with gaining financial and emotional independence, as well as developing intimate relationships with others. During this time Vaillant observed young men getting married, having children, and working hard to achieve at their jobs. Once they had solidified their personal identity and formed successful, intimate relationships, men in their 30s expanded their identity to include the world of work. In establishing a career identity, men at the end of young adulthood were able to transform their job or hobby into a career by demonstrating contentment, competence, and commitment. While Vaillant initially studied affluent men, he later investigated the developmental pattern of well-educated women and White youth from lower socioeconomic backgrounds. The results of these studies suggested that women and those from lower socioeconomic backgrounds experience a series of developmental changes similar to those described in his initial study (Vaillant, 2002; Vaillant & Milofsky, 1980).

Gould's Evolution of Adult Consciousness

Roger Gould (1972), like Erikson, Levinson, and Vaillant, also suggested that personality development continued into adulthood. Specifically, Gould proposed that adult personality development occurs through a series of six stages by which individuals move from childhood consciousness to adult consciousness. Childhood consciousness is characterized by dependence and reliance on caretakers to provide basic needs and a sense of safety and security. Adult consciousness, on the other hand, involves independence from caretakers, a greater sense of competence, self-understanding, and self-reliance. During each stage of development, individuals abandon childhood myths (i.e., false assumptions that are developed in childhood), begin to confront reality, and raise their level of self-awareness. Gould's first two stages of development occur during young adulthood. The first stage, "leaving the parents' world," begins in late adolescence and involves confronting the childhood myth that young adults will always be dependent on their parents and must accept their belief system. In particular, young adults in this stage shift from a position of dependence on their parents to developing the confidence and skills needed to care for themselves and effectively make decisions about life. Young adults begin to form their own opinions and belief systems that are independent of their parents' values. Young adults may also feel they do not belong in the family any more as they struggle to be independent and learn to rely on people outside of the family for support. As individuals move into their mid-to late 20s, they progress through Gould's second stage of development, "I'm nobody's baby now." This stage involves confronting the childhood myth that if young adults move through life playing by their parents' rules, mustering strength and determination, they will reap benefits. Individuals now feel a strong sense of autonomy, but they are still learning how the world works and must come to realize that people who play by the rules are not always rewarded. Life is not fair and justice may not prevail. Young adults must also come to accept that there is no correct or best way to go about things. Finally, in this stage, young adults learn to commit to adult roles and responsibilities (e.g., being a spouse, having a child, being an employee).

Allport's Dimensions of Maturity

Gordon Allport (1961) believed that adult personality development was characterized by increases in psychological maturity. Allport, unlike Erikson and other emotional-social

TABLE 14.1 ✦ ALLPORT'S SEVEN DIMENSIONS OF MATURITY

Dimension	Description
Extension of the self	Mature adults are able to develop meaningful relationships with persons outside the family, as well as to take on occupational, leisure, and/or civic activities that have true significance for an individual. It is important to note that involvement in relationships and activities involves moving from a sense of obligation to one of personal interest as adults mature.
Relating warmly to others	Adult maturity involves a readiness for intimacy and an ability to develop personal relationships that are characterized by mutuality, empathy, and reciprocity. Individuals must be ready not only to commit to others, but also to be willing to nurture and maintain these intimate relationships.
Emotional security	This dimension is comprised of four qualities: self-acceptance, emotional acceptance, frustration tolerance, and confidence in self-expression. Mature individuals are able to fully accept who they are as people, including their weaknesses. They are also able to acknowledge that emotions, both the good and the bad, are part of the normal human experience. They are not afraid of their emotions, do not let their emotions control their lives, and are able to cope with life's frustrations in a healthy manner.
Realistic perception	Mature individuals are able to perceive the world around them accurately and do not distort their perception of reality to selfishly meet personal needs.
Possession of skills and competencies	Allport believed that all individuals possess a particular skill. Mature adults strive to hone this skill and are driven to express their competence in a skill through engaging in some type of activity, taking pride in their work/accomplishments.
Knowledge of the self	Maturity involves possessing self-insight. In particular, knowledge of one's self involves knowing what one can do or not do, as well as knowing what one ought to do.
Establishing a unifying philosophy of life	Mature individuals are able to develop their own life's purpose based on personal ideals and values. They also develop and implement personal goals based on their philosophy of life, and are able to cope with failures and challenges to meet such goals.

developmental theorists, did not delineate specific stages of personality development. Instead, the development of maturity is viewed as an ongoing process that involves overcoming the obstacles present with each phase of life. Allport identified seven specific dimensions of maturity that emerge in adulthood. The seven dimensions include: (1) extension of the self; (2) relating warmly to others; (3) emotional security; (4) realistic perception; (5) possession of skills and competencies; (6) knowledge of the self; and (7) establishing a unifying philosophy of life. Table 14.1 provides a description of each dimension of maturity. Note that age alone is not a guarantee of maturity. Being 50 years old does not ensure that you are any more mature than you were at age 25. Instead, maturity is nurtured through honing effective coping methods for dealing with life's frustrations and let-downs, as well as the ability to appreciate your achievements and successes.

Mental Health in Young Adulthood

For the general population, young adulthood is a time when the problem behaviors of adolescence dissipate and overall mental health improves. However, the occurrence of psychological disorders (e.g., major depression, schizophrenia) increases. In any given year, experts estimate that anywhere from 14% to 20% of young adults have a diagnosable mental illness (O'Connell, Boat, & Warner, 2009) and nearly 75% of all mental disorders are diagnosed by age 24 (Kim-Cohen et al., 2003). This spike in mental illness during early adulthood may be related to the many demands young adults face. Moving out of one's parents' home into an apartment, starting college and/or a career, and taking on responsibility for one's own well-being can be a liberating experience, but many young adults may find the real-world pressures that come with leaving the safety and security of adolescence to be overwhelming (Schulenberg & Zarrett, 2006). The fear and anxiety of not being able to "make it" in the world may spur the onset of mental illness.

Young adults who suffer from mental illness may struggle to achieve the developmental tasks and achievements associated with early adulthood. They are at higher risk for dropping out of college, abusing substances, being unemployed, having unplanned pregnancies, and having a criminal record (Gralinski-Bakker, Hauser, Stott, Billings, & Allen, 2004; O'Connell et al., 2009). Additionally, young adults with mental health issues have difficulty establishing healthy interpersonal relationships, achieving financial independence, and they experience feelings of loneliness as well as low self-worth (Gralinski-Bakker et al., 2005). While the impact of mental illness on young adults' social and emotional development can be devastating, mental health service utilization drops from adolescence to early adulthood. Teens comprise 13% of outpatient service usage and 38% of inpatient residential care, as compared to 10% and 18% of young adults, respectively (Gralinski-Bakker et al., 2004). Likewise, Mojtabai and Olfson (2008) found that less than one-fourth of college-age adults with mental illness seek treatment. For a professional counselor, half the battle in providing services to this population will be finding creative ways to reach out to young adults and encourage them to seek out professional help. Let us turn our focus now to some of the common disorders that may develop in young adulthood.

Depression

Depression involves a significant degree of sadness over an extended period of time. Depression is one of the most common mental health disorders in the United States, and the incidence of this disorder increases during young adulthood. In fact, it is estimated that one in four adults experience a depressive episode between the ages of 18 and 25 years (Kuwabara, Van Voorhees, Gollan, & Alexander, 2007). The prevalence of depression in early adulthood may be associated with the transition from adolescence to adulthood. As previously mentioned, young adults must confront many challenges as they move toward adulthood, and they may experience increased stress as they work to achieve independence, form intimate relationships, and begin a career. Such pressures may inhibit young adults' ability to cope and lead to a depressive episode. They may also fail to successfully accomplish these major tasks, which can lead to distress and depression. Women are at increased risk of being depressed and are nearly twice as likely as men to be diagnosed with depression. Black women are also 1.6 times more likely to experience depressive symptoms than their White counterparts (CDC, 2014). Several environmental risk factors have also been associated with the onset of depressive symptoms. These include minority stress (e.g., from racial discrimination, heterosexism, sexism), lower socioeconomic status, lower educational levels, having to care for children, and being a single parent with the dual responsibility of maintaining employment and managing a household. In fact, a recent study has shown that minority stress, specifically the experience of heterosexism, was a strong predictor of depression and suicidal ideation in LGBT individuals (Kelleher, 2009). Finally, genetics can increase one's risk of depression, as a person is more likely to have a depressive episode if a family member has been diagnosed with the disorder. Depression may significantly affect daily functioning for a young adult, as they are more likely to experience marital issues, sexual dysfunction, substance abuse, parenting problems, and chronic absenteeism from work than their non-depressed peers (Kuwabara et al., 2007).

Fortunately, depression is treatable, typically involving a combination of antidepressant medication and counseling.

Schizophrenia

Schizophrenia is a chronic and severe mental disorder that is characterized by a breakdown in thought processes and perceptions. This psychotic disorder triggers debilitating symptoms such as delusions, hallucinations, blunted affect, and avolition (i.e., lack of desire to work toward goals). Approximately 1% of the U.S. population has schizophrenia, but those with a parent or sibling with schizophrenia have approximately a 10% chance of developing the disorder (Regier et al., 1993). The onset of schizophrenia ordinarily occurs in early adulthood. Symptoms typically emerge between 20 and 28 years of age in men, and around 26 to 32 years of age in women. Individuals with schizophrenia often have difficulty maintaining long-term employment and establishing relationships. Depending on the severity of symptoms, individuals may also have trouble accomplishing ordinary daily tasks of living. No cure for schizophrenia exists, but symptoms of this disease can be managed effectively through antipsychotic medication and counseling. People with schizophrenia can benefit greatly from individual and/or family counseling, self-help groups, and residential treatment programs. These treatment options can help individuals with schizophrenia live meaningful and rewarding lives in the community.

Addictions

Alcohol abuse and dependence is one of the most prevalent substance use disorders in the United States, with 18 million Americans diagnosed with an alcohol use disorder (National Institute on Alcohol Abuse and Alcoholism, 2013). Alcohol use disorder, as defined by the DSM-5 (American Psychiatric Association, 2013), is a long-term condition characterized by compulsive drinking, increased tolerance, the presence of withdrawal symptoms when alcohol is not present in the body, failure to reduce alcohol use, and interference with daily life. Individuals tend to drink the heaviest in their late teens and early 20, with the onset of alcohol dependence peaking around age 21. It is estimated that at least once a year 46% of young adults consume more alcohol than the recommended daily limit (i.e., two drinks for men and one drink for women) and 14.5% consume more than the recommended weekly limit (National Institute on Alcohol Abuse and Alcoholism, 2006). Engaging in heavy drinking behaviors places young adults at high risk for developing alcohol-related disorders. Grant et al. (2004) found that White males from age 18 to 29 were at the highest risk for alcohol dependence, but noted that alcohol abuse in minority young adults was on the rise, particularly for Black males, Asian females, and Latino males. Heavy drinking in young adults is also associated with increased illicit drug use. As mentioned in the beginning of this chapter, illicit drug use, like heavy drinking, peaks around age 20 years and declines sharply throughout adulthood. Treatment options for alcoholism and other substance disorders include detoxification (i.e., removal of the substance from the body), therapeutic treatment and counseling (e.g., residential rehabilitation facilities, outpatient counseling), and relapse prevention treatment (e.g., Alcoholics Anonymous).

Establishing Intimate Relationships

A critical developmental task of young adulthood is the establishment of intimate relationships. Intimate relationships require individuals to be able to engage in self-disclosure, be empathetic toward others and attentive to others' needs, and demonstrate mutual respect and positive regard. Forming relationships with others also entails self-awareness, conflict-resolution skills, effective communication skills, and the ability to commit to another person.

Young adults must also learn to balance their need for intimacy with independence. They face the challenge of establishing an autonomous identity while developing friendships and romantic relationships that require relying on others. Recall from Erikson's developmental theory that the inability to form intimate relationships can be detrimental to young adults' emotional development. These individuals may seek out or be referred to counseling because they feel depressed or isolated. Young adults may also seek out counseling services if they have difficulty balancing independence and intimacy. In this section, two expressions of intimacy in young adulthood are explored: friendship and love. In addition, interpersonal attraction and attachment are discussed.

Friendship

Friendships play an important role in the lives of young adults. Over 90% of young adult women and 88% of young adult men report they have a best friend of the same sex (Blieszner, 2009). In young adulthood, friendships are often developed through work or parenting activities, and we often seek out friends who are experiencing similar life events. Friends tend to be less stable during this time due to the transient nature of young adulthood. Most individuals leave friends behind to pursue educational opportunities or take a new job; others may relocate to be closer to a potential spouse or partner. Over the course of young adulthood, the number of friends we have and the amount of time spent with friends gradually decreases. Single young adults are more likely to rely on friends to meet their social needs than married adults or couples with children (Carbery & Buhrmester, 1998). While friends may be few and fleeting as individuals progress through young adulthood, friends play an important role in the happiness and well-being of young adults. For instance, friendships can provide emotional support to young adults during the transition period between leaving their parents' home and starting a life with a romantic partner (Collins & van Dulmen, 2006). Young adults also report that living with a group of friends during this time provides much-needed support after a bad day at work, a fight with parents, or a break-up with a romantic partner (Heath & Cleaver, 2003).

When compared to men, women tend to have more intimate relationships and demonstrate more emotional intimacy with a close friend (Boden, Fischer, & Niehuis, 2009). Women are more likely to engage in self-disclosure, sharing their experiences, thoughts, and feelings. They also provide emotional support to friends, listening at length to what their friends have to say. Men typically share information and activities, but confide less in their friends (Rosenbluth & Steil, 1995).

With as many as 76% of young adults using instant messaging or texting and 45% of young adults' time online being spent at social networking sites, a discussion regarding the impact of technology on friendships is imperative. Social scientists and media journalists alike have expressed worry over young adults' increased use of the Internet and other

Think About It 14.2

As a college counselor and professor, I have noticed an increased use in smart phones over the past few years. It seems that nowadays clients and students are engaged in texting, social media, selfies, and video streaming rather than paying attention to what is happening in the moment. For instance, college student clients sit in the waiting room and use their phone instead of engaging with those around them. My students are more likely to spend their breaks in class on their phones rather than talking with classmates. What impact do you think technology and social media are having on young adults' social development. Does it facilitate or hinder their ability to form intimate relationships with people? What role do counselors play in helping young adults develop and maintain meaningful relationships in this increasingly technological era?

social media to establish and maintain friendships. Many believe that Facebook, Twitter, and other modern technologies (e.g., email, instant message, text messaging) do not allow young adults to create the same meaningful and long-lasting relationships that face-to-face communication permits. Several studies (e.g., Kraut et al., 1998; Moody, 2001) have also found that high levels of Internet use are associated with a decrease in a person's social circle and increases in depression and emotional loneliness (i.e., a sense of emptiness brought on by the absence of intimate relationships).

While the use of social media may negatively affect the development of intimate relationships in young adulthood, a few research studies have highlighted the benefits of using technology to form and maintain friendships. Cummings, Lee, and Kraut (2006) studied young adults who were transitioning from high school to college and found that email and instant messaging were useful in helping participants to maintain their high school friendships. In fact, engaging in computer-mediated communication appeared to prevent disruption in friendships more than in-person and phone communication for participants. Cummings et al. suggested that using computer-mediated communication (e.g., email, instant messaging) to maintain friendships contributed to a positive quality of life for young adults as they transitioned to college. Also, Ellison, Steinfield, and Lampe (2007) found that the use of Facebook to establish and maintain friendships may be beneficial for college students with low self-esteem, who otherwise might have shied away from initiating communication with or responding to others. Thus, it is not clear whether the use of technology to develop and sustain intimate relationships is helpful or harmful to young adults. Counselors should therefore consider every client's case individually, as electronic communications may contribute to feelings of isolation and depression for one client, while increasing another client's well-being amidst the transitionary period of young adulthood.

Love

Love is an integral component of intimate relationships. While we normally associate the term love with romantic relationships, close friendships in early adulthood are often founded on mutual affection and devotion. In this section we will consider three widely identified types of love: romantic love, affectionate love, and consummate love.

Romantic and Affectionate Love

Customarily, love has been divided into two broad categories: romantic and affectionate love. **Romantic love**, also referred to as passionate love, is often associated with being "in love" with someone. This type of love involves complex emotions, such as passion, anger, joy, jealousy, and fear; it is also linked to sensual feelings, infatuation, and sexual desire (Berscheid, 2010). In fact, Regan (1998) found that most laypersons believe individuals cannot be "in love" with another unless they find the person sexually desirable. **Affectionate love**, also referred to as companionate love, is described as the type of love you feel for a close friend or family member. Grote and Frieze (2005) described affectionate love as "a comfortable, affectionate, trusting love for a likable partner, based on a deep sense of friendship and involving companionship and the enjoyment of common activities, mutual interests, and shared laughter" (p. 275). Scholars believe that affectionate love forms the basis for many intimate relationships, and that while passionate love predominates in the early stages of a romantic relationship, affectionate love sustains the relationship in the long term. For example, Grote and Frieze found that affectionate love was more highly related to relationship satisfaction, perceived importance of the relationship, and feelings of closeness in married adults than romantic love. College students also indicated that affectionate love was more important to relationship satisfaction than romantic love.

Consummate Love

Robert Sternberg (1986), who developed the triangular theory of love, proposed that love was not simply romantic or affectionate, but was comprised of three main dimensions: passion, intimacy, and commitment.

- *Passion* involves feelings of sexual desire and physical attraction toward someone.
- *Intimacy* involves emotional feelings of warmth, caring, and trust in a relationship.
- *Commitment* involves the intent to maintain the relationship over time, despite the occurrence of hardships.

Consummate love, according to Sternberg, is the most complete form of love; it occurs when all three dimensions of love—passion, intimacy, and commitment–exist in a relationship. We all aspire to achieve consummate love, but it is difficult to maintain the three components long term. Romantic love, the presence of intimacy and passion, often characterizes the early stages of most romantic relationships. Over time, however, feelings of passion may subside and affectionate love, the presence of intimacy and commitment, increases in romantic relationships. Some couples may experience fatuous love, the presence of passion and commitment, and decide to marry after a passionate, whirlwind romance. Others may be infatuated with one another, the presence of passion and absence of intimacy and commitment, in a short-lived romance. Romantic partners may also experience empty love over time, the presence of commitment and absence of passion and intimacy. For example, parents might decide to stay committed to their relationship for the sake of their children long after their passion and affection for one another have faded. Finally, relationships may involve only intimacy and feelings of liking someone, and may not be romantic at all. Mathematically speaking, if Liking = Intimacy alone, Infatuation = Passion alone, and Empty Love = Commitment alone, then combinations of these basic processes lead to more complex love processes: Intimacy + Passion = Romantic Love, Passion + Commitment = Fatuous Love, Intimacy + Commitment = Compassionate Love; thus, Intimacy + Passion + Commitment = Consummate Love.

While Sternberg's theory of consummate love provides counselors with insight regarding love and how it is manifested in intimate relationships, it is important to note that how young adults in the United States define love is significantly shaped by cultural values. For instance, middle-class young adults seek love that involves lifelong commitment and faithfulness (Swidler, 2001). However, the degree to which one values commitment and faithfulness in intimate relationships may be partially dependent on cultural factors such as gender and sexual orientation. Meier, Hull, and Ortyl (2009) found that women value lifelong commitment and faithfulness more than men, and sexual minorities value lifelong commitment and faithfulness less than heterosexual individuals. Heterosexual women were found to value lifelong commitment and faithfulness the most. Young adults, on the whole, tend to have broadly similar ideas as to what love entails; however, our expectations and values regarding love in intimate relationships are significantly influenced by our intersecting identities.

Attraction, Attachment, and Mate Selection

Passion, commitment, and intimacy are key ingredients to a successful, long-lasting romantic relationship, but what initially draws two people together? Is it a romantic pick-up line, a warm smile, or a nice gesture? In this section, key elements of attraction and attachment are considered that have the power to turn two strangers into lifelong lovers.

Interpersonal Attraction

Interpersonal attraction refers to the attraction between two people that leads to the development of an intimate relationship. Attraction arises from our desire to form and maintain close, affectionate relationships with others. Three major factors have been found to influence the degree to which a person is attracted to another. These include *proximity, similarity,* and *physical attractiveness.* The physical distance between people is one of the strongest predictors of whether or not they form a relationship. Consider the findings of a classic social science study by Festinger, Schachter, and Black (1950) that examined the formation of friendships in student housing at the Massachusetts Institute of Technology (MIT). Student residents were randomly assigned to 17 different on-campus dorms; over time, the researchers noticed people who lived near each other were more likely to become friends than those who lived a greater distance apart. In fact, students who lived on the same floor were more likely to be friends with those who lived next door than with students who lived a few doors down. One is also more likely to fall in love with someone who is geographically close than someone who lives miles away. Think about how most couples you know met. They were most likely living in the same city/town, went to the same university, or worked for the same company. People are simply more likely to meet and interact with those who live nearby. Social scientists also believe that proximity plays a role in attraction due to the fact that the more people see someone or something, the more people like it (i.e., the "mere exposure" effect).

Attraction between two people reflects the familiar saying "birds of a feather flock together." As a general rule, we tend to be attracted to people who are similar to us. Researchers used to believe that individuals with complementary personalities were attracted to one another because it enhanced the probability that one's needs would be met (De Raad & Doddema-Winsemius, 1992). For instance, a frugal spender might be attracted to the spontaneity of a partner who spends money on a whim, and the spender may appreciate having someone who is cautious with spending money. Persons may be occasionally drawn to their "opposites," but this attraction usually is often short-lived and rarely develops into a serious intimate relationship. Instead, mate selection, especially in heterosexual couples, is enhanced by similarity in demographics, physical appearance, attitudes, interpersonal style, social and cultural background, personality, interests, and social skills. Several studies have reported that partners in same-sex relationships may not be as similar as heterosexual couples in relation to ethnicity, age, and SES (Jepsen & Jepsen, 2002; Rosenfeld, 2007). Nevertheless, partners who share some similarities are assumed to be attracted to each other as they validate each other's beliefs and assumptions about the world (Morry & Gaines, 2005). Additionally, similarity between individuals may reduce the occurrence of conflict and increase relationship satisfaction (Lutz-Zois, Bradley, Mihalik, & Moorman-Eavers, 2006; Morry & Gaines, 2005).

Physical attractiveness is the final factor that plays a role in interpersonal attraction. In general, we tend to be drawn more to those who are attractive than to less attractive individuals (Sprecher, 1989). Attractive individuals are assumed to be happier, more intelligent, and more successful than those who are less attractive. While good looks may take you far in the dating game, not everyone places equal value on attractiveness when selecting a potential mate. Research demonstrates that men place more importance on physical attractiveness than do women (e.g., Sprecher, Sullivan, & Hatfield, 1994). Women, on the other hand, express more interest in a partner's level of education and financial resources. It is important to note that both genders consider neither physical attractiveness nor financial resources to be the most important attribute of a potential mate. Instead, men and women generally desire a partner who is intelligent, honest, and caring (Impett & Peplau, 2006).

Adult Attachment

The concept of attachment was first introduced in Chapter 4 as a bond that develops between an infant and a caregiver. Recall that caregiver sensitivity toward and attention to the infant's needs determines whether the infant will become securely or insecurely attached to the caregiver. Securely attached infants are able to explore the world around them, returning to the caregiver to obtain comfort and security when they feel uncomfortable or stressed. While romantic relationships differ significantly from parent–child relationships, adults strive to form attachments to significant others in order to fulfill their emotional needs. Like infants, some adults form secure attachments to their romantic partners, whereas others form insecure attachments. The types of attachments formed in adult relationships are largely influenced by early relationships with caregivers. Several studies have demonstrated that young adults who were securely attached in their romantic relationships described being securely attached to their parents during early childhood (e.g., Shaver & Mikulincer, 2009). Early experiences with caregivers affect the way people view the world. People create expectations about how people behave and the way they treat others. These expectations then influence how people relate to others in the intimate relationships formed.

Adult attachment styles refer to unique patterns of thinking, feeling, and behaving in intimate relationships that are influenced by early attachment experiences with caregivers. Four different adult attachment styles have been identified by researchers that reflect the degree to which adults (1) avoid intimacy and being dependent on others, and (2) experience anxiety about being rejected and/or abandoned by others (Fraley & Shaver, 2000). The four attachment styles include:

- *Secure attachment:* Secure people have low anxiety and avoidance, believing that their partner will be kind and attentive to their needs. These individuals are comfortable with relying on others in an intimate relationship.
- *Preoccupied attachment:* Preoccupied people have high anxiety and low avoidance. They desire to form intimate relationships with others, but are very afraid of being rejected. Accordingly, preoccupied individuals may need constant reassurance from their partner that they are loved.
- *Fearful-avoidant attachment:* Fearful-avoidant individuals have high anxiety and high avoidance, believing that they will ultimately be rejected. This distrust of others causes these individuals to avoid growing close to others and forming intimate relationships.
- *Dismissive-avoidant attachment:* Dismissive-avoidant people have low anxiety and high avoidance. They believe others are unreliable and, as a result, tend to be self-sufficient. These individuals are also not concerned with whether they are accepted by others.

Over half of all adults (60%) describe themselves as securely attached in their relationships (Mickelson, Kessler, & Shaver, 1997), and most prefer a securely attached partner (Zeifman & Hazan, 2008). Being a securely attached adult has numerous benefits. Securely attached adults are more likely than those with insecure attachments to be satisfied with their relationships, form long-term intimate relationships characterized by trust and commitment, and have an easier time forming friendships. Insecure individuals, on the other hand, may be more likely to suffer from a number of health-related issues, including chronic pain, headaches, stroke, heart attack, high blood pressure, and ulcers (e.g., Maunder & Hunter, 2001; McWilliams & Bailey, 2010). In addition, insecure attachments in adulthood have been linked to depression (Bifulco, Moran, Ball, & Bernazzoni, 2002). Attachment styles remain somewhat stable over the lifespan, but as counselors it is important to remember that adults do have the capacity to change. Forming an intimate relationship with a partner who is supportive, caring, and attentive to one's needs can help an insecure adult gain self-confidence, learn to trust others, and feel secure.

Young Adult Lifestyles

Today young adults have more flexibility in their lifestyle choices. Marriage is but one choice in a sea of lifestyle options, and the societal stigma attached to lifestyles that are alternatives to marriage is decreasing. Young adults no longer have to aspire to having a spouse, two kids, and a dog. They can choose to live alone, cohabitate with a partner, or live with someone of the same sex. In this section, several of the lifestyle options available to young adults are explored.

Singlehood

Many of today's young adults are choosing to live alone. While 95% of adults do eventually marry, the number of single young adults has sharply increased in recent years. Approximately 73% of men and 63% of women under age 35 years reported being single and never married in 2002, as compared to 64% of men and 52% of women in 1980 (Goodwin, McGill, & Chandra, 2009). Rises in the number of single adults may be attributed to: (1) society's increasing acceptance of the choice to remain single in young adulthood, and (2) young adults' decision to postpone marriage in order to pursue educational and career opportunities. Young adults may also choose to remain single and delay marriage because they enjoy the freedom of singlehood, have concerns about separation and divorce, are searching for an ideal mate, or are dealing with unresolved issues from past relationships.

Single young adults may enjoy several advantages revolving around having the freedom to essentially do as one wishes. Single individuals are able to make personal life and career choices without having to consider a partner's or child's needs. They have financial autonomy, may lead a spontaneous lifestyle, and are free to pursue their own hobbies and interests. Although singlehood provides freedom and independence, it can also be lonely. Soons and Liebroer (2008) found that individuals who are single had the lowest level of well-being when compared to young adults who were dating, cohabitating, or married. Being single may make it difficult for young adults to find their niche in a society where it is still expected that individuals will eventually settle down, marry, and raise a family. Single young adults may feel pressured to get married as they approach middle adulthood, and can experience discrimination if they choose to remain single. Single, never-married women reported experiencing more discrimination (e.g., felt less respected by others, received substandard service at restaurants, were called names such as spinster, bachelorette) than married women. Similarly single, never-married men were more likely to report that they were treated rudely, not viewed as smart, and characterized as dishonest than married men (Burne & Carr, 2005). DePaulo (2006), furthermore, noted that single adults earn less than married adults, have fewer work-related benefits, and are treated inequitably regarding income tax policies and automobile insurance.

Cohabitation

Rates of **cohabitation**, living with a sexual partner outside of marriage, in the United States are dramatically increasing. In 2007, 4.85 million unmarried couples were living together, which is more than 10 times the number of couples (439,000) who were reported to be cohabitating in 1960. Today, nearly half of all women between the ages of 15 and 44 years report having lived with a romantic partner without being married. Cohabitation is especially prevalent in early adulthood, and many young adults may view living with a partner before marriage as an opportunity to determine whether they are compatible with their partner, avoid a bad marriage, and decrease the risk of getting a divorce. In fact, cohabitation precedes over half of all first-time marriages. However, couples who live together before marriage experienced lower marital satisfaction and a decreased quality of married life (Jose, O'Leary, & Moyer, 2010). They were also more likely to separate and have higher rates of divorce than those who did not cohabitate prior to marriage (King & Scott, 2005; Whitehead & Popenoe, 2004).

While over half of all couples who cohabitate are married within five years, some young adults view cohabitation as a permanent lifestyle and are not interested in marriage (Wilson & Stuchbury, 2010). These individuals may not want to deal with the legal ramifications and commitments that accompany marriage. It may also be easier to legally dissolve a cohabitation relationship than a marriage. Most cohabitation relationships are transitory, and in the United States less than one in 10 of these relationships last five years. Rates of cohabitation are higher among young people who have less education and lower income, as well as those who are less religious and have parents who are divorced (Bumpass & Lu, 2000).

Regardless of the reasons for cohabiting, young adults who choose to live with a partner outside of marriage face many challenges. Individuals who cohabitate may experience parental or societal disapproval of their lifestyle choice. A study by Eggebeen (2005) showed that cohabitating young adults often did not receive emotional support from their parents and were less likely to turn to their parents in a time of need than adults who were married. Unmarried individuals who live together do not have the same legal privileges as those who are married; they have limited rights when it comes to purchasing a house or property, filing taxes, and dissolving the relationship. These challenges are likely to place additional strain on a couple's relationship and may lead to maladaptive ways of coping. For example, both men and women in a cohabitation relationship are more likely to report problems with alcohol than married or single individuals. Cohabitating women also report an increased incidence of intimate partner violence than married women (Brownridge, 2009). Children with unmarried parents are more likely to receive poor parenting, experience child abuse, and have behavioral disorders (DeKlyen, Brooks-Gunn, McLanahan, & Knab, 2006).

Marriage

The institution of marriage in the United States has changed dramatically over the past 80 years. One of the most noticeable changes involves a significant decline in the number of young people who are marrying. In the 1960s, approximately 80% of young adults ages 25–34 were married, but in 2009 the overall marriage rate dropped to 45% for this age group. The decline in young adult marriage rates may be due in part to their choice to postpone marriage. In 2010, the average age for a first marriage in the United States peaked at 28.2 years for men and 26.1 years for women, whereas the average age for a first marriage in 1980 was 24 years for men and 21 years for women. The postponement of marriage and overall decline in marriage rates may mirror changes in how today's young adults view marriage. A century ago marriage was seen as the beginning of adulthood, as it offered financial stability, a sense of identity, and an opportunity to raise a family. Young adults in the 21st century, on the other hand, believe that one must complete many of the critical developmental tasks of young adulthood before getting married. Most desire to marry, but want to establish themselves in a career and achieve financial independence before settling down. They also view traditional marriages with fixed gender roles as nonviable in today's society and aspire to create an individual identity separate from their marital role, through pursuing their own careers and interests (Fussell & Furstenberg, 2005).

Most adults do eventually marry. In fact, 81% of men and 86% of women will marry before age 40 years (Goodwin et al., 2009). Marriage rates in the United States, however, do vary according to race/ethnicity, socioeconomic status, and educational level. For example, in 2008 Asian, Hispanic, and White women were twice as likely to be married for the first time as African-American women (U.S. Census Bureau, 2010a). Individuals with a college degree are increasingly more likely to marry than those with a lower level of education. Finally, African-American men who live below the poverty line are less likely to marry than middle-class African-American men (Goodwin et al., 2009). The average length of marriages has risen in recent years. Three out of four couples (75%) married after 1990 reported celebrating a tenth anniversary, which was 3% higher compared to couples married in the 1980s when divorce rates peaked. Scholars believe this increase is due to individuals postponing marriage. This allows men to complete their college degree and become financially stable and mature when they say "I do." More than half of the couples in the United States have been married at least 15 years and a third for 25 years (National Center for Family and Marriage Research, 2010).

Marital Roles and Responsibilities

The transition to married life brings about major changes in young adults' lives. One of these changes involves adapting to new roles and responsibilities. Individuals must learn and adapt to marital roles. Such roles may include initiating affection and sex, being the spiritual leader, resolving marital conflicts, or planning social and recreational activities.

Couples must also decide how to manage their finances, as well as negotiate familial and religious obligations. Aside from these larger roles and responsibilities, newlyweds have to determine how to divide household labor and the tasks of daily living. Gender roles and expectations have always played a significant role in the division of household labor among married couples, but over the past several decades these expectations for men and women have shifted. According to a survey conducted by Amato, Booth, Johnson, and Rogers (2007), both men and women have less conservative gender attitudes than they did in 1980. Specifically, most men surveyed believed their spouse should assist in earning an income and, in turn, husbands should take on more housework responsibilities. Similarly, women expressed a belief that husbands should be responsible for a larger share of household chores and assist more with child care. Despite the shift in gender attitudes over the last two decades, women, even when employed full time, are responsible for the bulk of day-to-day housework and child care. The number of hours women spend on housework has been nearly cut in half since 1960, and the amount of time men spend doing housework has doubled in the past 40 years (Bianchi, Milkie, Sayer, & Robinson, 2000). As a result, the average husband is currently responsible for a third of all housework.

Sex and Marriage: Dealing with Infidelity, Sexual Dysfunction, and Infertility

In addition to adapting to new roles and responsibilities, young adults must also negotiate sexual activity after marriage. Although married couples have sex more often than singles, the frequency of sex may decline after marriage for couples who were cohabiting prior to "tying the knot." Face-to-face interviews with married men and women between ages 18 and 59 reveal that only about a third had sexual intercourse more than once a week (Laumann & Michael, 2001). Married couples do, however, report being more emotionally satisfied from engaging in sex than single or cohabiting individuals (Waite & Joyner, 2001).

It is difficult to know how many married individuals engage in extramarital sex. While the general media reports that up to 60% of men and 40% of women have engaged in sex with someone other than their partner, research suggests that it may actually be a lot less common. For example, a national survey conducted by Whisman and Snyder (2007) found that 6% of women reported engaging in extramarital sex within the past year. Likewise, Smith (2006) reported that only 3% of married individuals had a sexual partner other than their spouse in 2002. The occurrence of extramarital affairs is most prevalent in young adults and, over the past 15 years, rates of infidelity among individuals aged 18–25 have steadily increased (Atkins & Furrow, 2008). Husbands are twice as likely to engage in extramarital sex as their wives, although infidelity rates indicate that men and women under age 40 had similar rates of infidelity between 1991 and 2006 (Smith, 2006). In addition to gender and age, factors associated with an increased risk of engaging in an extramarital affair include personality traits like narcissism, psychoticism and low conscientiousness, degree of marital satisfaction, length of marriage, and opportunity.

The disclosure of an extramarital affair can be devastating for a couple and is a common presenting problem in couples counseling. Betrayed spouses may experience an extreme loss of personal or sexual confidence, have a poor self-image, feel abandoned, and have a decreased sense of belonging. They may also feel angry and betrayed, and experience the need to "get back at" or do justice to their spouse by leaving the relationship. Couples counselors report that extramarital affairs often damage the marital relationship beyond repair. For example, one study found that, as a result of infidelity, 34% of relationships ended in divorce; 43.5% of marriages were preserved, but soured by the experience; 6% of marriages remained intact, but were considered empty and the couple was uncertain whether they would remain together in the future; and only 14.5% of marriages remained intact, experiencing improvement and growth (Charny & Parnass, 1995).

Not all married couples are sexually exclusive; some may, in fact, welcome extramarital sexual relationships. **Open marriages** refer to marriages in which both partners agree that the other may engage in sexual relationships with other individuals. Partners in open marriages do not view these extramarital relationships as infidelity. Instead, these marriages are built on openness and mutual trust. While the research on open marriages is dated, most studies concluded that these marriages, similar to traditional marriages, have both positive and negative aspects. Most partners found their open marriages to be emotionally and sexually satisfying, but some reported feelings of guilt and jealousy, as well as difficulty balancing time between their spouse and extramarital partner (Buunk, 1980, 1981). Some couples may also engage in swinging or partner swapping. **Swingers** are partners in a committed relationship who mutually agree to engage in sexual activities with other like-minded couples as a social activity. Swinging can occur at informal social parties, swingers clubs, or through online social networking sites.

Sexual functioning, which peaks during early adulthood, is an important part of couples' health and well-being. Normal sexual functioning for men and women typically begins with a desire to have sex and/or a longing to express love, feel emotionally closer, and share physical pleasure. This leads to a state of sexual arousal and enjoyment of a sexual experience which may or may not terminate with an orgasm. Unfortunately, sexual dysfunction in the United States is a widespread problem affecting many men and women. It is estimated that 43% of women and a third (30%) of men suffer from sexual problems (Laumann, Paik, & Rosen, 1999). **Sexual dysfunction**, in general, refers to a multidimensional health issue that results from biological, psychological, and interpersonal factors. Due to the psychological nature of some sexual disorders, the DSM-5 provides an overview and diagnostic criteria for several sexual dysfunctions.

The DMS-5 (APA, 2013) defines a sexual dysfunction as a disturbance in sexual desire and response cycle that causes distress and impairment. Common sexual problems include sexual interest/desire dsyfunctions, sexual arousal disorders (e.g., erectile dysfunction, genital arousal dysfunction), persistent sexual arousal dysfunction (e.g., premature ejaculation), orgasmic dysfunction, dyspareunia, vaginismus, and sexual aversion. Several risk factors have been associated with sexual dysfunction in men and women. In particular, individuals with chronic diseases such as diabetes and heart disease experience increased levels of sexual dysfunction. An individual's mental health plays a role in sexual dysfunction. Psychological disorders (e.g., depression) are associated with a decreased sex drive and sexual arousal disorders. Sexual dysfunction is also a common side effect of psychotropic medications. Increased anxiety and stress levels can affect an individual's ability to become sufficiently aroused and reach orgasm. Finally, interpersonal factors may also influence an individual's level of sexual functioning. Bancroft, Loftus, and Long (2003) found that women's emotional well-being was related to the amount of distress reported during sexual activities. Women who felt emotionally close with their partner were less likely to report distress during sexual activity than those with low emotional well-being. Sexual dysfunction often has a significant impact on the quality of a couple's relationship. It may be emotionally distressing for both partners, leading to disruption in the relationship and marital discord.

Infertility is another issue that some young adults may have to face. It is estimated that 7% of all couples experience **infertility**, the inability to conceive a child after 12 months or more of trying without contraceptive use. Fertility in women decreases in their late 20s. For men, age is less of a factor in fertility, but the ability to reproduce does decline by their late 30s. As men and women postpone marriage and the start of a family to pursue educational and career opportunities, infertility has become more widespread. Major causes of infertility are biological, and men and women are equally likely to be the source of fertility issues [American Society for Reproductive Medicine (ASRM), 2011]. The primary cause of infertility in men is a low sperm count. For women, infertility may be caused by blocked fallopian tubes, failure to produce viable ova, or a disease of the uterine lining. In women over 30 years of age, deterioration of the ova due to age is a major cause of infertility. The inability to conceive can be extremely disappointing for a couple. They may struggle with feelings of inadequacy and embarrassment, become depressed, or experience increased anxiety (Clay, 2006). In some cases reproductive issues can be fixed with surgery. Other couples turn to reproductive technologies such as *in vitro* fertilization and donor insemination to help them successfully conceive a child.

Martial Satisfaction

Marriage is hard work! Marriage ushers in a series of challenges. Couples must negotiate daily chores and make key decisions about their life together: who cleans the dishes or cuts the grass, where to live, how to manage finances, how to resolve conflicts, with which in-laws the holidays will be spent. Despite these challenges, marriages can be both satisfying and successful. In particular, a couple's degree of happiness with marriage is determined by their sensitivity toward one another, their ability to be empathic, and their communication and conflict resolution skills (Clements, Stanley, & Markman, 2004). Surprisingly, educational level, how long the couple has known each other or dated before marrying, and whether they cohabitated before marriage have little or no impact on marital success. Another factor of successful marriages is an egalitarian relationship. Amato (2007) found that couples who shared the responsibility in making key decisions reported more marital happiness, less conflict, and were less prone to divorce. Finally, couples who engage in premarital counseling are more satisfied with their marriage and less likely to divorce than couples who did not attend counseling (Stanley, Amato, Johnson, & Markman, 2006). People who are happily married lead longer and healthier lives than those who are divorced or dissatisfied with their marriage. They experience less physical and emotional stress and have fewer psychological problems.

Gay/Lesbian Relationships

Between 40 and 60% of gay men and 45 to 80% of lesbians report being in a committed, romantic relationship. Nearly a third of these couples have lived together for 10 or more years. However, many people may have misconceptions about gay/lesbian relationships, assuming that one partner in the relationship is masculine and the other feminine, or that gays or lesbians have multiple sex partners and rarely enter into a committed, monogamous relationship. Indeed, in many ways gay/lesbian couples are very similar to heterosexual couples. As well-known marriage and family therapists John Gottman and Robert Levenson (2003) observed, "Gay and lesbian couples, like straight couples, deal with every day ups-and-downs of close relationships" (para. 3). Mounting research evidence indicates that gay/lesbian couples are, on average, just as satisfied with their relationships as heterosexual couples (e.g., Gottman & Levenson, 2003; Kurdek, 2001), with satisfaction being relatively high at the beginning of a relationship and decreasing over time (Kurdek, 1998). Gay men and lesbians, in general, report positive feelings regarding their partner and describe themselves as happy in the relationship. Not surprisingly, both heterosexual and homosexual relationship quality is predicted by the same factors: personality characteristics, communication and conflict resolution styles, and perceived level of support for the relationship from family and friends (Kurdek, 2006).

Additionally, homosexual couples have the ability to, and do, build intimate, long-lasting relationships; however, when compared to married heterosexual couples, gay and lesbian couples may be at a slightly higher risk for dissolving their relationship. In particular, female same-sex relationships may dissolve sooner than male same-sex relationships (Carpenter & Gates, 2008). Kurdek believes that same-sex couples are not necessarily less stable, but must endure without the institutional supports that married heterosexual couples have.

Gay and lesbian couples are markedly different from heterosexual couples in many ways. One notable difference between homosexual and heterosexual couples is the division of household labor. Homosexual couples, unlike heterosexual couples, do not assign household labor based on gender stereotypes (e.g., husband cuts the grass and wife cooks the dinner). Instead, members of gay and lesbian couples are more likely to negotiate the division of tasks and attempt to accommodate partners' diverse interests, skills, and schedules (Kurdek, 2006). Gay and lesbian couples also tend to resolve conflict better than heterosexual couples. Gottman and Levenson (2003) found that homosexual couples are more likely to remain positive during a disagreement, using fewer controlling emotional tactics and taking negative comments less personally. A final difference between homosexual and heterosexual couples relates to relationship support. Gay and lesbian couples are less likely to receive support for their relationship from family members as compared to heterosexual couples. In particular, families may refuse to accept the same-sex couple and may end emotional or financial support. Same-sex couples often must rely on friends for support and encouragement. Same-sex couples may also face the absence of legal, social, political, economic, and religious support for their relationship. In much of the United States, gays and lesbians are still fighting for the legal recognition of their unions and the right to adopt children. As of 2015, 36 states permit same-sex marriage.

Despite the lack of familial and institutional support, same-sex couples can be healthy and happy if they receive high levels of support from friends (Kurdek & Schmidt, 1987). A final difference between same-sex and heterosexual couples concerns the practice of monogamy. Male same-sex couples have been found to practice sexual monogamy less than female same-sex couples and heterosexual couples. According to researchers, sexual monogamy is viewed as separate from emotional faithfulness in male same-sex couples (Kurdek, 1991), and that being faithful to one's partner emotionally is more important than sexual exclusivity (Adam, 2006). These findings suggest that the practice of monogamy is shaped by gender, sexual orientation, and the intersection of these characteristics.

Parenthood

Beginning a family is a significant developmental task that often occurs in early adulthood. For many young adults, the decision to become a parent is planned in advance and coordinated with the couple's financial situation, but it may be a complete surprise to others. Regardless, the arrival of a child marks a major transition in the lives of new parents. While it is a time of excitement, joy, and wonder, new parents may also feel anxious and overwhelmed by their new roles. In this section the transition to parenthood and how having children affects a couple's relationship is further explored. Nontraditional paths to parenthood will also be considered by looking at parenting for gay/lesbian couples and single parents.

The Transition to Parenthood

Today people in the United States are having fewer children and choosing to start a family later in life. In 2005, the average age of a mother at the birth of a first child was 25, as compared to 21 years of age in 1970 (Martin et al., 2009). Young couples may prefer to delay pregnancy until they have achieved educational and career goals, and are financially stable. The age of a first-time mother does, however, vary with ethnic background. For example, in

2006 the average age of Asian-American and Pacific Islander new mothers was 28.5 years, compared to American-Indian and Alaska Native women, who were just under 22 years of age when their first child was born. It is also important to note that voluntary childlessness has increased dramatically over the last few decades (Chancey, 2006).

The onset of parenthood can be quite stressful for both members of the couple, placing strain on the couple's relationship. Marital satisfaction typically declines after the birth of a baby. Young couples with infants report lower satisfaction with the overall quality and intimacy of their marital life than childless couples (Schulz, Cowan, & Cowan, 2006). New parents must provide around-the-clock care to their new baby and find they have less time to show affection and engage in leisure activities with one another. Sexual intimacy may also decrease during this time as the exhaustion from providing care to an infant causes sexual desire to decrease. An increased workload, coupled with exhaustion and less time for intimacy, can trigger marital conflict and disagreements (Nomaguchi & Milkie, 2003). Marital conflict may also ensue over disagreements regarding the division of child and household responsibilities. Although most mothers now work outside the home, they are still largely responsible for the care of children and the home. The unequal distribution of domestic tasks may leave some women feeling overworked and underappreciated, and they may begin to harbor feelings of resentment and anger toward their spouse. Fathers today are more involved in raising their children and taking on household responsibilities than they were 45 years ago. In 2006, fathers spent twice as much time per week on household chores (9.7 hours) and providing child care (6.5 hours) than in 1965 (Bianchi, Robinson, & Milkie, 2006). As fathers become more involved in providing child care, couples may discover they endorse different parenting styles and practices. These differences may cause additional friction between the couple as they try to negotiate the best way to raise their child.

The demands associated with parenting can take an emotional toll on individuals. Men and women raising children are more likely to have higher levels of depression than individuals without children (Evenson & Simon, 2005). High levels of parental stress are also associated with child abuse (Haskett, Ahern, Sabourin Ward, & Allaire, 2006). Parents are more likely to abuse their children when they have a history of being verbally or physically aggressive, were abused in childhood, have substance abuse issues, struggle with mental illness, experience domestic violence, and/or perceive their child to have behavioral problems (Barth, 2009; Hazen, Connelly, Kelleher, Landsverk, & Barth, 2004; Jones, Macias, Gold, Barreira, & Fisher, 2008; Smith, Johnson, Pears, Fisher, & DeGarmo, 2007). As mandated reporters, counselors should be aware of these warning signs as they interact with children and their parents, and be prepared to provide resources and community referrals to parents who are struggling. For a comprehensive list of child abuse warning signs and symptoms, counselors should see Child Welfare Information Gateway (2007). Counselors should also be prepared to report any suspicion of child abuse to Child Protective Services (CPS).

While the transition to parenthood can be difficult for couples, not all couples experience declines in marital satisfaction. New parents who demonstrate their affection and appreciation for one another, and who refrain from showing disappointment and reacting negatively toward their partner, are able to maintain higher levels of marital satisfaction (Shapiro, Gottman, & Carrere, 2000). Supportive spouses who demonstrate a sense of partnership and commitment to mutual caretaking also act as a buffer against martial dissatisfaction. Couples who have realistic expectations of parenthood may weather the stress of the transition better than those with unrealistic expectations. They understand that the arrival of a child creates additional responsibilities and restricts the amount of quality time the couple will spend together. Finally, participation in a professionally led parenthood group that focuses on parenting and relationship issues may assist couples in transitioning to their new roles as parents and decreasing the stress that accompanies the arrival of a child (Schulz et al., 2006).

Nontraditional Paths to Parenthood

There are many paths to parenthood, and the transition to being a mother or father does not have to occur within the context of a heterosexual marriage. Individuals can be single parents, or they can cohabitate with a partner of the same or opposite sex. In this section, parenthood from the perspectives of gay/lesbian couples and single parents is explored.

Gay/Lesbian Couples

Today, many gay and lesbian couples are choosing to become parents. In fact, approximately 20% of same-sex couples do have children. The path to parenthood for same-sex couples may involve having children from a previous heterosexual relationship, choosing to adopt a child, receiving donor insemination, or surrogacy. While our society has questioned whether having two moms or two dads is optimal for a child's development, research shows that gay and lesbian parents are just as devoted and capable as heterosexual parents, and that the children of same-sex parents generally are well adjusted (Tasker, 2005; Wainright, Russell, & Patterson, 2004). Same-sex parents and their children may, however, face homophobia and societal disapproval, which can lead to feelings of self-doubt and ambivalence about parenthood (Bos, van Balen, & van den Boom, 2007). Despite these barriers, same-sex couples with children report greater interpersonal satisfaction than same-sex couples who remain childless (Shechory & Ziv, 2007). They are also more likely to divide child care and household tasks equally than heterosexual couples. Gay couples also have greater financial resources due to their combined salaries than lesbian or heterosexual couples.

Single Parents

Growing up in a single-parent household is increasingly common for many children in the United States. In 2007, there were approximately 13.7 million single parents in the United States, who were raising 21.8 million children (26% of U.S. children) (Grall, 2009). The U.S. Census Bureau (see Grall, 2009) also reported that the majority of single parents are women (84%) who are divorced (45%) or never married (34%). Nearly 80% of single mothers are gainfully employed, though a third of employed mothers work part time. Only 16% of single parents are fathers, and over half (57.8%) of single fathers are divorced or separated. Ninety percent of single fathers are gainfully employed, and 71% of those fathers work full time. As a result, very few (12.9%) single fathers and their children live in poverty, as compared to the nearly 30% of single mothers who live in poverty with their children. Poverty rates are higher among single parents who are young (i.e., under 30 years of age), Black, and have never been married.

Single parents often face more barriers to raising their children than do married parents. They often have fewer financial resources, minimal coping resources, and increased responsibilities. Specifically, single parents are responsible for child care, maintaining a household, and providing economically for the family. As a result, single parents may struggle to balance child care with their careers. Some single parents must also work more than one job to make ends meet, which limits the time they spend with their children. The stress and extra responsibilities of single parenthood can have a negative impact on the functioning of both the parent and the child. For instance, Chairney, Boyle, Offord, and Racine (2003) found that single mothers were more likely to suffer from depression than married mothers. Single mothers often experienced isolation, having little involvement with friends and family, and were less likely to have a strong support system, which contributed to their depression.

Growing up in a single-parent household is associated with poor academic performance and increased behavioral problems in children. Children in both single-father and single-mother families are outperformed academically by children from two-parent families (Lee & Kushner, 2008). Children from single-parent families are also more likely to receive less parental monitoring and to make decisions without consulting a parent. As a result, these children are more susceptible to peer pressure, exhibit higher levels of delinquency and problem behavior, and display higher rates of adolescent substance abuse and smoking (Griffin, Botvin, Scheier, Diaz, & Miller, 2000). While being raised by a single parent can negatively affect a child, children who are raised by a single parent in multigenerational households fare equally well academically as children raised in a two-parent family (Deleire & Kalil, 2003). The presence of grandparents can provide additional financial support for the single parent and assist with child care, increasing the access a child has to parental figures.

Divorce and Remarriage

Within the past 10 years the number of couples divorcing in the United States has steadily declined compared to the divorce rate in the 1980s and 1990s. Still, rates of divorce are high. Approximately one in five adults in the United States has been divorced (Kreider, 2005), and 50% of all marriages currently end in divorce. Rates of divorce are more prevalent in:

- People with a lower income and fewer of the resources that are needed to establish a household (Martin & Parashar, 2006),
- Young adults who marry in their late teens and early 20s (Raley & Bumpass, 2003),
- Couples who rely solely on each other for emotional support (Coontz, 2006), and
- Women whose parents divorced when they were children (Whitton, Rhoades, Stanley, & Markman, 2008).

Divorce is also more likely to occur if one or more of the following is present in a couple's relationship: alcoholism, mental health problems, domestic violence, infidelity, or inequity in the division of household tasks. Most marriages that end in divorce do so after seven to eight years. Hence the phrase "the seven-year itch," or desire to seek out intimate relationships outside of marriage. Most couples do not divorce because they have become bored, as implied by the "seven-year itch" phrase. A study that detailed the accounts of 130 divorced women found that the most frequently cited reasons for divorce were incompatibility and a lack of emotional support (Dolan & Hoffman, 1998). Additional reasons may include spousal or child abuse, a lack of career support, infidelity, a breakdown in communication, and differences in priorities and expectations.

The breakup of a marriage can be a particularly painful time for a couple. Divorce may result in reducing one's standard of living, disputes of personal property and finances, relocating to a new residence, and changes in relationships with family and friends. Men and women may also experience declines in physical and mental functioning due to the stress of a divorce. In particular, individuals may have low self-esteem, decreased feelings of happiness, increased psychological distress, and feel socially isolated (Amato, 2000). Conversely, the end of a highly conflicted and/or abusive marriage may bring a sense of relief and increase an individual's long-term well-being.

Despite the hardship associated with divorce and the ending of a marriage, many adults form new intimate relationships and remarry. In the United States, one out of every three marriages is a remarriage (Kreider, 2005). Individuals also tend to remarry rather quickly, with half of all remarriages occurring three to four years after a divorce (Family Watch, 2011). Typically, men remarry earlier than women, and men with higher incomes are more likely to remarry than those with lower incomes.

People who remarry face many challenges. Remarried couples are often unstable and are more likely to divorce in the first few years of the remarriage than first-marriage couples (Waite, Luo, & Lewin, 2009). Adults in remarriages may also be dealing with mental health issues, such as depression and alcoholism. Remarriage may involve the blending of two families, and couples may experience additional stress as they adjust to the stepparent role.

Women report more difficulty raising stepchildren than their own biological children (MacDonald & DeMaris, 1996). Stepparenting may be especially difficult if the stepchildren are older. The new blended family does, however, eventually provide a warm and loving environment for all of its members. The family becomes an integrated unit, and a strong alliance is formed between the couple in order to ensure that all family members' needs are met. Several additional benefits are associated with remarrying. For example, remarriage may improve the financial status of one or both partners, and the new marital arrangement is often more egalitarian than the first marriage (Waite et al., 2009).

SECTION II: Career Development

A central task of young adulthood is beginning a career. In addition to forming intimate relationships, finding a partner, and starting a family, young adults invest much time and energy into choosing a vocation, receiving the training needed to qualify for a particular vocation, and establishing a career. The tasks associated with finding and maintaining a career are often stressful and may lead a young adult to seek career or personal counseling (see Case Example 14.1).

➤ CASE EXAMPLE **14.1**   BONITA.

Bonita is a 19-year-old sophomore at a four-year college majoring in chemistry. She is seeking counseling at the on-campus counseling center because she has noticed a steady decline in her grades over the past two semesters, and she has also been feeling depressed for the past few months. Bonita believes she is not smart enough to major in chemistry and describes the course material as being "way over her head." She can no longer keep up in her classes and is really worried about how her slipping grades will affect her chances of being accepted into a medical school. Bonita also worries that if she should fail to go to medical school she will let her family down. She is a first-generation college student and feels a lot of pressure to complete college and have a career.

Young adults can face numerous challenges in establishing a career that provides financial stability, satisfaction, and happiness. These challenges often cut across family and personal issues. It is important for counselors to understand career development in young adulthood and how cultural and personal circumstances affect the process of establishing a career for young adults. This final section of the young adulthood chapter examines how young adults choose a career, options for vocational training, and the workforce transition. The process of career development for women and minorities and how young adults balance work and family are also explored.

Selecting a Career

The selection of a career in young adulthood is often a complex process. It requires young adults to know themselves (e.g., skills, values, interests) as well as information about the world of work. Individuals must also use the personal and work information they gather to make a decision about which career to pursue. This subsection explores the factors that affect an individual's career decision and the process young adults go through to select a career.

Factors That Affect Career Selection

Many career theories highlight the importance of personality in understanding why people choose certain careers. One such theorist is John Holland (1997), who proposed six different personality and work environment types: realistic, investigative, artistic, social, enterprising, and conventional. Holland also believed that people had preferred ways of

TABLE 14.2 ✦ HOLLAND'S PERSONALITY TYPOLOGIES AND RELATED OCCUPATIONS

	Personality Types					
	Realistic	Investigative	Artistic	Social	Enterprising	Conventional
Description	Possess mechanical and athletic abilities; enjoy working with tools, machinery, and objects; prefer dealing with things rather than people	Possess analytical, mathematical, and technical abilities; enjoy working work alone and solving problems; prefer to work with ideas	Possess innovative and creative abilities; enjoy emotional expression and creating unconventional works; prefer to work with ideas rather than people	Possess interpersonal skills in mentoring, teaching, and healing; enjoy helping people and have a concern for the well-being of others; prefer to work with people	Possess leadership and persuasion skills; enjoy being influential and being involved in politics; prefer to deal with people	Possess organizational, mathematical, and clerical skills; enjoy working indoors and organizing things; prefer to deal with numbers
Related Occupations	Mechanic, electrician, firefighter, laboratory technician, forest ranger, police officer, truck driver	Academic professor, pharmacist, mathematician, physicist, technical writer, meteorologist	Actor, artist, composer, fashion designer, poet, cartoonist, comedian	Counselor, teacher, social worker, speech therapist, physical therapist, pastor	Politician, sales manager, lawyer, company CEO, real estate agent, entrepreneur	Administrative assistant, accountant, bookkeeper, court clerk, bank teller

interacting with their work environment and should match their personality type to their work environment. In other words, a social individual may choose an occupation, such as sales or counseling, that allows the opportunity to interact with and help people. On the other hand, a realistic personality type may be drawn to professions that deal more with machinery and tools (e.g., mechanic) than with people (see Table 14.2). If individuals were able to successfully match their personality and interests with a career, Holland believed they would do well in their chosen vocation and be satisfied with their career choice. Research that spans the past few decades has indeed found Holland's assertions to be true. The results of multiple studies show that a good fit between an individual's personality type and job characteristics predicts job satisfaction, performance, stability, and personal well-being (e.g., Holland, Gottfredson, & Baker, 1990; Spokane & Cruza-Guet, 2005).

In addition to personality traits, a person's interests, skills, and values affect vocational choice. **Career interests** refer to preferences that individuals have for particular life activities (e.g., writing, working on cars, solving math problems). Individuals may verbally *express* their interests in a conversation or a class, or their interests may become *manifest* through activities they engage in. For example, an individual who enjoys art may attend a gallery showing. Most of us dream about getting paid to do what we love and, for young adults, the consideration of personal interests is important in selecting a career. Young adults also take their skills and abilities into account when making a career decision. Long gone are the childhood dreams of becoming a professional baseball player or ballerina. Instead, young adults realize they must also have the skills and talent needed to turn their interests into a viable career.

At the beginning of this section, we saw that Bonita had an interest in chemistry, but may not have the aptitude or skills needed to successfully complete college courses in the discipline. Like Bonita, many young adults may find that they lack the skill set needed to achieve a specific career. Their decision to pursue a particular career may depend on whether or not they are capable of obtaining certain skills, the type and availability of training needed to obtain the skills, and how determined they are to complete such training. For instance, in Bonita's case, she must determine her level of motivation to complete the chemistry degree, and her willingness to hire tutors and obtain additional academic support to ensure her success. While most career skill sets can be learned, others are innate. Some are just born with an inclination toward solving complex math problems or composing music. As young adults grapple with the reality of making a career choice, it is important to realize areas where they excel, as well as those where they do not.

Finally, a person's work values play a large role in the career selection process. **Work values** reflect what a person needs to be present in the work environment in order to find satisfaction on the job. The majority of young adults, who have just begun to explore potential careers, tend to value the extrinsic rewards of work (e.g., salary, job security, social status). As they move through the career selection process, individuals often begin to realize that they also have intrinsic (e.g., expressing creativity, further learning through work) and altruistic (e.g., helping others, contributing to the betterment of society) values that need to be met by a work environment. In addition to learning about personal work values, it is helpful for young adults to prioritize each value. An important piece of the career selection process is knowing which values can be compromised and still lead to happiness on the job, and which cannot. Ultimately, job satisfaction ensues when the work environment is congruent with central work values.

To consider only personality traits and preferences in choosing a career severely underestimates the impact of cultural factors on the selection process. Put simply, career choices do not merely reflect a combination of personality typologies, skills, interests, and values, but are the result of other forces that interact with these individual characteristics. One major determinant of career choice is socioeconomic status. Young adults are influenced by the occupational achievements and ambitions of those around them (e.g., friends, family, mentors). As a result, those who grow up in the middle class are likely to pursue middle-class, white-collar occupations (Roe, 1957).

Socioeconomic status may also determine the work values of young adults. Those in the middle class often strive to find an occupation that is personally fulfilling and provides a sense of identity, whereas young adults from disadvantaged socioeconomic backgrounds are more concerned with the extrinsic rewards of work, such as salary or job security. Young adults interviewed by Chaves et al. (2004) reported that they had received obvious messages from their families that the primary goal of work was to earn a paycheck. Consider the case of John in Case Example 14.2.

➤ CASE EXAMPLE **14.2** JOHN.

John is 19 years old and just received his GED a couple of months ago. He is from a blue-collar family in which most of the men in his family worked in manual labor. Following in his father's footsteps, John currently works as an auto mechanic at a local garage and feels that it is his duty to work hard to provide for his family. He just had a baby with his live-in girlfriend. Though he views work as a means to earning a much-needed paycheck, John is often bored at this job and dislikes manual labor. He finds it difficult to stay engaged at work and dreams of having a job that he likes. His supervisor has noticed John's frequent "slacking" on the job and has told John that he needs to shape up. John sought career counseling because he fears that he may be on the verge of losing his job. During counseling sessions, John expresses that he is extremely dissatisfied with his job, but needs to keep it in order to provide for his newborn child. He would love to have the opportunity to receive additional vocational training or go back to school; however, he cannot afford to do so. How can you help John with his dilemma?

It is important that counselors be cognizant that clients may face several barriers in pursuing a job or career that is fulfilling and matches their individual personality, values, and interests. While a client may have high aspirations concerning a career, factors such as socioeconomic status, race, and situational issues (e.g., having a child at an early age, criminal behavior) do affect the degree to which a young adult is able to work toward and achieve vocational goals (Broderick & Blewitt, 2014). Counselors must help clients navigate their career paths, while attending to the very real need to earn a paycheck. It is important to note that supportive relationships with friends and family or a counselor can provide a sense of hope to young adults that they will achieve their career aspirations and improve their chances of upward mobility.

Another factor that influences career selection is gender. As early as age 3 people receive strong cultural messages regarding gender-appropriate occupations (Gottfredson, 1996). Such messages sometimes influence thinking that women are supposed to be teachers and nurses, while men are supposed to be doctors, lawyers, and CEOs of companies. While we receive these cultural messages early in life, they are still fully present in the career selection process in early adulthood. Consider, for example, that women make up nearly one-half of the workforce but only a quarter of those in the science and engineering occupations (National Science Foundation, 2002). Research further suggests that parents' gender-stereotyped beliefs leave a long-lasting impression on children and the careers they choose. For instance, Bleeker and Jacobs (2004) found that maternal gender stereotypes early in a child's life were related to math and science self-efficacy two years after finishing high school, and that maternal beliefs in a child's ability to succeed in a math career were related to career choice in young adulthood. Women are also more likely than men to choose careers with a relational and altruistic focus (Su, Rounds, & Armstrong, 2009). In particular, women are over-represented in caregiving fields such as nursing, social work, and education (Weisgram, Bigler, & Liben, 2010), while men remain dominant in science, technology, engineering, and math (Landivar, 2013). While increased awareness of the impact of gender on career choice in the past two decades has led counselors and other helping professionals to encourage men and women to seek nontraditional career paths, gender stereotypes still remain a key determinant of career choice in young adulthood, and they are a more powerful predictor of vocational interests than race/ethnicity, age, or educational level (Fouad, 2002).

The Career Selection Process

Career theorists have many ways of conceptualizing the career selection process. One of the most popular and widely used career selection processes in career counseling is derived from trait and type theory. Trait and type theorists, such as John Holland, believe that the process can be reduced to three steps: (1) self-understanding, (2) information about the world of work, and (3) integration. In step one, young adults focus on gaining self-understanding. They work to ascertain their personality traits, interests, skills, and values. Some may talk with mentors, friends, and family members to increase their knowledge, while others may take objective assessments (e.g., interest inventories, self-directed search). The second step involves learning about the world of work, which may include information related to education and training, salary and benefits, work environment, job duties, and employment outlook. Young adults can find this information through government websites, computer-assisted career guidance programs, career books, informational interviewing, job shadowing experiences, volunteerism, and internships. The final step of the career planning process, from a trait and type perspective, is for young adults to integrate their self-understanding with information learned about the world of work. Individual traits must be "matched" with the characteristics of specific occupations.

One major limitation of using the trait and type method of career selection is that it perpetuates the assumption that choosing an occupation is a one-shot deal. Young adults often feel pressured to choose the "right" major and career, believing that this choice will determine the rest of their lives. In fact, people's interests, values, and skills change as they age, and many will make a career change at some point during their lifetime. Counselors should dispel this myth when working with young adults who are in the process of selecting a career.

One career approach that may be particularly useful to young adults who are selecting a career is planned happenstance. **Planned happenstance** theory is the work of John Krumboltz and his associates (e.g., Krumboltz, 1979; Mitchell, Levin, & Krumboltz, 1999) and recognizes the importance of unplanned, chance events in people's vocational lives. Unlike trait and type theory, Krumboltz believes it is not necessary to plan your career in advance. Instead, young adults should take advantage of the unplanned social, educational, and occupational events that come their way.

To illustrate the role of planned happenstance in career selection, let us consider the case of John again. Suppose during his counseling sessions, the counselor de-emphasizes matching personal and work characteristics to make a single career decision. Instead, the counselor teaches John to keep his options open, take calculated risks, and begin taking actions outside of the counseling session that will lead to a more satisfying vocational and personal life. Specifically, the counselor encourages John to capitalize on unplanned, chance events. One day John is working at the garage and strikes up a conversation with a customer. The customer is a landscaper and is looking to hire. John does not know anything about landscaping, but expresses interest in working for the customer. The customer offers him the job. A year later, John is still working at the landscaping job and has even taken a few horticulture courses; he is much more satisfied with his career. As you can see, John's vocational path was significantly influenced by a chance event (i.e., meeting the customer at his garage), and because off his willingness to take a risk (i.e., taking the job without training) he has a fulfilling career.

Vocational Preparation in Young Adulthood

College is increasingly important in the vocational path of many young adults and one of the most prevalent types of vocational preparation. Nearly 70% of all high school graduates attend two- or four-year colleges [National Center for Education Statistics (NCES), 2007]. While most college students attend four-year, degree-granting institutions, the number of students attending two-year community colleges is increasing (Seftor & Turner, 2002). Students enrolled in community colleges, when compared to those attending four-year universities, tend to be older, female, minorities, from low-income backgrounds, and live independently from their parents. They are also likely to maintain full-time employment while attending school part time (Horm & Nevill, 2006). College enrollment in the United States is affected by gender, race, and socioeconomic status and the intersection of these characteristics. Female enrollment in higher education has increased significantly in the past few decades. Women now make up over half (57%) of all undergraduate students in the United States and are more likely than men to earn a master's degree (59% to 41%; NCES, 2007). Socioeconomic status and race affect young adults' access to higher education. For example, in 2005, 81% of high school graduates from high-income families enrolled in college immediately following graduation, as compared to 53.3% of those from low-income families. However, the number of minorities attending and graduating from institutions of higher education is increasing. More than half of all Latino and Black students who finished high school go directly to college, and minority students now account for 50% of the increase in bachelor's degrees awarded (NCES, 2007). While attending two-year and four-year academic institutions is increasingly common, only one in four young adults who enroll in college actually receive a degree after five years (Horn & Berger, 2004). Black and Native American students are still at increased risk of dropping out of college before graduating (Aud, Kewal-Ramani, & Frohlich, 2011). While the factors associated with lower rates of retention for minority students are complex, the stress associated with minority status, along with feeling unsupported and disconnected, may contribute greatly to dropping out of college. Increased minority retention rates can be mitigated; research has demonstrated that minority students who experience academic validation and are involved in academic and social activities are often successful in their academic pursuits (Hurtado, Cuellar, & Guillermo-Wann, 2011; Pascarella & Terenzini, 2005).

For most college students vocational training is a priority. Young adults often enter college in order to increase their chances of securing a "good job" and enhancing earning potential. College students are interested in receiving practical career training in college. Choosing a major and selecting an occupation often define young adults' college experiences. College presents young adults with an opportunity to try out different career options with relatively little cost and, as a result, most college students switch their major at least once (Herr, Cramer, & Niles, 2003). The selection of a major can affect the likelihood that a young adult will be successful in college; therefore, it is important that college counselors assist students with career planning and selection. Data from the Bureau of Labor Statistics (BLS, 2011) demonstrate that college does indeed pay off in the long run for young adults. In 2010, individuals with a bachelor's degree earn approximately $20,000 more per year than those with a high school diploma and were more likely to be employed. The college experience not only improves young adults' career opportunities, but also facilitates intellectual and critical thinking, and increases the likelihood of leading a healthy adult life and having a successful marriage.

Nearly a third of all high school graduates do not enroll in a two- or four-year academic institution immediately following graduation. These young adults are known as the "forgotten half" (William T. Grant Foundation Commission on Work, Family, and Citizenship, 1988). Much like those who pursue a college degree, these noncollege young adults desire to have a meaningful job that offers good pay and opportunities for advancement. Unfortunately, the career opportunities for young adults in the United States with only a high school diploma are somewhat limited, and the vocational training system for those who are not college bound is largely disorganized and undervalued.

Many vocational training options do exist for young adults who are not college bound, including vocational education, apprenticeships, and the military. **Vocational education**, which is also known as career and technical education (CTE), prepares young adults for nonacademic careers related to a specific trade (e.g., plumbing, masonry). The skills taught in vocational education programs are pragmatic, labor-intensive, and directly applicable to the trade. Vocational education is available at both the secondary and postsecondary level, and may be provided by a community college, career training college, or trade school at the postsecondary level.

While vocational education has traditionally focused on blue-collar trades such as mechanics, welding, or plumbing, changes in the labor market over the past 50 years have sparked diversification in the training programs offered by schools. Today, young adults can receive the training and certifications needed to begin a career in information technology, tourism, medical information and technology, and human resources, to name a few.

Many high school students have access to modern-day apprenticeships through school-to-work programs. **School-to-work programs** are found in high schools across the nation, and they combine a classroom-based education with practical work experience. Students enrolled in these programs generally receive the opportunity to learn valuable job skills through a co-op or internship experience. School-to-work programs, therefore, rely on collaborative relationships between local school districts and community businesses to provide vocational training to young adults.

For some young adults, enlistment in the U.S. Armed Forces is an optimal way to receive career training. The U.S. military offers a variety of career paths for enlisted youths and provides classroom training in addition to field instruction. Service members also receive educational benefits that include federal tuition assistance. While a good number of vocational training opportunities exist for noncollege-bound young adults, they often face significant barriers when trying to obtain information about vocational preparation for jobs and careers that do not require a college degree (Broderick & Blewitt, 2014). It is important that counselors realize the college route may not be ideal for all young adults. Consequently, counselors must be familiar with alternative types of vocational training in order to provide young adults with a variety of career options. Specifically, Rosenbaum and Becker (2011) recommend that noncollege young adults receive extensive vocational counseling that includes information regarding postsecondary vocational training opportunities that lead to technical certificates or associate degrees, as well as participation in apprenticeships and work-based learning.

Transitioning to the Workforce: Finding Job Satisfaction and Establishing a Vocational Identity

Young adulthood is not only a time for exploring careers and receiving vocational training, but it also involves transitioning to the workforce. Donald Super (1953), a career development theorist, described how the transition to employment unfolds in young adults. Super believed that career development is a lifelong process. His life-space career theory delineated five successive stages that are accompanied by a series of developmental tasks. According to Super, adolescents and young adults begin to explore careers, gather occupational information, crystallize their career alternatives, specify an occupational choice, and actively pursue appropriate vocational training and/or work experiences. By their mid-20s, most young adults complete their vocational training and begin transitioning to the workforce. Super believed that this transition propelled young adults into the establishment phase of career development. In the establishment phase, which lasts until mid-adulthood, individuals launch a career by starting a job in their chosen occupation. Initially, young adults must work to meet the job requirements, become competent, and establish a positive reputation as a productive employee. If young adults are able to succeed in their job position, they may advance to a position with added responsibility and increased pay. In addition to job performance, young adults who are new to the workforce must also find ways to achieve job satisfaction and work to develop a vocational identity.

REFLECTION 14.2 ALL DEGREED UP AND NO PLACE TO WORK

My own transition to the workforce from college was very stressful. I operated under the false assumption that having a four-year college degree would make it easy to secure a job that would pay me enough to live on my own. Instead, I was unable to secure employment immediately following graduation and had to move back in with my parents. It quickly became apparent that I lacked the training and work experience I needed to secure the jobs that appealed to me. I also did not have a strong professional network or any job search skills. It took more than half a year for me to secure my first postgraduate job. During that time, I became very disillusioned with my educational and career choices and, overall, was dissatisfied with my life. [~SC]

Job Satisfaction

The transition from school to work can be a difficult and unsettling experience for many young adults. Like me, many young adults may be dissatisfied with their jobs and even their career choices. Young adults, in fact, experience less job satisfaction (i.e., how content individuals are with their job) and more vocational distress than older workers (Career Vision, 2005). A number of factors may account for the high rates of job dissatisfaction in young adulthood. Many young adults are overly optimistic about the world of work. They may believe that it will be easy to find a high-paying job that provides security, allows for the application of the skills learned in vocational training, and provides a sense of meaning and satisfaction. In reality, individuals in their 20s tend to work in low-wage, low-skill positions with frequent job turnover (Hamilton & Hamilton, 2006). In fact, the employment rate (54%) for young adults between the ages of 18 and 24 is at an all-time low, and young adults who are employed full time have recently experienced a significant drop in weekly earnings (Pew Research Center, 2012). As a result, young adults may be disillusioned and dissatisfied with their jobs. Young people may also find that their educational training did not sufficiently prepare them to enter the workforce. In the United States, higher education strongly focuses on academic knowledge rather than vocational skills. They must attain and maintain a job position with little understanding of what it takes to be a successful employee. Finally, for some young adults the transition to the workforce can be disappointing because their job fails to match their interests, skills, and personality. Only 30% of today's young adults view their current job as a career, while nearly half of young people report that they took a job they did not want in order to pay the bills (Pew Research Center, 2012). These individuals may return to school for more education and training. Job dissatisfaction can lead to burnout and negatively affect young adults' professional and personal functioning. They may experience high levels of job stress, extreme fatigue, alienation, and feelings of depression. Job dissatisfaction has also been associated with increased absenteeism, poor physical health, increased job turnover, and more complaints (Schmidt, 2007).

Work and the Development of Self-Concept

Frequently at social events, when meeting for the first time, acquaintances are curious about what others do for a living. For most, work plays a central role in people's lives and shapes who they are as individuals. Perhaps no one has emphasized the relationship between work and self-concept more than Donald Super. Super (1953) recognized that an individual's **vocational self-concept** develops from experience and changes throughout the lifespan. A person's vocational self-concept emerges from one's broader sense of identity and includes ideas about which characteristics of the self are congruent with the requirements of an occupation. For example, an individual who does not see himself as being good at school may choose to pursue an occupation that requires vocational training rather than a college degree. Vocational self-concept is determined by two factors: (1) one's perception of personal and psychological characteristics (e.g., believing that you are not good at school), and (2) one's appraisal of life circumstances and the barriers associated with these circumstances (e.g., not having money to attend college, lack of family support). Thus, career decisions are not influenced only by how one defines oneself, but also by the beliefs of one's family and friends, and the resources to which one has access. Young adults entering the workforce often choose jobs that are congruent with their existing self-concept. A vocational self-concept then begins to emerge as young adults continue to define themselves through their work experiences. Therefore, the self-concept facilitates career development in young adulthood and, at the same time, is a product of it.

While the self-concept plays a key role in the career development process of young adults, some may have very little understanding of self and have difficulty separating their self-concept from the expectations of family, friends, and society. The central role of a counselor is to help young adults answer the question "Who am I becoming and how shall I express my emerging self?" Often young adults enter counseling asking what the expectations of friends, family, and society are for their vocational lives. In turn, counselors must assist young adults to construct their own vocational self-concept that is grounded in external expectations, rather than authored/dictated by them.

Career Development for Women and Ethnic Minorities

The presence of women and ethnic minorities in the workplace is rapidly increasing. The U.S. Department of Labor (2011) predicts that women and minorities will enter the workforce at higher rates than White men by 2018. Increasing diversity in the labor force requires counselors to be sensitive to the vocational needs of minority workers, understand differences in the career development paths of minority workers, and acknowledge the barriers that minority workers face.

The career development path for women is notably different from that of their male counterparts. Men tend to follow a linear career development path in which they first try out a variety of different jobs and then launch into a stable, long-term career. For women, the path of career development may not be as linear and often involves interruptions. For example, women who begin a career early in young adulthood may later decide to marry and have a family. They may leave their career to be a full-time homemaker while they raise children, and return to the workforce when the child-rearing responsibilities are less pressing. Other women may establish their career and take on a second career as a homemaker, raising their children while working full time; this career development pattern is often referred to as the "double-track career pattern."

The **double-track career pattern** is increasingly common among women today. Compared to 1950, when 88% of women with children under age 6 were full-time homemakers, more than 62% of mothers with preschoolers were employed full time in 2002 (Cohany & Sok, 2007). Still, family and child-rearing concerns are central to a woman's career development at nearly every stage. Women place greater priority on their caregiver responsibilities than on their role as a breadwinner (Vermeulen & Minor, 1998). As we discussed earlier in the chapter, working women still take on more of the child care responsibilities and household tasks than men. Women also have lower expectations for career success, underestimating what they can achieve in their vocational lives (Matlin, 2004), and low self-efficacy beliefs about their ability to succeed in nontraditional careers (Watt, 2006). As a result, they often do not consider pursuing, or drop out of, nontraditional career fields (e.g., engineering, physics, mathematics). Today's women also face wage and workplace discrimination. Men still make more money than women, with women earning 77 cents on the male dollar. Women who are employed in male-dominated career fields are more negatively evaluated for their work than their male counterparts. Those who are successful also experience the glass ceiling and are only able to advance so far on the corporate ladder. For instance, only 15 of the Fortune 500 companies are headed by women.

To date, the majority of what we know about career development is based on studies examining White, middle-class individuals. We have much less knowledge about the career development of individuals from diverse racial and ethnic backgrounds. Gysbers, Heppner, and Johnston (2009) point out that most career development theories are rooted in six fundamental tenets that do not necessarily apply to minority populations. These six tenets are (1) universality, (2) individualism and autonomy, (3) affluence, (4) myth of meritocracy, (5) salience of work in people's lives, and (6) linearity. In order to provide effective services to diverse clients, it is imperative that professional counselors realize:

1. Career development theories cannot be universally applied and do not adequately explain the experiences of individuals from diverse backgrounds.
2. Career decisions that promote autonomy and are based on individual desires and needs are not always valued by collectivistic cultures. A person's career development path may be determined more by family and the community than by the individual.

3. Not all individuals have the economic means to pursue a career that fulfills their personal interests and goals. Ethnic minorities among the poor and working class place more emphasis on finding a job that pays for basic needs (e.g., food, clothing, shelter).

4. Hard work does not ensure one will have a prestigious job, be wealthy, and accumulate resources. Instead, success is largely contingent on privilege and an individual's access to resources (e.g., financial resources, family support). Working-class minorities are not poor because they are lazy, but rather because they face institutional, political, and economic barriers, as well as discrimination.

5. Work may not play a central role in a person's life and define who they are. For some individuals, family, church, civic, or leisure activities may be more meaningful than what they do for a living.

6. The career development process may not be linear for racial and ethnic minorities.

Similar to women, racial and ethnic minorities face discrimination in the workforce. Racial and ethnic minorities are less likely to graduate from high school and complete a four-year college/university education than Whites (U.S. Census Bureau, 2007). They lack confidence in their academic abilities, face familial disapproval, and lack the economic resources needed to pursue higher education (McWhirter, 1997). While ethnic minorities have the skills and training required to be successful in the workforce, they often believe they will be rejected and devalued at work (Gloria & Hird, 1999). Relatedly, racial and ethnic minorities earn less than their White counterparts, even when educational status is accounted for. Many minorities anticipate facing sexual and ethnic discrimination in the workplace. Counselors play a critical role in helping to rectify the social inequalities faced by women and racial/ethnic minorities. It is imperative that counselors provide culturally relevant counseling and career services, understand the barriers faced by these populations, acknowledge the presence of discrimination in the workplace, and work to empower women and minorities by providing clients access to a variety of educational training and career opportunities.

Balancing Work and Family during Young Adulthood

As young adults are establishing a career and adjusting to the workforce, they are also adjusting to their new roles as spouses and parents. Trying to juggle work and family responsibilities is not easy for young adults, especially in families where both parents work or families that are headed by a single parent. The number of dual-earner families has increased in recent years and, though difficult, they can have several advantages over single-earner families. Two incomes can provide the financial resources needed to support a family and promote the establishment of an egalitarian relationship between spouses. However, dual-earner spouses can experience **role overload**, having more family and work demands than time needed to fulfill them, and conflicts between work and family responsibilities. Given that working women are responsible for the majority of child care and household tasks, they are more susceptible to the stress of balancing work and family needs. Women who experience role overload are more likely to have diminished well-being, be dissatisfied with their work and marriage, and experience mental health issues (Pearson, 2008). Having a flexible job, the opportunity to work from home, and/or time off from work to care for a sick child can reduce the strain on dual-earner families. Additionally, access to affordable, quality child care and after-school programs allows men and women to pursue their career goals and raise a family without having to choose one over the other.

Summary

Young adulthood is a developmental period that marks the transition from adolescence to adulthood. In young adulthood, many of the identity issues individuals faced as adolescents have been resolved. Therefore, young adults are able to invest in establishing intimate relationships with partners, friends, and family, and achieve the developmental milestones often associated with this developmental period (e.g., starting a family, managing a home). During young adulthood, significant energy is also invested into selecting and starting a career, achieving job satisfaction, and striving for work–life balance. The achievement of such tasks ushers in a variety of social/emotional and career development changes.

According to Havighurst (1952), successful adaptation to adulthood involves completing a series of developmental tasks in young adulthood. Such tasks often include selection of a mate, learning to live with a partner, starting a family, raising children, managing a home, starting an occupation, and assuming civic responsibilities. Successful development depends on both completion and timing of these tasks. Individuals who are off time with regard to the social clock may experience difficulty in their developmental trajectory due to the negative consequences associated with going against the societal norms that dictate the age by which certain life events should occur.

One of the major developmental tasks of young adulthood involves the establishment of intimate relationships. Erik Erikson (1963) asserted that the establishment of intimate relationships involves having a genuine concern for another's needs and a willingness to sacrifice one's own needs at certain times. Individuals who fail to form intimate relationships risk becoming socially isolated. Young adulthood encompasses the establishment of both friendships and long-term, romantic relationships. According to Sternberg (1986), long-term relationships are sustained by consummate love. Consummate love involves passion, intimacy, and commitment. Our ability to form and sustain intimate relationships is also dependent on attachment styles. Adult attachment styles are influenced by early relationships with primary caregivers and reflect the degree to which adults avoid intimacy and being dependent on others, and experience anxiety about being rejected or abandoned by others (Fraley & Shaver, 2000).

Levinson (1986), like Erikson, believed that changes to an individual's life structure occur as the person encounters the key developmental tasks of young adulthood. Young adulthood, according to Levinson, is characterized by exploration, opportunity, and the accomplishment of financial independence, marriage, parenthood, and starting a career. While young adulthood is generally viewed as a time when opportunity and optimism abound, the occurrence of psychological disorders actually increases. This spike in mental illness may be attributed to the many developmental tasks and life demands that young adults face.

Young adults today experience more freedom and flexibility with regard to their lifestyle and vocational choices. The number of single young adults has increased sharply in recent years. Likewise, cohabitation rates are also increasing dramatically, as many young adults choose to live with a sexual partner outside of marriage. Marriage rates in young adulthood have declined, as many young adults prefer to establish themselves in a career and achieve financial independence before settling down. Similarly, young adults are choosing to have fewer children and start a family later in life.

In addition to forming intimate relationships, finding a partner, and starting a family, young adults devote much of their time to choosing and establishing a career. The career development process in young adulthood often begins with the selection of a career. Individuals must gain knowledge about themselves and the world of work in order to make a career decision that will lead to long-term satisfaction. Young adults spend time exploring their vocational interests, abilities, values, and occupational characteristics. They must also learn to take advantage of unplanned social, educational, and occupational events in order to create vocational opportunities for themselves. In addition to career exploration, young adults invest in vocational preparation opportunities to prepare for their future careers. Most high school graduates will attend two- or four-year academic institutions, but young adults can also pursue training through vocational education or school-to-work programs. Young adults not only choose a career and receive vocational training, but also must make the transition to the workforce. A successful transition to the workforce involves achieving job satisfaction and developing a vocational identity. As individuals transition to the workforce and establish their career, they may experience conflict between work and family obligations. Young adults often strive to find a balance between work demands and family responsibilities.

Middle Adulthood: Physical and Cognitive Development

By Robin Lee, Jennifer Jordan, Michelle Stevens, and Andrew Jones

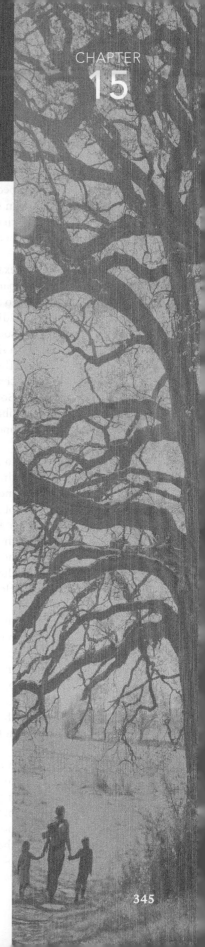

In the past decade, middle adulthood has been redefined by society. No longer is middle adulthood considered to be the beginning of the aging process; rather, it is recognized that this group of people may be entering an exciting chapter in their lives. Middle adulthood can be an incredibly rich stage of life, with a variety of life experiences. Many in middle adulthood are raising children; others are enjoying grandchildren. Some are rediscovering their partners or significant others after years of focusing on children or careers. With the momentous developments in medical technology, many in middle adulthood are finding ways not only to delay aging, but also to prevent it in some ways. While some in middle adulthood may face negative changes to their physical health, they can also experience significant positive changes in all areas of development including physical, cognitive, and social/emotional. People currently in middle adulthood have experienced a wide variety of social events that have defined them, from the civil rights movement to the women's movement, as well as the development of technologies we all use today. All these significant experiences have created a rich developmental stage of life—middle adulthood.

An Overview of Middle Adulthood in Contemporary America

The odyssey continues into middle adulthood, which is typically defined as occurring somewhere from the mid-30s to 40 up to approximately 60 to 65 years old. While we can assign specific chronological years to this developmental stage, it is a difficult task to understand the sheer complexity of this stage in life. Currently, middle adulthood describes a group of people ranging from Baby Boomers to Generation X. Because these two age groups differ in so many areas (e.g., different generational characteristics, upbringing, education, experiences), trying to develop a cohesive understanding of this socioculturally diverse group becomes a challenge.

Due to changes in our society, middle adulthood covers a wide range of lifestyles. For example, it has become more common for those in middle adulthood to become first-time parents. To better understand this age group, let's compare the two generations. According to Strauss and Howe (1992), **Baby Boomers** were born between 1944 and 1964, and so in 2015 they were between the ages of 50 and 70. Historically, there were at least three major social movements that happened during the maturation of those in this age range that had a significant influence on our society. The Vietnam War changed how wars were viewed. The civil rights movement changed how we related to each other. The women's movement changed the basic functioning of the family. Due to the unique experiences of the Baby Boomers, they are often considered to be a on a wide continuum of belief systems, from liberal to conservative. Baby Boomers are typically considered optimistic, independent, and idealistic.

Those born from 1964 to about 1984 are referred to as **Generation X**, often referred to as Xers. Although the Xers did not directly experience the major social movements, they were no less influenced by them. As Xers aged, the effects of two of the major social movements became apparent. As mothers began to join the workforce, the beginnings of the latchkey kid phenomenon (children who cared for themselves after school) and a distinct focus on self-reliance and independence emerged. While Xers did not witness the civil rights movement, they were able to negotiate race relations within schools, neighborhoods, and communities. Xers are considered to be less socially conscious than their Baby Boomer counterparts, yet are just as independent and self-reliant (Strauss & Howe, 1992).

While there are major differences between the experiences of these two generations, the commonalities are apparent as well. Because both groups experienced these social movements, albeit one directly and the other indirectly, this has allowed for a certain level of mutual understanding. However, the chronological ages of these two groups place them in the same developmental stage of life. In addition, the universality of many of the developmental tasks provides a more cohesive understanding among members of these groups. Counselors need to consider not only the developmental tasks of this age group, but also the influence that generational characteristics may have on how they approach the tasks at hand.

Although there are many developmental theories, few directly address middle adulthood. For example, Erik Erikson (1950, 1963, 1982) defined the developmental crisis in middle adulthood as generativity versus stagnation. According to Erikson, the task of helping a younger generation develop successful lives is defined as generativity. The other side of the continuum is stagnation, described as when a person is left feeling as if one has done nothing to help the next generation. Some changes in middle adulthood are inevitable, and therefore are considered primary aging. Other age-related changes are due to disease, lack of care given to health, or poor environmental conditions; these changes are considered secondary aging.

"Forty is the new 30" or "50 is the new 40." You may have heard these statements made by a midlifer. While this may be an attempt to maintain a youthful outlook, the physical changes in middle adulthood are unmistakable. For many, such changes may be gradual. For others, changes in appearance may seem to occur overnight. No matter how a person begins to pay attention to physical changes in middle adulthood, these changes are inevitable.

Growing, Maintaining, and Managing Losses in Health and Fitness

One change that Western society has experienced in recent years is an attempt to stop the aging process. Plastic surgery has become a booming industry, with over 13.1 million cosmetic procedures performed in 2010, an increase of 5% over the previous year [American Society of Plastic Surgeons (ASPS), 2011]. Procedures to change one's appearance have moved from serious hospital procedures (e.g., breast augmentation, liposuction) to less invasive outpatient techniques (e.g., Botox injections, chemical peels). According to the ASPS (2011), botulinum toxin (i.e., Botox) injections increased by 12% in 2010. Botox is an injectable substance designed to block nerve impulses, which temporarily paralyzes the muscles and causes skin to appear smoother and more refreshed. Although people spend a significant amount of money to "stop the clock," physical changes are universal. Although inevitable, these changes can be affected both positively and negatively by lifestyle and genetic makeup.

External Aging

Physical Appearance

Wrinkles, gray hair, baldness, and changes in weight are just a few of the physical changes that people in middle adulthood may experience. Visible changes are the defining signs of aging. Although physical changes may vary among people, they are also universal. Wrinkles are caused by changes in skin structure. Skin can begin to show wrinkles and sag due to fat and collagen loss in the tissue. Wrinkles can become more prominent due to smoking and sun exposure. The effects of excessive sun exposure can also cause age spots to develop. To deal with skin changes, there are several cosmetic procedures available such as injectables (e.g., Botox), chemical peels, and microdermabrasion (i.e., removing the top layer of skin in order to stimulate new growth).

Hair turns gray, then possibly white, due to a lack of production of pigment in hair. In addition, hair may begin to thin. Hair loss or alopecia is typically linked to genetics. Androgenic alopecia (AGA), or male/female pattern baldness, is most common. According to the American Hair Loss Association (AHLA) (2010a), AGA accounts for 95% of all male pattern baldness. One myth that continues to be perpetuated regarding male pattern baldness is that it is linked genetically to the mother's side of the family, which is not the case. For men, baldness typically begins on the top of the head and can progress toward complete baldness. Women can also be susceptible to hair loss or thinning. Hair loss in females can be linked to hormones, childbirth, malnutrition, infection, surgery, or stress (AHLA, 2010b).

Many people spend significant amounts of money on hair products to keep the gray away or to grow new hair. However, although many men spend time, money, and energy to deal with baldness, others have begun to embrace their new appearance, even opting to shave their heads completely rather than have various patches of hair.

Weight gain can be a problem in middle adulthood due to changes in metabolism, poor diet, and even pregnancy. According to the Centers for Disease Control and Prevention

(CDC, 2011d), approximately one-third of U.S. adults (33.8%) are obese. One sobering statistic is the costs related to weight issues. The CDC reported that in 2008, $147 billion was spent on medical costs associated with obesity. Geographically, the southern states had a higher prevalence of obesity (30%). By ethnicity, African-Americans have the highest rates of obesity (44%), compared to Mexican-Americans (39%), all Hispanics (38%) and non-Hispanic Whites (32%). Being overweight also has a significant effect on how people perceive their health, especially in middle adulthood. White females who are overweight tend to rate their health much lower than other groups (Zajacova & Burgard, 2010).

This negative view can in turn lead people to spend large amounts of money on weight-loss programs. Americans spend approximately $40 billion annually on weight-loss products and programs. Although there have been many studies comparing weight-loss methods, the research varies on how effective these methods are. However, most groups recommend a balanced diet of lean meats, fruits and vegetables, and whole grains, while limiting saturated and trans-fats, cholesterol, salt, and sugar.

Although people may be gaining weight in middle adulthood, they can actually lose height. According to the National Osteoporosis Foundation (NOF, 2011), bone development peaks between 18 and 25 years of age, meaning this is the point when the maximum amount of bone has developed. Beyond this point, bone density begins to decrease, often to the point where **osteoporosis** can develop, a condition in which the bones become more porous. The Office of the Surgeon General (U.S. Department of Health and Human Services, 2004) has reported that the prevalence of osteoporosis will increase due to the aging of our population. By the year 2020, half of all Americans over age 50 will be at risk of hip and skeletal problems due to osteoporosis.

Women are more susceptible to osteoporosis than men. According to NOF (2011), 10 million Americans over the age of 50 currently have osteoporosis, and 8 million (80%) of these are women. Anyone with osteoporosis is at an elevated risk for broken bones and fractures. Regular exercise can help address both potential weight gain and bone problems. Weight-bearing and muscle-strengthening exercises are recommended to improve bone density. Examples of weight-bearing exercises include aerobics, dancing, hiking, and jogging. Examples of muscle-strengthening exercises include lifting weights or using exercise bands. Non-impact exercises such as yoga and Pilates can improve both areas as well.

Muscle

As people age, their muscle mass can begin to deteriorate, which is called **sarcopenia**. Along with sarcopenia, a 12% to 15% loss in strength-length occurs per decade, beginning in middle adulthood (Cooper et al., 2012). Although in the past it was believed that this deterioration was inevitable, evidence shows that exercise (e.g., strength-training exercises such as squats, push-ups, and lunges) can prevent some of the loss.

Senses

Vision

Changes in vision typically begin around age 40 years of age. Decline in vision may happen gradually for most. One reason for this decline is the deterioration of dynamic accommodation within a person's eye (Lockhart & Shi, 2010). When a person needs to move a book or newspaper an arm's length away in order to see the words clearly, it may be quite a shock. This is due to a condition called **presbyopia**, which is when there is an inability to focus on objects at a close distance. Many people find themselves buying their first pair of reading glasses during middle adulthood. In addition, a decline in the ability to adapt to sudden changes in light or dark conditions can emerge. By the time someone has reached 40 years of age, approximately half of the rods in their eyes have dissipated (Bonnel, Mohand-Said, & Sahel, 2003). The purpose of the rods (i.e., black and white receptors) is to help us see when light is dim. This is one of the reasons people begin to experience problems driving at night. Whether it is the first sign of decline in vision or more chronic vision problems, glasses that are necessary simply to read may transition into a need to wear glasses for all occasions. In this case, glasses with bifocal lenses (i.e., glasses with two separate sections for seeing distances both close and far) may be required. The good news for those in middle adulthood is that glasses have become more fashionable in recent years. They no longer just signal one's advancing years, but can now be considered a fashion choice!

Hearing

According to the American Speech-Language-Hearing Association (ASHA, 2013), age-related hearing loss is called presbycusis. Although hearing does decline during middle adulthood, it is more important to note that extraneous variables can affect hearing as much as aging. According to the CDC (2011f), hearing loss due to occupational hazards is the most common work-related injury in the United States; there are an estimated 22 million U.S. citizens with work-related noise hazard injuries. In addition, approximately $240 million is spent on workers compensation because of hearing loss disabilities. Another extraneous variable that can affect hearing includes personal listening devices. In 2005, ASHA issued a warning regarding the effects of personal listening devices on hearing; if not used properly, such devices can damage hearing. ASHA (2006) indicated that approximately 10 million Americans have experienced hearing loss from excessive noise exposure, which will continue to increase as more people use these devices. ASHA recommends keeping the volume of personal listening devices at low levels, avoiding continued listening, taking frequent breaks, and wearing headphones as opposed to ear buds. In addition, ASHA (2013) recommends that if you answer yes to two or more of the following questions, you should consider a hearing test conducted by an audiologist:

- Do you have a problem hearing over the telephone?
- Do you hear better through one ear than the other when you are on the telephone?
- Do you have trouble following the conversation with two or more people talking at the same time?
- Do people complain that you turn the TV volume up too high?
- Do you have to strain to understand conversations?
- Do you have trouble hearing in a noisy background?
- Do you have trouble hearing in restaurants?
- Do you have dizziness, pain, or ringing in your ears?
- Do you find yourself asking people to repeat themselves?
- Do family members or coworkers remark about you missing what has been said?
- Do many people you talk to seem to mumble (or not speak clearly)?
- Do you misunderstand what others are saying and respond inappropriately?
- Do you have trouble understanding the speech of women and children?
- Do people get annoyed because you misunderstand what they say?

Other Senses

Changes may occur to both taste and smell as people age. Taste buds, which allow us to distinguish bitter from sweet and salty from sugary, can change over time. The way we perceive sweet and sour tastes does not change as we age. However, aging does affect our ability to taste things that are salty and bitter (Winkler & Garg, 1999). Taste buds typically regenerate every 10 days. In the early 40s, this regeneration process slows, thus affecting taste senses. Women's taste buds may be less affected than men's due to estrogen levels that increase with age.

REFLECTION 15.1 THE MIDDLE-AGED MOM

I do not think I am aging well. While my physical health is great, biologically I am not pleased with several aspects of aging, most of which is based on pure vanity. I have no conditions, no pain, and no signs of inability to maintain the same pace as in earlier years. Yet there are some minor physical changes that are irritations more than anything. I now need reading glasses to read everything! I even bought a glasses chain, albeit a very stylish one. I once had an incredible metabolism when I was younger; that no longer exists, and therefore weight is always an issue. After having two children, my body has changed in ways I can't fix with diet or exercise. The worst part is the wrinkles. I've invested lots of money in facial care products, with no results. At this point, I begin to recognize that all the time I spent in the sun using baby oil with iodine to get that awesome tan was not such a good idea. Sunscreen will be a priority with my kids. While there are a few things I would change, there are some positive aspects. First of all, I have more money to fix those physical irritations (e.g., facials, Botox). Second, a few years ago I had a successful endometrial ablation, which eliminated my menstrual cycle. Beyond eliminating the monthly annoyance, it also improved my and my husband's sex life. This brings me to another positive physical change—sex. I am more comfortable with sex than ever before, which is great! [~PM]

Smell can also change with age. After the age of 60, some may notice more loss in their sense of smell. Since food flavors are detected in the nose, this may cause the taste of food to change and be less appetizing.

Reproductive System

The **reproductive system** is made up of the organs responsible for reproducing. In middle adulthood, the reproductive system begins to see the same degree of changes as since adolescence. During adolescence, the reproductive system matures to the point that a human can reproduce. In middle adulthood, the reproductive system eventually loses the ability to reproduce. This process is called **climacteric**. Although most people later in middle adulthood are unable to reproduce, it is important to note that with advances in technology, particularly related to assisted reproduction technology (ART), both women and men are able to reproduce later than ever. ART involves fertility treatments, in which both eggs and sperm are manipulated by surgically removing eggs from the ovaries, combining with sperm, and returning the fertilized egg to the womb. However, ART does not include techniques where only sperm are manipulated or egg production is stimulated by use of medications. Due to ART, women as old as 70 have been able to have children. Recently, a woman in India, Rajo Devi Lohan, gave birth at 70 years of age. Although she successfully gave birth to a child, she experienced complications that have made her unable to care for the child, thus calling into question the ethics of ART (Fox News, 2010).

Women's Reproductive Health

There are several reproductive health issues with which middle-aged women deal. According to the CDC (2009), approximately 20 million U.S. women have had a **hysterectomy**, which involves the surgical removal of the uterus. Other than cesarean section, a hysterectomy is the second most commonly performed surgery in reproductive-aged women. Hysterectomies are typically performed due to uterine leiomyoma (i.e., fibroid tumors), endometriosis (i.e., tissue that normally lines the inside of the uterus grows outside the uterus), or uterine prolapse (i.e., stretching and weakening of the muscles and ligaments that provide support for the uterus, causing the uterus to drop into the vaginal cavity). An alternative to a hysterectomy is an endometrial ablation, which is a surgical procedure undertaken to remove the uterine wall. This procedure is typically recommended for women with heavy vaginal bleeding during monthly periods. The ablation will typically either lighten the period or end it altogether. An ablation is not recommended for women wishing to become pregnant, those who have uterine cancer, or those who are past menopause.

Menopause is one of the more universal reproductive health issues for women, occurring when a woman's period stops completely for 12 months. Menopause typically happens between the ages of 45 and 55, although it can occur earlier in some women. During menopause, the hormones estrogen and progesterone begin to decrease. Menopausal women often experience symptoms such as hot flashes, sleeplessness, mood changes, fatigue, rapid heartbeat, or nausea. Hot flashes are one of the more common symptoms. Smoking can increase the severity and likelihood that women will experience hot flashes during menopause (Gallicchio et al., 2006; Sievert, Obermeyer & Price, 2006). On the other hand, women who engage in frequent and intense exercise, at least twice a week, report fewer hot flashes than women who are less active (Kandiah & Amend, 2010). Although most women do not need treatment for these symptoms, others find it necessary to deal with the effects of menopause. Treatments can include natural alternatives such as eating healthy, exercising, and controlling stress to more extreme treatments such as **menopausal hormone therapy** (MHT), which is when women take estrogen and progesterone to deal with the symptoms of menopause. Although research regarding the risks of MHT is unclear, the U.S. Food and Drug Administration (2009) approved the use of MHT to deal with menopause symptoms. One key recommendation is that a low dose be used to avoid any severe side effects such as stroke, breast cancer, or other complications.

Men's Reproductive Health

Unlike women, men's reproductive health is less affected by age. While women can have rapid declines in hormone levels during middle adulthood, men have a more gradual decline. Men's testosterone production tends to decline by approximately 1% per year. And although men do begin to lose sperm count, they are still able to reproduce later in life. In fact, similar to Rajo Devi Lohan, the woman from India who gave birth at 70, it has been reported that one of the oldest fathers to date also lives in India. Ramajit Raghav fathered a child at 94 years of age with his wife, Shankuntala Devi, age 52 (*New York Post*, 2010).

Although men are able to reproduce well into middle adulthood, and even late adulthood on occasion, some men voluntarily choose to end their ability to reproduce by having a vasectomy. A **vasectomy** is a surgical procedure considered to be a form of male birth control that will sterilize a man, preventing him from releasing sperm during ejaculation. A vasectomy is typically an outpatient procedure that may take less than 30 minutes. In this procedure, the vas deferens (a narrow tube connecting the testicle to the urethra) is sealed by either clamping or cutting, thus preventing sperm from mixing with semen and ejaculating through the penis. Vasectomies are almost 100% effective, with only 1 to 2 women out of 1000 becoming pregnant after their partner has a vasectomy. Another advantage is that a vasectomy is more cost-effective and has fewer complications than a female tubal ligation (i.e., having the "tubes tied").

One of the most significant changes men may experience during middle adulthood is **erectile dysfunction** (ED) or impotence, which is the inability to obtain and maintain an erection firm enough for sex. ED is the most common sexual problem reported among men (Lindau et al., 2007). Although erectile problems can be common, the problem may need to be addressed when it happens frequently. Because sexual arousal is connected to so many different systems (physical, mental, social), the cause of ED is difficult to determine. Causes may include illness and medical conditions, social habits such as smoking and alcohol use, or stress and depression. ED can also be a predictor of more serious, life-threatening diseases. For example, men who have ED are at a greater risk of heart disease (El-Sakka,

Morsey, & Fagih, 2011). There are several treatments for ED, the most common being oral medications. Medications such as sildenafil (Viagra), tadalafil (Cialis), or vardenafil (Levitra) are specifically developed to treat ED. These medications increase nitric oxide in the body, which is a chemical produced naturally in the body that relaxes muscles, thus increasing blood flow to the penis, allowing for an erection in reaction to sexual stimulation.

Sexuality

Although middle adulthood typically means the end of the ability to reproduce, it certainly does not mean the end of a healthy sex life. In the mid-1960s, Masters and Johnson (1966) revolutionized how we view sexuality, particularly as related to older adults. Masters and Johnson found that older adults are perfectly capable of having a fulfilling sexual life as they age. Although a healthy sex life is possible, there are some important changes to note. First of all, for men, it may take longer to achieve an erection. In addition, it may take more time for men to recover from an orgasm, thus allowing for a subsequent erection and orgasm. This is called the refractory period. For younger men, it may take 15 to 20 minutes. For older men, it may take more like 24 hours. For women, the vaginal walls begin to thin, thus causing the lubrication process to slow. Vaginal lubricants may help in minimizing any discomfort. One of the major benefits of the sex life of men and women in middle adulthood is the fact that they do not have to be concerned with birth control, "times of the month," or unwanted pregnancy. This may allow for more freedom to initiate sex when the opportunity arises.

Other Organ Systems

Many of the body's systems are affected by age. This includes all major organ systems, including the cardiovascular, nervous, respiratory, and urinary systems. Some, like the cardiovascular system, may be more affected by age than others. Nonetheless, we see both primary and secondary changes in all systems.

Cardiovascular System

The **cardiovascular system** is designed to provide the body with the blood, oxygen, and nutrients it needs to function. In middle adulthood, the function of the cardiovascular system is challenged due to a build-up of fat deposits, cholesterol, and calcium that leads to plaque developing in the arteries, a process called atherosclerosis. When the plaque begins to harden, the arteries narrow, restricting the flow of blood. Because of this, the heart has to work harder to pump blood, which results in **hypertension** or high blood pressure. There are other factors that can contribute to hypertension, including obesity, smoking, stress, too much salt in the diet, and lack of exercise. It is important to monitor hypertension in middle adulthood because it has no obvious symptoms and can go untreated. If hypertension goes undetected and untreated, it can lead to a heart attack or stroke. Making changes that focus on secondary aging issues can prevent cardiovascular problems. By exercising regularly, controlling stress, maintaining a good diet, and avoiding tobacco, a person can reduce the risk of hypertension and heart disease.

Respiratory System

The **respiratory system** is designed to deliver oxygen to the body. While there may be little change to the respiratory system in middle adulthood, changes have already occurred during one's 20s and 30s. The function of the lungs changes because the muscles and tissues begin to lose their ability to expand and contract. During one's 40s, **vital capacity**, the amount of air the lungs can inhale and expel, begins to diminish. Environmental factors can have the biggest effect on the respiratory system. The delicate tissue of the lungs is directly connected to the outside environment, which is affected by anything you breathe. For example, people breathe in germs, smoke, and other harmful substances, which can damage the lungs. Diseases of the respiratory system include lung cancer, asthma, influenza (flu), and COPD (emphysema and chronic bronchitis).

The American Lung Association (ALA, 2011b) described several warning signs which would require medical evaluation: prolonged chronic cough or shortness of breath, labored or difficulty breathing, chronic mucus production, wheezing, coughing up blood, and chronic chest pain. One of the most important recommendations to maintain and/or improve the respiratory system is to avoid smoking. The ALA (2011a) reports that the major cause of lung cancer and COPD is cigarette smoking. Approximately 400,000 people die each year from tobacco-related disease, which makes it the most preventable cause of death. In the United States, smoking-related illnesses cost over $193 billion in 2004, which included almost $100 billion in health care costs alone. The damage from smoking begins immediately, with the first cigarette, causing a loss of lung elasticity. Typically, the lungs expand when inhaling and then return to the original state because of the elastic tissues lining the inner wall. Smoking damages the elastic tissues through continued deposits of tar, which permeate and affect the function of the lungs, thus making it more difficult to exhale. This condition is called **emphysema**. However, the good news is that as soon as a person quits smoking the body immediately begins to repair the lung damage.

Urinary System

Food allows the body to receive the nutrients it needs to function. However, after the food is processed, waste is left in the blood and bowel. The urinary system is designed to eliminate waste from the body, eliminating on average a quart and a half of urine daily. The urinary system includes the kidneys, ureter, bladder, sphincter muscles, and urethra. The effects of age include a lessening of the elasticity of the bladder, which decreases the organ's ability to retain or expel urine from the body. Because of this, urinary infections may become more common due to the bladder's inability to empty successfully. In addition, the muscles of the ureters, bladder, and urethra can lose strength.

For men, the urinary system may be affected by the enlargement of the prostate gland, which is called benign prostatic hyperplasia (BPH). According to the National Institute of Diabetes and Digestive and Kidney Diseases (NIDDK, 2010), more than half of men in their 60s report symptoms of BPH, and as many as 90% of men over 70 years report symptoms. The most common symptoms are more frequent urination, particularly at night, an interrupted or weak stream, and leaking or dribbling. According to the CDC (2012a), 16% of men will be diagnosed with prostate cancer, and about 3% of all men will die from prostate cancer.

For women, a common urinary system problem is urinary incontinence (UI), which is involuntary loss of urine. This loss of urine can be as minor as losing a few drops while coughing or running, or it can mean losing a large amount, which can often be embarrassing. UI can be due to pregnancy, childbirth, or menopause. Although UI is most common in women, it also occurs in men. It is important to know that all types of incontinence are treatable at any age. Treatments include behavioral treatments (e.g., bladder retraining, kegel exercises) and surgery.

Health Concerns

One aspect that begins to change in middle adulthood is the realization that aging is occurring. Prior to this stage, the majority of people may not have experienced any health concerns that caused them to recognize their vulnerability. Younger people may not necessarily consider the effects their choices have on their health later in life, thus causing them to make poor decisions that can dramatically alter their physical health in middle and later adulthood. The reality is that in middle adulthood, physical health concerns are inevitable. Injuries can occur that would not have occurred in early years. In addition, what would have been minor injuries can have a major impact on performance. For example, a back injury may result in a trip to the doctor for medication or even long-term disability. Although health concerns do begin to have more of an impact on overall health in middle adulthood, one does not need to assume that all those in this stage of life are "sickly." Middle adulthood usually is a stage of good health.

Illness

There are two types of illnesses to consider: acute and chronic. **Acute illness** is defined as conditions that develop quickly but are usually temporary. Examples of acute illnesses are the common cold, influenza (flu), stomach or abdominal problems, and rashes or skin injuries. Acute illnesses are also typically isolated to one part of the body, can be treated, and may require less care due to their temporary nature. While there may be little difference in how those in middle adulthood may respond to acute illness, there is a dramatic difference in their susceptibility to chronic illness. **Chronic illness** is a condition that has developed over time, and is typically persistent and not completely cured. Examples of chronic illness include heart disease, cancer, stroke, and diabetes. According to the National Center for Chronic Disease Prevention and Health Promotion (NCCDPHP, 2011), 70% (1.7 million per year) of all U.S. deaths are due to chronic diseases. According to NCCDPHP (2010), the four most common causes of chronic disease are "lack of physical activity, poor nutrition, tobacco use, and excessive alcohol consumption" (p. 1). Chronic diseases are affected by both nature (genetics) and nurture (environment).

Heart Disease

Although heart disease may not have been a concern for most people prior to middle adulthood, based on statistics from health organizations, it certainly should become one. According to the CDC (2011c), heart disease is the leading cause of death for both men and women. The most common form of heart disease is coronary heart disease (CHD) or coronary artery disease. CHD is a result of plaque buildup inside the coronary arteries, which supply blood to the heart muscle. This buildup is called **atherosclerosis**, which can occur over time and may ultimately cause a heart attack. The CDC (2011c) reports that every 34 seconds, someone has a heart attack in the United States.

A term given to a set of characteristics that increase a person's risk of heart attack and premature death is **metabolic syndrome**, or syndrome X. These risky characteristics, which include high blood sugar and insulin levels, high blood pressure, low HDL cholesterol or good cholesterol levels, and a large waistline, are both genetic and environmental factors. Those in middle adulthood should also be aware of whether or not their parents have suffered from heart disease. Children whose parents have suffered from heart disease are more likely to experience heart-related issues throughout their lives (Lloyd-Jones et al., 2004). Although heart attacks should be of concern in middle adulthood, it is important to recognize that they can be prevented or treated with changes in lifestyle, medications, or surgery. Cardiac CT scans, echocardiography, and enzyme-blocking drugs are some of the medical devices at the forefront of preventing death related to heart disease (Weisfeldt & Zieman, 2007).

Cancer

While heart disease is the leading cause of death in adults, cancer is the second leading cause (CDC, 2010a). There are many types of cancers. Although this is not a complete list, some of the more common cancers are breast, cervical, colon, lung, ovarian, prostate, and skin cancer. According to the CDC, the most common type of cancer is skin cancer. While melanoma can have a genetic link, most skin cancers can be prevented. Sun exposure, particularly exposure to UV radiation, is the most common cause of skin cancer. In addition, most skin cancers can be treated effectively, although melanoma can be more dangerous. While skin cancer is the most common form of cancer, lung cancer is the deadliest. The CDC reports that lung cancer kills more people than any other type of cancer, and this is true for both men and women. Risk factors include smoking (including secondhand smoke), exposure to substances like asbestos or radon gas, and family history. One positive trend is that the number of new cases of lung cancer and deaths from lung cancer in men have decreased over the past few years, probably due to a decline in smoking. Unfortunately, reports indicate that new cases and deaths from lung cancer have increased in women.

For women, breast cancer is the second most common type of cancer next to skin cancer, and breast cancer is the leading cause of death due to cancer in women. According to the American Cancer Society (ACS), "the chance that breast cancer will be responsible for a woman's death is about 1 in 36 (about 3%)" (2011a, p. 9). The ACS also reports that in 2011 approximately 230,480 women were diagnosed with invasive breast cancer, 57,650 were diagnosed with noninvasive breast cancer, which is the earliest form of breast cancer, and approximately 39,520 women died from breast cancer.

In 1982, the Susan G. Komen Race for the Cure organization was started by Nancy G. Brinker, whose sister, Suzy, died from breast cancer at the age of 36 after a three-year battle. By hosting the Komen Race for the Cure, the organization has raised almost $2 billion to help fight breast cancer and has partnered with many businesses and corporations to continue their efforts to focus attention on breast cancer.

Although breast cancer is rare in men, it does occur. According to the National Cancer Institute (2011), less than 1 out of every 100 cases of breast cancer is diagnosed in men. According to the ACS (2011b), prostate cancer is a very common cancer in men, second only to skin cancer. The ACS estimated that some 240,890 men were diagnosed with prostate cancer in 2011, and almost 34,000 died from prostate cancer.

➤ CASE EXAMPLE **15.1**   CONNECTION BETWEEN PHYSICAL AND MENTAL HEALTH.

Clinically, one of the most important considerations in middle adulthood is physical health due to the initial decline during this stage. Because of the many changes in physical health, counselors should consider ruling out health-related conditions and diseases as the cause of a client's mental health concerns. Depression can be associated with many conditions or illnesses such as hormone imbalance, menopause and perimenopause, diabetes, and cardiovascular disease. Anxiety can manifest with many chronic illnesses, possibly related to the illness itself, any treatment required, as well as simply having to navigate the challenging and often frustrating health care system. If left untreated, mental health issues can affect the efficacy of medical treatment for illnesses and diseases. Thus, it is crucial to communicate with the client's primary care physicians when counselors suspect an illness or disease is the cause of mental health concerns. Many primary care physicians are becoming more aware of the relationship between mental health and physical complaints and may be supportive of treating mental health concerns by prescribing psychotropic medications, encouraging counseling, and readily communicating with counselors (Riba, Wulsin, & Rubenfire, 2012).

Risk Factors to Health

There are several risk factors that can significantly affect a person's health, including smoking, alcohol, obesity, and poor nutrition.

Smoking

Most would agree that smoking is clearly hazardous to a person's health, perhaps more so than other risk factors. The CDC (2011b) offers some startling statistics regarding smoking:

- The adverse health effects from cigarette smoking account for an estimated 443,000 deaths, or nearly one of every five deaths, each year in the United States.
- More deaths are caused each year by tobacco use than by all deaths from human immunodeficiency virus (HIV), illegal drug use, alcohol use, motor vehicle injury, suicide, and murder combined.
- Smoking causes an estimated 90% of all lung cancer deaths in men and 80% of all lung cancer deaths in women.
- An estimated 90% of all deaths from chronic obstructive lung disease are caused by smoking.

Since 1964, the U.S. Department of Health and Human Services, Office of the Surgeon General (2010a) has issued a report regarding the health risks of smoking. According to this report, there is no safe type or amount of smoking. Any tobacco exposure, even minimal or secondhand, is harmful. This report offers strong language regarding smoking that should be considered. "Damage from tobacco smoke is immediate ... smoking longer means more damage ... cigarettes are designed for addiction and there is no safe cigarette" (p. 1) are all strong statements that clearly indicate the problematic nature of smoking. The CDC (2011b) reports that smoking causes the following cancers: acute myeloid leukemia, bladder cancer, cancer of the cervix, cancer of the esophagus, kidney cancer, cancer of the larynx (voice box), lung cancer, cancer of the oral cavity (mouth), cancer of the pharynx (throat), stomach cancer, and cancer of the uterus.

Although the statistics related to smoking are harsh, it is important to note that it is never too late to quit smoking. The CDC (2011e) offers information about smoking cessation, describing smoking as a chronic condition that may require multiple attempts to quit. According to a report by Fiore et al. (2008) and published by the U.S. Department of Health and Human Services, titled *Treating Tobacco Use and Dependence: 2008 Update,* there are currently more former smokers than there are current smokers. This report focused efforts on providing information to help people quit smoking. In addition, the CDC (2004) offers information about the positive effects of quitting on a person's health. Within 20 minutes after smoking that last cigarette, the body begins a series of changes that continue for years.

- 20 minutes after quitting: Heart rate drops.
- 12 hours after quitting: Carbon monoxide level in the blood drops to normal.
- 2 weeks to 3 months after quitting: Heart attack risk begins to drop; lung function begins to improve.
- 1 to 9 months after quitting: Coughing and shortness of breath decrease.
- 1 year after quitting: The added risk of coronary heart disease is half that of a smoker's.
- 5 years after quitting: Stroke risk is reduced to that of a nonsmoker's.
- 10 years after quitting: The lung cancer death rate is about half that of a smoker's. The risk of cancers of the mouth, throat, esophagus, bladder, kidney, and pancreas decreases.
- 15 years after quitting: The risk of coronary heart disease is back to that of a nonsmoker's.

Alcohol

Although alcohol use is common in our society, it can have negative effects on health. While it is very clear that smoking affects the body, alcohol has broader effects. The health risks of alcohol include both immediate and long-term risks. Immediate risk includes traffic accidents, intimate partner violence, risky sexual behaviors, or alcohol poisoning. More long-term effects include liver disease, cancer, hypertension, depression, anxiety, and personal problems such as lost jobs and family problems. Other problems with alcohol are binge drinking, heavy drinking, or excessive drinking. According to the CDC (2011a), a standard drink for adults is a 12-ounce beer, a 5-ounce glass of wine, or 1.5 ounces of liquor such as rum, vodka, or whiskey. Binge drinking is defined as four or more drinks at one time for women and 5 or more drinks for men. Heavy drinking is defined as more than 1 drink per day for women and more than 2 drinks per day for men. Excessive drinking is a combination of the two.

Obesity

Obesity has become more of a risk factor for adults in recent years. Obesity is defined as 20% over a person's normal weight. It is typically measured by examining body mass index (BMI), which calculates a person's body fat. A normal BMI is between 18.5 and 24.9. When a person is considered obese, the BMI is over 30. Overweight is defined as a BMI of between 25.0 and 29.9. It is estimated that over 97 million people in the United States are either overweight or obese. This is roughly one-third of the U.S. population (CDC, 2011d).

Obesity is a health risk because it can lead to heart disease, hypertension, type 2 diabetes, and cancer. According to Finkelstein, Trogdon, Cohen, and Dietz (2009), the annual price tag of medical costs due to obesity is about $147 billion dollars. Obesity is a complex disease with multiple causes. Causes of obesity can be linked to both genetics and environment, and from metabolic problems and lack of exercise. According to a report developed by National Heart, Lung, and Blood Institute (2000) titled *The Practical Guide: Identification, Evaluation, and Treatment of Overweight and Obesity in Adults,* assessment and management are the key aspects of dealing with obesity. This report suggests that treatment should include (1) assessment, which determines the degree of obesity and risk, and (2) management, which includes reducing excess weight, maintaining the lowered body weight, and controlling risk factors.

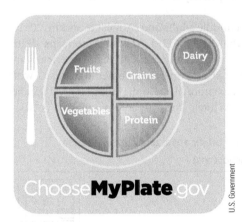

Figure 15.1 USDA recommendations for daily caloric intake.

Poor Nutrition

Poor nutrition can be a problem at any age. As with the other health risks, poor nutrition can lead to obesity and other diseases. The U.S. Department of Agriculture (USDA) makes recommendations for daily caloric intake (see Figure 15.1). The recommendations are based on two types of lifestyles: sedentary or active. Sedentary is defined as an activity level that includes only normal daily activities. Active is defined as "physical activity equivalent to walking more than 3 miles per day at 3 to 4 miles per hour, in addition to the light physical activity associated with typical day-to-day life" (USDA, 2010, p. 14). For sedentary lifestyles, the USDA (2010) recommends 1800 daily calories for women aged 31 to 50 and 2200 calories for men. For active lifestyles, 2200 daily calories for women and 3000 for men are recommended.

Eating Disorders

In addition to obesity and poor nutrition, the number of women presenting with eating disorders has increased in treatment facilities. Although limited, research indicates that eating disorders are not limited to adolescent girls, but are also found in women over age 50 years (Gagne et al., 2012; Mangweth-Matzek et al., 2006; Midlarsky & Nitzburg, 2008). Eating disorders bring unique challenges for women who are also dealing with life stresses such as family, career, and changing bodies. In addition, the body becomes less resilient with age, making it more difficult to recover from eating disorders. Women may be less likely to share issues related to eating disorders with their health care professionals, thus making diagnosis and treatment difficult.

Minorities and Health

As is often discussed, the demographics of U.S. society will be changing in the future. According to the U.S. Census Bureau (2011a), what are currently considered minority populations will increase in numbers, with the non-Hispanic White population decreasing as a percentage of the total U.S. population. Groups such as Black, Asian and Pacific Islander, American Indian, Eskimo, and Hispanic-origin populations will increase in numbers and as a percentage of the U.S. population (see Figure 15.2). The Black population will double in size to 62 million by 2050. By 2020, the Asian and Pacific Islander population will triple in size, increasing to 41 million by 2050. The Hispanic-origin population will increase by 60% between 2030 and 2050. With these increases in numbers, our society faces challenges regarding our physical health. Minority groups generally have more health concerns due to lack of access to good health care, genetics, and environmental factors. One potential reason for this is that minorities are less likely to participate in physical exercise and more likely to eat unhealthy diets.

This difference is seen even more clearly in middle adulthood (August & Sorkin, 2011). According to the Office of Minority Health at the CDC (2011a), African-Americans' death rates due to heart disease are 40% higher than among Whites, and African-Americans are 30% more likely to die of cancer, particularly African-American women diagnosed with breast cancer. African-Americans are seven times more likely to die from HIV/AIDS and six times more likely to die by homicide than Whites. The Hispanic population is twice

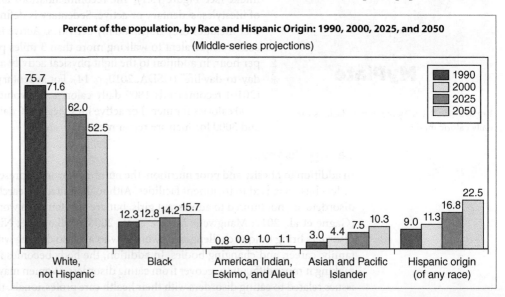

Figure 15.2 The changing demographics of the U.S. population.

as likely to develop diabetes as Whites, and often experiences higher rates of obesity and high blood pressure (CDC, 2011c). Native Americans and Alaska Natives are more likely to experience death caused by intentional injuries and suicide than Whites, and suffer higher rates of diabetes (CDC, 2011b).

Successful Aging

Throughout the odyssey of life there are many factors that affect the aging process. Health professionals typically agree on several aspects that can have positive influences on aging. Rowe and Khan (1998), the authors of *Successful Aging,* suggested three components to successful aging: avoiding disease and disability, engagement with life, and maintaining physical and cognitive health. Avoiding disease is basically a focus on prevention, which seems to be the trend in health care. In fact, one of the most significant changes to health care occurred in March 2010 when President Barack Obama signed into law the Afford-able Care Act. One significant part of the new legislation was a focus on prevention. In June 2010, President Obama signed an executive order creating the National Prevention, Health Promotion, and Public Health Council (U.S. Department of Health and Human Services, 2013) with the mission to develop policies and make program recommenda-tions that would improve prevention strategies in health care. In June 2011, the council published its 2011 Annual Status Report. Some of the key elements of the council's focus included:

- Prevention is important at every stage of life; the strategy should emphasize a life-stages approach.
- Addressing health disparities needs to be a central theme and should be elevated from a priority to a strategic direction.
- Health is influenced by many factors outside of a doctor's office; the strategy should include the importance of a cross-sector approach.
- The strategy should convey the importance of community-focused, community-led prevention efforts.
- There are many innovative efforts across the United States where health is used as a cri-terion in program planning and policy development. This approach should be reflected in the strategy. (p. 3)

More specific recommendations of the council included focusing on medical technolo-gies, tobacco control, obesity prevention, HIV-related health disparities, and better nutri-tion and physical activity. See Table 15.1 for more specific programs and recommendations (National Prevention Council, 2011).

Think About It   15.1 Getting Older Leads to Feeling Younger

According to data gathered from the MIDUS study, most Xers *feel* younger than their actual age. This is referred to as age identity. Age identity is the age people *feel* they are as opposed to their actual chronological age. Age identity that is rated younger than one's actual age starts to be seen around the age of 30 years and peaks as late as 70–74 when individuals rate their age identity as 13 years younger than their actual age! In other words, a 70-year-old grandmother *feels* as if her age is 57. Another interesting result is that most people's ideal age happens to be around 40 years of age, which marks the beginning of middle adulthood. Ideal age is the age an individual desires to be. The reasons for this discrepancy in age identity can be psychological, cultural, or just chalked up to our desire to be younger. In any case, discrepancy between actual age and age identity is the one thing most Xers have in common (Westerhof, 2008).

TABLE 15.1 ✦ NATIONAL PREVENTION, HEALTH PROMOTION, AND PUBLIC HEALTH COUNCIL, 2011 ANNUAL STATUS REPORT

Department/agency	Program/strategy/initiative
Department of Agriculture	Healthier U.S. School Challenge
	Healthy food financing, food access
	Release, implementation, and communication of the 2010 Dietary Guidelines for Americans
	New performance standards for campylobacter and salmonella
Department of Education	Promise Neighborhoods
	Green Ribbon Schools
	Carol M. White Physical Education Program
	Safe and Supportive Schools Program
Federal Trade Commission	We Don't Serve Teens (alcohol consumer education initiative)
	Interagency Working Group on Food Marketed to Children
	Initiative to facilitate availability of generic drugs
Department of Transportation	Safe Routes to School Program
	Partnership for Sustainable Communities
	National Distracted Driving Initiative
Department of Labor	Campaign to prevent heat illness in outdoor workers
	Distracted Driving Initiative
	Hazard awareness of formaldehyde-containing hair-smoothing products
	Outreach and education initiatives including the Health Benefits Education campaign
Department of Homeland Security	Anthrax 101 training
	Medical countermeasures—points of dispensing team training
Environmental Protection Agency	Lead Risk Reduction Program
	Protecting People and Families from Radon: A federal action plan for saving lives
Office of National Drug Control Policy	Reducing prescription drug abuse
	The National Anti-Drug Youth Media Campaign
	Drug Free Communities Support Program

U.S. Government

A second aspect of successful aging is active engagement in life activities, which includes continuing to connect with others and engaging in productive activities. Relationships with others can prevent isolation and can continue to provide significant meaning for those who are moving into another phase of life. One aspect midlifers may have to deal with is a child leaving the home. Empty-nest syndrome can be negative for some parents, leaving one feeling empty and lost after children leave the house. Others may respond positively, allowing more focus on reconnecting with one's spouse, partner, or significant other. Some midlifers may find more time to focus on enjoyable activities that were once impossible to fit into life's busy schedule. In addition, after children leave the home, midlifers may find

REFLECTION 15.3 THE MIDDLE-AGED ATHLETE

I have considered myself some type of an athlete my entire life, an OK basketball player in high school who managed through pure determination to make a junior college team in Nebraska, where my hopes of a pro career died a sudden death. Later in life I turned to running, mostly 5-Ks and 10-Ks, with a few longer runs such as half and full marathons here and there. I even completed a few shorter triathlons, most done in the spirit of having fun or just to see if I could do them. As I moved into middle age, several things began to happen both physically and mentally. Physically I began to realize that my body does not react, recover, or perform as easily as it did when I was younger. Mentally I began to realize that my peak years for ticking off the bucket list items and meeting personal time goals may be limited. My experience has been that being a middle-aged athlete has given me the focus and drive to outperform the younger me. In middle age I am limited in time and my body does not recover as quickly as it did when I was younger, so it forces me to prepare for events in a much smarter manner. As I have aged I have tackled more challenging and longer events and have been able to keep posting best times . . . the older I get. My fastest marathon time was on my 25th try, my longest run was 32 miles as a 46-year-old, and my fastest Ironman time was after six attempts. Although I do not subscribe to the "you are only as old as you feel" mindset, I do believe that us "middle-agers" are a bit smarter and wiser than our younger selves, and all of my experience proves you do not have to hang up your quest to get better at 40. [~CK]

themselves with more disposable income than in the past, thus allowing them to consider leisure activities and travel.

A final aspect of successful aging is a continued focus on cognitive and physical health. The most important elements of physical health are good nutrition and exercise. As discussed previously, a diet rich in lean meats, vegetables, and fruits is recommended at any life stage, but particularly as we age. Our focus should not only be on caloric intake but on water balance as well. In addition, consideration should be given to additional vitamin supplements including vitamin B6, folic acid, vitamin B12, vitamin D, and antioxidants such as vitamins A, C, and E, beta-carotene, and selenium. Exercise is also critical at every stage. Levels of activity remain consistent throughout a person's lifetime, and those who are active earlier in life are more likely to continue to remain active as they become older (Freidman et al., 2008). As we age, our focus should be on aerobic exercise, which can include activities such as walking, jogging, and dancing. Strength training through weightlifting can also be beneficial to improving muscle strength and endurance.

As we transition from physical elements of aging toward other areas such as cognitive and psychological health, one of the most important myths that needs to be addressed regarding physical health is the idea that changing years of bad choices will not be helpful. In fact, research indicates that it is never too late to begin making better choices that can improve your health.

SECTION II: Cognitive Development

Conventionally, it was thought that cognitive development did not continue past early adulthood. However, in the most comprehensive study regarding cognitive development across the lifespan, the Seattle Longitudinal Study (SLS) by K. Warner Schaie in 1996, this long-held belief was debunked. Schaie studied adult cognitive functioning in over 500 adults ranging in age from their early 20s to their late 90s. He monitored them in seven-year intervals beginning in 1956. The focus of the research was to determine individual as well as generational differences in basic mental functioning. Schaie found that the mental abilities of inductive reasoning, spatial orientation, vocabulary, and verbal memory had modest gains from young adulthood to middle adulthood before peaking for both men and women. These results suggested that during middle adulthood people are performing at their fullest potential in more sophisticated and complex mental abilities (Schaie, Maitland, Willis, & Intrieri, 1998).

Individual Variations

Cognitive function varies from individual to individual. Such factors as physical and mental illness, smoking, menopause, stress, and environmental stimuli can adversely affect one's cognitive functioning (Jarvis, Thompson, & Wadsworth, 2003). Stine-Morrow, Parisi, and Morrow, and Park (2008) found that those adults who continue to use their skills and challenge their intellectual functioning are more likely to keep their intellectual functioning intact longer. They also stated that those in higher SES categories, people with more flexible personalities, and those with intellectually challenging relationships also maintain their cognitive level of functioning longer.

Male and Female Variations

Willis and Schaie (1999) found that women scored on average at least one-half a standard deviation above their previous scores on spatial orientation, verbal memory, and vocabulary at midlife. Men reach their peak cognitive performance levels prior to women in midlife, though the increase was not as significant as for women. However, women showed a decrease in perceptual speed before men did. It has also been found that declining levels of estrogen put women at a higher risk of memory loss and possible dementia. Women tend to score better on verbal tasks and perceptual speed, with men performing higher on spatial skills. Interestingly, cohort models have shown differences in women from one cohort to the next in the increase in cognitive functioning across mental abilities, pointing toward the women's liberation movement having resulted in more women in education and the workforce (Ardila & Rosselli, 2011).

Information Processing

Reaction Time/Speed of Processing

Reaction time, also known as psychomotor speed, refers to the time it takes to make a specific response. Salthouse (2000) found that speed of reaction time begins to slow in the early 20s and progressively continues to slow as one ages, varying by the task being performed. He concluded that what declined was the speed with which one needed/decided to respond. It has also been found that during middle adulthood, experience and practice overcompensate for decreases in reaction time, meaning that reaction time may be slower but fewer mistakes are made (Zimprich, Hofer, & Aartsen, 2004).

Attention

Attention is the amount of information a person can take in at one given time. Attention involves focusing on pertinent information and ignoring superfluous material, while at the same time being flexible about the demands of the situation. Several types of attention have been studied, and not every type is influenced to the same degree by the aging process (Rogers, 2000). **Selective attention** is the ability to restrict awareness to a limited number of stimuli while ignoring other distractions. In middle adulthood selective attention is maintained for tasks that are familiar to a person, yet unfamiliar tasks and those requiring two or more features show age-related deficits (Cansino, Guzzon, Martinelli, Barollo, & Casco, 2011). Cansino et al. also found that older adults were more likely to benefit from cuing in these tasks than younger adults. **Focused attention** involves concentration and does not show any decline with age in midlife. **Sustained attention** presents mixed results: Rogers (2000) concluded that age-related decline is most likely due to other aspects of the tasks which may decline with age. **Attention switching** or **divided attention** is the ability to switch between two tasks simultaneously, such as reading a book and listening to the radio. Age has not been found to be a factor in simple tasks, but the more complex the divided task becomes the more decline is seen with age. Practice was shown to reduce the decline.

Memory (Short and Long Term)

Short-term memory, also known as **working memory**, is a structure in which information is stored briefly and then sorted out before being transferred to long-term memory. Everyone has a limited amount of working memory; however, with age comes a slight decline, though not as dramatic as was once thought. In general, the older one gets, the more overloaded they become when processing more and more information in too short a time (Prull, Gabrieli & Bunge, 2000).

Long-term memory can be broken down into two types: implicit and explicit. **Implicit memory** is the unconscious recollection of information learned at a given point in time. **Explicit memory** is the conscious recollection of previous experiences or information. Long-term memory can be further subdivided into episodic and semantic memory. **Episodic memory** deals with remembering information or events one has experienced from a specific time or event. It includes things such as remembering where you are going or where you put something. Older adults tend to have more problems with episodic memory, especially when stressed or under pressure. **Semantic memory** involves the basic information learned in school, such as historical facts and concepts; it often increases over the lifespan. Regarding semantic memory, older adults generally test as well as younger adults. However, though research suggests that semantic memory remains intact and even increases over time, older adults often report difficulty retrieving previously learned material. Studies have supported the notion that older adults do have more retrieval failures than younger adults and are slower to retrieve words from the semantic memory (Dixon, De Frias, & Maitland, 2001).

Practical Problem-Solving/Expertise

Practical problem solving refers to everyday situations and complications and how to deal with them appropriately. People in midlife excel in the area of practical problem solving due to their higher levels of expertise, their use of integrated knowledge, and their increased organizational skills. They have an improved capacity to translate their current skills and knowledge when encountering new problem-solving tasks.

Wisdom

Miščević (2012) reported that characteristics of wisdom often are identified in middle-aged adults, finding them to be more related to personality features than to cognitive abilities. Those who are wise seem to have a deeper understanding of reality and the meaning of life, and recognize what is good for them and others. Martin, Jäncke, and Röcke (2012) consider the development of wisdom to be one of the advantages of getting older. McKee and Barber (1999) attribute wisdom to the loss of illusions. As people age they experience stress, pain, and suffering that triggers self-reflection and personal growth. Both are factors attributed with wisdom.

Fluid and Crystallized (Comprehension) Abilities

Fluid intelligence is the ability to think and reason abstractly and solve problems. This ability is considered independent of learning, experience, and education. Fluid intelligence has been shown to decrease with age, but not until around the age of 60. **Crystallized intelligence** involves learning from past experiences and knowledge, such as reading comprehension and vocabulary. This type of intelligence increases with age as one accumulates new knowledge and understanding.

➤ CASE EXAMPLE **15.2** UNDERSTANDING COGNITIVE IMPAIRMENT.

When cognitive impairment is noted at midlife, the counselor should examine the client's lifestyle to determine risk factors such as smoking, menopause, stress, and physical or mental illness. Do not conclude that age is the only factor contributing to mental decline. In particular, counselors should be aware of any cognitive impairments caused by affective disorders that may have an impact on middle-age clients. Another issue counselors should keep in mind is that adults in midlife may become concerned about loss of short-term memory known as episodic memory, which deals with remembering where they were going or where they put things. This is typically not an early indicator of Alzheimer's disease as many people fear, but is more a sign of daily stress and pressure.

Midlife and Mental Illness

While issues may be very clear and are often universal in other areas affecting middle adulthood development (e.g., physical changes, cognitive development), mental illness and mental health are not. Some people may lead very mentally healthy lives with no major issues that develop. Others may find themselves facing unexpected mental health concerns as they age. Because of the varying results of research conducted in this area, it is certainly hard to predict who may avoid mental illnesses and who may not.

Aldwin, Spiro, and Levenson (1989) conducted a longitudinal study to determine changes in mental health as a person ages. The researchers found little variation in psychological symptoms reported with age, consistent with previous research (Robins et al., 1984). Aldwin et al. found that the total incidence rates of practically all psychological disorders dropped by age 45, including those related to substance abuse and schizophrenia. On the other hand, Calvete, Camara, Estevez, and Villardon (2011) reported that women were more depressed than men and reached a depressive peak in middle adulthood. A more recent study on mental health and aging suggested that a peak in psychological stress and mental disorders in midlife was due to income levels, not age (Lang, Llewellyn, Hubbard, Langa, & Melzer, 2011). Those in higher income groups appeared to be immune from this increase during the middle adulthood years.

Given the contradictory findings in the literature, one theme does stand out regarding mental health in middle adulthood: Of all the mental disorders, depression is the most common form of mental illness for adults of all ages (Ponterotto, Pace, & Kaven, 1989). Monroe and Simons (1991) explained depression through a diathesis/stress model of psychopathology, which is used to help define behavior based on either genetic factors (nature), life experiences (nurture), or in combination. In this model, depression is viewed as a result of the interaction between a person and their environment. Individual factors such as personal resources, stressful life events, and social environment influence depressive symptoms. Middle-aged people often report the highest levels of stress (Matud, 2004). However, stress alone does not predict mental illness, although it does influence how people behave. Men tend to externalize problems (Stapley & Haviland, 1989), while women are inclined to internalize problems, often ruminating to the point of depression (Kuehner & Huffziger, 2012). People who employ better coping strategies are much less likely to suffer from depressive symptoms. Aldwin and Levenson (2001) suggested that the actual process of dealing with the changes in middle adulthood may help people establish better coping skills. That is, individuals in middle adulthood may develop anticipatory coping strategies that can help prevent some problems from occurring.

According to data from the MIDUS study, physical appearance plays a role in the way those in middle adulthood view their perceived control at work. Baby-faced Xers feel more constrained in their life and less control in their workplace. How attractive an Xer feels plays a role in perceived control at work. If Xers feel attractive, they will also feel a greater sense of control. This is seen more in women but is also evident in men. Also, the more health problems someone in middle adulthood has, the lower their perceived control at their workplace. In terms of gender, women in midlife feel as if they have greater control at their place of employment than do men (Andreoletti, Zebrowitz, & Lachman, 2001).

> **Think About It   15.2**
>
> What additional mental disorders are prominent in middle adulthood? How will you approach the treatment of older adults differently from adolescents and young adults?

Summary

Middle adulthood is described as the age range from the mid-30s to about the mid-60s; currently this is Generation X and the Baby Boomers. Despite the similar ages of the baby boomers and the Xers, they are vastly different. The Vietnam War, civil rights movement, and women's movement influenced not only developmental growth but also interpersonal relationships.

The aging process is universal and is evident for everyone. However, Western society has developed a strong desire to stop the aging process by means of Botox and plastic surgery. If untreated, sagging skin and sunspots appear as aging occurs. Hair will begin to thin and turn gray in both men and women. Weight gain is common, along with loss of height, which can lead to osteoporosis. With aging also comes a loss of muscle mass (sarcopenia) and a deterioration of the senses. Most commonly, presbyopia, or the inability to focus on close objects, develops around the age of 40. Hearing loss is another common part of the aging process, though most hearing loss in middle adulthood is due to occupational hazards. The sense of smell also begins to deteriorate over time, affecting the taste of food. The sense of taste will degenerate for salty and bitter, but the ability to taste sweet and sour remains stable.

During middle adulthood the reproductive system goes through a process of climacteric, the loss in the ability to reproduce. With advances in technology, men and women are able to have children later into the aging process through assisted reproductive technology (ART). Between the ages of 45 and 55 women experience the cessation of menstruation, called menopause. Men, on the other hand, lose testosterone at a much slower rate and continue to be fertile well into their later years.

However, a common problem men face in middle adulthood is erectile dysfunction (ED), known more commonly as impotence. Sexuality continues to develop in middle adults; there is no longer the burden of unwanted pregnancy or menstruation, allowing for more sexual freedom.

Primary and secondary changes occur in all systems, including the cardiovascular system. Due to lifestyle choices and biological predispositions, atherosclerosis and hypertension are some common cardiovascular problems faced during middle adulthood. The respiratory system primarily changes during the 20s and 30s; however, during middle adulthood the lungs' vital capacity begins to diminish. In order to help with diminished lung capacity, middle-aged adults are encouraged not to smoke, which helps to prevent emphysema. Men in particular show changes in the urinary system with the development of benign prostatic hyperplasia (BPH), an enlargement of the prostate gland. Women sometimes develop urinary incontinence (UI) or uncontrolled loss of urine.

With aging comes a variety of health concerns besides the normal decrease in biological functions. Injury in middle adulthood becomes harder to recover from and may lead to more long-term disability. Heart disease is the leading cause of death; a common form of heart disease seen in middle adulthood is coronary heart disease (CHD). Cancer is the second leading cause of death in middle adulthood, the most common type being skin cancer. There are also many risk factors that negatively impact health during middle adulthood. Smoking is responsible for about one out of every five deaths in the United States. Alcohol is responsible for risky behavior with immediate risks and long-term conditions such as hypertension, liver disease, depression, and anxiety. Obesity is a risk factor because it contributes to hypertension, heart disease, type 2 diabetes, and cancer. Poor nutrition is another risk factor that can be prevented by a healthy lifestyle and proper diet.

Risk factors are especially important when looking at disease through a multicultural perspective. Demographics are shifting, with the non-Hispanic White population decreasing and the former minorities increasing. African-Americans, Hispanics, Native Americans, and Alaska Natives have much higher rates of heart disease, cancer, obesity, and intentional injury/suicide.

Avoiding disease and disability through prevention is a current trend in health care and an important choice in aging successfully. Having an actively engaged lifestyle that consists of engaging with others can prevent isolation and foster fulfillment. Good nutrition and exercise help maintain a healthy physical and cognitive self, helping to increase successful aging.

Complex mental abilities are performed at a higher level during middle adulthood. Cognitive function varies from person to person; however, those who actively use their skills tend to keep their intellectual function longer. Men reach their cognitive peak before women, who reach theirs during middle adulthood. However, women who have declining levels of estrogen are at risk for memory loss and dementia. Reaction time and processing speed tend to decrease with age. Older adults also have difficulty manipulating working and episodic memory, but semantic memory is maintained and can increase over the lifespan. Due to higher levels of expertise, knowledge, and organization, practical problem-solving skills excel in middle adulthood. Wisdom increases along with fluid and crystalized abilities.

Mental illness is represented in middle adulthood by a variety of factors. Women are more likely to reach a depressive peak in middle adulthood. Overall, mental illness and psychological disorders begin to drop off at the age of 45. Mental disorders are more likely due to income levels than to age. Middle adulthood typically sees the highest stress levels. Men are prone to externalize problems, whereas women are prone to internalize problems; without proper coping mechanisms this can lead to severe depression.

Biologically, middle age appears to present a decrease in organ function and an increase in medical concerns. Psychologically, middle-aged adults are shifting to a new role, with more sexual freedom and healthier options. Healthy lifestyles become increasingly important during middle adulthood as they can help counteract the natural aging process.

Middle Adulthood: Social/Emotional, Family, Career, and Spiritual Development

By Robin Lee, Jennifer Jordan, Michelle Stevens, and Andrew Jones

M iddle adulthood brings about myriad social and emotional developmental changes; it is a transition between being the younger generation and beginning one's adult life and being the older generation and slowing down. This stage within the lifespan introduces new situations: establishing a career, raising children, caring for the older generation, and preparing for retirement. Middle adulthood describes a developmental stage that often gets "stuck" and overlooked but given greater responsibility. Is this the cause of the "midlife crisis"? Does the "midlife crisis" really exist? Middle adulthood also presents different challenges and opportunities such as maintaining marital relationships, ending them, or beginning new relationships. But relationships change because the self-concept of a middle adult is often one of confidence and insecurity.

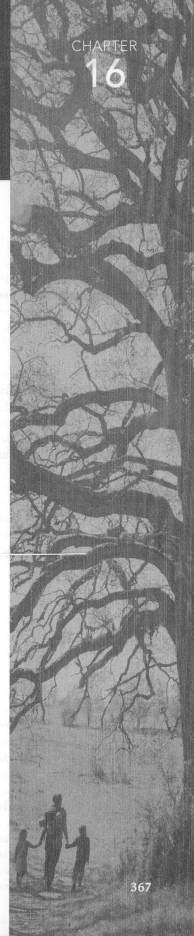

SECTION I:	Social/Emotional Development

Middle adulthood comes with changes that relate not only to biological and cognitive issues, but also to social and emotional issues as well. There are questions about whether a "midlife crisis" exists, how we might best approach midlife transition issues, and what the effects are of gender differences related to midlife transitions.

Midlife Transition Issues

The Sandwich Generation

Middle-aged adults are often referred to as the **sandwich generation**. Though it has multiple meanings, this term is often used to describe those who are "stuck" between the responsibilities of their parents' generation and their children's generation. Some of these responsibilities result in providing care for both their adolescent and adult children as well as their aging parents. With Americans living longer and starting families later, the number of middle-aged adults who find themselves in the sandwich generation is on the rise.

One out of every eight Americans aged 40 to 60 is raising a child and caring for a parent at home (Pew Research Center, 2008). Further, 7 to 10 million Americans are caring for their aging parents from some distance away (U.S. Census Bureau, 2011a). It is estimated that 16 million Americans find themselves "sandwiched" between two generations, contending with raising their children while caring for an aging parent. In 25 years, there will be 60 million Americans between the ages of 66 and 84, many of whom may be in need of full- or part-time care.

Many adults in the sandwich generation provide a majority of the in-home long-term care services for their aging family members, disabled adult children, and other loved ones. Much of the long-term care provided by middle-aged adults includes providing assistance with activities of daily living, coordination of medical services, administration of medication, and financial, legal, and mental health assistance. Common concerns of the sandwich generation include:

- Balancing roles between caring for children and aging parents.
- Delineating time limits and boundaries of caregiving roles.
- Maintaining a healthy personal relationship with a significant other.
- Creating time for oneself.
- Finding resources.
- Maintaining financial stability.
- Maintaining positive mental and emotional health.

Although it is typical for women to care for both children and their aging parents, there is also an increase in the percentage of men who find themselves in the caregiving role. An important issue to be raised is the increased incidence of rural families providing care services for their aging parents. Providing care services in this situation can be difficult because the caregivers may find themselves isolated from professional, financial, or other supportive services and care networks. These caregivers may also find themselves isolated from other caregivers, informal support, and family members. Both urban and rural caregivers are at risk of burnout, increased amounts of stress, and depression.

As mentioned above, adults in the sandwich generation may report an increased amount of mental and emotional stress associated with the elevated level of responsibility, lack of resources, financial strain, and increased need to balance multiple roles. Counselors should focus on assisting clients in the sandwich generation with building resilience and establishing strategies to equally share caretaking responsibilities with fellow adult siblings

When attempting to conceptualize what a midlife crisis looks like, several examples may come to mind. A middle-aged man who suddenly decides he wants to change careers, a middle-aged man who abruptly realizes that he no longer has anything to offer his marriage, or a middle-aged man who runs away with a much younger woman in his brand new red sports car. Now imagine that this person is a woman. These examples raise the question: midlife crisis or normative crisis? What do you think?

and significant others (Riley & Bowen, 2005). Additionally, taking a proactive approach to identifying resources and establishing preventive measures such as crisis planning and involvement in support groups or respite care is a practical and helpful way to work with these adults.

Midlife Crisis: Life Events or Normative Crisis?

Middle adulthood brings such significant life changes that a "midlife crisis" is a concept we have all heard about and may widely accept as fact. A common definition of a **midlife crisis** is a difficult transition period occurring around the age of 40 (Wethington, 2000). The term midlife crisis can be rephrased as a midlife transition that also includes some positive aspects. Although this period in life can be accompanied by serious unhappiness, it can also mark a period of remarkable growth. This transition period tends to occur around significant life-changing events, such as a child graduating college or the passing of an aging loved one. Although when the term midlife crisis is discussed, the immediate thought tends to be of a middle-aged man buying a red sports car, both men and women experience this transitional period, and it manifests differently in men and women. Men are more likely to measure their worth by their job or career accomplishments, while women tend to validate themselves through their close relationships. In the case of a midlife crisis, the woman is likely to reevaluate her roles as a wife or mother.

However, there has been a significant amount of debate over whether or not a midlife crisis exists or if this stage is simply a normative transitional period in life. Some of the argument involves different perspectives on what constitutes a midlife crisis, as well as when this crisis might occur. Vaillant (2002) reported slow and steady changes rather than a "crisis." The MIDUS participants (see Figure 16.1) reported transitional points that were considered major changes in their lives and how they handled these major changes, while only a small

The responsibility of helping my mom remain in this world healthy and capable of caring for herself along with help from others was a very rewarding one. It took a lot of energy and determination to shuffle a job, raise a daughter, and care for an ailing mother all at the same time. Finishing college during midlife added another layer of stress. However, looking for a new way to enjoy life and having a sense of wholeness enabled me to take on many different responsibilities at one time period. Also, knowing that I would be sustained by my spiritual beliefs helped me understand that I could do all the things. Although my mom has since passed, I know that she enjoyed her life and knew that she was loved by her family up until her battle with cancer ended. I was able to maintain a good relationship with my daughter and complete my master's degree during Mom's illness. I know that support from my siblings and close friends around me contributed to surviving that difficult time. Nonetheless, I am grateful to have had the opportunity to care for and grow closer to my mother in the evening of her life. [~VG]

In 1989, the John D. and Catherine T. MacArthur Foundation Research Network on Successful Midlife Development (MIDMAC) was developed to study middle adulthood, which at the time was one of the least studied stages of life (MIDMAC, 2006). MIDMAC is an interdisciplinary research group, composed of various disciplines such as medical and psychology professionals, with the primary purpose of identifying "the major biomedical, psychological, and social factors that permit some people to achieve good health, psychological well-being, and social responsibility during their adult years" (Research Network on Successful Midlife Development, para. 3).

The primary research study was called the National Survey of Midlife Development in the United States (MIDUS). The instrument used, the Midlife Development Inventory (MIDI), was developed by the group and designed to measure "patterns, predictors, and consequences of midlife development in the areas of physical health, psychological well-being, and social responsibility" (Research, para. 1). The MIDUS survey was a national comprehensive study involving approximately 7000 respondents throughout the United States. The study included a brief telephone interview followed by a self-administered questionnaire. In addition, the study included more extensive research on siblings and twins, and five in-depth investigations on stress, social responsibility, daily experiences, psychological experiences, and personal and social well-being. Other research sub-projects included studies to ensure representation of ethnic and racial minorities in urban areas, and several longitudinal studies.

The results of the extensive study were a book published in 2004 titled How Healthy Are We?: A National Study of Well-Being at Midlife. The book summarizes the study as well as provides summaries of key findings organized by topics.

Based on the success of the original research, the Institute on Aging at the University of Wisconsin–Madison was awarded a grant from the National Institute on Aging to continue the research. What resulted was longitudinal follow-up research of the MIDUS respondents called MIDUS II.

All the research conducted has provided the most comprehensive information about middle adulthood to date. Topics addressed include: living arrangements, social networks and support, childhood experiences and family background, social participation, occupational history, religion and spirituality, financial situation, mental and emotional health, quality of spousal/partner relationship, self-rated physical health, information on parents, chronic conditions, information on children and parenting experiences, health symptoms, psychological factors (personality, sense of control, goals, well-being, perceived discrimination), disability and functional limitations, and health beliefs and practices. In addition, assessments included individual differences based on age, gender, socioeconomic background, marital status, and race/ethnicity. MIDUS II provided longitudinal information over a 10-year period on areas such daily stress and reactions to it, in-depth cognitive evaluations, comprehensive biomarker assessments, and neuroscience assessments.

For more information, visit the following websites: MIDMAC at http://midmac.med.harvard.edu/; MIDUS at http://www.midus.wisc.edu/.

Figure 16.1 Results from the MIDUS study.

percentage of participants reported what they would consider to be a midlife crisis, attributing the changes to life events rather than to age. Some theorists consider middle adulthood to be the time when individuals take the time to review their goals and their accomplishment or non-accomplishment of those goals, while perhaps making significant changes in order to fulfill their goals and dreams. Different theorists have proposed various points in this transitional period. Erickson focuses on the struggle occurring during generativity and stagnation, while Levinson views this period as a transition as opposed to a crisis. Another perspective supports the idea that this transitional period of life is determined by environmental and personal experiences. A majority of MIDUS study participants reported that most life changes or turning point events, such as career concerns and marital issues, actually occurred in early adulthood.

Theories of Psychosocial Development

Levinson's Theory of the Seasons of Life

A more concentrated view of psychosocial developmental based on the sequence of life is Levinson's theory (Levinson, Darrow, Klein, Levinson, & McKee, 1978). This theory calls into question the order of the life course. Like Erikson's theory, Levinson's theory is founded on stages, but in Levinson's theory the stages are considered to be seasons. Early adulthood (the 20s) serves as an exploratory period in which one discovers the possibilities of living as an adult. The 30s are a period heavily focused on family and career development. The middle adult years (the 40s) are a period of reevaluation of one's life goals as well as evaluation of how one envisions oneself over the remainder of their lives. Each season consists of a transition period, followed by a stable phase in which individuals tend to make crucial life-changing decisions. Middle adulthood is entered into as a transitional period in which one reevaluates the successful attainment of early life goals.

Some of these life-changing decisions may include a change in relationship status and major career changes. Levinson's theory is based on his research involving in-depth interviews with forty 35–45-year-old men, then later interviewing 45 women 35–45 years of age across various occupational subgroups. A key component of Levinson's theory is the **life structure**, the fundamental configuration of an individual's life. An individual's life structure is molded by their social and physical environment, as well as religion, race, occupational status, and socioeconomic status. During the reevaluation of their life goals, individuals undergo four primary developmental tasks (see Figure 16.2).

Peck's Tasks of Ego Integrity

In an attempt to more clearly define the image of late adulthood, Robert Peck (1968) suggested that personality development in aging people is occupied by three major developmental

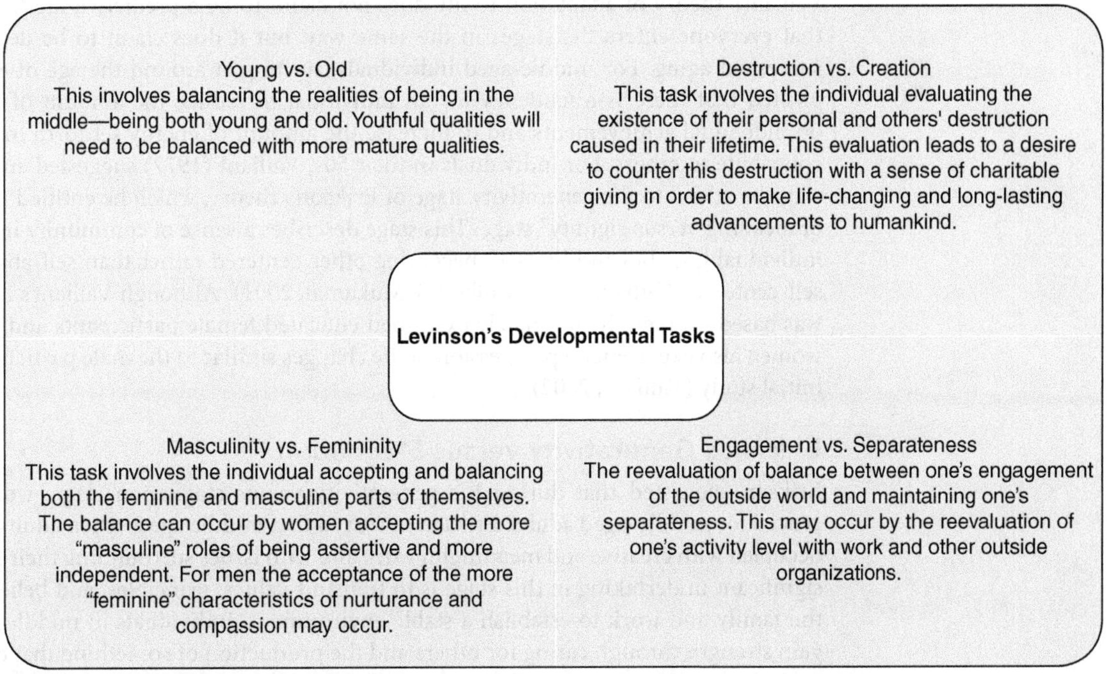

Young vs. Old
This involves balancing the realities of being in the middle—being both young and old. Youthful qualities will need to be balanced with more mature qualities.

Destruction vs. Creation
This task involves the individual evaluating the existence of their personal and others' destruction caused in their lifetime. This evaluation leads to a desire to counter this destruction with a sense of charitable giving in order to make life-changing and long-lasting advancements to humankind.

Levinson's Developmental Tasks

Masculinity vs. Femininity
This task involves the individual accepting and balancing both the feminine and masculine parts of themselves. The balance can occur by women accepting the more "masculine" roles of being assertive and more independent. For men the acceptance of the more "feminine" characteristics of nurturance and compassion may occur.

Engagement vs. Separateness
The reevaluation of balance between one's engagement of the outside world and maintaining one's separateness. This may occur by the reevaluation of one's activity level with work and other outside organizations.

Figure 16.2 Levinson's developmental tasks.

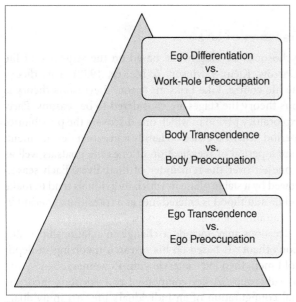

Figure 16.3 Peck's developmental tasks.

tasks or challenges. Peck's first developmental task is **ego differentiation versus work-role preoccupation**. In working on this task, it is suggested that people must redefine themselves in ways that do not relate to their work roles or occupations. Some of the ways in which aging people redefine themselves are through increased contact with family and friends, and giving back to the community, which is just as satisfying as their previous work life. Peck's second developmental task is **body transcendence versus body preoccupation**. In this task, it is suggested that aging individuals must learn to cope with and move beyond changes in physical capabilities that accompany the aging process. As a result, aging individuals must emphasize the offsetting benefits of cognitive, emotional, and social powers. Peck's third developmental task is **ego transcendence versus ego preoccupation**. In this task, it is suggested that aging individuals must begin to cope with the reality of their coming death in the wake of the loss of significant others, siblings, friends, and loved ones (see Figure 16.3).

Vaillant's Theory of Adaptation to Life

Vaillant (1977) conducted a longitudinal study involving about 250 men born in the 1920s, following many throughout their lifetimes. In Vaillant's conclusions he suggests that a person's life course is shaped by meaningful relationships with important people. Vaillant evaluated how the men altered themselves to adapt to life situations. This developmental theory of adulthood focuses on the progression toward maturity in an individual's life. Vaillant's theory of adaptation to life does not claim to be a predictive model, assuming that everyone enters the stages in the same way, but it does claim to be descriptive of successful aging. For middle-aged individuals, starting at around the age of 40, Vaillant posited that there is a tendency for an individual to reduce the amount of time spent on individual achievements and to increase the amount of energy set forth to create and contribute to others. For individuals in their 50s, Vaillant (1977) suggested an additional stage be added to the generativity stage of Erikson's theory, which he entitled the "keeper of meaning versus rigidity" stage. This stage describes a sense of community in which the individual goes beyond himself, becoming other centered rather than self-absorbed and self-centered (Vaillant, 2002; Vaillant & Mukamal, 2001). Although Vaillant's initial study was based on men, he ultimately examined educated female participants and found that women also experience a progression of life changes similar to the male participants in his initial study (Vaillant, 2002).

Erikson's Generativity versus Stagnation

Erikson suggested that during the generativity versus stagnation stage, work is most crucial for middle-aged adults. Erikson observed that middle age is when adults tend to be occupied with creative and meaningful work and with issues surrounding their family. The significant undertaking in this stage is to transmit values, principles, and beliefs through the family and work to establish a stable environment. Individuals in middle adulthood gain strength through caring for others and the production of something that contributes to the betterment of society. This concept of giving back is **generativity**. In contrast lies the fear of becoming stagnated and self-absorbed by way of inactivity and meaninglessness.

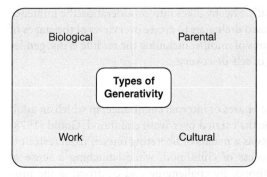

Figure 16.4 Erikson's generativity vs. stagnation stage.

With adult children beginning to transition out of the home, as relationships and goals shift direction, middle-aged adults may be faced with major life changes, and struggling to find new meanings and purposes in life. If these transitions are not met with a sense of reevaluating meaning and purposefulness, middle-aged adults can become self-absorbed and stagnate.

Generativity versus stagnation (Erikson, 1950) allows individuals to strive to reach generativity by attempting to generate something that makes an impact on society by ways of giving back to the next generation. Along with family, career and work are extremely important during this stage (see Figure 16.4). It is important for individuals in this age group to create or nurture things that will exist beyond their lifetime. Generativity may be achieved by raising children or making a constructive difference that benefits other people and society as a whole.

During generativity versus stagnation, feelings of worth and achievement often amount to success, while having a superficial and uncommitted involvement in society often amounts to a sense of failure. This sense of failure leads to stagnation. Stagnation occurs if an individual becomes self-absorbed and uninterested in others once life goals are achieved, such as having successful relationships or marriage, raising a family, and having a successful career.

When a counselor is working with a client experiencing concerns related to middle adulthood, the counselor has an opportunity to encourage and empower the client to use the skills they already have. Due to the tendency of people in middle age to believe more in themselves, the counselor may be able to help the client build upon their self-acceptance, strong sense of autonomy, and ability to control external activities.

REFLECTION 16.2 FINDING FULFILLMENT THROUGH SERVICE

As my child became an independent adult and moved out on her own, I had more free time in which I was able to give back to my community. I became involved in volunteering at my local hospital and spending more time with people at my church. I also helped tutor children for an after-school program at a local agency. I had a sense of fulfillment when I was able to help young people know that they could do anything they put their minds to. I believe that showing young people that individuals have the ability to care for family and others helps them to have a more rounded understanding of growing up and being successful. [~FS]

Gail Sheehy

Sheehy's original work, *Passages* (1976), discussed the developmental process as one that continues from 18 through 50 years of age. *Passages* consists of a collection of life stories of couples that establish Sheehy's theory that times of crisis are inevitable and necessary for developmental growth. Sheehy postulated that each developmental passage is accompanied by predictable crises and that the passages are the same for male and females, although the effects are different.

Sheehy describes **marker events** as those concrete events that happen in a person's life. However, each developmental stage is not defined by those concrete occurrences, but by the process that occurs within the phases. Sheehy also discussed four areas of perception that will undergo subtle changes. The first area of perception is the interior sense of self as it relates to outside individuals. The second is the proportion of safety to danger an individual experiences in life. Perception of time is the third area of perception, in which one views time as being either in abundance or in shortage. The final perception is of experience, or one's sense of being alive or stagnant. These perceptions are facilitators of the decisions one makes in life. Sheehy discussed "life accidents" as events that individuals are powerless to prevent, such as war, mental illness, the death of a parent, child, or significant other, or a genuine threat to the individual's life. Finally, Sheehy takes into consideration the influence of generation and social change. Sheehy used dialogues to create overviews of the stages of life. *Passages* summarized some expectations of midlife, including the midlife crisis, gender identity, sexual issues, and an abundance of self-discovery.

Gould's Developmental Theory

Gould's developmental theory charted the phases of internal cognizance, in which an adult discharges several misconceptions and myths carried over from childhood. Gould (1978) discussed the adult developmental process as a means of liberating oneself from restraints acquired in the early developmental process of childhood, while launching a sense of personal identity in middle to late adulthood. By challenging and confronting the misconceptions and false security of early development, the adult develops a higher level of awareness of self. Gould's theory describes stages of personality development associated with specific age periods. This awakening of awareness involves the adult developing a sense of urgency to attain his life goals and the realization of the limitation of time. The development process is also a period where the adult experiences a realignment of life goals, as well as developing an acceptance of life's reality as he approaches adult maturity.

In keeping with the theme of debunking childhood misconceptions, Gould proposes that transformations that occur in sequential, age-related stages lead the adult to resolve assumptions related to relationship with parents, level of independence, the idea that life is simple and controllable, and the existence of real evil and mortality (see Table 16.1). Further, the transitions involve shifting from a childhood consciousness that is dependent on external regulations and parental protection to an adult consciousness that leads to interdependence, higher self-competence, internal regulations, and a profound understanding of one's self. Throughout one's 30s, the adult turns inward toward a better understanding of self. During one's 40s, an acceptance of mortality arises, allowing the adult to experience a feeling of freedom, a sense of self-acceptance, and responsibility for herself.

TABLE 16.1 ✦ GOULD'S DEVELOPMENTAL STAGES

Age	Stage
16–22	▪ Leaving the parents' world
22–28	▪ Getting into the adult world
28–34	▪ Questioning and reexamination
35–45	▪ Midlife decade
43–50	▪ Reconciliation and mellowing
50+	▪ Stability and acceptance

U.S. Government

Maslow's Self-Actualization Theory

Maslow (1965) defined **self-actualization** as the act of experiencing life in its fullness, in a vivid, selfless manner. This experience involves the person becoming completely absorbed in something without defenses or self-consciousness. Maslow's self-actualization studies focused on "happy" people. Maslow posited that individuals have an innate urge toward healthiness or self-actualization. However, it is noted that in order for an individual to feel unrestricted enough to desire this level of actualization, the individual's basic needs must be met first (Maslow, 1968).

There are eight steps to achieving self-actualization. The first step involves experiencing life fully. Being completely absorbed in an act allows the individual to live vividly and selflessly. The second step is to take risks. Taking risks as opposed to choosing safety fosters progress and growth. Step three involves the emergence of the self. It is positive to shut out external clues to what "should" be thought or done, rather than what the individual truly feels. The fourth step suggests that honesty will lead to responsibility. Step five suggests that it is in the person's best interest to disregard outside judgments. Step six involves the use of intelligence to complete things soundly. Step seven involves making peak experiences more likely, and removing misconceptions and fabricated notions to lead to the acknowledgment of what the individual is truly capable of accomplishing. Finally, step eight involves self-exploration and self-discovery, where the individual recognizes his defenses, which leads to the eventual release of those defenses.

Self-Concept

With the changes that occur in middle adulthood, it is necessary to discuss the degree to which self-concept is affected by these changes. Life experiences and varying abilities result in personality changes throughout the lifespan. Several qualities in individuals predictably increase during middle adulthood, including self-acceptance, autonomy, and environmental mastery.

People in middle adulthood tend to believe in themselves more than during early adulthood. There is a tendency for middle-aged adults to recognize both their positive and negative qualities. There is also an increase in self-perceived autonomy as middle-aged adults view themselves as more concerned with self-proclaimed principles. During middle adulthood, people also tend to view themselves as higher in environmental mastery, of being able to effectively manage a multifaceted assortment of tasks. The term **environmental mastery** refers to the ability to control various external activities. Individuals with a high sense of environmental mastery tend to feel competent in managing the environment and making effective use of opportunities in their surroundings. An individual who feels they experience a low sense of environmental mastery expresses difficulty managing day-to-day events, feels unable to alter their surrounding context, lacks awareness of surrounding opportunities, and lacks a general sense of control as it relates to the world around them.

A study by Van Aken, Denissen, Branje, Dubas, and Goossens (2006) examined the stability of personality change in middle adulthood as related to adaptation to midlife concerns. Most research indicates that personality is stable throughout adulthood; however, Costa and McCrae (2006) posit that personality development is a characteristic of both change and stability. The Van Aken study attributes personality change to the interactions between the person's individual characteristics and environmental factors. The researchers found that personality change was moderately stable, while small reliable changes in personality were found. Fathers in the study experienced personality change related to life satisfaction, work stress, and perceptions of the internalization of problems by their adolescent children. Mothers in the study experienced change in personality as it related to their life satisfaction only. The results may suggest that the change in personality is associated with how well an individual adapts to middle adulthood concerns. An overall feeling of life satisfaction and acceptable contentment with the roles of worker and parent led to personality maturation throughout middle adulthood.

REFLECTION 16.3 LIFE SATISFACTION

Being in middle adulthood overall is a great time in my life. I feel more confident, worry much less what other people think, and trust myself more. I have created a life in which I am satisfied in my career and am financially stable, lifting much unneeded stress from my life. I am at a place where I want to try new things and reach out of my comfort zone a little. I have struggled with some minor health-related issues such as a decrease in my energy level and a loss of libido. I was tested and found to have extremely low testosterone levels and was placed on hormone replacement therapy. This treatment was not hugely successful for me, so I have invested more of my time into eating healthier, using supplements, and exercising. Overall, this has been a less stressful and more enjoyable time in my life. I am more assertive in taking control of my happiness and doing what is best for me. [~JJ]

Gender Identity

It is noted throughout the psychological literature that there is an increase in masculine traits in women and feminine traits in men during the middle adulthood years. This movement in the direction of androgyny is consistent with Levinson's theory: a need to fulfill changing roles and cope with possible stress related to these new roles. Women often experience an increase in confidence and assertiveness, while men often experience an increase in sensitivity and consideration. Due to fewer gender restrictions in middle age, there is a tendency for men and women to explore characteristics typically displayed by the opposite gender. This convergence of gender is noted in research by Bulanda (2011). Biological, cultural, and psychoanalytic factors are possible explanations for this crossover of gender identity. The biological factors involve a decrease in hormonal levels and a decline in sex hormones, while women show an increase in masculine traits and men experience an increase in traditionally feminine traits. Even in diverse cultures, cultural norms tend to be less restrictive and supportive of the blurring of traditional sex roles, when it pertains to gender identity during middle adulthood. It is posited by Bulanda that the concept that individuals have both feminine and masculine characteristics is consistent with psychoanalytic thought, and that social pressures push people to conform to society's standards in order to gain a sense of belonging in society as a whole.

Intimacy and Marriage

Marriage and intimate relationships in midlife are significantly different from marriage and intimate relationships in earlier developmental stages in life, and for several reasons. One factor is the amount of time invested in the relationship. Due to the higher rates of remarriage, it is plausible that a couple may have been established for only a few years. Generally, however, midlife couples have been married or partnered for more than 10 years and upward of 30 years (Hollist & Miller, 2005). As a result, most midlife couples have survived the early years of marriage and partnership, which involve the highest risk of divorce (Bramlett & Mosher, 2002). One of the perks of marriage in midlife is a greater sense of social well-being. According to data gathered from the MIDUS study, married couples have greater social well-being than couples who live together but are not married (Shapiro & Keyes, 2008). Additionally, transition issues such as entering parenthood have already been encountered. It is also suggested that midlife couples have an established relationship history which may result in the formation of meaningful patterns of relating to one another (Miller, 2002).

Outside influences may also affect marriage and intimate relationships in middle adulthood. Life experiences in general may contribute to an increased sense of endurance as it relates to tolerance of hardships in relationships. Many life changes such as adult children leaving the home (empty nest), possibly caring for parents, and other role changes can both positively and negatively affect how middle-aged couples' relationships change.

Same-sex couples and gay, lesbian, bisexual, and transgendered middle-aged individuals may have several varying developmental experiences related to the limitations regarding same-sex marriage in the United States. Currently, most states issue marriage licenses to same-sex couples.

In regard to the psychological impact of the limitations regarding same-sex marriage, many same-sex couples and GLBT individuals report reduced psychological well-being. The resulting negative effects include an increased amount of depressive symptoms and higher negative affect (Riggle, Rostosky, & Horn, 2009). GLBT individuals observe that their relationships are generally undervalued when compared to heterosexual relationships. This devaluing includes placing barriers on reaching relationship goals due to implementation of laws and policies that limit marriage rights to same-sex couples (Frost, 2011).

Additionally, same-sex couples report conflict in their intimate relationships related to additional stress caused by limitations on same-sex marriage. Some of the additional stress results in relational conflict and negative interactions and experiences with their partners (Lannutti, 2013; Maisel & Fingerhut, 2011).

In spite of negative experiences with legislative restrictions, GLBT individuals in long-term committed and legally recognized relationships report a lower level of psychological concerns and a greater level of psychological well-being than GLBT individuals not in long-term committed or legally recognized relationships (Riggle et al., 2009). When reporting less psychological stress, there were lower incidences of internalized homophobia, depression, and stress. When discussing the increased level of psychological well-being, there were reports of having a feeling of purpose and adding meaning to one's life. Similar to the positive effects of marriage in heterosexual relationships, long-term commitment and legal recognition of same-sex relationships adds positive benefits to the psychological well-being of the individuals and the couple as a whole.

REFLECTION 16.4 DADDY AND "DADDY OTHER ONE"

I've spent my life trying to "prove" I was normal. Now I'm 53 years old and finding that proving to others I am "normal" is no longer a priority. Having been lucky enough to build a life with my partner Ed, the past 19 years have been a wonderful experience. We started as two, trying to prove to others that we were a couple of guys who were in love and could contribute to society. If we did contribute, then how could they not believe we were worthy of their respect and accept us as equals?

Luckily, we have been blessed to share our lives with two wonderful souls that God put on this Earth for us. One of the most extraordinary blessings in our lives was the opportunity to adopt two children. They have given us the ability to overcome any obstacle and have shown us total unconditional love. Our two sons, Jack and Brad, give us experiences of wisdom. From their pure hearts and unconditional love, we see every day that we have a purpose, which is to ensure they grow up knowing how special, unique, and loved they are.

I was so afraid when we adopted them that we could not give them what they would need to make it in this world. Our lives would change. We would have sleepless nights and never have time for us again. My mother, my friends, and coworkers gave their opinions. None were good. I looked each of them in the eye and asked if they were pregnant or their spouse was pregnant, would they give the child up or abort it? It was difficult to consider that they were thinking that two gay guys, particularly their son, friend, or coworker, should not raise a child, but I'm sure some were. Our commitment to both of our sons began before they were born, and once we made the commitment there was no turning back, period!

It is quite humorous now, looking back at our concerns. No mom in the house, how could the boys be normal? How are we, and the boys, going to deal with the stigma of two dads? Two old guys raising two young boys . . . what would people think? I guess all of those concerns were valid at the time as we were navigating uncharted waters, at least for us. Now I am concerned that we make sure our sons grow to be confident, loving, empathetic adults who are comfortable with not only themselves but able to find their God-given passions in life and pursue them. The hell with what anyone else says!

We all have our loads to bear, our crosses to carry. As a parent I now want to dedicate my life to setting an example for my sons that the world is theirs and any deficit they perceive in themselves is self-inflicted. I want to help them figure out how to overcome obstacles. We all are different but similar. And there is no one, and I mean NO ONE, who is better than anyone else.

I learn every day from my sons. They teach me, and remind me what life is truly about. I always remember that I am here for them before worrying about myself. We will still have opportunities to grow and learn, though some opportunities are not such positive lessons. We experienced an incident where a man called Ed, my partner, a "faggot." Yes, the kids heard him. We all learned from this experience. We also learned from the parent who would not let her son call Jack at home because he lives with two "queers." These were hard lessons for our sons. But we have been dealing with that our entire lives. The key is to make sure it is a positive learning experience for all of us, showing them that it is best to respect others who are different. Again, through all that we are learning and through both good and bad, nothing trumps the hug, the honest look, the smile, and the words "I love you Daddy Rich" or "I love you Daddy Other One" (Jack's chosen name for Ed). Such is the life of middle-aged gay dads, which include homework, extracurricular activities, etc., plus the continued legal papers that we have to constantly update to protect us as a family. [~RW]

Important Relationships and Friendships

Experiencing intimate relationships in middle adulthood is a crucial component that leads to satisfaction, happiness, and self-admiration. Middle-aged adults tend to be more selective in picking friends in this phase of life. The selection process is based more on mutual pleasure than for supportive reasons. As with friendships across the lifespan, middle-aged men tend to be less expressive than women in their friendships. Women report a larger number of friends than men; they also report more emotional support gained (Antonucci, Akiyama, & Takahashi, 2004).

Stress

Stress can be defined as a normal physical response to events that cause an individual to feel threatened or upset in some way (Sutin, Costa, Wethington, & Eaton, 2010). How people interpret and cope with stress can depend upon their stable characteristics. Also, these interpretations change throughout the lifetime. One's level of education plays a part in one's experiences with stress. According to data retrieved from the MIDUS study, those who are more educated have fewer and less severe stressors than those who are less educated (Almeida, Neupert, Banks, & Serido, 2005). **Coping** is referred to as any way to handle stress. **Stress** is any internal or external force in the world that affects the individual. People respond to stress in ways that affect the environment as well as themselves. Stress is typically viewed as a negative experience; however, from a biological standpoint stress can be a neutral, negative, or even positive experience.

Some external stress factors include major life changes, relationship difficulties, caretaking responsibilities, financial problems, and role overload. Internal factors determine the body's ability to respond to, and deal with, the external stress-inducing factors. Some internal stress factors include physical health, eating habits, emotional well-being, and sleep patterns. Internal factors determine the body's ability to respond to, and deal with, the external stress-inducing factors.

Theories of Stress

Hans Selye (1985) focused on the internal aspects of stress, postulating that a stress response can result from various types of stressors. Selye noted three phases that people who undergo a prolonged state of stress experience: alarm, resistance, and exhaustion. Together, this group of stress reactions is referred to as the general adaptation syndrome (GAS). The first stage, the alarm reaction, is similar to the fight or flight response and is accompanied by neurological and physiological responses. The second stage, resistance, is a constant state of arousal. If a prolonged exposure to the stressor exists, a high level of pituitary gland hormones (ACTH) is present, which may disrupt homeostasis and damage internal organs. Last is the exhaustion stage, which occurs after prolonged resistance in which the body's reserve energy is dissipated and physical malfunction is likely. In humans, it is in the stage of resistance when many diseases are precipitated or caused by stress occur. Examples of these diseases of adaptation include insomnia, high blood pressure, cardiovascular disease, kidney disease, and headaches.

Type A Personality

There is a strong relationship between cardiovascular disease and stress. Friedman and Rosenman (1974) noted two personality types with different risks of cardiovascular disease. People with **Type A personality** characteristics are more likely to develop cardiovascular disease than people with Type B personality. Some characteristics of Type A personality individuals include extreme competitiveness, intense anger, hostile tendencies, restlessness, being overly aggressive, and frequent impatience. In contrast, people who display characteristics related to **Type B personality** may tend to be calm, easygoing, relaxed, and not often hurried.

Coping Skills in Adult Life

When combating stress, adults of middle age tend to focus on and identify with the positive components of transition and stress (Sutin et al., 2010). Also, because of an increased amount of life experience, middle-aged adults tend to be less impulsive, thereby postponing actions needed to combat the stressful situation. Another coping skill noted among individuals in middle adulthood is the anticipation of crisis and stress-related circumstances, leading to an increased amount of planning on the individual's part to address stressful situations should they arise. It is reported that humor is often used as a coping skill, along with an increase in confidence level and experience. Middle-aged adults also tend to integrate and accept their strengths and weaknesses more than younger adults.

Techniques for Dealing with Stress

A significant way to combat the effects of stress is by engaging in exercise. The U.S. Department of Health and Human Services suggests exercising three or more times a week in order to increase longevity and overall health and reduce stress. Regular exercise can reduce stress over the short and long term (Rimmele et al., 2008). Aerobic exercise may help to provide a positive physical outlet that facilitates the release of built-up tension, while low-intensity exercises can have a more soothing effect.

Optimism

An optimistic approach to life may also provide middle-aged individuals a means of staying healthy and combating stress. A study of more than 340,000 people published in *Proceedings of the National Academy of Sciences* (Taylor, 2010) found that feelings of adjustment and well-being improve as one enters middle adulthood. It is noted that levels of stress are reduced as well as incidents of worrying and anger. An increase in levels of happiness and pleasure was reported by respondents.

REFLECTION 16.5 COMBATING STRESS IN MIDLIFE

The first thing that comes to mind about dealing with stress is hindsight. It was not until I was in the years of aging that I experienced how important it is to exercise, have good eating habits, and administer self-care. The things that I have incorporated into my life to combat stress are walking three miles a day at least five days out of the week and meditating. As I exercise, I listen to a book on tape, or music; and depending on where I am mentally, it will be soothing music or music that gets my blood flowing and helps to pick up the pace.

Another important factor is that I am surrounded by a wonderful array of people who encourage and support me whenever needed. Strong, healthy relationships play a vital part in my life in those moments when stress is overwhelming. A spiritual relationship and prayer is by far my most important remedy in dealing with my stress. Fellowshipping with others, participating in praise and worship, and hearing the Word helps me to get my life in perspective and reduce my everyday stresses. [~JC]

Middle Age and Attachment

It has been suggested that patterns of attachment relate to emotional experience in middle age; for example, middle-aged men with secure attachments tend to experience more joyful relationships. The attachment styles of middle-aged adults vary based on emotional context in relation to social origins, emotional experiences, and the variety of roles of men and women (Consedine & Fiori, 2009).

Fearful avoidant personality types are often found in both younger and older generations. However, in middle age populations this attachment style causes an increase in negative affect and poor relationships. Secure relationships in middle age promote security and predict lower levels of anxiety, depression, and hostility (Consedine & Fiori, 2009).

Intra- and interpersonal dynamics have direct effects on particular emotions of middle-aged adults, specifically with grief and loss. Middle-aged adults who experience more death in their lifetimes are more likely to develop avoidant attachment styles. Anxiety itself begins to decline in middle age, but men in particular will experience higher levels of anxiety than women, especially due to interpersonal loss (Consedine & Fiori, 2009).

Personality in Middle Adulthood

Through the middle adulthood years, personality traits remain fairly stable. The stability can be marked by the concept of possible selves, which can be defined as a representation of what one hopes to be in the future. Longitudinal, cross-cultural, and cross-sectional research has discussed personality characteristics as remaining stable across the lifespan. The Big 5 personality traits (see Table 16.2) represent the most basic dimensions of personality: (1) neuroticism, (2) extraversion, (3) agreeableness, (4) conscientiousness, and (5) openness to experience (Costa & McCrae, 2006). A majority of these longitudinal studies report that these personality traits remain fairly fixed after the age of 30 years.

TABLE 16.2 ✦ THE BIG 5 PERSONALITY TRAITS

Neuroticism
- These traits include the tendency for the individual to experience negative emotions such as excessive worrying and being unpredictable, erratic, self-absorbed, overly emotional, and vulnerable. These individuals tend to be over-sensitive and nervous.

Extraversion
- These traits include being energetic, affectionate, outgoing, talkative, and assertive. These individuals tend to enjoy the company of others and are outgoing and passionate.

Agreeableness
- These traits include being friendly, compassionate, empathic, compliant, and trusting. These individuals tend to be generous and affectionate.

Conscientiousness
- These traits include being organized, reliable, accountable, ambitious, and self-controlled. These individuals tend to be efficient and self-disciplined.

Openness
- These traits include being open to experience, creative, insightful, and liberal. These individuals tend to be inventive and curious about new ideas.

Role Expectations and Family Developmental Issues

Most worthwhile odysseys present unique challenges, and this can be true for the middle adulthood stage of the lifespan, when several family developmental issues may arise. These family developmental issues may result in changes related to role expectations, thus impacting the level of stress faced by adults in midlife. Some of these issues may include family adjustments to crises, grandparenthood, parent–adolescent interaction, launching periods, caring for aging parents, and marital issues.

Family Adjustment to Crises

A family crisis is any demand placed on a family that causes stress (Lamanna, Riedmann, & Riedmann, 2006). Examples of stressors that may cause a family crisis include the birth or addition of a family member, loss, and indistinct losses. Additional stressors that may lead to a family crisis are stress-related responsibilities around caring for loved ones. Daily living activities and role shifts can also trigger stress for families. As a family undergoes a crisis, three distinct stages are seen: adaptation, disorganization, and recovery.

In the adaptation stage the family may function in much the same way as the family was functioning before the crisis. Interestingly, some members of the family may continue to function on a comparable or even a higher level during the adaptation. During the disorganization period, the functionality of the family system declines, and traditional roles and routines become distorted and jumbled. There is an increased level of anger in the family dynamic. The final phase, recovery, is where the family has the opportunity to begin the establishment of new behaviors. Every family experiences crisis differently. Some families fail to recover from stressful times of crisis, while some families are quite resilient. It is important to note that some families do not recover; instead, they dissolve. Others are able to stay intact, but function on a much lower organizational level. Still other families are able to bounce back while matching the level of support and functionality that existed before the crisis.

Grandparenthood

One of the joys for many middle-aged adults is becoming a grandparent. There are several styles of grandparenting, including: involved grandparents, compassionate grandparents, and remote grandparents. Involved grandparents are vigorously involved in their grandchildren's lives and have clear hopes for the grandchild's behavior. Compassionate grandparents are calm, providing camaraderie and support to their grandchildren. Remote grandparents tend to be aloof and uninvolved in their grandchildren's development. These grandparents are disconnected and withdrawn from their grandchildren.

Empty Nest and Boomerang Generation

Another family development issue occurs when adult children leave the home, creating an empty nest. Though gaining a sense of freedom caused by having an empty nest is usually looked forward to by parents, this event can lead to issues related to reestablishing an identity outside of raising children. Some negative feelings associated with the empty nest are isolation and depression.

An external factor that may affect marriage and intimate relationships in middle adulthood is the return of adult children to the parents' home, referred to as the boomerang generation. During difficult economic times, it is common for adult children to reestablish residency with parents. According to the Bureau of Labor Statistics (2010), 15.6% of 20–24-year-olds are unemployed versus 8.7% of adults over the age of 25. The return of adult children often indicates sociological, demographic, and economic difficulties that may affect the parent–child relationship as well as the parents' marital satisfaction during middle adulthood. Mitchell (1998) found that such returns do not generally result in dissatisfaction or conflict. Additionally, Mitchell concluded that when the returning children are close to achievement in their adult roles, provide additional support, and are more independent, a greater level of parental satisfaction is found.

Divorce

Some of the life changes mentioned above may force couples to reevaluate the progression of their relationship and make adjustments accordingly. If this reevaluation and adjustment is not made, divorce becomes a likely possibility for middle-aged couples. Though the statistics on divorce show a greater number of divorces occurring within the first 5–10 years of marriage, only about 10% of couples experience a divorce after 20 years of marriage (U.S. Department of Health and Human Services, 2010b). Although divorce at any age is painful and distressing, greater coping and problem-solving skills may help people in middle age to adjust to divorce with more ease than a younger adult.

Divorce rates rise as the number of times an individual marries increases; thus, the divorce rate is higher for remarried individuals (U.S. Department of Health and Human Services, 2010b). It is possible that divorce is more widely accepted in our society, as the divorce rate during middle adulthood is higher than it has been in generations past. People are more individualistic than they used to be and often choose their own personal happiness over their marriage. Divorce is more accepted now than it used to be, and couples in Western cultures often divorce when passionate love subsides, because romance and passion are highly valued in our society. Societal stress on families is another reason divorces during middle adulthood are on the rise.

Children and Divorce

The adjustment process for children of divorce can be lengthy and tumultuous. This process can place the children of these families at a greater risk for a multitude of emotive and responsive problems. Occurrences of these issues often emerge well before the actual divorce. These concerns may include both externalizing and internalizing behaviors (Taylor, Purswell, Lindo, Jayne, & Fernando, 2011). Divorce often affects parent–child dynamics regardless of the age of the child. However, researchers note that preteens who experience the divorce of their parents are more likely to display antisocial behaviors (Strohschein, 2005), while teenagers were more likely to encounter academic issues (Lengua, Wolchik, Sandler, & West, 2000). There are several adjustment issues that may affect family dynamics as well. Some of these issues include decreased amounts of financial, social, and emotional resources. While undergoing this adjustment period, children may experience a sense of abandonment (Ängarne-Lindberg, Wadsby, & Berterö, 2009), rejection, isolation, and depression. An increase in stress may lead to a higher incidence of conflict and a lower incidence of positive communication interactions between parent and child. Despite the negative effects of divorce on family dynamics, strong parent–child relationships can counterbalance the effects divorce has on the family.

Remarriage

Most people remarry or repartner within two to five years after divorce. Research suggests that divorcees who reestablish relationships after divorce ordinarily experience a positive personal adjustment to their new life experiences (Blekesaune, 2008; Wang & Amato, 2008). Men are more likely to remarry, while many women do not remarry as often. The likelihood that women remain unmarried increases if women are custodial parents of children. The decision to remarry becomes complicated with the presence of children. Challenges involving partner selection and partner/child introductions are common experiences for divorced parents.

Coping with Role Expectations and Family Developmental Issues

It is important for counselors to be aware of additional ways of combating stress resulting from developmental issues and increased role expectations. It is possible that the above-mentioned family developmental issues may induce stress in adults in middle adulthood as well as their families. As previously mentioned, adults in midlife tend to use a different set of coping mechanisms to combat this stressful time than adults in earlier stages of life. These coping mechanisms include preventive planning, increased use of optimism and humor, spirituality, and an increased level of self-care. Counselors should encourage clients dealing with such life issues to seek social and emotional support from their peers and loved ones, as well as encouraging resilience through the promotion of confidence and self-efficacy.

SECTION III:	Career Development in Middle Adulthood

Job Satisfaction/Dissatisfaction

Typically, midlife is a time when people evaluate their career satisfaction and personal happiness. A common stereotype holds that this period of time represents a crisis for some, often referred to as a "midlife crisis." However, current research does not validate the notion of a crisis at midlife. Hunter (2011) found that both men and women in middle age were more satisfied with their jobs than young adults. However, rapid changes in technology are demanding that people learn new skill sets just to remain proficient in their current positions. Now more than ever, keeping up and learning new skills is imperative to keep skills from becoming obsolete or irrelevant. People in midlife who make fewer changes and advances in their skill set are more dissatisfied in their careers (Spector, 1997).

Kawada and Otsuka (2010) reported that white-collar, middle-aged workers were both intrinsically and extrinsically more satisfied than their younger, blue-collar counterparts. Intrinsically, white-collar, middle-aged workers feel more competent in their positions and have a stronger sense of perceived control, leading to added confidence and satisfaction. Extrinsically, middle-aged workers tend to hold more senior-level positions, resulting in higher salaries and prestige within an organization.

Changing Careers at Midlife and Unemployment

Currently, countless factors may lead to career change at midlife. Fewer workers are changing careers now than in earlier years due to boredom, wanting to follow a passion, or having the financial security to try something new. Instead, changes in the economy, death of a spouse, divorce, outsourcing, and technology (just to name a few) have mandated many midlife career changes. Those who can voluntarily change do so based on a reevaluation of their life and satisfaction with their careers. They also may be reacting to their children leaving home and their partner returning to work, allowing them the freedom to take more financial risks than in the past.

In the current state of the economy it is more likely that career change at midlife is involuntary, most likely resulting from being laid off or fired. Research from the John J. Heldrich Center for Workforce Development at Rutgers (2009) found that one-third of the unemployed are in middle adulthood. For those in middle age, the average length of

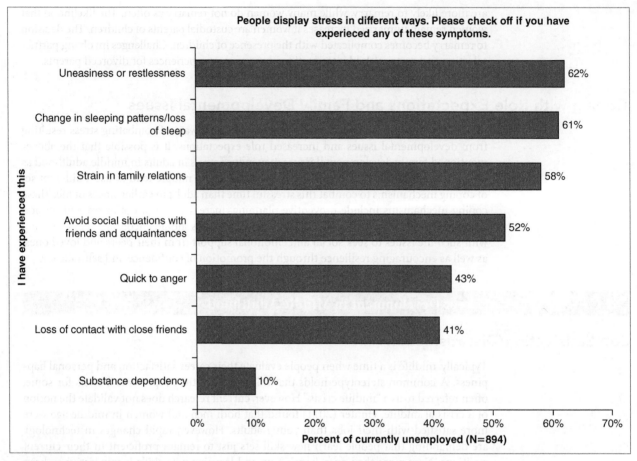

Figure 16.5 Percent of unemployed reporting psychological symptoms.
Source: U.S. Department of Labor, 2010.

unemployment is 34 weeks. Due to financial insecurity and lack of opportunity, those in midlife are looking at new careers, using their existing skill sets or going back to school or to training programs to gain new skills. People finding themselves forced into career change often experience myriad psychological symptoms such as depression, anxiety, anger, helplessness, hopelessness, and stress (U.S. Department of Labor, 2010) (see Figure 16.5).

Adult Learners, Returning Students

Hatch, Feinstein, Link, Wadsworth, and Richards (2007) found a correlation between continued education in middle adulthood and higher verbal ability, verbal memory, and verbal fluency. They propose that the benefits of this correlation can be seen in increased social integration, well-being, and a delay of cognitive decline in later life. With the many benefits of returning to school at midlife there are also many stressors that require a tremendous amount of support for the middle-adulthood student.

Support for returning students comes from a variety of areas in one's life: family, school, job, church, and other social networks. Family and friends play a large role in supporting a student's return to school at midlife, especially for those people returning to school who have a full-time job and are raising children or supporting aging parents. Sharing in household chores and child-rearing responsibilities as well as supporting and encouraging the educational pursuits of the student at midlife go far in aiding their educational success.

Universities have seen a dramatic increase in online, weekend, and evening courses leading to the support of midlife workers returning to the educational domain. Various workplaces offer financial support and incentives as well as flexible scheduling to accommodate workers returning to school. This benefits both the workers and the companies, ensuring continued skill development, job security, and employee retention.

➤ CASE EXAMPLE **16.1** EXPLORING CAREER ISSUES IN MIDDLE ADULTHOOD.

The literature shows that midlifers in white-collar positions are more satisfied in their careers. Developmentally, this is a normal time for people to reassess their career choice and to explore alternatives. This is also a time to examine the negative impact that job loss or forced career change may have on your clients. Those in this category may experience depression, anxiety, anger, helplessness, hopelessness, and stress. Helping clients explore alternatives in the workforce or pursuing continuing education is crucial. In addition, helping clients identify leisure activities they enjoy can lead to increased mental well-being. What are some approaches you think might be particularly helpful to use with midlife career changers? What resources are available to help them make use of the many educational opportunities now available to all adult learners?

Women in the Labor Force

In 2010 the U.S. Department of Labor reported that 46.7% of all women over the age of 16 were in the work force. The peak for women in the workforce is in middle adulthood for women, especially married women, as opposed to early adulthood for men. Middle adulthood is a time when children leave home and women have more time to pursue a career.

Male/Female Differences

In spite of the number of women in the workforce the ratio of women's to men's earnings, for all occupations, was 81.2% in 2010. Men on average have more salaried, higher-level executive positions and job status. Social changes over the past few decades are reducing these margins as well as breaking the barriers between traditionally male- and female-stereotyped positions. More and more men are staying home to raise the family while women pursue careers in the workforce. Men are becoming nurses and secretaries; women are becoming pilots and CEOs (Mott, 1998; Wentling, 2002).

Interestingly, the average family now has two working parents, resulting in dual-career or double career households. A **dual-career household** is one in which both partners have individual careers that are not sacrificed by the other or by the family. In turn, a **double career** is when one partner takes on a career outside the home and additional duties such as household responsibilities and child-rearing. Usually, this burden still rests predominantly on the female in the household (Townsend, 2001).

Leisure Activities

In a New Zealand study of midlife adults' leisure, Gray (2011) found that 86% of the participants were satisfied with how they spent their leisure time. People tend to remain consistent across their lives as far as what leisure activities they pursue. The intensity of the activity may dissipate with age, but the interest generally stays the same. Midlife adults with higher levels of education and income were found to be more active than those with less education or income.

The benefits of leisure during midlife are substantial; they include an increase in health and mental well-being. Studies on leisure in the middle adulthood years have determined that leisure activities that included physical activity at least twice a week were associated with a reduced risk of dementia and Alzheimer's disease, and increased overall well-being. Leisure activities can lower the risk of mortality, reduce stress, and stimulate positive mental

REFLECTION 16.6 LEISURE ACTIVITIES IN MIDLIFE

As a younger man I always looked at people in middle age and envied them. They seemed to have a lot of toys and did the things I couldn't afford. Now that I am in middle age, I have made that happen for myself. I am at a place of financial security which allows me to do the things of which I once dreamed. I can travel, go deep-sea fishing, and explore other interests. I can take care of my family and include them in the things I love. I do feel that I am stuck in a career that is not very satisfying to me, yet have traded that for financial security because I can't bear the thought of starting over and giving up all the other things I love. I feel it is worth the sacrifice and am happier now than I have ever been. [~BJ]

health in women. A lack of leisure pursuits during middle adulthood was related to depressive symptoms, underlining the importance of including leisure activities with self-care and social support (Lu, 2010).

Planning for Retirement

The period of time prior to retirement is known as the preretirement phase. This occurs at different points of time for each individual due to issues related to finances, social supports, and work history. Planning for retirement can elicit different feelings from different people. Some welcome the idea, looking forward to exploring their interests and spending time with friends and family, while others fear the prospect. Of course, planning is recommended in order to facilitate an optimal transition into the retirement years (Warr, Butcher, Robertson, & Callinan, 2004).

The steps one takes during middle adulthood directly affect when one can retire. For instance, women who have taken time off to raise children often push their retirement age back many years. Economic recessions influence retirement plans of many middle-aged adults. Studies show that finances are the most explored issue relating to retirement during the preretirement phase. Without proper financial support the options for retirement are diminished. In 2011 the first Baby Boomers reached retirement age. The Social Security system has been stretched and will continue to struggle, making retirement planning more difficult for subsequent generations. Already the impact on retirement due to lack of finances is being seen in the Baby Boomer group. A recent AARP survey found that 40% of boomers plan to continue working indefinitely (Roper, 2011).

SECTION IV: Spirituality in Middle Adulthood

As in other aspects of development, one's spiritual life goes through different phases during the aging process. Understanding these developmental stages has become critical for counselors. The Association for Spiritual, Ethical, and Religious Values in Counseling (ASERVIC, 2009) has included understanding of these spiritual development models as part of their newly revised competencies.

There are six stages of faith (Kelcourse, 2004). The majority of adults fall in the fifth stage, **conjunctive faith**. In this stage, one has developed personal beliefs about spirituality that are not based solely on what one has been told throughout life. Religion and spirituality become more concrete than in previous stages. To put this stage in a broader context, adults begin to come to terms with things outside of spirituality, such as children leaving home and the stark reality of death. A mark of conjunctive faith is a greater awareness of one's spiritual life as well as acknowledgment of aspects of religion that one may never fully understand. The ability to have open-minded conversations with others from different religions is also seen in this stage.

People's spiritual exercises and religious activities undoubtedly have an influence on their lives. This impact is usually perceived as a positive one. For middle-aged adults, a stronger sense of spirituality can also lead to a greater sense of psychological well-being. Spiritual rituals, whether they include religious activities such as attending a church service or engaging in a daily activity such as praying, lead to higher levels of psychological well-being (Greenfield, Vaillant, & Marks, 2009). There are fewer instances of depression among individuals who are religious or spiritual (Murphy & Fitchett, 2009; Young, Cashwell, & Shcherbakova, 2000).

Although the inclusion of spirituality in life is usually seen as positive, some can experience negative aspects of spirituality. A form of obsessive-compulsive disorder called **scrupulosity** can be seen in individuals who take religious activities to extremes, such as constant worry over sin or rituals like prayer that are taken to an unhealthy level (Ciarocchi, 2009; Miller & Hedges, 2008). As with any other mental health concern, not addressing scrupulosity can have a negative influence on development.

Intersectionality

Aspects of diversity in the developmental process of middle adulthood is presented to acknowledge differences and similarities between the experiences of adults in this developmental stage based on race, class, gender, sexuality, and other aspects of diversity. These aspects of diversity are related to development in many ways. It has been noted in this chapter that there are differences based on gender and race related to biological changes in middle adulthood, as well as gender differences in cognitive development, such as the prevalence of certain diseases and disorders. With respect to psychosocial development, there are many social and cultural differences that may impact how one experiences developmental changes. One of these differences includes one's view of caretaking responsibilities. For instance, if a person has been raised in a collectivist community, that individual is more likely than an individual raised in an individualistic community to take on the caretaking responsibilities for an aging parent. Also, women are more likely than men to physically undertake the caretaking responsibilities for aging parents, while men are more likely to undertake the financial caretaking responsibilities. It is important to note that there are a variety of differences affected by diversity in many aspects of middle adulthood, ranging from gender and ethnic differences in biosocial development, to gender differences in intimacy and role expectations. Finally, differences within groups as well as differences among groups should also be taken into account when considering the intersection of diversity and biosocial, cognitive, and psychosocial development in middle adulthood.

Summary

Middle adulthood is defined as the period from the mid-30s to approximately 65 years of age. This developmental stage currently contains two generational age groups: Baby Boomers and Generation X ("Xers"). The two groups have commonalities and distinctive characteristics that set each apart from the other. Baby Boomers are typically considered optimistic and idealistic. People from Generation X are viewed as more logical and practical. However, both groups are very independent and self-reliant. While there are similarities, there are developmental differences in experiences. Baby Boomers may be nearing the end of their careers and child-rearing, considering retirement, and enjoying grandchildren. Xers may have as much as a decade or two of work left and may be in the midst of raising children. Baby Boomers directly experienced some of the most significant social movements in the past 50 years (the Vietnam War, civil rights and women's movements), while the Xers experienced these indirectly. These common social experiences allow for a more cohesive understanding of the group.

There are many transitional issues experienced throughout the midlife developmental period. Some middle-aged adults are referred to as the sandwich generation, which refers to adult children who are raising their own children while caring for their aging parents. One out of every eight Americans aged 40–60 falls into the sandwich generation experience. Some common concerns of sandwich generation caregivers are balancing roles, delineating boundaries, maintaining healthy relationships, and maintaining positive mental and emotional health. Another transitional issue presented is the question of the midlife crisis. There are varying perspectives on the midlife crisis. Erikson emphasized the struggle occurring during generativity versus stagnation, while Levinson interprets this period as a transition rather than a crisis. Another perspective on the midlife crisis is one that proposes that this transitional period is affected by environmental and personal experience.

There are several theories of psychosocial development pertaining to middle adulthood. Levinson's seasons of life theory is a concentrated view of psychosocial development based on the sequences of life. Peck's tasks of ego integrity attempt to more clearly define the image of middle adulthood through three major developmental tasks or challenges. These developmental tasks include ego differentiation versus work-role preoccupation, body transcendence versus body preoccupation, and ego transcendence versus ego preoccupation. Vaillant's adaptation to life theory concluded that a person's life course is shaped by meaningful relationships with important people. Individuals in their 40s tend to reduce the amount of time spent on individual achievement, and an increasing focus on contributions to others; individuals in their 50s tend to increase the sense of community by becoming other centered rather than self-centered.

In Erikson's developmental theory, the generativity versus stagnation stage is most closely related to middle adulthood, suggesting that adults tend to be occupied with creative and meaningful work, along with issues surrounding their family, and gain strength through giving back to others and contributing to the betterment of society. If this transitional period is not met with a sense of reevaluating self-meaning, then middle-aged adults enter stagnation. Sheehy suggested that the developmental stages individuals encounter are passages that are accompanied by predictable crises. Sheehy proposed that the passages are the same for men and women, but may result in differential effects. Gould's adult development theory charts the phases of internal cognizance, in which an adult discharges several misconceptions and myths carried over from childhood. In Gould's theory of development, individuals in middle adulthood develop a sense of acceptance of mortality, leading to a feeling of freedom, a sense of self-acceptance, and responsibility for oneself. Maslow defined self-actualization as the act of experiencing life in its fullness, which involves an individual becoming completely absorbed in something without defenses and self-consciousness.

There are significant issues related to gender identity, marriage, intimate relationships, and stress that occur in middle adulthood. There is an increase in masculine traits in women and feminine traits in men. There may be an increase in confidence and assertiveness for women, while there is an increase in sensitivity and consideration for men. Marriage and intimate relationships in midlife are significantly different than in earlier developmental stages of life. These differences include the amount of time invested in the relationship and a greater sense of social well-being, satisfaction, happiness, and self-admiration. Also, because of an increased amount of life experience, middle-aged adults tend to be less impulsive, postponing actions to combat stressful situations.

In terms of family development issues in middle adulthood, there are several that may impact a middle-aged individual, including a family crisis (e.g., birth or addition of a family member, loss), becoming a grandparent, having an adult child leaving the home or returning, and divorce. The divorce rate during middle adulthood is higher than it has been in generations past. One possible explanation for this is that people are generally more individualistic and choose their own personal happiness over their marriage.

During this developmental stage, people may face career challenges as well. Evaluation of career satisfaction and personal happiness is typically done during midlife. Many factors can come into play when contemplating a career change or retirement. Changes in the economy, death of a spouse, divorce, outsourcing, and technology are found to be the leading causes. Due to financial insecurity and lack of opportunity, those in midlife are looking for new careers using their existing skill sets, going back to school, or attending training programs to gain new skills.

Planning for retirement can elicit diverse feelings. Some welcome the idea, looking forward to exploring their interests and spending time with friends and family, while others fear the prospect. Without proper financial support, the options for retirement are slim. The impact on retirement due to lack of finances is being seen in the Baby Boomer generation, as a recent AARP survey found that 40% of Baby Boomers plan to continue working indefinitely (Roper, 2011).

Regarding spirituality in middle adulthood, the majority of adults fall in the fifth stage (conjunctive faith) of the six-stage model of spirituality. In this stage, an individual has developed their own beliefs about spirituality that are not based solely on what they have been told throughout their lives. Religion and spirituality become more concrete than in previous stages. Middle-aged adults begin to come to terms with things outside of spirituality, such as children leaving home and the stark reality of death.

Later Adulthood and Old Age: Physical and Cognitive Development

By Cecile Yancu, Debbie Newsome, Joseph Wilkerson, and Shannon Mathews

Globally, the population is aging. Those 60 years and older have increased from 8% of the total population in 1950 to 11% in 2011 and are expected to reach 22% by 2050. Among the elderly, the 80 years and over group is also growing exponentially. In the United States, the leading edge of the "Baby Boomer" generation, a large cohort of people born between 1946 and 1964, has reached the age of Medicare and Social Security. Although population aging raises important challenges for every society, the good news is that while people are living longer, they are also living healthier for more years of life. With the help of modern medicine, a healthier lifestyle, and a cleaner environment, older people are often able to delay debilitating illness until shortly before death. As a result, our ideas about growing older have evolved from it being a time of social withdrawal and frailty to a period of vitality, community engagement, and tackling challenges head on. Older people are now seen by many as a valuable social and economic resource capable of contributing to the economy in myriad ways, from volunteerism to skills experience to consumer power.

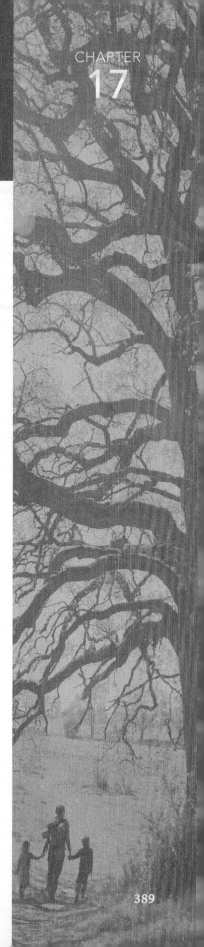

SECTION I: Physical Development

As the title of this book suggests, the stages one encounters throughout the life course reflect an odyssey, a type of journey with a beginning, a middle, and an end. Those who reach the end of the journey in old age probably do so because they were lucky enough to steer clear of harm's way and fortunate enough to come from genetically healthy parental stock. From this transitional perspective, later life and old age represent the inevitable conclusion of the voyage. For most, it is a period of reflection and assessment of a lifetime's worth of accumulated experience. It is also a time for adjustment and accommodation to an onslaught of physical, social, and emotional changes, some of which are more easily adapted to than others.

REFLECTION 17.1   RUBY REMEMBERS

"Life is not a dress rehearsal so I may as well enjoy it while I'm here. It's not that every day is a good day—far from it. I do know that if I don't look in the mirror it's hard to believe that I'll be 91 next month." When asked if she had any advice for the students who would read this book, Ruby answered without hesitation. "No! We all age differently. We all went through different things getting here."

Ruby has been through a lot in her 91 years. Like many of her generation, she married at age 17, moving from her family home to her husband's. She has lived through war, relocation, financial hardship, and loss; 15 years ago she lost her husband of nearly 60 years. For the last 10 years of her husband's life she was his primary caregiver as he struggled with a debilitating combination of angina and congestive heart failure. The weaker his heart got the less he was able to do for himself. On good days when he was able to walk they could leave the confines of the apartment and enjoy the day. On the bad days, he had too little strength or too much chest pain to move from room to room. "Those were the hardest days; to see him like that, gasping for breath. His heart was suffocating." Ruby said that she had no real friends to speak of because there wasn't time. "When he needed the rest, I would go out for a walk and do bit of shopping. In his last two years there were a lot of ambulance trips to the hospital. The doctors had trouble controlling his pain. But during that time our relationship changed. We became friends. We talked—oh, how we talked. In the last two weeks before he died we talked day and night." At the end of June he died. He was 89 years old.

Ruby said a mix of despair, detachment, and overwhelming grief consumed July and August after he died. And, although that memory is a blur, she vividly recalls waking up one morning in September and saying to herself, "There has to be a future; but it's only going to happen if I build it myself. I have to learn how to live on my own." Her first independent steps led her to volunteer at the same hospital that looked after her husband. She started with two days per week, and 14½ years later she still works two days a week at the same hospital. Asked why, she said, "It's the breath of life to be needed, to be useful. And they were good to him." The year after her husband died, Ruby signed on for one day a week to work as a docent at the museum. She remained with the museum for 10 years, confiding that the only reason she gave it up was the subway steps. "I hated to leave the museum. The work was wonderful. I got to meet all kinds of interesting people. But getting there was exhausting."

How does she spend her time now? Ruby said that on Mondays she works a three-hour shift in angiography, assembling patient packages for the nurses, making up treatment beds, helping patients by giving them warm blankets, sometimes answering questions, but mostly talking with them. Later in the week she puts in four hours with medical imaging. She walks with patients to their appointments, listening to their fears and talking with them. "I'm afraid to go out in the snow and the ice. That's when I take a taxi to work." Clearly she loves the work and is dreading the day when she won't be able to do it any more. When she's not at work she shops and cooks.

"It's hard being 90, because I'm slow. Everything becomes harder. My strength is gone. I have to ask for help and it's degrading. Sometimes people say 'yes' and sometimes they say 'no'; they wouldn't help me with my groceries or they shut the building door in my face. The ice and the wind are hard. I'm always afraid that I'll fall. The best thing about being 90 is my functional ability. I can still volunteer. I'm still useful!" [~CY]

Living Longer, Living Healthier

Ninety-two-year-old Maude is chatting in the front yard with two of her neighbors.

Maude: I take 12 pills a day—three for my diabetes, two for my cholesterol, two for my blood pressure, a baby aspirin, two for my back pain, and two for who-knows-what!

Dani-Ella (age 85): That's nothing. Before he passed, my Harry told me that if I live carefully I should have enough money to get by on until I die. After the letter I got from my accountant yesterday I best be dying tomorrow.

Esperanza (age 82): I have three children, all retired now, seven grandchildren who can't find decent jobs, and four great grandchildren, including little Linda here.

At that moment Linda tugs on her grandmother's shirt and says, "Gran, what did mama mean when she said that these were your golden years?"

Perhaps growing older is not easy. Bodies change inside and outside, minds take a little longer to process information, friends and family scatter across the globe or die off, and the geography of one's social world shrinks as self-confidence begins to erode. The good news is that people can expect to live longer, healthier lives than their grandparents. The brain has the potential to keep growing in response to cognitive challenges, and even if people cannot travel with the same ease and energy as at 50 years of age, the Internet makes it possible to keep up with events, news, friends, and family.

It is important for health professionals who are counseling, caring for, or nursing older adults to understand that despite the increased risk of physical, cognitive, social, and functional challenges associated with aging, many "seasoned citizens" continue to view themselves as engaged and productive members of society. Even those living with multiple chronic conditions report well-being and satisfaction at being able to participate in social roles and daily living activities (Anaby, Miller, Eng, Jarus, & Noreau, 2011). All of this is to say that common stereotypes of older people as frail, passive, and characterized by multiple losses are just that—stereotypes. Many of today's elders embody extensive strengths in the form of remarkable adaptability, resilience (Wozniak & Jopp, 2012), and experience.

Ask 10 different people "How old is old?" and chances are that 10 different answers will emerge. That is because society does not have a set definition for "old age." Typically, the concept of *old* is most often associated with people over the age of 65 (or 67). In the United States, this perception is reinforced by the minimum age at which people may receive certain government entitlements (Snaedal, 2011), such as Social Security and Medicare. In other words, age 65 signals an individual's transition from middle age to senior citizen.

As with any other social construct, however, ideas about what it means to be old vary over time and across cultures. All cultures have norms about what is appropriate behavior at various stages in the lifespan. A century ago the face of aging was characterized as the rocking-chair generation, those who stepped aside to make room for the next generation. Today, older people represent a dynamic and growing segment of the population, many of whom enjoy a wide variety of interests, ranging from grandparenting to travel to second careers to skydiving. For example, despite being wheelchair bound, former President George H. W. Bush celebrated his 90th birthday with a skydiving jump over Maine (Dooley, 2014).

One factor that influences ideas about old age is our predictions about **average life expectancy** (ALE). Although highly sensitive to statistical changes related to rates of infant and maternal mortality, wars, and infectious disease epidemics, ALE has increased dramatically since 1900 in both developed and developing nations. Prior to 1900, being middle aged meant one was anywhere from 14 years old to the mid-20s, and late life hovered around age 40 depending on your social class. The science of paleopathology confirms that between c. 4000 and 400 BCE, wealthy ancient Egyptians could expect to live to between 40 and 50 years; those who were poorer fared less well, usually dying between the ages of 25 and 30 (David & Zimmerman, 2010). Although it varies by race/ethnicity, gender, and region,

TABLE 17.1 ✦ AVERAGE AMERICAN LIFE EXPECTANCY FROM BIRTH IN 2010

	White	African-American
Female	81.3	77.2
Male	76.5	70.2

Source: U.S. Census Bureau data for 2010. U.S. Census Bureau (2011), *Statistical Abstract of the United States: 2012* (131st ed.), Table 104: Expectations of Life at birth, 1970 to 2008, and projections, 2010 to 2020. Retrieved from http://www.census.gov /compendia/statab/

an American born in 2010 is likely to live to about 79 years of age. Table 17.1 provides some average lifespan estimates as of the 2010 U.S. Census.

The bulk of this increase in ALE is attributable to (1) improvements in public health, such as sanitation laws, vaccinations, and clean water; and (2) reductions in infant and child mortality (Olshansky et al., 2005). As a result, the number of Americans aged 65 and over is expected to swell from 40.0 million in 2010 (13.1% of all Americans) to 72.1 million by 2030 (19% of the population) [Administration on Aging (AoA), 2011], with those 85 and older growing at an even faster rate (Peltz, Kim, & Kawas, 2010). By 2020, the 85 and older population is expected to reach 6.6 million people, up from 5.5 million in 2010 (AoA, 2011). Table 17.2 shows the states that have the largest proportion of persons aged 65 and over.

Broken down by race/ethnicity, census data show that the structure of American aging is also shifting. In 2010, racial minority elders accounted for 20% of the aging population and are projected to grow to 24% by the year 2020 (AoA, 2011). In other words, by 2020, nearly one in four people over the age of 65 years will be an ethnic minority elder. Table 17.3 summarizes recent changes in racial groups within the U.S. population; Table 17.4 summarizes the nations that are experiencing the largest shifts in aging populations.

On average, women typically outlive men. In 2010, there were 23.0 million older women as compared to 17.5 million older men (AoA, 2011). Not surprisingly, older men are much more likely to be living with someone than are older women. Out of the 11.3 million non-institutionalized elders, only 3.2 million men lived alone. The rest were women who lived alone.

TABLE 17.2 ✦ STATES WITH THE LARGEST PROPORTION OF PERSONS AGED 65+ AS A PERCENT OF TOTAL POPULATION, 2010

Rank	State(s)	Age 65+	Age 85+
	U.S. total	13.0	1.8
1	Florida	17.3	2.3
2	West Virginia	16.0	1.9
3	Maine	15.9	2.2
4	Pennsylvania	15.4	2.4
5	Iowa	14.9	2.5
6	Montana	14.8	2.0
7	Vermont	14.6	2.0
8	North Dakota, Puerto Rico	14.5	ND 2.5; PR 1.7
9	Arkansas, Delaware, Rhode Island	14.4	AK 1.8; DE 1.8; RI 2.5
10	Hawaii, South Dakota	14.3	HA 2.2 SD 2.4

Source: Administration on Aging (AoA) Census Data and Population Estimates. U.S. Population by Age: July 1, 2010. Populations for states by age group percentages—April 1, 2010. Retrieved from http://www.aoa.gov/aoaroot/aging_statistics /Census_Population/census2010/Index.aspx

TABLE 17.3 ✦ PERCENT CHANGE IN POPULATION AGE 65+ BY RACE/ETHNICITY (2000 AND 2010)

Group	2000	2010
White, not Hispanic	83.7	80.0
African-American, not Hispanic	8.0	8.4
Native American, not Hispanic	0.4	0.4
Asian, not Hispanic	2.3	3.4
Native Hawaiian/Pacific Islander, not Hispanic	0.1	0.1
Two or more races, not Hispanic	0.5	0.8
Hispanic	5.0	6.9

U.S. Government

Source: Administration on Aging (AoA), Census Data and Population Estimates. U.S. Population by Age: July 1, 2010. 65+ minority population comparison using Census 2000 and Census 2010. Retrieved from http://www.aoa.gov/aoaroot/aging _statistics/Census_Population/census2010/Index.aspx

TABLE 17.4 ✦ NATIONS LEADING THE GLOBAL AGING BOOM: AGE 65+ YEARS AS A PERCENT OF TOTAL POPULATION

Country	% of population in 2010
Japan	23
Germany	20
Italy	20
Greece	19
Austria	18
Bulgaria	18
Latvia	18
Portugal	18
Sweden	18
United States	13

World Bank

Source: The World Bank. Population age 65 and above (% of total). Retrieved from http://data.worldbank.org/indicator /SP.POP.65UP.TO.ZS

Although the future is uncertain, it is conceivable that many of those children born in the 21st century will live long enough to blow out 100-plus candles on a birthday cake (Vaupel, 2010). A report from the U.S. Census Bureau found that by December 2010, almost 72,000 Americans were classified as **centenarians** (i.e., people who are alive and at least 100 years of age), with that number expected to increase to over 600,000 by 2050 (U.S. Census Bureau, 2011d).

From a policy perspective, the global population aging trend represents a double-edged sword—a blessing and a challenge. As a resource, the large numbers of people surviving into old age and beyond comprise a generation of individuals capable of significant social contributions. Equally important, they also represent major consumers of both products and services and contribute to the global economy. On the other hand, population aging places additional burdens on the existing social welfare system (Christensen, Doblhammer, Rau, & Vaupel, 2009); and because aging is often associated with functional limitations and disability, it will likely tax available health care systems and society's ability to provide

REFLECTION 17.2 SO YOU WANT TO LIVE TO BE 100!

"Bessie and I have been together since time began, or so it seems. Bessie is my little sister, only she's not so little. She is 101 years old, and I am 103. People always say they'd like to live to be one hundred, but no one really expects to, except Bessie. She always said she planned to be as old as Moses. And, when Bessie says she's going to do something, she does it. Now I think Moses lived to 120. So I told Bessie that if she lives to 120, then I'll just have to live to 122 so I can take care of her." (Delany, Delany, & Hearth, 1993, p. 5)

care (Potter, 2010). As it stands, almost 3.5 million American elders were living below the poverty line in 2010 (AoA, 2011).

The Times, They Are A-Changin'

Almost every society uses cultural norms to regulate the flow of people into and out of more or less valued statuses on the basis of age. One of the most striking ways in which today's older people differ from earlier generations of elders is in their social visibility. Commonly referred to as Baby Boomers, this generation of 76 million Americans was born after World War II, between 1946 and 1964 (Dohm, 2000). The Boomers, as they are known, represent an **age cohort**, a group of people set apart from earlier or later generations. Socially, Boomers are seen as a group marked by change, challenge, and transformation (Leach, Phillipson, Biggs, & Money, 2008). During the 1960s, 1970s, and 1980s the United States saw the introduction of the birth control pill and with it, sexual freedom and the burgeoning HIV/AIDS epidemic, widespread protests against the Vietnam War, a second wave of feminism, the civil rights movement, and growing concern about government ethics after the Watergate incident.

This was a generation not content with the status quo. They wanted social change and fought for it. Not surprisingly, age has done little to dampen their passion for change. For example, in 1998, Pfizer carefully orchestrated a new sexual revolution among older men after discovering that a drug originally developed as part of an ongoing search for heart disease medicine had the unexpected side effect of erectile stimulation (Tiefer, 2006). Since the prevalence of erectile dysfunction increases with advancing age, there was a willing and eager market for Viagra™ (Tur-Kaspa, Segal, Moffa, Massobrio, & Meltzer, 1999). At the same time the hit comedy series *Sex in the City*, about four sexually active New York women, empowered women's sense of sexuality and heighted men's performance anxiety (Tiefer, 2006). The end result was a medication that almost overnight morphed into a cultural icon and yielded at least a billion dollars in annual sales in 2005.

Physical Changes in Later Adulthood

Changes in the Physical Body

Must we get old and die? Why? The good news is that if you are a Prokaryotes bacterium (Lowenstein, Shubert, & Timofeeff, 2011) or Bristlecone pine (Bale et al., 2010) you probably do not have to worry about such questions because your ALE is in the range of thousands of years. The human lifespan, however, is considerably shorter. **Lifespan** is the average length of time that members of a population or species will live (all things being equal). Lifespan should not be confused with life expectancy. Although ALE has clearly increased (to 85 years) since 1900, one cannot say the same for maximum longevity (lifespan). Among humans the difficulty in determining lifespan is directly proportional to the intricacies of unearthing verifiable records of a birth date (Perls et al., 2002). One reason that age verification is problematic is that a reliable system for reporting national, regional, or local aggregate death records did not exist until Sweden developed it in 1861 (Vaupel, 2010). Still today, the process of determining extreme age is costly and cumbersome. In the pre-Internet era, document retrieval was a labor-intensive process of culling through public, private, and parish records. Age verification requires that all archival documentation (e.g., birth records, census data, military service history) confirms the same date of birth (Wilmoth, Skythe,

> **REFLECTION 17.3** DON'T TAKE IT FOR GRANTED
>
> "Prevention is cheaper and easier than repair," shared a 76-year old active African-American woman. She went on to say that she only now understands what her grandmother told her years ago. According to grandma, "You begin to die the day you are born." What she meant was that you need to treat your body like a temple from the start because it is too damn difficult to play catch-up! [~CY]

Friou, & Jeune, 1996). Between 1990 and 2005, scientists confirmed 15 **supercentenarians** who had reached 115 years (Jeune et al., 2010). Until her death in 1997 at the age of 122, Madame Jeanne Calment was the "certified" oldest human (Maier, Gampe, Jeune, Robine, & Vaupel, 2010).

Although science has yet to fully explain why people age, researchers do know that aging, senescence, and death represent a failure of the human body's homeostatic dynamics. In humans, the aging process is an incredibly complex mix of biology and environment. The systemic breakdowns related to the aging process are probably influenced by thousands of genes (Perls et al., 2002). Environmental conditions, such as smoking, sun exposure, and chronic alcohol consumption, also accelerate the natural aging process (Guyuron et al., 2009). Taken together, this means that for some, age-related change is minimal; for others, aging involves significant functional decline and loss.

The interaction between genetics and environment also occurs at the population level. Humans are diverse in their cultural habits, lifestyle choices, economic conditions, education, and social networks. This means that although one may be predisposed to heart disease or diabetes through hereditary traits, environmental conditions affect the age at which the condition may manifest (if at all), all based on available resources and choices. For example, prior to the link being made between chronic sun exposure and skin cancer, it was common for people to spend hours outdoors unprotected from harmful ultraviolet rays. Today, people know better.

Finally, the gene–environment interaction associated with aging also occurs at the organism and cellular levels (Cevenini et al., 2010). Again, the rate and severity of decline in different organ systems vary greatly based on heredity, diet, exercise, and living conditions. For example, skin may degrade at a different pace than one's heart or liver depending on exposure to multiple environmental factors, such as sun or pollution. In summary, aging is a biological event that begins at birth and ends at death, while old age is a social construction, an idea people invent and reinvent to meet society's needs.

From a social perspective, the effects of biological aging must be viewed in context. Humans possess a remarkable ability to develop adaptive strategies to compensate for age-related changes. Since many changes, especially those early in the aging process, are gradual and subtle losses, people often adapt to their environment without even realizing it. Observe the way an older person leans on the supermarket cart while shopping. It serves the dual purpose of holding groceries and mimicking a walker—one that does not scream out that this person is old and feeble. Tables, kitchen counters, and bathroom vanity tops become the "new home" for items that would otherwise require reaching or bending to be put away. Clutter becomes the new normal.

Strategies for coping with functional decline vary from replacing worn-out knees to installing home modifications such as grab bars near tub and toilet areas, and even home security systems. Such innovations enable frail elders to remain in their homes. A recent two-year, randomized control study showed that although functional decline occurred in both elder groups, it was significantly slower in the treatment group (Wilson, Mitchell, Kemp, Adkins, & Mann, 2009). Table 17.5 provides some facts about the aging process and diseases.

Physiological Theories of Aging

Every 24 hours people get one day older. But what does that mean exactly? In 1951 the United States successfully eliminated "old age" as a cause of death when state and

TABLE 17.5 ✦ AGING IS NOT A DISEASE!

Aging is a process that:

- Is universal. All members of a species experience the phenomenon.
- Results in measurable physiological decline.
- Is progressive, with losses being gradual over time.
- Is intrinsic in that it cannot be self-corrected by the organism. We are not programmed to grow new hearts or brains.

Disease(s) can be:

- Damaging to the organism.
- Progressive over time.
- Intrinsic.

However, disease(s) are not universal! For example, not everyone will develop Alzheimer's with aging.

REFLECTION 17.4 LIVING WITH PROGERIA

Although she looked perfectly normal at birth, her growth was severely stunted at 12 months. Over the next five years her hair, eyebrows, and lashes all but disappeared. Her skin was sheet thin and marked by age spots. She walked with the bowed legs of an equestrian, but had never ridden a horse. In her little girl fairy tales she was a princess waiting for a handsome knight on horseback to rescue her from the clutches of the evil queen. But riding a horse in the real world would have been far too dangerous because of her paper-thin bones. Her unusually large forehead was offset by a tiny jaw. This gave her the appearance of little old lady. By the time she had reached the age of 6 she was statistically middle aged. Despite it all, Kennedy, like her older sister, went to school, played dress-up, gossiped with friends, and dreamed about her future. She lived to see her 20th birthday. Three days later Kennedy succumbed to the congestive heart failure typical of those like her who live with progeria. [~CY]

federal reporting agencies adopted a standardized list of 130 underlying and contributing causes for demise that did not include death by old age. Although it remains unclear how age-related physiological changes affect longevity, aging is known as a major risk factor for countless chronic and terminal diseases, such as cardiovascular pathologies (Warner, 2011). Such connections are particularly evident in human **progeroid conditions** (i.e., progeria, Werner's syndrome), where premature and accelerated aging is accompanied by increased risk for cardiovascular disease and cancer (Kirkwood, 2011).

Evolutionary Aging Theories

Wear and Tear Theory

Perhaps the most pervasive belief is that a body simply wears out over time (Mitteldorf, 2010). The idea underlying the wear and tear theory is that humans are homeostatic beings who survive by keeping internal systems in balance (Williams, 1979). Challenges related to day-to-day survival result in chronic stress. This stress sends the body into a continuous cycle of damage and repair. Despite the environmental improvements in public health (i.e., clean water and immunizations), increased access to health care, and biotechnological advances (i.e., medical equipment designed for early detection of disease and damage) that slow down degeneration, the cumulative damage eventually outpaces the body's ability to repair itself efficiently (Mittledorf, 2010). Simply stated, the body is a lot like a car. It operates at peak efficiency when all of its vital components are in good running order. Eventually, however, parts wear out from repeated use. Although this theory has merit, it fails to account for the fact that the body often responds to stressors by getting stronger. After all, isn't that the underlying principle of resistance training? This suggests that wear and tear alone is not enough to explain aging.

Systems Biology of Aging

Kirkwood (2011) counters the idea of simple wear and tear by conceptualizing systems biology in which the body's innate drive for homeostasis leads it into an evolutionary response mode of error correction. Physiological errors are corrected through micro-adjustments. The basis for Kirkwood's theory is that as multicellular beings we are made up of both reproductive and non-reproductive tissue (soma), with the latter being less important to species survival. In this model, most, but not all, damage is efficiently repaired. In other words, bodies were cleverly designed to protect reproductive cells. For the body to marshal resources in this way, it sacrifices the less important soma tissue. This leaves soma vulnerable to deterioration.

Kirkwood's theory assumes that the primary cause of aging is irrevocably tied to a natural selection process that pushes it into making instinctive choices about which damage or problem to tackle first, similar to the way an emergency-room physician might triage victims

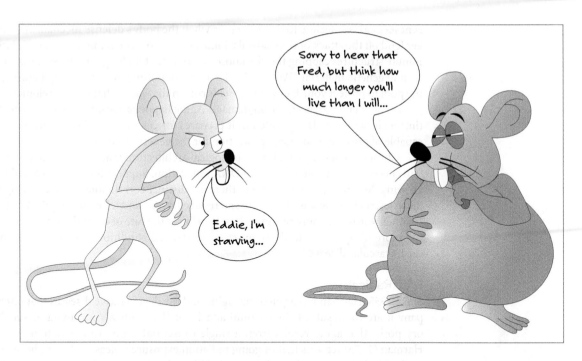

of a multicar accident. Basically, soma damage accumulates because the body has directed its intake of caloric energy to repair or enrich reproductive tissue as a way to ensure survival at a reasonable cost compromise. Thus, the systems biology perspective on aging argues for a genetic imperative for survival that dictates how the body's limited repair resources will be expended based on a metabolic cost-benefit analysis. Some say that the flaw in this theory is that it argues for increased caloric energy to satisfy both repair and reproduction demands (Mitteldorf, 2010). If this single-cause theory were the case, then overweight and obese individuals should live longer and age slower than underweight people. However, this assumption is completely at odds with the caloric restriction effect, a robust finding that is related to increased lifespan in rodents and nonhuman primates (Warner, 2011).

Caloric Restriction

The **caloric restriction** effect, also known as the dietary restriction theory, is based on the idea that limiting calories extends lifespan. Controlled animal studies in rodents and chimps strongly suggest that a 30–40% decrease in caloric intake equates to stronger, healthier subjects with greater physical endurance and that are more resistant to age-associated tissue damage and diseases (Warner, 2011). What remains unclear is whether this effect is reliable. Recent evidence in the form of a long-term, control-group study of rhesus monkeys casts significant doubt on the life-extending effects of caloric restriction (Mattison et al., 2012). Even if caloric restriction proves reliable, one must ask whether the effect is attributable to the quantity or the quality of calories consumed. It is also not yet clear whether the caloric restriction effect translates to humans to the same extent that it does to animals. Early evidence in the form of a six-month randomized control study of 46 moderately overweight but otherwise healthy adults suggests a modest benefit to caloric restriction (Meydani, Das, Band, Epstein, & Roberts, 2011). All of this means that one should probably pass on the bacon, but not deny oneself the occasional brownie. Especially since dark chocolate in moderation is good for health (and your psyche).

Damage-Based Theories

A cycle of cell death and replacement is a natural part of the aging process (Warner, 2011). The problem occurs when the cycle is interrupted. Damage-based theories argue that

senescence (i.e., decline to death) occurs when the body's defense mechanisms can no longer fend off the attack of free radicals, injuring DNA or damaging telomeres. **Telomeres** are minute structures capping the chromosomes that contain long repetitive sequences of non-coding genetic material (Warner, 2011). Think of putting on a swim cap before going into the pool to protect your hair from the chlorine in the water. That is what telomeres do. They protect our gene warehouse from damage. Aging happens because a telomere shortens each time a chromosome is replicated as it prepares for cell division. Eventually, it is no longer capable of providing adequate protection for the genetic material inside.

Chromosomes are vital bits of biological architecture that bind together complex proteins necessary to prevent errors in DNA replication. Support for damage-based theories is growing. Mounting evidence shows there are distinct correlations between living healthier lifestyles, such as increased exercise and reduced stress, and telomere length (Warner, 2011). In other words, the more one exercises, the slower the rate of degradation of telomeres, and the more likely one is to delay onset of age-related conditions, such as Alzheimer's and cardiovascular disease.

Free Radicals

Since 1955, Harman has argued that aging and the degenerative diseases that often accompany it are the result of the harmful attacks of "free radicals" on living tissue. This theory posits that aging results from a single cause: radiation. This radiation is all around. Harman (1955) reasons that ongoing radiation exposure unleashes free radicals that result in chemical changes at the cellular level. Although it is among the most commonly known theories of aging, evidence is building against it. Recent rat studies have found that subjects with high levels of oxidative stress from free radicals are living to the ripe old rodent age of 23 months, which is the same length of time as the controls (Lapointe & Hekimi, 2010).

Mitteldorf (2010) builds on this new evidence to suggest that "aging cannot be explained as a process of accumulated damage ... refusing to be tamed by simple, unifying hypotheses" (p. 325). After all, how logical is it to assume that senescence and its accompanying army of age-related diseases is the product of a single cause, given the complex design of animal biology? Now that something is known about "why" senescence occurs, what happens "when" people get older?

Health, Illness and Functionality in Later Life

Regardless of what promises the late-night infomercials make, bodies and minds will show signs of aging with the passage of time. Things one could do with ease a decade earlier begin to require a little more effort, a little more time, and often a lot more mental planning. The decades of stressors on the body accumulate to the point where one more event, (e.g., a fall) may trigger dramatic consequences for one's ability to function efficiently and remain independent. Although improvements are possible with rehabilitative therapy, when older, improvements often come in small, subtle steps rather than large, noticeable leaps of progress.

Health in Later Life

Older people typically experience one or more concurrent chronic illnesses. Fries (1980) coined the term **compression of morbidity** (COM) to describe the way chronic illness seems to be highly concentrated in the last years of life. Now, more than 30 years after proposing the COM paradigm, Fries, Bruce, and Chakravarty (2011) confidently point to numerous physiological, cognitive, psychological, and medical studies linking healthy lifestyles with a compression of morbidity and disability into a shorter period before death, meaning that with a little preventive care one can have more active, healthy years.

Among both Americans and Canadians, about 75% of those 65 and older report at least two chronic conditions, and about one-third report three or more chronic conditions

(Schoenberg, Bardach, Manchikanti, & Goodenow, 2011). Having multiple chronic conditions complicates both self-care and medical care in several ways. Signs and symptoms of one disease may mask or otherwise alter evidence of another. This makes diagnosis problematic. Similarly, treatment for one condition can interfere with the treatment, or alter the severity, of other illnesses. At the very least, the co-morbid patient may be at greater risk for adverse drug effects by taking multiple medications including self- and other-prescribed over-the-counter (OTC) treatments. For this reason health care providers should regularly conduct "brown bag" inspections. This is where older patients come in for a medications check-up, having put all their medications, both prescribed and OTC, into a single receptacle, giving physicians an opportunity to reduce the risk of adverse events.

As mentioned earlier in this chapter, it is important to remember when working with older people that aging itself is not a disease. People typically do not die of old age. They die from disease and illness. Unfortunately, when laypeople confuse the two, essentially attributing a disease's symptoms to "old age" and therefore inevitable and natural, they may wait too long to report a problem to their health care provider. This is where one's social support network is invaluable. Regular contact with family and friends makes it possible to observe change and suggest a visit to one's health care provider (see Case Example 17.1).

> CASE EXAMPLE **17.1**   KENJI.

At 70 years of age, Kenji retired from the company where he'd spent the last 52 years working his way up from copyboy to managing editor of the newspaper. About a year into retirement, his wife, Sumiko, worried that he was spending too much time in bed, sleeping fitfully. He had also developed a big belly for the first time in his life. When he was up and talking, he complained about neck pain. Sumiko insisted that Kenji see a doctor. After ruling out physiological causes for the symptoms, the doctor prescribed a low dose of an antidepressant, despite Kenji's protestations that he was not depressed and was just getting old. Within six months, Kenji was back to his normal personal routine and began to volunteer at the local youth shelter to fill his time.

The Aging Body

As one ages, changes occur in bodily systems. For example, a body's ability to control blood pressure and regulate fluids diminishes. Hair loses pigment, causing it to turn gray as the chemical proteins in the hair root slow down with age. Once they stop working completely, gray hair becomes white (Quadagno, 2011). Among men, who are genetically predisposed to it, the gene–testosterone interaction can lead to baldness, in some as young as their 20s and 30s. Whereas hair growth typically decreases on the scalp, facial hair (e.g., above the lip) increases in older women, and in the eyebrow, nostril, and ear areas in aging males. Skin becomes less elastic because collagen decreases. The thinning dermis leads skin to take on a translucent appearance. Once called "liver spots," lentigo is those patches of darkened skin where melanin accumulates into shallow pools just beneath the skin's surface. Those tiny expression lines around the mouth and eyes become more pronounced.

Botox anyone? Although a wrinkled complexion and gray hair are hardly fatal conditions, the desire to retain a youthful appearance has become a big business, totaling almost $17.7 billion dollars in sales worldwide in 2008 (Abjullah, Nasreen, & Ravichandran, 2012). On a more serious note, the most common form of cancer, skin cancer, typically appears around age 50, although the triggering damage likely began years before with sun exposure (Quadagno, 2011).

Eye and vision changes also occur with age. The protective tears that should generate each time one blinks decrease as the lachrymal gland slows down. The problem is that tears are necessary to cleanse and lubricate eyes. Without them people are more likely to experience dry, burning, "tired" eyes. When germ-ridden hands rub "tired eyes," the chances for infection increase. The eye environment itself also changes as the lens thickens with age, and the vitreous humor, the agent in which the lens floats, becomes more opaque, combining to distort one's ability to focus on objects (Quadagno, 2011). Night vision decreases, with such changes often leading older people to drive less after dark.

The most common vision disorders in older people are age-related macular degeneration (AMD), glaucoma, cataracts, and presbyopia. Presbyopia happens to most people, some earlier and others later in life. **Presbyopia** refers to the decreasing ability of the eye's lens to focus on close objects as it becomes less flexible, such as reading material with smaller print. It is most easily corrected with bifocal glasses or contacts. **Age-related macular degeneration** is the leading cause of irreversible blindness among those over age 50, affecting more than 1.75 million Americans (Barak, Heroman, & Tezel, 2012). It is a disease that occurs within the pigmented tissue of the retina, the area that makes one's central vision possible. Although substantial progress has been made in treatment techniques in the last decade, we are miles away from a clinically accepted protocol. **Glaucoma**, a rise in pressure leading to optic nerve damage, is treatable with varying degrees of success if caught early enough. **Cataracts**, where the normally clear optic lens becomes progressively cloudier, affect the quality of light filtering into the retina and can be surgically corrected or repaired with a laser.

Think about how often you exposed yourself to loud music, a great sound system at a concert, at the movies, the machinery we use, etc. (see Table 17.6). The hearing process sounds simple enough: Sound waves travel into the ear, bounce off the eardrum, causing it to vibrate, and the vibration sends a signal to the brain for interpretation. The problem is that the equipment nature designed to accomplish this task is delicate. A single exposure to intense noise, such as an explosion or too many years of loud music and headphones can lead to noise-induced hearing loss. Is it preventable? For the most part, yes; at the very least noise-induced hearing loss is amenable to commonsense risk reduction, for example, with judicious use of earplugs.

As one ages, the intricate structure of the auditory landscape begins to break down. One in three Americans over the age of 60 and 50% of those over 85 suffer from some degree of hearing loss (http://www.nidcd.nih.gov/health/statistics/Pages/quick.aspx). Hearing loss can have significant social consequences, ranging from abandonment and isolation to endangering one's safety through, for example, not hearing the warning from a smoke

TABLE 17.6 ✦ CONSEQUENCES OF AUDIBLE TRAUMA

Audio-impact Level	Decibel Level	Source
Death of hearing tissue	180	Being too near an explosion
Painful	150	Fireworks at 3 feet
	140	Firearms, jet engine
	120	Jet plane take off, siren, rock concert
Extremely loud	110	Maximum output MP3 player, chainsaw
	90	Subway, passing motorcycle
Very loud	80–90	Blow-dryer, food processor
	70	Busy traffic, vacuum cleaner
Moderate	60	Typical conversation, clothes dryer
	50	Moderate rainfall
	40	Quiet room
Faint	30	Whisper

Source: Adapted from www.noisyplanet.nidcd.nih.gov/parents/athome.htm

detector. Although hearing aids can help, they are costly and often uncomfortable. Despite significant technological advances in hearing aid mechanics, they remain inherently flawed because they amplify all sound for the wearer, including the ambient noise. As one friend put it, "When I'm in a restaurant, the sound of a piece of dropped cutlery hitting the floor sends shards of pain piercing through my head."

Taste and smell are two distinct senses that often work together. For example, when fully functioning they act in tandem to enhance the pleasure of food and drink. The smell of freshly baked bread or coffee brewing can stimulate salivary glands, preparing one to eat. Just as smell can excite the appetite, it can also warn of danger and keep people socially acceptable by telling them when they need a shower. With age comes a loss in our ability to detect odor, especially in men (Quadagno, 2011). Although we know that older people report a loss of taste sensitivity, its cause remains unclear. It may be related to degradation of the taste buds themselves, or the brain's ability to receive and interpret taste bud information. Either way, a diminished sense of smell or taste can lead to poor nutrition or overuse of seasonings (e.g., salt).

In later life, people's sense of touch becomes less sensitive. The same things that lead one's face to show age, the thinning, drier dermis and lack of collagen, can cause fingertips to become less sensitive to interpreting what they touch. Age is also often accompanied by a reduced sensitivity to pain (Quadagno, 2011), possibly stemming from poor blood circulation, diabetes-related nerve damage, neurological conditions, or certain drugs and medical treatments.

The muscle, bones, and connective tissue that provide a structural framework for the body, protecting its inner resources and enabling us to move through space, undergo a cascade of changes in later adulthood. Muscle strength typically decreases with age. However, it is not certain whether the decreases stem from age, inactivity, poor nutrition, disease, or side effects of medication. What is known is that loss of muscle strength varies not only among people, but also within an individual's muscle groups (Sousa, Mendes, Abrantes, & Sampaio, 2011). Moreover, exercise programs for healthy older individuals can to some extent rehabilitate muscle performance. Cartilage, the material that keeps joints lubricated and flexible, degrades and decreases with age. This causes joints to lose their ability to adapt to repetitive stress and typically leads to joint pain.

Bone mass peaks in the mid-30s. Gradually after that, bones' ability to remodel breaks down faster than it can repair itself. Today, some 10 million Americans over 50 years of age have osteoporosis, and another 34 million Americans show evidence of significant bone loss (Price, Langford, & Liporace, 2012). In **osteoporosis**, bone density becomes sponge-like and porous. The bones' outer walls thin and weaken. Once a woman reaches age 50, the odds of her dying from a fractured hip are equal to those of her lifetime risk of dying from breast cancer. In its later stages, the osteoporotic individual may show a pronounced curving of the upper back and/or spine (sometimes called a dowager's hump), report significant pain in the back, neck, and shoulder, and grow shorter (Quadagno, 2011). Falls are often the result of a hip fracture rather than the other way around. Although men can experience osteoporosis, it is far more prevalent in women. The most recent evidence points to nutritious food choices, weight-bearing exercise, and supplemental use of vitamins D and K, calcium, magnesium, silicon, and boron as the best defense against the damage related to bone loss (Price et al., 2012). Although osteoporosis is medically treatable with drugs, the side effects of medication may be problematic (Rizzoli, 2011).

Reproductive system changes affect men and women very differently. Although women pass out of their childbearing years during their 40s, men retain the capacity to father children well into old age. **Menopause** in women refers to the end of menses. It comes in stages, beginning with perimenopause and premenopause, the stages at which symptoms first appear (e.g., irregular periods). During menopause a woman's monthly menstrual flow discontinues, she no longer releases monthly eggs from her ovaries, and her production of estrogen and progesterone declines.

It is this slowing down of hormonal production that is primarily responsible for the myriad of postmenopausal symptoms that many women notice. Though women vary in the ways they experience menopausal symptoms, the more common complaints are hot flashes and night sweats. The hormonal decrease prompts a loss in the body's temperature regulation mechanism. Other complaints include mood swings, fatigue, and a thinning and drying of the vaginal lining, making intercourse more painful. For years a very public debate played out in the medical community over the use of hormone replacement therapy (HRT) for women who complained of menopausal symptoms. In its favor, HRT eliminated hot flashes/ night sweats and kept the vaginal environment lubricated and elastic. However, HRT has also been related to increased risk of heart disease, stroke (Quadagno, 2011), and some cancers.

While some partners may disagree, there is no clear empirical evidence that male menopause exists. The prostate gland enlarges, causing decreased flow through the urethra. This presents as a frequent urge to urinate but a reduced ability for the bladder to empty itself. Although sperm cells continue to form, making fatherhood theoretically possible into one's 70s and 80s, blood flow to the penis declines progressively, making sustained erection difficult. Viagra (Tiefer, 2006) and similar drugs have addressed erectile dysfunction (ED), the other complaint most commonly associate with male aging. As the commercials on television boast, one pill as needed or a smaller daily dose and men will not have to worry about ED again, unless of course their erection lasts more than four hours. For that, one should seek immediate medical attention.

Changes in the cardiovascular system occur in the heart muscle, the valves through which it draws in and ejects blood, arteries, and blood vessels. Damage anywhere along this system interrupts blood flow, thereby starving the body's cells of oxygen and other nutrients and interfering with its ability to discharge waste products (Quadagno, 2011). The heart muscle itself atrophies over time. This reduces the heart's ability to pump blood evenly throughout the body. A relatively simple fix for this problem is surgical implantation of a pacemaker, a device designed to prompt the heart to beat regularly. With age, the arteries and vessels also lose some of their elasticity, just as the skin does. Given the amount of fat consumed by the average North American today, the arteries also become clogged. While the loss of elasticity is a natural phenomenon, clogged pipes reflect a disease process. And both negatively affect the amount of consistent blood flow throughout the body, causing sometimes dangerous changes in pressure that can lead to a heart attack or stroke. Physicians typically use a multipronged approach to treat cardiovascular damage and disease. Treatment protocols include surgical intervention; for example, a damaged valve can be replaced with a pig or mechanical valve. For a coronary bypass, a surgeon may use healthy leg arteries to replace one, two, three, or four coronary arteries that are blocked or otherwise damaged. Another less invasive technique is for the surgeon to insert a coronary catheter equipped with a balloon to open a blocked artery. The surgeon then implants a stent to keep the artery open. Other treatment protocols include an array of drugs and lifestyle changes by the patient.

Although the aging brain experiences structural and biochemical changes, these do not necessarily alter one's behavior or ability to process and recall information. Studies have shown that by continuously challenging the brain, new dendrite growth is possible. Physically speaking, the brain's dendrite growth decreases with age as the production of brain proteins and neurons slows down. Depending on the extent and location of the structural changes within a moderately healthy brain, the individual's functional ability may be affected to a greater or lesser degree. For example, the cerebellum to some degree controls body movement and balance (Quadagno, 2011). Since this area of the brain loses 25% of its cells with aging, an older individual's risk for falls due to impaired motor ability increases with age.

Functionality in Later Life

Personal control over the conduct of activities of daily living, both instrumental activities of daily living and personal care activities of daily living, combined with mobility are crucial to

Think About It 17.1 Being 65 and Beyond

Now that we are living longer, healthier lives, how we spend that extra time means developing a new identity as a retiree. Some people may be disciplined enough to develop a "retirement strategy" before-hand. Whether one develops new hobbies, pursues an education, or engages in volunteerism, the critical factor is learning how to give meaning and structure to a life no longer organized around paid employment. What does one do when a career is no longer the heart and soul of one's identity?

the older person's ability to maintain independence and mini-mize risks for institutionalization, quality of life deficits, and premature mortality. Studies indicate that one of the strongest predictors of diminished physical capacity and increased risk for multiple morbidities in older people is long-term physical inactivity (Fielding et al., 2011). In 2010 about 37% of older Americans reported having some type of functional limita-tion, for example, with hearing, vision, cognition, or ambula-tory skills (AoA, 2011). The impact of such limitations varies widely depending on the older person's coping skills and sup-port system (Yancu, 2011). For example, studies show a strong correlation between functional limitations and self-reported health status (AoA, 2011). Those individuals age 65 and over who reported fewer limitations were also less likely to rate their overall health status as poor, in contrast to those with more severe disabilities. More importantly, however, for many older persons functional limita-tions represent a threat to cherished independence, and by extension to their quality of life.

SECTION II: Social Aspects of Physical Aging in Society

Although the psychosocial and emotional aspects of aging will be discussed in greater depth in the next chapter, it is difficult to think about functional aging without at least briefly con-sidering how elders are integrated into modern society. Despite studies showing that as people transition into later life they are more prone to activity limitation and concomitant restrictions in social engagement (Levasseur, Desrosiers, & Whiteneck, 2010), the sheer volume of global aging means that "contributory (useful) aging" is a social imperative. In other words, it makes no sense to consider functional health in aging without also including social functioning.

Social Structures, Status, and Roles

The patterns of social relationships in everyday life form **social structures**, the organizational concepts about how society works. Social positions within the social structures are organized in hierarchies of relative status based on influence and power. **Social status** may be either earned during one's lifetime (e.g., a doctorate) or ascribed at birth (e.g., gender). Thus, an individual will occupy a combination of statuses, some more valued than others. **Social roles** provide a frame-work that informs behavioral expectations aligned with the rights and obligations of each social status. Simply put, social roles guide social interactions that correspond to social status. Keep in mind, however, that status and role are socially constructed, flexible, fluid, agreed-upon ideas that change with the needs of society.

Think About It 17.2 Build an 80-Year-Old Person

Reconstruct the life an 80-year-old person by identifying at least 10 social roles that (s)he likely filled throughout life. Remember that roles include those that are both achieved and ascribed. Next, rank the roles by social status. What combinations of statuses are possible? What resources, rewards, and obligations go with the status combinations? In what way(s) are the roles and statuses different at age 80 than they were at 25 or 45 years old?

Social Theories of Aging

Social gerontological theories of aging provide a basis for examining the social environ-ments of older individuals and their effect on society. At the individual level, social roles represent participatory activities available to older people that offer a sense of purpose (e.g., volunteering, working for pay or personal development) (Heaven et al., 2013). At the macro level the increase in the aging population represents a new social norm, one that intersects

REFLECTION 17.5 BEWARE OF RETIRED HUSBANDS UNDERFOOT

It was a second marriage for both Edith and Walt. She was in her mid-70s and he in his early 80s. They had both been widowed after relatively good first marriages. She had always been a homemaker. After her first husband, Frank, died, she lived alone for 10 years until she met Walt. The difference this time around is that he is a spouse who is home full-time. This presented a set of challenges that neither was prepared to handle. Edith, only half joking, announced one day that she'd agreed to "for better or for worse but NOT FOR LUNCH!" This meant that both had to find a way to give each other space. In other words, each had to adapt their behaviors and beliefs about marriage. How would you help Walt and Edith adjust to their new living circumstances? [~CY]

with every segment of society including personal support systems, a growing target market for pharmaceuticals and other products, and a vital source of unpaid (volunteer) labor.

From a context of role transitions, aging reflects a period of life that is characterized by losses, such as diminished functional and cognitive abilities, a shrinking social and physical world, dependence on children for support, and loss of identity through retirement. For many older workers, age-related changes render the workplace a more challenging environment because of vision and hearing loss, diminished strength and endurance, and problems with balance. Nevertheless, many say that if given a choice, they would choose a phased transition, preferring to work fewer hours as an alternative to full retirement (Potter, 2010).

Today, average North Americans may find themselves spending 15–20 years in retirement (Adams & Rau, 2011). Many vital older individuals find that this period of withdrawing from the paid labor market provides an incentive to reinvent oneself through taking on new projects, community engagement, and enjoying more leisure activities. For those with some degree of economic stability, this means that the greatest gain in later life is having the freedom to decide how to spend one's time. For those without the financial resources, some form of paid work remains a necessity for survival.

Although retirement may sound great in theory, the truth is that humans need a sense of purpose, a reason to get out of bed in the morning. For those who do their homework and prepare for retirement, the transition becomes a shift in, rather than a loss of, occupational status. An added benefit of remaining active is that studies continue to show that older people who maintain their social ties after retirement, or who cultivate new ones, retain cognitive abilities longer than those who are isolated and lonely (Ristau, 2011). In this situation, however, women may have the advantage over men because females generally have a more highly developed sense of social competency.

REFLECTION 17.6 WHAT NEXT?

Over the course of the 15 years Eddie Mae was the primary caregiver for her mother and father; most of her days were spent visiting the local nursing home where they resided. She split her day between the memory care unit looking after her mother, who suffered from Alzheimer's, and the nursing home unit where her frail and much older father was housed. Much of her time was devoted to many of the tasks usually performed by the certified nursing staff, such as bathing, dressing, and feeding her parents. When her parents died, just two years apart, she felt lost for several months. As she described it, "I realized no one needed me any more and I simply didn't know what to do. My life has been spent caring for others; my six kids, my parents, and the kids at work [i.e., she worked 30 years with developmentally disabled adults]; I was sad about my parents' death and about not being needed any more." She eventually responded to a request for volunteers at her local church and began to volunteer her time with their after-school program. "The church has always been where I'd go when I didn't know what to do, so it seemed to make sense to start there and help."

For the last seven years, Eddie Mae has worked every day in her church's after-school program. During that time, she has progressively become more and more involved in the program, adding to her responsibilities each year. On a typical day she arrives at 2:00 pm, sets up classroom space, organizes snacks, ensures supplies are stocked, meets with tutors and helps to coordinate volunteer assignments, monitors clean-up, and supervises pick-ups. She enjoys being a part of a team, feeling needed, and contributing to her church community.

When asked about why she volunteered every day and why she is so involved in the program, Eddie Mae answered, "I thought I would just do one or two things, but the more I was here, the more I wanted to help, and the kids are great. I just love helping them." Ultimately, Eddie Mae has found a sense of purpose, being a functioning, contributing member of the community. Moreover, it is a symbiotic relationship because she gains a sense of well-being knowing she is connected to the human race. She is also a great structural boost to the faith-based program, which like many other community agencies could not function without the help of volunteers. [~CY]

➤ CASE EXAMPLE **17.2**   CASE STUDY CONTRAST.

At 79, a divorced, white male with multiple age-related illnesses spends most of his time obsessing over his medications and organizing visits to his many physicians. Socially, he retired at age 62, effectively severing ties with his master status, his corporate identity, of 40 years. Although he interacts with friends weekly, his personal hygiene and functional abilities suffer on those many days he spends alone. By choice, he remains largely detached from the social world, preferring to observe through social networks on the Internet and through television news. The end result is that his vitality, physical health, and cognitive abilities are rapidly deteriorating to the point where he will soon need to consider assisted living.

Next month she will celebrate her 90th birthday. Despite myriad health problems ranging from adult-onset diabetes to severe osteoporosis, she continues to remain active and alert. A widow for 13 years, she still volunteers at the local hospital twice a week. She stays current watching the nightly news and keeps herself impeccably groomed. Overall, she takes care of herself and is able to live alone quite comfortably. Where he accepted or even welcomed old age, she acknowledges getting older but rejects old age as a limiting factor.

Socialization is a lifelong process whereby individuals learn social norms, customs, practices, values and beliefs, and, most importantly, role expectations. These are learned through interactions with others. Numerous theories have been generated to explain socialization in later life. This volume of proposed theoretical frameworks shows the challenge of balancing the positive and negative perceptions about the intersection of social locations that older individuals inhabit today. Are older Americans a burden, an asset, both, or neither? Added to the multidimensional nature of the role of elders in society is the difficulty of distinguishing between accurate reflections of age-related biopsychosocial changes and distorted views or stereotypes of older people (Loeckenhoff et al., 2009).

The top five theoretical frameworks commonly used to explain the relationships between elders and society are called life course perspective, life-span developmental theories, role theory, exchange theory, and person–environment/ecological theories of aging (Alley, Putney, Rice, & Bengston, 2010). For a brief description of each theory see Table 17.7.

Refining an Understanding of Aging in Society

When it comes to contemporary perceptions of aging in society, a growing body of evidence finds that the views that older people hold of themselves, and the way that others see them, differ both *within* and *across* cultures (Loeckenhoff et al., 2009). In a study of college students' perceptions of aging in 26 countries, across six continents, Loeckenhoff et al., found

TABLE 17.7 ✦ KEY SOCIAL THEORIES OF AGING

Perspectives/theories	Description	Roots
Life course perspective	A group of theories that links social disadvantages to biological aging; builds on the idea that social institutions provide a structural basis for organizing society; people fit into assigned roles over the course of a lifetime depending on the needs of the society.	Cain, L. D., Jr. (1964). Life course and social structure. In R. E. L. Faris (Ed.), *Handbook of modern sociology* (pp. 272–309). Chicago, IL: Rand McNally.
Lifespan developmental theories	A group of theories that propose control as the key theme; builds on the idea that humans (from birth to old age) want to exert control, especially primary (environment) control over behavior–environment activities.	Heckhausen, J., & Schulz, R. (1995a). A life-span theory of control. *Psychological Review, 102,* 284–304.
Role theory	Based on the idea that work/employment is the central activity in human lives; retirement represents a loss of social identity and marks the onset of social isolation; builds on a belief that the roles we play define us, shape self-concept and behavior according to social norms.	Parsons, T. (1942). Age and sex in the social structure of the United States. *American Sociological Review, 7,* 604–616.
Exchange theory	A group of theories modeled on a cost-benefit view of social interaction, exchange theory is used as a way to explain decreased interaction between the generations; based on the idea that people continue to engage in activities and relationships that they find in some way rewarding; conversely, they withdraw from high-cost activities and relationships.	Dowd, J. J. (1975). Aging as exchange: A preface to theory. *Journal of Gerontology, 30,* 584–594.
Person–environment theory (PET) & Ecological theory of aging (ETA)	Both theories are based on the idea that sound person–environment fit has important consequences for healthy aging; builds on the importance of internal and external resources to ameliorate the stresses that accompany misalignment between the individual's needs and the environment in which he or she lives.	PET: Kahana, E. (1978). A congruence model of person–environment interaction. In M. P. Lawton (Ed.), *Theory development in environments and aging.* New York, NY: Wiley. ETA: Lawton, M. P., & Nahemow, L. (1973). Ecology and the aging process. In C. Eisdorfer & M. P. Lawton (Eds.), *The psychology of adult development and aging* (pp. 619–674). Washington, DC: American Psychological Association.

Summarized from source: Alley, D., Putney, N., Rice, M., & Bengston, V. (2010). The increasing use of theory in social gerontology: 1990–2004. *Journal of Gerontology B: Psychology and Social Sciences, 65B*(5), 583–590. Theories were ranked by the authors according to frequency of publication in the eight major aging and sociology journals between 1990 and 2004.

some cross-cultural consensus on the basic patterns of attitudes about biological aging and the declines in cognitive abilities. This suggests a more global-level agreement about perceptions of aging and age-related changes.

Intersectionality

Today, having minority-group status is recognized as having an impact on the aging experience (van Wagenen, Driskell, & Bradford, 2013). We use the term **intersectionality** to explain this phenomenon. In intersectionality theory, inequalities stem from mutually reinforcing systems in which race/ethnicity, gender, and age are social facts, arrangements that vary as a function of each other and not fixed or discrete categories that simply add or subtract (dis)advantages (Yancu, 2011). In other words, social structures, such as race, class, gender, and sexual orientation, interact with elder status in such a way that they foster experiences of privilege in some circumstances and oppression in others. For example, in many societies women's lower social location leaves them more vulnerable to poor health outcomes. Intersectionality argues that race/ethnicity, class, or elder status accounts for added variability for women based on unequal opportunities and variable access to resources.

How does intersectionality operate in real-world experiences? A recent study of successful aging among LGBTs found that of the 22 older adults interviewed, most reported having been marginalized across the life course because of their sexual orientation (van Wagenen et al., 2013) The study's authors are quick to point out that because their sample was largely homogenous (i.e., mostly white, highly educated, primarily lesbian), participant experiences probably differ in important ways from "less-educated, LGBT elders of color, bisexuals and transgendered elders" (p. 12). Seen in this light, the consequences of having had experiences or encounters with two or more forms of discrimination over a lifetime mean that we need to go beyond thinking about the impact of aging in society at the macro level to consideration at the individual level as well.

> **Think About It   17.3**
>
> How might the everyday experiences of privilege and oppression differ among older women of color relative to older white women or of older low-income women compared to middle-class older females? Keep in mind that age amplifies differences because longevity brings with it more time and therefore more opportunities to encounter inequalities related to race/ethnicity and gender.

Ageism

The view of older individuals is generally positive; older individuals are seen as active adults who contribute to society. However, ageism does exist. **Ageism** is prejudice and discrimination directed against older adults. Ageist stereotypes are patronizing and harmful. At their most benign, perhaps such attitudes portray older adults as "sweet," "harmless," and "helpless." At their worst, these stereotypes can lead to infantalization of older individuals, where even well-meaning others treat the adult as if the he or she was a helpless child. Such action can deprive older individuals of their right to self-govern their activities and behaviors, which in turn can lead to loss of self-esteem, and possibly contribute indirectly to decline in cognitive and/or physical function.

Successful Aging

The concept of successful aging came to the forefront when Rowe and Kahn published *Successful Aging* in 1989. According to Rowe and Kahn, aging and vitality owes more to lifestyle choices than to heredity. Their core argument is that successful agers are those individuals who possess better-than-average physiological and psychological characteristics, and that aging research should redirect its focus to health promotion and disease prevention. A decade later, Rowe and Kahn (1997) refined their definition to specify avoidance of disease and disability, preserved physical and cognitive function, productivity, and community/social engagement. Their groundbreaking work resulted in a reframing of geriatric and gerontological research. Gerontological approaches now stress life satisfaction, social functioning, and psychological reserves as primary components (Franklyn & Tate, 2008). Biomedical research now focuses more on cognitive, physical, and functional abilities. Trends toward healthy, active aging are supported by:

- Continued paid and unpaid employment opportunities.
- Public policy initiatives for training and education.
- Preventive health care.
- Multi-tiered residential options (e.g., age-friendly cities, in-home care, assisted living, full-support care).
- Naturally occurring retirement communities (NORCs), either in neighborhoods or buildings, where most residents are older and have either migrated to or aged in the place, making supportive services easier to coordinate.

From a biomedical perspective the three key elements of successful aging are: low risk of disease and related functional limitations, high cognitive utility, and active engagement in the social world (Franklyn & Tate, 2008). More recent studies have added the more subjective domains of spirituality and self-perceived health. Qualitative studies show self-acceptance and the ability to address challenges are linchpins of successful aging (Reichstadt, Sengupta, Depp, Palinkas, & Jeste, 2010). Reichstadt et al. also inquired about which interventions could facilitate successful aging. Responses focused on three points.

- Providing information tailored to help older individuals make informed decisions about understanding and preparing for major life changes. Such specifics would act to reinforce coping strategies.
- Help older individuals develop a network of programs and support systems.
- Help older individuals develop and engage in meaningful activities. (p. 572)

The successful-aging concept means that while ALE has increased, so too has the length of time spent in relatively good functional health. Aging is often associated with disability (Potter, 2010). Many studies have reported that at least 20 to 25% of people over the age of 65 have at least one disability. However, a careful reanalysis of the available data for eight industrial nations found that the prevalence of elder disability was effectively reduced by the use of supportive services, both public and private, coupled with increased access to assistive technologies (e.g., mobile telephones, home monitoring systems, modifications such as raised toilet seats, grab bars, and mobility aids) (Jacobzone, 2000), and age-friendly city design, according to a World Health Organization (WHO) guide to age-sensitive urban (re)planning. For a detailed description of WHO's (2007) guide to age-friendly cities around the world, see http://whqlibdoc.who.int/publications/2007/9789241547307_eng.pdf.

One of the main complaints about Rowe and Kahn's (1989) ideal of successful aging is that very few older people actually meet the criteria (McLaughlin, Connell, Herringa, Li, & Roberts, 2010). This has implications not only for public policy and planning, but also for generating flawed assumptions about what is intrinsically important to an older population. A recent study of ethno-racial and gender differences in affective suffering among community-dwelling elders found that depression-risk factors varied in important ways both by gender and by race/ethnicity (Yancu, 2011). Put another way, not everyone shares the same access to resources and opportunity; nor do they experience poverty, racism, wealth or prestige in the same way, especially after a lifetime of experience. For example, although women are more likely to face chronic health and social burdens across the life course because of their marginalized status relative to men, studies show that the influence of the gender burden differs between women of color and women who are White. When asked, older people identified successful aging as attitude/adaptability, security/stability, health/wellness, and engagement/stimulation (Reichstadt et al., 2010).

SECTION III: Cognitive Development

The fear most often expressed when we think about growing older is loss of the ability to live independently (Park & Bischof, 2013). Many normal cognitive changes may occur during late adulthood, in addition to pathological aging processes such as Alzheimer's disease or other dementias (Clay et al., 2009). The aging brain is characterized by both structural and functional changes; functional changes may reflect attempts to compensate for age-related declines (Drag & Bieliauskas, 2010). Cognitive development in later life is multidimensional and is often associated with incremental changes in the areas of intellect, processing, language, problem-solving, and learning (Richards & Deary, 2005). Age-related cognitive declines occur in specific domains, and can generally become more pronounced as the cognitive demands grow in complexity. Tasks, such as recall, that require strategy initiation in combination with effortful processing tend to be more age-sensitive than the more automatic processes such as recognition (Drag & Bieliauskas, 2010).

Aging is associated with differential patterns of decline in cognitive function. For instance, decline varies from person to person and is influenced by demographic factors including lifestyle and health-related factors (Ferdous, Cederholm, Kabir, Hamadani, & Wahlin, 2010). Many older adults may not show evidence of cognitive decline, while others may experience varying degrees of severity. Among older adults who experience cognitive decline, it is generally more pronounced in functions such as working memory, reasoning, episodic memory, and spatial orientation (Sander, Werkle-Bergner, & Lindenberger, 2011).

The good news is that active, cognitive, and functional reserves within the aging brain strongly suggest that changes or declines may be modifiable at *all* stages of the life course, even in later life (Richards & Deary, 2005). Although older brains may have less neuroplasticity than younger ones, evidence suggests that engaging in challenging leisure activities that stimulate memory and reasoning (e.g., problem-solving in a social setting) may delay cognitive decline (Park & Bischof, 2013). Even those who are genetically predisposed to Alzheimer's disease because they carry the apolipoprotein E allele (APOE ε4) appear to benefit cognitively from participation in leisure-time physical activity (Woodard et al., 2012). Table 17.8 highlights differences between cognitive decline and dementia.

A wide array of techniques and interventions are available to compensate for declines in later life, when and if they occur. Many older adults effectively use selective optimization compensation (SOC) to accommodate loss. This technique maximizes existing cognitive skills by prioritizing (selecting) valued activities to increase gains (optimization) and minimize losses (compensation) (Freund, 2008; West & Hastings, 2011).

Cognitive aging is a complex and multidisciplinary area of focus, requiring a far more comprehensive treatment than the scope allowed within this chapter. Because cognitive aging affects cognitive abilities in a number of distinct domains, select domains and abilities will be discussed next.

TABLE 17.8 ✦ MILD VERSUS MAJOR COGNITIVE DECLINE. WHAT'S THE DIFFERENCE?

	Mild Cognitive Impairment	Dementia
Symptoms	Problems with memory, language, and other primarily instrumental daily living activities	Progressive global decline of cognitive function in multiple domains (e.g., memory plus 1 additional area) such as comprehension, learning, or (spatial, temporal, or geographic) orientation
Impact	Often severe enough to be noticed by others, but not severe enough to interfere with routine daily life.	Symptoms are severe enough to disrupt daily life (e.g., interfere with instrumental and/or personal-care activities of daily living)
Diagnostic tools	e.g., Mini-Mental State Examination (MMSE); Montreal Cognitive Assessment (MoCA); Memory and Aging Telephone Screen (MATS)	Definitive diagnosis is done postmortem to detect plaque and tangles in the brain. Premortem, the patient's physician will evaluate cognitive skills, changes in personality, behavior, memory, etc.; may also order lab work to rule out conditions that mimic Alzheimer's symptoms (e.g., dehydration, thyroid problems, or B-12 deficiency).

Summarized from: Mayo Clinic Staff. (2013). *Diagnosing Alzheimer's: How is Alzheimer's diagnosed?* Retrieved from http://www.mayoclinic.org/diseases-conditions/alzheimers-disease/in-depth/alzheimers/art-20048075

Intellectual Variations

Intelligence: Fluid versus Crystallized

Intelligence refers to the mind's ability to function, or the "theoretical limit" of an older individual's performance (Hooyman & Kiyak, 2011). In the aging population, intelligence can be influenced by genetics, physical health, education, sensory decline, complexity of work, and vascular disease (Clay et al., 2009). From a functional perspective, intelligence is primarily associated with older adults' abilities in problem solving, verbal, and social competence. The two primary types of intelligence associated with aging are fluid intelligence and crystallized intelligence. **Fluid intelligence** is associated with a biologically determined ability to creatively make sense of our world, is independent of learned or acquired knowledge, and shows a linear decline with age (Tranter & Koutstaal, 2008). For example, suppose a person is driving home the usual way but there is an accident ahead and traffic is stopped for miles. Fluid intelligence enables that person to say, "If I get off at the next exit I may encounter more traffic lights but will still be home before it gets dark."

Crystallized intelligence is knowledge acquired through experience or education and can be maintained into late adulthood (Ferdous et al., 2010). For example, imagine that you and your friends just enjoyed a lovely meal at a restaurant to celebrate someone's birthday. The bill arrives at the table and you take on the responsibility of adding in the appropriate tip, subtracting the birthday dinner, and splitting the cost over the remaining members of the group. This requires crystallized capability.

Although the application of accrued knowledge and related abilities is not likely to decline until around 70 years of age, processing speed has been shown to decline beyond the late 20s to early 30s (Sander et al., 2011). In other words, the older one is the longer it may take to pay that restaurant bill for your friend's birthday celebration. Among seniors the ability to formulate a quick response to a question or rearrange facts is associated with fluid intelligence. Activities related to vocabulary or technical ability reflects crystallized intelligence. Both areas are highly influential in intellectual performance during late adulthood.

Factors Affecting IQ in Later Life

A measure of performance in these areas is customarily conducted using standardized testing of intelligence quotient (IQ). Theoretically, an IQ test can measure an older individual's ability in comparison to other individuals within the same cohort or chronological age group. Even as they age, older adults in general maintain relatively high stability of intellectual function, especially in crystallized intelligence (Gow et al., 2011).

Sensory declines can distinctly influence cognitive function and therefore affect performance on IQ tests and memory. Visual and auditory functioning are two sensory systems associated with intellectual performance (Clay et al., 2009). Declines in sensory systems affect the ability to take in, encode, manipulate, and store information. In essence, sensory declines act as a barrier to fluid abilities. Visuospatial abilities such as visuospatial attention, visuospatial memory, and visuospatial orientation can also decline with age and hinder an older adult's IQ test performance compared to a younger counterpart (Drag & Bieliauskas, 2010).

It is not all bad news, however. Strategies to improve or mitigate sensory impairment can ultimately improve cognitive performance. For example, cataract surgery may help with long-term maintenance of speed of processing, and could result in improved memory function or prevent age-related decline in cognitive abilities (Clay et al., 2009). Moreover, there is a positive relationship between levels of education and performance on cognitive tasks including block design, verbal fluency, and digit span. Simply stated, higher education levels correlate with better cognitive performance (Langa et al., 2009).

Memory Change

Late adulthood often brings changes in the process of retrieval, or recalling stored information. On a neuronal level, successful memory performance relies on a dynamic interplay among sensory-specific, multimodal association, and executive control regions of the brain. Most of the executive control regions involved in processes related to attention, selection, and optimization of memory representations are located within the frontal lobe, which may change structurally and functionally with age (Sander et al., 2011).

Attention and working memory are fundamental for selecting and maintaining behaviorally relevant information. Not only do both processes closely intertwine at the cognitive level; but also they tap into similar functional brain circuitries (Stormer, Passow, Biesenack, & Li, 2010). Older adults experience decreases in information processing, which influences cognition (Borella, Carretti, & De Beni, 2007). Functional decline in working memory capacity (i.e., ability to both simultaneously manipulate and store information) is also a commonly identified age-related change (Stine-Morrow, Miller, & Hertzog, 2006). Speed of processing and working memory can be readily influenced by the amount of time available and the pace required for related cognitive tasks. As individuals age, information processing occurs at a progressively slower pace, especially when it is has a multi-stimulus base. Moreover, taking in information can become problematic for older people because of increasing difficulties filtering out irrelevant information, despite retention of the ability to retrieve important information from long-term memory. Overall, throughout late adulthood, one's ability to selectively process information is subject to considerable change.

One critical aspect of human cognition is the ability to selectively attend to relevant issues and ignore irrelevant information in the physical environment and in mental representations (Stormer et al., 2010). During the course of healthy aging, the ability to ignore irrelevant information declines substantially; in the presence of chronic illness or pathological decline, this process is only compounded. Inability to filter irrelevant information or diminished ability to process at an appropriate rate makes the understanding of context a challenge for older adults. Deficiency in regard to the comprehension of context can influence an aging individual's perception of a situation and reaction to it.

Aging by itself does not lead to a global memory decline. However, it does affect specific domains of memory differently (Drag & Bieliauskas, 2010). A summary of variation in the types of memory and the extent of age-related decline follows.

- *Implicit memory* is automatic memory without conscious awareness. This memory is relatively stable across the life course and remains more intact than *deliberate memory* (i.e., trying to recall information) (Drag & Bieliauskas, 2010).
- *Associative memory* refers to binding mechanisms that form links within and between memory traces in the brain at different levels of complexity (Sander et al., 2011). Problems creating and retrieving links between pieces of information are an age-related deficit commonly experienced by older adults.
- *Remote memory* is very long-term recall. Despite the persistent myth that seniors remember the past better than recent events, remote memory is not any clearer than recent recall for seniors.
- *Prospective memory* is remembering to do planned activities in the future (Drag & Bieliauskas, 2010). Such remembering often relates to either time-based (e.g., remembering to meet someone at 6:00 pm) or event-based (e.g., remembering to meet someone after dinner). Older adults, in general, do better on event-based tasks rather than time-based tasks. There is more forgetfulness associated with prospective memory as people age. This form of memory requires self-initiated retrieval, as one needs to "remember to remember" as one ages. This ability can be complicated by the fact that internal cues and self-initiated processes become less reliable with age.

- *Autobiographical memory* is memory related to the self or one's own personal events (Fivush, 2008). Autobiographical memory goes beyond just recalling or recounting events to including evaluative and interpretive information associated to meaning or emotionality of the events. Older adults best recall their adolescent and early adulthood experiences in comparison to later life experiences. Autobiographical memory is often related to life transitions or major decisions such as getting married, going to college, having a first child, and starting a career. These experiences may have been more emotionally charged events across the life course, so they are remembered better. They become part of a person's life story, and are remembered often.

Language Processing

Sociologically speaking, language, whether oral, written, or by gesture, represents the symbolic representation of thoughts and ideas. In effect, language develops when cultures attach meaning to objects and ideas and then pass along shared meanings through generations. A dollar is only a dollar because socially we have agreed that a smallish, greenish piece of paper with Mr. Washington's picture on it represents some trade value. The intrinsic value of language is that it acts as glue holding social groups together, providing a mechanism for shared ideas.

Current perspectives on language skills view comprehension and communication as products of a coordinated array of processes that operate on acoustic signals to produce a symbolic representation of meaning (Stine-Morrow et al., 2006). Language is connected to higher mental processes. Language proficiency depends on one's ability to organize, plan, and monitor ideas, all of which mediate an individual's cognitive or affective activity (Lapkin, Swain, & Psyllakis, 2010).

Among older adults the majority of language difficulties stem from retrieval challenges rather than a loss of semantic information (Drag & Bieliauskas, 2010). The ability to find the right word(s), plan what to say, and determine how and when to say something are age-sensitive language processing abilities. Although older adults may have difficulty finding the right word or experience the tip-of-the-tongue phenomenon, they likely retain an intact knowledge of semantics and the ability to comprehend linguistic rules. In fact, semantic memory actually increases with age.

Evidence of language processing problems often emerges with speech pattern changes during later adulthood. Speech in later adulthood may be characterized by greater use of pronouns, unclear references, slowed speaking, frequent pausing, and increased difficulty with word selection. As a result, older adults may increasingly display more hesitations, false starts, sentence fragments, and word repetitions. This reflects an adaptive attempt to simplify speech as a means to maximize retrieval of information.

Problem Solving

Problem solving abilities decline in late adulthood. Nonetheless, older adults are better at solving problems they think are under their control. Problem-solving skills may be related to intact abilities to prioritize areas of control. For example, seniors make more rapid decisions in areas of health, as that is an area where many seniors feel a greater sense of efficacy.

Wisdom

The accumulation of factual knowledge and wisdom throughout the life course is relatively stable (Drag & Bieliauskas, 2010). Wisdom is associated with practical knowledge, ability to reflect on and apply that knowledge, emotional maturity, listening skills, and creativity in a way that helps others. Wisdom does increase with age. It comes about as people address more difficulties in life and are forced to find various means to adapt to change. Those with wisdom tend to have better education and are physically healthier.

Cognitive Interventions

Cognitive interventions can have some positive effect on cognitive abilities. Although age-related decline in cognition can occur, behavior interventions can enhance cognitive function (Hertzog, Kramer, Wilson, & Lindenberger, 2008). While cognitive intervention may increase cognitive performance, the use of specific, targeted cognitive training may be limited to trained abilities (Drag & Bieliauskas, 2010). Tailored cognitive strategies such as mnemonic strategies or use of lists/notes can produce improvements in performance for older adults (Lövdén, Bäckman, Lindenberger, Schaefer, & Schmiedek, 2011). Cognitive training and practice-oriented strategies can target a variety of cognitive processes, such as working memory, executive functions, or a combination of processes from various domains of functioning. Some training-induced performance gains may decrease with age; however, it is important to employ interventions that allow older adults to retain their level of abilities for as long as possible.

Lifelong Learning

Cognitive function is strongly associated with education or continued levels of learning. Education across the life course can influence abilities in late adulthood. For example, in the memory domain education can affect memory performance on tasks with high strategic demands (Drag & Bieliauskas, 2010). As a result, education may be a useful strategy for preventing and minimizing declines. Older adults with high levels of education, social engagement, and activity maintain higher cognitive function when compared to less educated, isolated, and inactive seniors. Therefore, lifelong learning can radically influence cognitive functions in late adulthood, whether initiated through formal programs or individually.

Lifelong learning and continued education provide benefits such as exposure to new information, increased awareness of the world, and opportunities for social interaction with peers and others. Such benefits not only improve cognitive function, but also enhance quality of life. Older adult–centered programs for learning may include senior-oriented travel packages, participation in college classes, or elderhostel programs that encourage seniors to travel and participate in higher education programs across the globe. The opportunity to continue to grow and develop not only has positive effects on cognition, but also increases intergenerational exchanges that help shape a better view of later adulthood.

Factors Related to Cognitive Change

One school of thought is that although a distinct pattern of decline often occurs just prior to death, the severity may depend on choices made earlier in one's life course. Some scholars argue that factors such as education, degree of mental engagement, nutrition, leisure activity, and level of physical activity can influence cognitive performance in late adulthood (Drag & Bieliauskas, 2010). For example, some studies (e.g., Lövdén et al., 2011) suggest that an active lifestyle rich in mental, physical, and social stimulation positively affects cognitive performance and protects against cognitive decline and dementia. Others (e.g., Naqvi, Liberman, Rosenberg, Alston, & Straus, 2013) find little solid evidence for any benefit derived from existing pharmacologic agents; even worse are risks attached to use of therapies such as estrogen supplements and anti-inflammatory medications; and only weak evidence exists for the benefits of physical activity. At this point, the extent to which late adulthood is defined by *preventable* changes in cognitive abilities remains unclear. However, quality of life does likely depend on how seniors choose to spend those years and the resources (financial, physical, social, etc.) to which they have access.

SECTION IV: Dying, Death, and Bereavement

Dying: Not Always Easy to Define

> Through my years as a hospice doctor, I have learned that dying does not have to be agonizing. Physical suffering can always be alleviated. People need not die alone; many times the calm, caring presence of another can soothe a dying person's anguish. (Byock, 1997, p. xiv)

Of all human experiences, perhaps none is more universal, overwhelming, or finite than death. Ironically, a review of the literature on dying and death reveals that there is neither a reliable definition for biological death nor a clear understanding of attitudes and behavior patterns consistent with life-limiting illness (Kellehear, 2009). In part, this is because culture, a highly dynamic system for understanding human behavior, informs normal responses to health and illness, care and healing, and confronting mortality and coping with loss (Yancu, Farmer, & Leahman, 2010). In other words, culture normalizes the customs and rituals that formalize the relationships between the living, the dying, and the dead. Cultural diversity means that service providers are constantly challenged with having to recognize and respect the unique and specific influences each group brings to the caregiving relationships at the end of life.

Defining Death Then and Now

Death, what Shakespeare's Hamlet called "The undiscovered country, from whose bourn no traveler has returned," signifies the end of life as we understand it. The process of defining the precise moment it occurs, however, has changed over time with the advent of new biotechnologies. Ancient Egyptians believed that the loss of a heartbeat signified death, whereas Maimonides in the 11th century cited irreversible loss of brain function (Laureys, 2005). Nineteenth-century physicians thought death occurred at the moment of cardiopulmonary arrest (Kinnaert, 2009). By 1981, the Uniform Determination of Death Act, a collaboration between the American Medical and American Bar Associations, defined death as "either a permanent loss of cardiopulmonary function or whole brain function" (Appel, 2005, p. 641).

The heart stops beating; the brain stops processing information. Why does it matter whether it is one or the other? Ask anyone who has ever successfully given or received cardiopulmonary resuscitation (CPR) or used defibrillation paddles for resuscitation purposes. The idea of being declared dead while still alive is so compelling that it has generated a genre of horror films and curious inventions such as Russian Count Karnice-Karnicki's flag and bell apparatus designed to signal that the interred "deceased" was not really dead (Laureys, 2005).

Critics of the "brain death" standard oppose its inclusion in criteria for determining death, preferring instead *permanent loss of all higher brain function* (neocortical death) (Appel, 2005), because the concept of "whole brain death" leaves room for interpretation. Opponents cite procurement of "healthy" organs for transplant as the main reason to include brain death in the definition, pointing to postmortem studies of heart-beating donors with little or no evidence of structural brain damage at organ harvest (Verheijde, Rady, McGregor, & Murray, 2008).

Dying Is a Process with Death as the Endpoint

Triffletti (2010) describes his mother's last days and hours beginning on December 18 with appetite decline, mild bouts of delirium, and pain that is manageable at first. By Christmas day,

> [with] her body shutting down and aggressive pain management, she passed into a state of unresponsive[ness]. . . . Her hands were warm for hours as I sat beside. Then as her breathing became more agonal, her hands turned cool and cyanotic. Her eyes opened wide . . . and then she heaved her last breath. (pp. 39–40)

His mother finally died at 3:30 am on December 26.

TABLE 17.9 ✦ CHANGES TYPICAL IN THE FINAL DAYS AND HOURS OF LIFE

Category	Outward Symptoms
Energy decline	Feeling tired and drowsy; sleeping more; slipping in and out of consciousness
Reduced food and fluid intake	Loss of appetite; difficulty swallowing both solids and liquids; digestive and absorption problems
Changes in breathing	Breathing becomes less regular; breathing becomes noisier and may sound like a rattle because of a mucous buildup
Confusion and hallucinations	Medications and/or endocrine changes may lead to hallucinations and/or confusion; restlessness; anger outbursts
Chills in the extremities	Hands and/or feet may feel cold because of reduced circulation; skin may appear bluish (cyanotic) because of a lack of oxygen in the blood.

Source: National Health Service. (2012). *End of life care*. Retrieved from http://www.nhs.uk/Planners/end-of-life-care/Pages /changes-in-the-last-hours-and-days.aspx.

It is especially important for health care providers to recognize the onset of dying, partly because they may need to initiate final-decisions conversations and partly because about 55% of patients are not necessarily aware (or in denial) that they are indeed dying (Papadimos, Gafford, Stawicki, & Murray, 2014). People tend to think about death as an event; *one minute you are here and the next you're gone.* Death as instantaneous is often how it is portrayed in films and on television. For example, the news might report that the victim died at the scene of the accident or died of a drug overdose. However, for most people dying is an active process, engaging the physical body in addition to one's psychological side and social world. Table 17.9 provides indicators of the "shutting down" process.

Decisions, Decisions, Decisions!

Although society has yet to reach consensus on its definition, in a complex world, determinations of death have meaning well beyond the need for donor organs. Death certification affects family decisions about withdrawing life support, property distribution, and marriage termination (Appel, 2005), which in effect restructure the family.

The language of death and dying often adds to our uncertainty. The battery on a mobile phone "*dies*" and what is done? People recharge or replace it and bring the phone back to life. The fact that death is a series of physiological events (Cohen, 2012) taking place over a period of time is an important distinction because people now have a variety of ways in which to intervene in the dying process, be it through biological or mechanical organ replacement, electrical nerve stimulation, ventilator, or tube feeding. Imagine that a drowning man is pulled from the water. At some point before the rescue his brain was deprived of oxygen, causing brain damage and signaling his body to begin the shut-down process. But if he receives immediate medical treatment we can keep most if not all of his vital organs alive. Although medical personnel can keep his body alive, technology does not currently exist to reverse the damage to his oxygen-starved brain. Think of a line of standing dominos. Knock over the first one and each one after that knocks down its neighbor in a cascade effect. But take away just one domino so that the one in front can no longer reach its neighbor, and the process is, in effect, interrupted. Philosophically, the question is: "Has the action taken lengthened life expectancy of the drowning man or prolonged his dying process?"

Perhaps nowhere is the question of defining death more pressing than in cases of persistent vegetative state (PVS). Once called *coma dépassé* (death of the nervous system), and later *irreversible coma,* individuals in this state are clearly not dead, yet neither are they alive because of irreversible brain damage (Kinnaert, 2009). Clinically, the person "living" in a PVS likely retains some degree of brain stem function responsible for respiration and heartbeat, but has lost higher cortical function, the ability to think and feel. In other words, PVS refers to a clinical diagnosis of someone who, although physically alive, is devoid of intellectual activity, sensation, and social ability for at least one month (Laureys, 2005). For the family, PVS can be especially difficult because the patient's eyes are typically open and they often retain some motor activity, all of which gives the appearance of being less ill than they truly are. Unlike death, however, PVS can in certain circumstances be reversed, either spontaneously or through treatment. In cases where PVS persists beyond three months for nontraumatic or 12 months for traumatic injury, the patient's diagnosis changes to a permanent vegetative state. Table 17.10 provides key criteria used to differentiate brain death and PVS.

Choices, Decisions, and Conversations: Where and How We Die Today

In 1969, Kübler-Ross wrote that the more "we are making advancements in science, the more we seem to fear and deny the reality of death" (p. 7). She went on to argue that dying today has become more isolated, mechanized, and dehumanized. Unfortunately, physicians still lack the ability to accurately predict imminent death in the short term, tending instead to overestimate a patient's likelihood of survival (Papadimos et al., 2014).

Prior to the increase in ALE in the early 20th century, death was so omnipresent that it was treated as a family matter. People typically died in their own homes close to family, friends, and the familiar. By the 1950s, death was reconceived of as a "medical problem" entrusted to the care of physicians and nurses within the confines of a hospital (Lee, 2009) and, more significantly, separated from family and home. Today, death and grieving are hidden; approximately 50% of American seniors die in acute-care hospitals; many will spend their final moments in intensive care units (ICUs) and emergency rooms (Kompanje, 2010).

Advanced care planning (ACP) is viewed by many today as a way for terminally ill patients to direct treatments consistent with their personal beliefs, whether or not they have

TABLE 17.10 ✦ KEY CRITERIA USED TO DIFFERENTIATE BRAIN DEATH VS. PERSISTENT VEGETATIVE STATE

Key Criteria for Brain Death[1]	Key Criteria for PVS[2]
▪ Demonstration of coma	▪ No evidence of awareness of self, environment
▪ Evidence for cause of coma	▪ Inability to interact with others
▪ Absence of confounding factors (e.g., hypothermia, drugs)	▪ No evidence of sustained, reproducible, purposeful, or voluntary behavioral responses to visual, tactile, auditory, or noxious stimuli
▪ Absence of brainstem reflexes	
▪ Absence of motor responses	▪ No evidence of language comprehension or expression
▪ Apnea	▪ Intermittent wakefulness manifested by the presence of sleep–wake cycle
	▪ Sufficiently preserved hypothalamic and brain stem autonomic function to permit medically assisted survival
	▪ Bowel and bladder incontinence
	▪ Variably preserved cranial nerve and spinal reflexes

Summarized from the following sources:

[1]Quality Standards Subcommittee of the American Academy of Neurology. (1995). Practice parameters for determining brain death in adults (summary statement). *Neurology, 45,* 1012–1014.
[2]Multi-Society Task Force on PVS. (1994). Medical aspects of the persistent vegetative state. *New England Journal of Medicine, 330,* 1499–1508.

decision-making capacity (Dobbs, Emmett, Hammarth, & Daaleman, 2012). Advocates of ACP argue that the power to direct one's own death process is a fundamental human right. Today ACP involves more than completing a legal document. It is a process that includes multiple conversations, preferably reviewed over time with family, friends, spiritual advisors, and health care providers. Designed to document final wishes, the conversations should cover a range of topics from scope and range of treatment options to final disposition of the physical body and property.

In 20th-century America, both birth and death charted the same course of moving from the home into the hospital (Kompanje, 2010). Although both birth and death are natural events, medical advocacy has in effect normalized the idea that physicians should be present "in case something goes wrong." Death in the hospital means that it is sterile, hidden, and, for the patient, isolated from loved ones, who are left to grieve in silence (Lee, 2009). The fact that not everyone is willing to die in such an antiseptic environment led to the birth of the "Death with Dignity" and "Right to Die" movements.

One of the most notable names in the physician-assisted suicide movement is Dr. Jack Kevorkian, also known as "Dr. Death." In 1990, Dr. Jack Kevorkian used a machine he developed specifically for the purpose of assisting Janet Adkins, a 54-year-old Alzheimer's patient, to commit suicide. And a firestorm of controversy was unleashed on the American public. Ultimately, Dr. Kevorkian claimed to have assisted with about 130 deaths. A California court charged him with second-degree murder and illegal delivery of a controlled substance in 1999. He spent eight years in prison. For good or ill, the one thing that Jack Kevorkian can take credit for is making the conversation about how one die a public one.

Suicide and Older Adults

Evidence-based studies of effective suicide prevention in older adults are lacking (Erlangsen et al., 2011). According to the World Health Organization, high rates of elder suicide, especially among men, occur in the more developed nations (e.g., Canada, United States, Japan, European Union nations) (Fässberg et al., 2012). This is not a surprising finding in light of Durkhiem's (1897/1951) seminal work in the 19th century on suicide. Durkheim postulated that less developed nations tend to reflect what he called mechanical (less structurally complex) societies, and pointed out that the two factors most related to suicide are lack of social integration and anomie (lack of moral alignment with the larger society). Both of these conditions are more likely to occur in more highly complex societies.

Does Being Married Really Help?

The longer one lives, the more likely it is that physical, psychological, and social losses will add up. Although copious research shows that being married is associated with favorable health outcomes, especially for men, there is no reason to assume that the marital relationship is a positive one (Fässberg et al., 2012). It may be that a couple has stayed together because of a cultural dictate, or out of habit, fear of loneliness, or financial reasons. Seen in this light it is important to remember that the cumulative losses common in aging may challenge one's ability to remain socially integrated regardless of marital status.

What about Gender Differences?

Suicide ideation is a recognized indicator of depressive suffering. And affective suffering is prevalent among older adults. Years of research show that affective suffering is more

Think About It 17.4

An 88-year-old white male, a former blue-collar worker, has just lost his wife of 60 years. His functional limitations prevent him from walking one block and he no longer drives because of limited vision. His glaucoma also prevents him from easy computer use. When he and his wife bought their house, the neighborhood was family friendly, but today it is covered in graffiti and gang-ridden. He lives in California and his only daughter lives in New York City. Assess this client's suicide risk. Discuss the criteria you used to identify his risk of suicide.

prevalent among women than men (Luppa et al., 2012). Although explanations for higher rates of depressive suffering in females vary from physical to emotional to social-environmental, all ideas seem to assume that women are homogeneous (Yancu, 2011). This would mean that women are a generic group made more vulnerable to depression because they are biologically distinctive (sex) or have role-based commonalities (gender). Is this a flawed assumption? Recall that earlier in this chapter we talked about intersectionality, meaning that social factors such as race/ethnicity, class, and sexual orientation interact with age and gender (see Case Example 17.3).

➤ CASE EXAMPLE **17.3** ALL OLD WOMEN ARE ALIKE!

Imagine that you have been tasked with assessing five women ranging in age from 68 to 95 for suicide risk. What biases about homogeneity will you bring to the assessment? You have read the literature that concludes women are 2–3 times more likely to be depressed than men. The women are sitting together talking at the local senior center in a large city run by a neighborhood church.

Woman 1 is 68 years old, Caucasian, born and raised in the United States, twice divorced, and now married to a man 20 years her senior who needs constant care for middle-stage Alzheimer's. She has diabetes, osteoporosis, and painful angina.

Woman 2 is also 68 years old. She is a Latina originally from Cuba, having fled the country in 1959 when Castro took over. Although she grew up in relative socioeconomic privilege, she worked her entire life as a seamstress in the United States. She is a staunch Catholic, married to another Cuban refugee for 40 years, and has four children and six grandchildren, all still living in the neighborhood. She has uncontrolled diabetes.

Woman 3 is 74 years old. She is originally from Nagasaki, Japan, and remembers being 5 years old when the bomb dropped on her home. For some reason she never understood, she survived, though thousands did not. Emigrating to the United States as an adult, she eventually became a social worker. She never married. She's a breast cancer survivor but today is battling ovarian cancer.

Woman 4 is a 76-year-old African-American who grew up in North Carolina. Married for 25 years, she was widowed 10 years ago. She worked as a middle school teacher and continues to volunteer at the same school from which she retired 15 years ago. She sings with the church choir and stays fit by going to the local gym 4–5 days a week. Her only real health problem is long-term hypertension.

Woman 5 is 95 years old. A Caucasian and a Jew, she survived Auschwitz, a World War II German concentration camp, where she had been starved, beaten, and lived in a forced labor situation for two years. Her late husband, also a camp survivor, has been dead for 25 years. Together they previously owned a neighborhood grocery store and lived above it for years. After his death she volunteered in the community until she was no longer able to walk without a walker. She has congestive heart failure, diabetes, and arthritis.

1. Identify as many similarities and differences among these women as you can.
2. Which woman are you most concerned about as a suicide risk? Why?
3. Which woman are you least concerned about as a suicide risk? Why?

As can be seen with these diverse women, suicide prevention among older adults should span a range of considerations from the macro to the micro levels (Erlangsen et al., 2011). At a macro level it may be prudent to develop policies that address structural impediments to independence (e.g., having to rely on others for help to get around). At the median level, a more targeted intervention may focus on standardizing training for staff working with older adults to make them sensitive to the impact of loss (e.g., retirement, a driver's license, or continence). Micro-level prevention could mean individual referral to community and social resources, talk therapy, and identifying and treating underlying depressive suffering.

Hospice and Palliative Care

One alternative to the Dr. Death scenario is hospice and palliative care. **Hospice** is a program of care designed to provide support and comfort to patients and their loved ones when a life-limiting illness no longer responds to curative treatments (Yancu et al., 2010). It is important to realize that hospice is not always a brick-and-mortar building where individuals with terminal illnesses go to die. Hospice is a source for care that is by definition palliative, not curative, holistic rather than disease focused, and most importantly, patient centered. Hospice can provide a range of services, including physical pain management, spiritual support, and volunteers who come into the patient's home to provide assistance and social support.

Advance directives describes a series of forms that can be completed by individuals before they encounter a life-limiting illness. Included in the advance directives package is a Do Not Resuscitate (DNR) form and a "living will," a legal document that states the individual's wishes about heroic measures (e.g., ventilator, antibiotics, feeding tubes). This document goes into effect when the person is unable to speak for himself or when death is imminent. The health care power of attorney (HCPA) is designed to appoint a health care agent to speak on your behalf when the patient is incapacitated. The HCPA can be any competent adult who is not one's paid health care provider. He or she makes such decisions as starting/stopping life-prolonging measures and selecting treatment facilities. Finally, the physical order for life-sustaining treatment (POLST, or MOST depending on state of residence) is a relatively new legal document developed for seriously ill patients to endorse actionable medical orders. For more information about POLST, see http://www.ohsu.edu/polst/patients-families/faqs.htm; for MOST see http://www.ncdhhs.gov/dhsr/ems/dnrmost.html.

Grief, Bereavement, and Mourning

Suffering through loss is part of life. For older people, the accumulation of deaths (e.g., friends, family, pets) and loss events (e.g., physical function, cognitive skills) leaves them vulnerable to bereavement overload. Left unchecked, the stresses associated with loss have been related to increased morbidity and premature mortality for the surviving spouse or parent (Buckley et al., 2012) or escalating to pathological grief a condition characterized by debilitating symptoms (e.g., social withdrawal, intense yearning, somatic distress) (Miller, 2012). Table 17.11 differentiates among the concepts of grieving, bereavement, and mourning.

TABLE 17.11 ✦ DIFFERENTIATING AMONG BEREAVEMENT, GRIEF, AND MOURNING

Bereavement	This state of having suffered through a loss represents an objective experience (e.g., when someone close to them has died).
Grieving	The intellectual response to bereavement; painful emotions, actions, expressions (e.g., pangs of sadness and/or crying/sobbing mixed with periods of respite) that help a person come to terms with the loss of a loved one. The grief experience varies by culture and personality traits.
Mourning	This is the outward expression of loss and grief. Mourning includes rituals (e.g., wearing of specific colored clothing) and actions (e.g., gathering of loved ones to share the loss experience). Mourning, like grief, is informed by cultural traditions and personality.

Summarized from source: American Cancer Society. (2012). *Grief, mourning and bereavement.* Retrieved from http://www.cancer.org/treatment/treatmentsandsideeffects/emotionalsideeffects/griefandloss/coping-with-the-loss-of-a-loved-one-intro-to-grief-mourning-bereavement

It is reasonable to assume that some amount of grief will follow an emotionally charged loss. Healthy grief will likely vary and wane over time. In cases of normal grieving, social support is helpful in restoring one to pre-bereavement functioning levels within about 6–12 months; during the latter phase of this period, feelings of loss and sadness are still present in the background (Miller, 2012). Another source of support is hospice. Bereavement counseling for patients and loved ones falls under the domain of hospice care. The holistic model followed by hospice includes spiritual, psychosocial, and emotional services both before and after death (Barry et al., 2012).

Pathological grief refers to those who remain "stuck" in a state of intense grief (e.g., constantly preoccupied with their loss for a year or more to the point where it disrupts daily living) (Miller, 2012). Cognitive behavioral therapy with a mental health professional may be helpful at this point (Miller, 2012). However, it is important to remember that the grief process itself is inherently complicated by personality traits and by spiritual and cultural dictates. Caution around medicalizing grief is necessary (Rando et al., 2012).

Some Final Thoughts on Dying, Death, and Bereavement

Although studies show that end-of-life discussion is vital to compassionate end-of-life care (Kuhl, Stanbrook, & Hébert, 2010), most Americans are reluctant to talk about dying, death, and bereavement (Petasnick, 2011). As a result, people are often ill-equipped to navigate end-of-life care for themselves and loved ones (Considine & Miller, 2010). This may be a good time to recall the words of Dame Cicely Saunders (De Boulay, 1984), founder of the modern hospice movement:

> The greatest sorrow of the dying patient is the ending of relationships and responsibilities. We live in our interchange with others and as encroaching weakness leads to the change of roles . . . it is not hard to feel useless and humiliated. The family often takes readily the opportunity to repay debts of love and care but it is not easy to be perpetually at the receiving end of other people's concern and this must be given with sensitivity. This time can be used to heal bitterness and find reconciliation. (p. 229)

Summary

The average lifespan expectancy for individuals has increased dramatically since 1900, particularly in countries with sufficient medical care. The primary reasons people are living longer than ever before are attributable to more effective public health measures, with support from health care improvements and reductions in infant and child mortality (Olshansky et al., 2005). In this chapter, statistics were provided related to aging, taking into account the intersection of race/ethnicity, nationality, socioeconomics, sexual orientation, and gender, among other cultural characteristics. While aging, accompanied by declines in bodily functioning, is inevitable, many people who are living longer are living better. Older adults who have successfully navigated the developmental tasks outlined throughout this text are more likely to have established a firm foundation for successful aging (Baltes, 1997).

Physical changes that occur in later adulthood were reviewed; many of these are affected by environmental factors and genetics. The remarkable ability humans have to adapt to age-related changes was highlighted, as were different physiological and evolutionary theories of aging, including the wear and tear theory, systems biology concepts, and damage-based theories of aging. Although the theories differ, each is supported by research.

Next, the focus shifted to health, illness, and functionality in later life. As adults age, they often experience one or more chronic illnesses. However, because of the increased emphasis on prevention and wellness, older adults are much more likely to experience healthy, active lifestyles than ever before. With this in mind, we realize that aging has its physical drawbacks. Changes in body systems associated with aging include changes in blood pressure, vision, hearing, and skin elasticity. The senses of touch and taste tend to decline, and numerous age-associated changes occur in the body's structural support framework: bone mass, muscle strength, and connective tissues. Hormonal levels, which begin changing during middle adulthood, continue to decrease. Additional changes in the cardiovascular system, cognition, and ambulatory skills can be limiting. The effects of these limitations vary depending on older adults' coping skills and support systems (Yancu, 2011). Cognitive development and decline are important considerations when studying later adulthood. The aging brain is characterized by both structural and functional changes. Variations in cognitive functioning depend on a range of lifestyle and health-related factors. Many older adults may not show evidence of cognitive decline, whereas other individuals may demonstrate pronounced decline (e.g., individuals diagnosed with Alzheimer's disease or various forms of cognitive dementia). Cognition is complex, and factors such as crystallized and fluid intelligence, processing speed, and memory changes are all components of cognition that may be affected by the aging process. In general, education, mental engagement, nutrition, and levels of physical activity can influence cognitive performance in later adulthood. However, when organic factors destroy brain cells, the resulting cognitive deficits are medical in nature and are unlikely to be influenced by the above-mentioned preventive factors.

Although many do not want to think about the end of life, death is universal to the human experience. Death may come expectedly, at the end of a long life, or it may come as a result of illness, trauma, or other unexpected events. Though death is associated with aging, readers were challenged to think about their own views of death and dying. For example, when does "death" actually occur? In some instances, a person may be kept alive by medical intervention, even though he or she has experienced permanent, irreversible brain damage and the person is living in what is called a persistent vegetative state. It is important for older adults to engage in advanced care planning, giving them choices in making decisions regarding whether or not they want life-sustaining treatment when they are no longer able to speak for themselves.

In sum, laughter, wine, and chocolate; these were three things to which Madame Jeanne Calment attributed her longevity when at the age of 120 years and 164 days, she passed into the *Guinness Book of World Records* as the world's oldest human in 1995 (Guinness, 2014). Regardless of the cause, Mme. Calment's lengthy existence shows that humans have the potential to live more than 120 years. (She lived to see her 122nd birthday.) Now that we know how long we can live (longevity), it's time to focus on how we live (vitality) for a very long time!

Relationships and Psychosocial Aspects of Later Adulthood

By Debbie Newsome, Cecile Yancu, Joseph Wilkerson, and Shannon Mathews

This chapter discusses the ways social relationships evolve and change in older adults, as well as two important societal concerns: ageism and elder abuse. Next, socioemotional theories related to aging are introduced, as well as theories related to personality stability and change in older adulthood. A special focus involves ways older adults deal with adversity and what makes some older adults more resilient than others as they age. Finally, issues of spirituality and religion in later life are addressed.

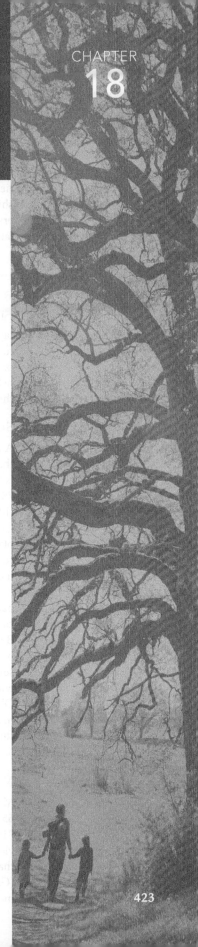

SECTION I:	Relationships in Later Adulthood

The degree and extent to which older adults are involved with their environment and other people in later adulthood is dependent on the social networks and support available to them. As individuals age, the need for social support often increases, making the relational ties that older adults form (or do not form) across the life course very significant. Relationships with spouses, siblings, adult children, grandchildren, friends, neighbors, and caregivers (informal and formal) can influence social, psychological, and physiological health in late adulthood.

The Changing Nature of Social Support Networks and Relationships as People Age

Older adults who have high-quality, diversified networks and social support have an advantage in late adulthood. Social support, both given and received, can positively affect cognitive function, mitigate adversity or negative life experiences, and lower risk of morbidity and premature mortality among older adults. This means that the quality of social relationships held in later life may be a key indicator of the needs and risks older adults may encounter as they age.

Sexual Relations

A prevailing stereotype about older adults is that they do not engage in sexual activity and that once late adulthood is reached the desire for sexual relations diminishes. The reality is that sexual interest remains well into late adulthood. In fact, only about 25% of men 75 to 85 years old and 50% of women 75 to 85 years old report a lack of interest in sex (McFarland, Uecker, & Regnerus, 2011). The physical pleasure and emotional satisfaction gained from sexual relations remain relatively high, with approximately 33% of older adults placing a high value on sex well into late adulthood (Laumann et al., 2006). Sexual activity retains multiple benefits for older adults, including cardiovascular stimulation, increased life satisfaction, and increased marital quality and duration.

The availability of partners and physical or functional decline strongly influence participation in sexual relations during late adulthood. Among older adults, widowhood can initiate the loss of sexual activity associated with partner loss, especially for women. Beyond partner loss, chronic conditions, physical decline, medication side effects, and mood impairment disorders may alter or terminate participation and/or lower desire for sexual relations (Lindau et al., 2007). For example, postmenopausal women who experience vaginal dryness may minimize or eliminate sexual activity due to painful intercourse. Older men with erectile dysfunction (ED) may also have diminished desire to participate in sexual relations, especially if available ED medications are contraindicated. Physical dysfunction, whether treatable or not, can also effect the self-concept and make an older adult feel less sexually desirable.

Marriage

Many older adults, particularly males, live with a spouse. In 2010, 56% of individuals aged 65 and older were married (U.S. Census Bureau, 2010a). Among these individuals, about 71% of older men were married, compared to 42% of older women. Being married provides protection across the life course, especially for women. For example, studies show that marriage increases the likelihood of good health and affluence across the life course (Grundy & Tomassini, 2010). A wide range of benefits are associated with marital status, including positive effects on individuals' economic well-being and mental and physical health (FamilyFacts.org, 2012). Marital status is also associated with lowered risk for health-related conditions, such as depression. Married older adults report less depression and greater life satisfaction when compared to their never-married and divorced counterparts. In fact, never-married and divorced individuals have approximately twice the premature mortality rate of those who are married (FamilyFacts.org, 2006; U.S. Department of Health and Human Services, 2007). Overall, compared to their single counterparts, married older adults tend to have better cognitive function, life satisfaction, and well-being. It may be that older couples benefit cognitively from continued learning within the marital relationship, because partners must learn to adapt to changing roles and expectations in order to preserve the functionality of the living arrangement.

Many older adults report satisfaction with their marital relationship and typically have marriages of longer duration compared to their younger counterparts (Grundy & Tomassini, 2010). For those married 20 or more years, the median age of husbands was 61 and the median age for wives was 58 (U.S. Census Bureau, 2011b). Recent evidence also supports the idea that marital history influences late life health for both partners, with long-term first marriages benefiting men and women more than post-divorce remarriages (Grundy & Tomassini, 2010).

Divorce and Remarriage

An increasing proportion of older adults are experiencing divorce in late adulthood. Divorced individuals 65 and older account for 22% of the older population, with approximately 10% of older men and 12% of older women being divorced (U.S. Census Bureau, 2010a). Divorce can negatively affect the economic, physical, and mental well-being of those in late adulthood. Divorce even appears to weaken or diminish altogether any marital benefits in the case of remarriage (Grundy & Tomassini, 2010). Generational social forces may result in older adults, more than their younger counterparts, experiencing a sense of personal failure and loss of identity in the face of divorce. This sense of loss and failure may be particularly acute for older women.

Parental divorce seems to also affect parent–adult child relationships. Divorce can affect intergenerational bonds within a family, weakening family ties between mothers and fathers and their adult children over time. Adult children of divorced parents may be less likely than children of married parents to provide support to their parents as the parents age (Lin, 2008). Beyond the emotional effects, divorce and remarriage can have negative consequences for adult children and their parental relationships, especially when it comes to financial support. Most often, older women who typically went into a marriage with fewer resources experience greater stress and economic consequences of divorce on parents.

Remarriage rates in late adulthood are relatively low, and they decline with age. However, older individuals who experience divorce are far more likely than widowed older adults to remarry. Remarriage after divorce for parents, especially older men, who are more likely to remarry, can create competing priorities, reducing their support to adult children (Lin, 2008). Additionally, while there is an obligation to provide support for aging parents, there is less emotional incentive to support stepparents, a clear consequence of divorce (Coleman, Ganong, & Rothrauff, 2006).

Widowhood

Approximately 28% of people 65 and older in 2010 were widowed (U.S. Census Bureau, 2010a). Census data show that older women accounted for 40% of the older adult population who had experienced the loss of a spouse, while older men represented only 13%. (The remainder of the sample who lost spouses was younger men and women.) One of the most robust findings of widowhood research is the high risk of premature mortality within 6–12 months after the spousal loss (Stimpson, Yong-Fang, Ray, Rajii, & Peek, 2007).

The loss of a spouse can radically alter late adulthood roles, resources, and sense of identity, especially for women. For example, for older women who have had long marriages, the loss of a spouse means the loss of a spousal role or identity as part of a couple. This loss may cause an overwhelming sense of loneliness or loss of self-esteem. Although the reasons remain unclear, widowhood mortality risk is higher among older men than women. Personality, age, sense of efficacy, and social support are factors that strongly influence how one adjusts to widowhood in late adulthood.

> CASE EXAMPLE **18.1** RHONDA.

Imagine you are a clinical mental health counselor who has some experience in gerontological counseling. A 78-year-old woman, Rhonda, presents for intake. She tears up a lot during the intake as she recounts the death of husband, Matthew. She and Matthew had been married for 45 years. Two years ago, Matthew was diagnosed with stage 3 lung cancer. Rhonda was his primary caregiver until he died two months ago. She says that her friends "drifted away" during the time she was caring for Matthew. The couple had no children, and Rhonda feels isolated and hopeless.

As her counselor, what additional information would you like to know about Rhonda? How would you assess for depression? How do you envision building rapport with her? What are some of the first steps you would take in helping her deal with her grief? How would you address her sense of hopelessness? What resources might help Rhonda as she attempts to build a future without Matthew?

Widowed women are economically vulnerable and susceptible to poverty after the loss of a spouse. The stressors associated with economic vulnerability can influence cognitive function and mental health. Frequently living alone, widowed older women are at particularly high risk for lowered mental health status due to reduced social support and a lack of compensatory resources (Gonyea & Hooyman, 2005). There is also an increased risk for poverty due to lack of financial assistance, which can lead to issues with depression or anxiety.

Among American ethno-racial groups, minority women may be particularly vulnerable because minority groups are at increased risk for both poverty and chronic illness. For example, older African-American women are more likely than White women to be living in poverty and unmarried or widowed, probably because of the gender gap in ALE (Gallant, Spitz, & Grove, 2010). Among Latinos, the risk of death related to widowhood is significantly higher for older Mexican-American men than for non-Hispanics; Mexican-American women are more likely to report a combination of depression (about the loss) and relief from caregiver burden (Stimpson et al., 2007).

Never Married with Children

Approximately 9% of those who have never been married in the United States are men and women 65 and older (U.S. Census Bureau, 2010a). In developed countries since the 1990s, there has been some increase in the number of women who are never married; however, this does not mean they are childless (Cwikel, Gramotnev, & Lee, 2006). Never-married individuals may age with a different set of skills and attitudes from other older adults. For example, many never-married older people develop compensatory relationships or strong reciprocal relationships within their extended family or family and friend networks. Older never-married individuals with children may rely more on adult children and the extended kin network to provide social support in later life than married individuals.

Ethnicity, economic status, educational attainment, and family dynamics are significant factors in determining the well-being of never-married individuals as they age. In fact, compared to other never-married women, more educated, never-married Caucasian women live the longest, healthiest (e.g., physical health, mental health) lives and are more likely to have continuous employment across the life course (Cwikel et al., 2006). Continuity of employment may have been a challenge for older women who had child care responsibilities or who were low wage earners throughout middle adulthood, thus shaping their economic and health risks in late adulthood. Historically, never-married mothers experience more stress associated with caregiving for family members, finances, and work–home balance (Umberson, Pudrovska, & Reczek, 2010). This may also shape the obligation of adult children to care for or support older never-married mothers.

Siblings

The sibling relationship is typically the longest-lasting relationship in older adults' lives, since approximately 80% of Americans spend at least one-third of their lives living with their sibling (Mikkelson, Myers, & Hannawa, 2011). These relationships in late adulthood are defined by shared history, increasing intimacy, and an egalitarian tone, which creates a relational context different from other relationships established across the life course (Myers & Goodboy, 2010).

Despite the involuntary nature of the sibling relationship, older adults value this relational tie, view it as a positive experience, and have a strong commitment to maintaining ties with siblings well into late adulthood (Mikkelson et al., 2011). Older men and women both perceive bonds with siblings to be of high importance, especially with sisters. The bond between sisters is seen as closer, and the closer the tie to a sister, the higher the elder's psychological well-being (Van Volkom, 2006). This may relate to the types of psychosocial support offered by sisters. Additionally, siblings are an extremely vital source of support during crisis, with an expectation of support and aid frequently expressed, even in the presence of strained relational dynamics. Siblings fulfill psychological and social needs for each other, such as psychological closeness and investment, the provision of instrumental support, emotional support, and acceptance or approval (Mikkelson et al., 2011). This type of psychosocial support given by siblings can enhance the quality of life experienced in late adulthood.

Friendships

Late adulthood can be characterized by shrinking social networks and social support related to the loosening of family- and work-related roles or responsibilities. Changes in life course roles can add to the significance of friendships maintained throughout later life. Individuals in late adulthood, similar to individuals in young adulthood, select friendships based on shared characteristics such as age, ethnicity, gender, and socioeconomic status. Therefore, opportunities to interact with peers or socialize, whether through community-based programs, religious affiliations, or social clubs, can be vital opportunities for older individuals to develop friendships.

Older adults gain intimacy, companionship, acceptance, and social connectedness from relationships with friends. Friends can be helpful in adapting to age-related changes; they can act as role models for individuals going through similar changes; they can influence one's sense of identity or self-efficacy; and they can provide emotional support (Stevens, Martina, & Westerhof, 2006). Having friends in later life can strongly influence older adults' mental and physical health as they age.

Adult Children

Relationships with children remain salient to parents' well-being throughout the life course (Greenfield & Marks, 2006). This importance is reflected in frequent contact and mutual exchange of support and affection between parents and adult children (Umberson et al., 2010). For example, more than half of adult children have daily contact with an older parent (Pew Research Center, 2006). A majority of adult children see or talk on the phone with an older parent at least once a week. The "linked lives" shared by older parents and adult children can profoundly affect many dimensions of an older adult's life (Umberson et al., 2010).

The quality of intergenerational ties and emotional closeness with adult children are associated with physical and psychological well-being in later life (Milkie, Bierman, & Schieman, 2008). For example, older adults who have poor relational ties with an adult child have higher levels of depression and a greater sense of loneliness in late adulthood. Negative treatment of aging parents by adult children is associated with more depression and anger in parents. The occurrence of negative events in adult children's lives, such as unemployment or divorce, can also have a negative effect on an older parent's psychological well-being.

Adult children can provide support, assistance with age-related declines, and resources to older individuals as they age. This is especially true for unmarried parents who may not have access to other informal caregivers (Pinquart & Sorenson, 2007). However, with the increase in multigenerational households, increased longevity, and stressors experienced by adult children, older adults also provide a significant amount of support and resources to their adult children.

Research suggests aging parents are more likely to give than to receive support from adult children, and those who provide financial and instrumental assistance to their adult children exhibit fewer depressive symptoms than other parents (Byers, Levy, Allore, Bruce, & Kasl, 2008). Individuals in late adulthood who own a home and are married or widowed (in comparison to those who are divorced) are more likely to provide assistance to adult children than to receive assistance from adult children (Grundy, 2005). Generally, older adults may provide support to adult children in the form of time, effort, and financial resources. Seniors who provide more support than they receive experience a higher level of life satisfaction compared to older adults receiving more support than they give.

The shared lives of older adults and their adult children suggest a link between living arrangements and parental well-being in late adulthood. Parents' gender may be an important consideration in terms of effects of co-residence on well-being (Umberson et al., 2010). For instance, co-residence with adult children is associated with decreased psychological well-being for mothers. Also, when care is needed for an aging parent, adult children (especially adult daughters) most frequently provide care. Therefore, many older adults live with the two-thirds of women acting as their informal caregivers (Pierret, 2006).

Declines or problems related to physical and mental health can influence living arrangements, psychological well-being, and assistance received and given by an older adult in late adulthood. Adult children's need for help due to problems regarding alcohol, emotional, school, work, or legal issues is associated with lower levels of psychological well-being for aging parents. This is especially true for unmarried parents.

Adult Grandchildren

During late adulthood, older individuals who are grandparents generally invest in future generations through various means of support, including the transmission of values, economic resources, and emotional support. A sense of legacy can influence the contributions and generational transfers experienced in late adulthood. As people live longer, economic pressures and increased demands for social support among family members trying to make ends meet may result in an increase in multigenerational households, contributing to the intergenerational exchanges experienced in late adulthood.

For a variety of reasons (e.g., drug use by and incarceration of their adult children), seniors in late adulthood are increasingly becoming custodial caregivers of grandchildren, an off-time or nonnormative grandparenting responsibility (Umberson et al., 2010). This will ultimately affect the types of relational ties older adults have as their grandchildren age. Grandparents caring for grandchildren experience challenges in housing, finances, work, and education that significantly disrupt retirement plans. Grandmothers caring for grand-children are likely to experience negative changes in health behavior, depression, and self-rated health than those who co-parent. This may ultimately affect the types of relationships seniors have with adult grandchildren, making these relationships more like a parent–adult child relationship.

LGBT Relationships

It is important to remember that older adults are as diverse in their sexual orientations, attitudes, and behaviors as younger individuals. Historically, there has been limited information in the research record regarding seniors who identify as lesbian, gay, bisexual, and transgendered (LGBT) [*Note:* Gay, lesbian, bisexual, and transgendered (GLBT) is also used in the literature to denote this group.] However, this group is estimated to represent approximately 3 million adults aged 65 and over (Knauer, 2009). LGBT Baby Boomers represent the first generation to live openly with regard to their sexual orientation and lifestyle preference, and it is suggested that the number of LGBT seniors will double by 2030.

Historically, the social stigma and consequences associated with being LGBT have created barriers within communities, caused disruptions in family relations, and hindered access to services. As a result, LGBT elders, when compared to other older adults, are more likely to be single, childless, estranged from their biological family, and reliant on families of choice, such as friends and other loved ones [LGBT Movement Advancement Project (MAP), 2010]. Only 10% of LGBT older adults have children, compared to 80% of their heterosexual counterparts (Knauer, 2009). Their reliance on selected families presents particular challenges with regard to social policies that prioritize only legal and biological kin relationships. This often results in restriction on the rights and privileges afforded to non-traditional caregivers or same-sex partners.

As members of a "socially and legally disfavored" group of older adults, LGBT seniors face distinct difficulties in late adulthood that affect their overall well-being (MAP, 2010, p. 4). Although the research is severely limited, the studies that do exist show isolation is a significant problem for this population (Knauer, 2009). One reason for this may be that the continued social stigma experienced by "out" individuals in late adulthood limits their ability to be socially involved in the communities in which they live. This may frequently be related to prejudicial treatment causing social isolation and unemployment. Ultimately, this could influence seniors' self-concept, social engagement, and risk for such conditions as depression or anxiety.

Community-dwelling and institutionalized LGBT seniors often report a fear of discrimination and lack of appropriate care as they age, directly related to their identification as LGBT individuals (MAP, 2010; National Senior Citizens Law Center, 2011). Many LGBT seniors, both in the community and in institutions, do experience differential care, with their needs being ignored or untreated. This only serves to compound the discriminatory care some may experience as a result of being aged.

The reliance of LGBT seniors on nontraditional caregivers and families of choice or fictive kin is a direct result of the marginalization many experience across the life course. Such compensatory networks, however, may leave LGBT seniors ineligible for assistance, supports, and resources provided to traditional caregivers and families. For institutionalized older adults, this frequently means a lack of privileges in regard to exclusion from visitation rights or decision making, which are instead assigned to traditional family members (National Senior Citizens Law Center, 2011). Existing policies and laws also fail to address other issues of access for this group. Thus, many do not experience the financial protections afforded spouses and survivors with regard to government programs such as Social Security. Such lack of protection in late adulthood directly affects access to resources necessary for successful aging.

Ageism and Elder Abuse

Ageism is a form of prejudice exhibited when people are categorized and judged based on their chronological age (Hays & Erford, 2014). Ageism was touched on in Chapter 17, but what follows is a more complete description of this form of prejudice and of how it is expressed. Ageism can reduce older adults' social and economic opportunities, damage self-respect, exacerbate health problems, and reduce the optimal potential of aging adults (Myers & Shannonhouse, 2013; North & Fiske, 2012). Ageism is peppered with stereotypes about older adults that are not based on fact. In reality, older adults are valuable members of society. Most have learned to adapt to life's changes, give back to their communities, and share wisdom that benefits younger generations (Newsome & Gladding, 2014).

Ageism is expressed in myriad ways, both subtly and blatantly. Oftentimes, people may not even be aware that they are expressing ageism. To illustrate, one manifestation of ageism is *elderspeak,* which is a condescending way of speaking to older adults. It often resembles baby talk, evidenced by simple sentences, exaggerated emphasis on phrases, a slowed rate of speech, and a higher pitch. Some people overuse terms like *dear, honey,* or *sweetie,* which can come across as patronizing. Understandably, older adults may react with resentment, anger, or self-doubt. Other examples of ageism include becoming frustrated or angry when driving behind older adults or standing behind them in the grocery store. As stated by Myers and Shannonhouse (2013), "Whenever people make choices and perform actions based on age, they may have succumbed to ageism" (p. 156).

Another form of ageism occurs in the workplace. Although legislation prohibits employers from discriminating against employees on the basis of age, companies often offer older workers "packages" providing financial incentives to retire. This practice occurs in spite of research findings suggesting that abilities and performance can continue to develop throughout our working lives and that new learning can occur at any age (Langer, 2009). Although some older adults experience conditions that may keep them from performing effectively (e.g., cognitive impairment, dementia, decline in health), many older adults perform as or more effectively than their younger counterparts.

It is important to examine our personal attitudes toward aging and older adults. In so doing, we can increase our efforts to combat ageism on personal and professional levels. **Elder abuse**, also called elder mistreatment or elder maltreatment, has developed into a significant social, public health, and criminal justice concern (e.g., Dong, 2014; Payne, Blowers, & Jarvis, 2012). Elder abuse includes "psychological, physical, and sexual abuse; neglect (caregiver neglect and self-neglect), and financial exploitation" (Dong, 2014, p. 153). Elder abuse can—and does—affect people of all ethnic backgrounds, social status, and gender. According to the National Center on Elder Abuse (NCEA, 2014), the following types of abuse are identified as the major categories of elder maltreatment:

- *Physical abuse*—Inflicting, or threatening to inflict, physical pain or injury on a vulnerable elder, or depriving them of a basic need.
- *Emotional abuse*—Inflicting mental pain, anguish, or distress on an elder person through verbal or nonverbal acts.
- *Sexual abuse*—Nonconsensual sexual contact of any kind, coercing an elder to witness sexual behaviors.
- *Exploitation*—Illegal taking, misuse, or concealment of funds, property, or assets of a vulnerable elder.
- *Neglect*—Refusal or failure by those responsible to provide food, shelter, health care, or protection for a vulnerable elder.
- *Abandonment*—Desertion of a vulnerable elder by anyone who has assumed responsibility for care or custody of that person.

It is challenging to determine the number of older adults who have been abused, primarily because much abuse goes unreported (Dong, 2014). National estimates "show that at least 1 in 10 older adults suffers some form of elder abuse, and many in repeated forms" (Dong, 2014, p. 154). Older women are at greater risk of experiencing abuse than are older men (Penhale, 2005). This may be largely due to the longevity experienced by women, making them a greater proportion of older adults in late adulthood. Older adults with various forms of dementia also are at higher risk for abuse than those without (Cooney, Howard, & Lawlor, 2006). Elder maltreatment crosses ethnic lines; however, the experience across cultures varies. Due to strong traditions of respect, obligation to care for older adults, and high disapproval of the maltreatment of elders, Asian, Hispanic, and Native American populations tend to experience lower rates of elder abuse (Sherman, Rosenblatt, & Antonucci, 2008).

Elder abuse is more likely to occur (e.g., is documented) among institutionalized older adults in nursing homes. High staff turnover, poor staffing ratios, overcrowding, stress, and minimal oversight contribute to elder maltreatment of nursing home residents (Payne & Fletcher, 2005). However, elder abuse occurs in domestic settings as well, and the abuse often goes unreported. Elder abuse is perpetrated by family members, friends, outside caregivers, peers, and strangers. With that said, most cases of elder abuse are instigated by known and trusted others, particularly family members, including adult children, spouses, and others (NCEA, 2014). Regardless of the setting, elder abuse can result in a tumultuous downward spiral, leading to an older adult's loss of mental well-being, independence, and in worst-case scenarios, loss of life (Burgess & Hanrahan, 2006).

Preventing elder abuse is a top priority worldwide (Dong, 2014). Education is key to prevention and early intervention. Although elder abuse is better understood today than it was two decades ago, knowledge and advocacy must be increased so that incidences of elder abuse are recognized, reported, and halted.

SECTION II: Psychosocial Aspects of Late Adulthood

Psychosocial Theories of Development in Later Adulthood

This section focuses on psychosocial theories of development in later adulthood. It is important to note that not everyone experiences developmental changes in the same way or at the same time. Furthermore, what may be true for a 65-year-old is likely to be quite different for someone in his or her 90s. Although some texts distinguish *young-old* (adults who are active physically, mentally, and socially) and *old-old* (elders who appear frail and show physical signs of decline), such a distinction, particularly when demarcated by age, is arbitrary and differs from individual to individual. In this section, four theories of psychosocial adjustment are described, recognizing that the process is not always linear and cannot be ascribed to a specific age. Noted theorists who describe psychosocial development in later adulthood include Erik Erikson, Robert Peck, James Fisher, and Gisela Labouvie-Vief.

Erikson: Ego Integrity versus Despair

Erikson (1963) understood psychosocial development in older adulthood as a conflict between ego integrity and despair. As individuals live their later years, much that was connected in the past comes undone on multiple levels. The tissues of the body weaken, physical relocation and others' deaths change relationships that included physical presence, involvement in community activities may decrease, and individuals live a great temporal distance from the past they remember. Lurking beneath all of these is the approach of the ultimate physical separation: death.

REFLECTION 18.1 IS ALBERT EXPERIENCING DESPAIR?

Albert's wife of 40 years died after a long battle with congestive heart failure. Albert spent the last five years of his wife's life as her sole caregiver, rarely accepting help from well-meaning friends. After her death, Albert was 78 years of age and felt that there was no reason to continue living. He found little joy in the activities he had enjoyed earlier in life, such as gardening and playing cards with friends. He disdained the concept of reaching out for help from the church, counseling, or antidepressant medication. In his own world of despair, he insulated himself from his community and spent his last two years of life watching TV, eating microwaved meals, and resenting the cards life had dealt him. [~DWN]

Faced with such powerful forces of disconnection and a limited future, some older adults struggle to develop and maintain a sense of coherence and of life's meaning. These people see time as too short, or feel helpless to correct or make meaning of past failures. They feel despair and are disgusted with themselves, which they may express as misanthropy and disdain for life. They may struggle with regrets, question their personal worth, and believe that the time they have left on Earth is too short to "make right" any poor decisions made in the past.

In contrast, many older adults are able to develop and maintain an overarching sense of ego integrity. They see the events of their past—successes, failures, and paths not taken—as meaningfully contributing to a unique life course. They are able to view life in the larger context of humanity and find increased contentment in recognizing who they are within that context (Berk, 2010). Such an attitude both requires and crystallizes the wisdom accumulated over the previous seven psychosocial stages. Jung (1965) articulates his experience of integrity in the final paragraphs of his autobiography, *Memories, Dreams, Reflections*, written late in his life:

REFLECTION 18.2 EXPERIENCING EGO INTEGRITY

Rosa, age 87, views life with optimism. Although her marriage dissolved 30 years earlier, she came to terms with the divorce and moved to the West Coast to be closer to her three adult children and her two aging siblings. She has been retired from her job as a nurse practitioner for many years. Even so, she continues to explore lifelong learning opportunities by being an active member of two book clubs, participating in community activities, and socializing regularly with family and friends. She enjoys life and states that she has "few regrets." She looks forward to what new paths lay ahead. [~DWN]

> I am satisfied with the course my life has taken. It has been bountiful, and has given me a great deal. How could I ever have expected so much? Nothing but unexpected things kept happening to me. Much might have been different if I myself had been different. But it was as it had to be; for all came about because I am as I am. (p. 358)

Reminiscence and Life Review

> It is through story that we embrace the great breadth of memory, that we can distinguish what is true, and that we may glimpse, at least occasionally, how to live without despair in the midst of the horror that dogs and unhinges us. (Lopez, 1999, p. 13)

One way that sometimes helps older adults develop ego integrity is the process of reminiscence. Simply stated, **reminiscence** is the recall of memories. People begin to reminisce early in life, experiencing daydreams of and nostalgia for past events (Haber, 2006). In later life, reminiscence is a means by which people recall, assess, and evaluate past events. According to Webster and McCall (1999), there are eight purposes of reminiscence, most of which are positive. Healthy purposes include identity formation, preparation for death, and problem solving. Social purposes of reminiscing include conversing and teaching others from past experience. However, reminiscing to fight boredom, revive bitter feelings, or avoid adjustment to loss by ruminating about the deceased can be dysfunctional and lead to despair.

Why do older adults often reminisce about their past more than their younger counterparts? Erikson (1963) believed that the process of recalling and taking stock of one's life experiences is essential to the development of ego integrity during the final stage of psychosocial development. Similarly, Atchley (1989) believed that reminiscence helps older adults to achieve a sense of **inner continuity** during the internal and external transitions of older adulthood. This strategy of using familiar methods to cope with changes provides a degree of competence and mastery that bolsters self-esteem. Narrative theories support the notion that we continuously (re)construct our identities over time by telling and retelling our life stories (Haber, 2006).

Life review is one activity that can further the therapeutic potential of reminiscence. During life review, people not only describe but also reflect on and evaluate their life experiences. They focus on themes like childhood, family, parenting, grandparenting, vocational choices, personal meaning and values, and experiences with aging and dying (Haber, 2006). Often family, caregivers, or groups assist individuals with life review by serving as an audience. Life review may occur in pairs or in groups, and as a structured or unstructured activity. It may be oral, written, or carried out using music or other expressive arts. For mental health caregivers, using structured life review as an intervention may seem less threatening and more familiar to older adults than other psychotherapeutic approaches (Haight & Haight, 2007; Weiss, 1995).

Life review has many benefits for older adults. It typically increases ego integrity, life satisfaction, and positive feelings, and decreases feelings of depression and despair (Bohlmeijer, Roemer, Cuijpers, & Smit, 2007; Stinson, 2009). MacKinlay and Trevitt (2010) demonstrated that a carefully facilitated reminiscence group can improve the quality of life and spiritual well-being of individuals with dementia. Beechem, Anthony, and Kurtz (1998) suggested that life review can help older adults gain a sense of control over their personal narratives, which is especially important as they lose other forms of control and independence. Assisted reminiscence can help older adults discover existential meaning as they reflect on the purpose of their lives and the place of their lives in a larger context (Haber, 2006). Finally, life review completed with family members can enrich both the storyteller and the listener, thus strengthening generational ties (Luepker, 2010).

➤ CASE EXAMPLE **18.2**   PLANNING FOR A LIFE REVIEW GROUP.

You are a counselor at an adult community retirement center. You have learned about the value of life review groups and would like to lead one at the retirement center. After consulting with a colleague, you decide that a life review group that includes family members would be especially helpful.

- What are some considerations to account for during the planning stage?
- Would you use a creative medium to facilitate group interaction (e.g., photographs, music, drawings)? What is an example of a creative intervention that might be helpful? What other interventions would you consider?
- Which do you think would be more effective—a structured group or an unstructured group?
- What are some ways family members can contribute to and benefit from the process?
- What outcomes would you hope to see after the life review group ends?

Peck's Tasks of Old Age

Robert Peck delineated three developmental tasks for individuals after retirement. These tasks provide a framework for successful aging (Kolb, 2008). The first task is **ego differentiation**, or enlargement of one's identity beyond one's former work role. Retired and retiring individuals may redefine their self-worth outside the work arena and begin to find satisfaction in non-work roles. Peck, whose theory was developed during the era when most women worked at home, viewed this as a particularly crucial transition for men. He acknowledged that women, whose primary work consisted of mothering and homemaking, experienced ego differentiation differently, and sometimes earlier than men. In contemporary times, both men and women often invest heavily in career, thus making ego differentiation a time when both genders find new or additional ways to affirm self-worth, often through ties with family, friendship, and community (Berk, 2010).

Peck's second task is **body transcendence**, or redefining happiness and comfort in terms of relational, mental, and creative activities with which the physiological declines of old age do not interfere. Individuals who accomplish this goal may experience as much physical unease as those who do not, but they enjoy life greatly rather than becoming preoccupied with their physiological distress.

Peck's final task is achieving a state of **ego transcendence**, which he describes in this way:

> To live so generously and unselfishly that the prospect of personal death—the night of the ego, it might be called—looks and feels less important than the secure knowledge that one has built for a broader, longer future than any one ego ever could encompass. (Peck, 1955, p. 48)

Older adults transcend their personal egos by purposefully and actively investing in relationships with the things and people that will go on after their own deaths.

Gerotranscendence

Erikson's widow, Joan Erikson (Erikson & Erikson, 1997), coined the term **gerotranscendence** as a developmental task that is associated with Peck's task of ego transcendence as well as Erikson's eighth stage of his psychosocial model of development. Adults experiencing gerotranscendence shift from a connection with the material world to a more transcendent, cosmically directed sense of connection (Degges-White, 2005). Gerotranscendence is marked by feelings of heightened inner calm and contentment. Older adults may turn inward, spending more time in self-reflection. Whereas some of the markers of gerotranscendence may be misidentified as psychological issues, Degges-White suggested that if the aging adult's withdrawal from social interaction is a personal choice, counselors and caregivers need to ensure that the client's right to choose to enjoy a time of extended solitude is respected. Although more research is needed to confirm the process of gerotranscendence, a large body of evidence supports the existence of this final stage of aging.

Fisher's Five Periods of Older Adulthood

Fisher (1993) developed his theory of older adulthood after interviewing 74 people over the age of 60. Fisher outlines five periods of older adulthood, some that are stable and others that are transitional. The first period is a continuation of middle age. For some older adults this means continuing to work and support themselves. For others, it represents the freedom to pursue retirement plans in the absence of work, including leisure and volunteering. For some, this period is carefree; for others, it is a time of growing concern over finances, health, and premonitions of a limited future.

The second period is initiated by voluntary and involuntary transitional events which end continuity with middle adulthood. Examples include the need to relocate, the death of a spouse, a physical illness or decline in ability, and the decision to retire or return to work part time. In each case, older adults feel a limiting effect of their age in some way, but preserve their autonomy. Some older adults begin to experience loneliness resulting from relocation or the death of a spouse or partner during this period.

In the third period, which is considered stable, older adults adjust to the transitional changes made in the previous period while maintaining relative independence. When possible, older adults continue to pursue their retirement goals from the first period, accommodating any new limitations. Some experience greater freedom, as when the death of a spouse frees an individual from caretaking responsibilities; for others, a similar loss limits freedom. Many older adults seek out and become involved with others in their age group for the first time, often in response to increasing loneliness. Others choose to volunteer, work, or join social service organizations as a way to stay active and socialize.

The fourth period, which is transitional, involves significant declines in independence. This period often is initiated by losses in health or mobility, by the death of a spouse, or by the loss or relocation of a caregiver. In each case, older adults must transition into an environment of greater dependence on others and adjust their activities and goals according to their environment and their abilities.

The fifth and final period is a stable one in which older adults live with limited mobility and largely depend on others for care. Some experience loneliness, having outlived friends and family, are unable to initiate visits, and are resigned to their limitations. Many, however, continue to grow, thrive, and learn during this period, overcoming various levels of disability and immobility and staying active.

Labouvie-Vief: Affect Optimization and Affect Complexity

Gisela Labouvie-Vief and her colleagues spent years researching ways in which individuals adjust to adversity and difficult life experiences while maintaining positive levels of affect and well-being (e.g., Labouvie-Vief, 2003; Labouvie-Vief, Diehl, Jain, & Zhang, 2007). They hypothesized that **cognitive-affective complexity** (i.e., coordinating positive and negative emotions into an organized self-description) increases from adolescence through middle adulthood and declines somewhat during later adulthood as certain cognitive skills diminish (Berk, 2010). However, older adults tend to compensate for declines in information-processing skills by developing increased affect optimization skills.

As the cognitive demands of integrating and blending positive and negative emotions become more difficult after middle age, some older adults learn to regulate emotion in different ways (Labouvie-Vief, 2003; Labouvie-Vief et al., 2007). Through the processes of **affect optimization**, older adults cognitively maximize positive emotions and dampen negative emotions. Through affect optimization, individuals are able to maintain positive emotions and psychological well-being in the face of major stressors such as bereavement, illness, and declines in independence.

Some older adults rely less on optimization strategies and continue to employ the differentiating function of **affect complexity**, which is often used in middle adulthood and also is evidenced in later adulthood. This more complex and cognitively demanding strategy helps individuals gain insight from emotions, maintain relative objectivity, form a distinct and historically situated sense of self, and realistically blend positive and negative emotions. People who employ this strategy report more negative affect than those who optimize, but they also tend to have greater perspective on these emotions.

According to Labouvie-Vief (2003), ultimately we may understand *affect optimization* and *affect complexity* as two poles on a spectrum of cognitive-affective strategies. As individuals age, they both optimize and differentiate in dynamic ways consistent with their changing cognitive abilities. Joan Erikson illustrates this dynamism in a reflective passage, written in late life:

> Love, devotion, and friendship bloom; sadness is tender and enriching....Looking back is engagingly memorable; the present is natural and full of little pleasures, immense joys, and much laughter....With whatever tact and wisdom we can muster, disabilities must be accepted with lightness and humor. (Erikson & Erikson, 1997, p. 9)

> **Think About It   18.1**

1. Think of Erikson's constructs of *despair* and *ego integrity* on a continuum. What older adults do you know who are much closer to experiencing ego integrity than despair? Who do you know that is on the opposite end of the continuum? As a counselor, how would you work with individuals who appear to be closer to despair than ego integrity?

2. Discuss ways that a counselor can use creative arts (e.g., photographs, music) to help older adults construct a *structured life review*.

3. Some theorists classify Joan Erikson's theory of gerotranscendence as the ninth stage of Erik Erikson's original theory. Others believe that it is fits better with Robert Peck's developmental tasks. What do you think? Do you know any senior citizens who appear to be experiencing gerotranscendence? Describe ways they exhibit this stage of development.

4. Fisher developed his five-stage theory of later adulthood development based on interviews with 74 adults. Research his theory to see if there is additional evidence to support it.

5. Discuss ways that affect optimization and affect complexity complement each other as adults age.

Effective emotional self-regulation differs from individual to individual, regardless of age. Certainly, there are "grumpy old men" (and women) just as there are "irascible teenagers." However, older adults' emotional perceptiveness and ability to cope with feelings before determining a course of action can benefit their ability to self-regulate and thereby maintain a sense of positivity and life satisfaction.

SECTION III: Work and Retirement

At what age does the average person retire? The answer, which frequently is the case with life development questions, is "It depends." A plethora of factors figure into the equation, including:

- Do I have the financial resources to retire?
- Do I have the physical ability to continue working?
- Do I work in a setting where layoffs are likely to occur?
- Do I want to continue working?
- Do I have the option to continue working?
- How does my spouse or partner feel about retiring?
- Do I want to stop work abruptly, or do I want to go through a phased retirement?
- To what degree is my personal identity connected to my working identity?

Consider the case of Susan and Michael (see Case Example 18.3).

➤ CASE EXAMPLE **18.3**   RETIREMENT: ONE COUPLE'S PERSPECTIVE.

I (DWN) recently interviewed a couple in their 60s, Michael and Susan. Michael had worked as a professional banker for 33 years when he was forced to retire due to company cutbacks. At that time, he was only 57 years old and had planned to work for several more years. He was not happy with the forced retirement, which was unexpected and brought his routine to an abrupt halt. He began walking daily to relieve stress. At the time, his wife Susan was still working in the public school system and did not plan to retire for three more years.

Five months after the forced retirement, Michael's company called him back. They needed his services. He negotiated an increased salary and worked with the company for three more years, when he retired by choice. Susan, who had been in the school system for 30 years, also chose to retire at that time. She loved her work but was ready for a life that provided more flexibility, independence, and time with Michael.

The couple described their "official" retirement as extremely rewarding. They had planned well financially and were able to travel, volunteer, remodel the house, and spend time with friends. When I asked them if retirement had redefined their sense of self-worth, both adamantly stated that it had not. Their views of self were not enmeshed in their work. Instead, they were satisfied that during their working years, "We did what we needed to do with integrity and with fairness." They said that they had no regrets about the past and were looking forward to the future.

Prior to retirement, both Susan and Michael had been caregivers for elderly parents. Caregiving was challenging and stressful, lasting over a course of five years. One parent had Alzheimer's and the other had many physical challenges. Both parents required a great deal of attention and care. According to Susan, she and Michael were "worn out" all the time. Working full time and serving as caregivers was stressful and physically demanding.

Susan gave Michael a lot of credit for his positive attitude, both during that difficult period and during the transition period afterward. He sees the glass as half full rather than half empty. Susan said that his attitude has rubbed off on her. Their faith and spirituality have deepened over time, as have their friendships. They are actively involved in their community and spend time helping older friends who need transportation assistance.

At the end of the interview, I asked the couple what advice they would give to people who are considering retirement. They shared the following:

- Pay off your house early.
- Plan financially.
- Figure out the things you like to do, and do them.
- Accept that retirement is a part of life. In some ways, it is a better stage of life—a second cup of coffee, so to speak.
- Enjoy freedom from the clock.
- Give your best to your job during your working years so that you can retire "guilt-free."
- Keep your mind, body, and friendships strong.
- Leave a legacy to your children by showing them what it means to work well and retire well.

After reading Susan and Michael's account, what are your initial impressions? What planning went into preretirement? How did involuntary retirement affect Michael, and how did its reversal impact the couple? In what ways did their socioeconomic status and intentional financial planning affect their adjustment to retirement? Often, older adults considering retirement may be in circumstances that differ significantly from Susan and Michael's. In many instances, older adults may not have sufficient resources to consider retirement. If an individual is dependent solely on government support, such as Social Security and Medicare, what does that mean in regard to quality of life? What if the individual develops a significant health problem that prohibits continued working, even though the income is needed? Or what if he or she is laid off in middle adulthood? Although it is not feasible to address each of these questions in this chapter, we want you to keep them in mind as you continue to read about working and retirement in later adulthood.

Retirement Trends

Before 1934, retirement was not even considered an option. People's lifespans were not as long, and it was assumed that individuals would work until it was no longer physically possible or until they died. In 1934, a railroad union sponsored a bill promoting mandatory retirement, and in 1935, the government established the **Social Security** program (Martin & Weaver, 2005). After the passage of Social Security, more people were able to retire. Indeed, retirement was considered mandatory for adults once they reached the age of 65. In 1950, the average man could expect to live another 13 years after retiring, and the average woman was expected to live at least 15 more years. In today's world, that number has increased substantially, and many seniors live 20 or more years after the age of 65 (National Institute on Aging, 2011). Social Security, which originally was designed to supplement older adults' income after retirement, is now expected to supply income for a group of adults who live considerably longer than they did when the program was implemented.

Mandatory retirement regulations in the United States were abolished in 1978 and 1986 by means of stepwise amendments to the Federal Age Discrimination in Employment Act (von Wachter, 2002). Although some older adults choose to retire when they are 65 or younger, others elect to remain in the workforce, either as full-time or part-time workers. The current economic climate has played a large role in that trend. Economic uncertainties, questions about whether the Social Security program will run out of money, and other financial factors, in addition to personal and professional factors, may mean that older workers will work for several years after the age of 65, due either to choice or to necessity. Currently, the age at which people working in the United States receive full Social Security benefits is dependent on their birth year. Full benefits were made available to adults born prior to 1938 when they turned 65. For adults born in 1960 or later, full benefits become available at the age of 67 (Social Security Online, 2012).

Making the Decision to Retire

Many factors influence an older adult's decision to retire. Affordability, physical health, occupational identity, the meaning attached to work, and living situations (e.g., single, married, partnered) are just a few of these factors. Sometimes retirement is voluntary. A person believes that it is time to end his current paid working life and transition into another phase of life. At other times, the decision is involuntary. An individual may be laid off or develop a health condition that makes continued working, at least in his or her current field, impossible. Sometimes retirees (voluntary or involuntary) take bridge jobs, either to make ends meet, or they find work that is more stimulating, or to pursue a job that is less physically demanding (Berk, 2010). A **bridge job** is a "bridge" between full-time work and retirement following a full-time career. It may be either full time or part time. It may be either an extension of one's career or a shift to something entirely different. For retirees, bridge jobs offer an opportunity to make a career move without pressure. It also serves as a means of connecting with other people, thus opening avenues for new friendships.

Adjusting to Retirement

There are many paths people can take when they reach their 60s. Some people choose to retire completely from full-time work. Others retire from their current work and choose bridge jobs or venture into a new field of full-time work. Some older adults choose phased retirement; they begin cutting down on time spent at work with a plan to retire completely at a selected point in time. Some seniors are laid off from their jobs, particularly during times when underemployment and unemployment are high. Still others retire from full-time work and then become involved in volunteer work, service projects, and other forms of non-paid work.

According to many gerontologists (see Santrock, 2011), older adults who adjust best to retirement are healthy, active, and educated. They are financially stable, have a supportive social network, and were satisfied with their lives before retirement. In contrast, seniors with financial burdens, health issues, and multiple stressors have more difficulty adjusting. For some older adults, leaving their profession represents a loss of identity and self-worth. They may feel that they no longer matter (Dixon, 2007).

Retirement represents a major life transition, which is a process rather than a single event. While there are many ways to consider patterns of adjustment, Nancy Schlossberg's transition theory, as it relates to older adults, is an important focus. According to **transition theory**, both positive and negative changes typically cause discomfort. When roles, routines, relationships, and assumptions change, it can be unsettling. It takes time to establish new paths, and as those new paths are established, people are in the midst of transition. There are no shortcuts to adjusting quickly. It takes time to adjust to a new way of living. During the transition process, people often grieve the lives left behind, flounder as they try out new paths, and then begin to integrate new ways of living with their integral sense of self (Schlossberg, 2011).

Schlossberg (2011) describes a set of four coping resources that help with transition periods. She calls this the 4S System:

- *Situation:* What is the person's situation at the time of transition? Are there other life stressors involved?
- *Self:* What inner strengths can the person draw on to cope with the situation?
- *Supports:* What supports does the person have during the transition time?
- *Strategies:* What specific methods of coping does the person use that will make the transition more navigable?

Schlossberg (2011) emphasizes the need to use multiple strategies flexibly in order to cope effectively. She suggests that when older adults look at the transition period related to retirement, it helps them to self-check the following: (1) Is my situation okay? (2) Are my supports in order? (3) Do I use several coping strategies effectively? (4) Am I resilient and optimistic? If all of the answers are "yes," the older adult will be able to manage the transition more effectively. If not, Schlossberg recommends taking time to figure out how to strengthen the areas that are weak. Often, personal or group counseling can be especially helpful at this juncture (Maples, 2009).

Group counseling for older adults can help identify common issues, concerns, and problems, as well as positive anticipations for the retirement transition. Maples (2009) described her work with six older professionals who had recently retired. She asked group members to identify topics for discussion around retirement. Group members identified several common themes that revolved around the broad topics of fear, apprehension, and confusion. The primary issue expressed was loss: loss of meaning, loss of identity, loss of structure, possible loss of a partner or spouse, and loss of the security of knowing what each day would bring. (In this group, financial security was not an issue, although for many older adults it would be.) The group met for eight weeks, and then decided to continue meeting afterward because of the positive outcomes members were experiencing. One of the members commented, "Since I now look forward to the end of my paid working life as another transition, of which I have had many [that were] successful, why should I fear this one?" (Maples, 2009, p. 34).

Does Ethnicity Affect Adjustment to Retirement?

According to one source (Kail & Cavanaugh, 2010), "There has not been much research examining the process of ethnicity as a function of retirement" (p. 567). However, late-life transitions such as retirement have been found to promote greater social connectedness via family, church, and community among older African-Americans and Latinos. It is likely that African-Americans and Latinos identify themselves as much or more with these groups than with their occupations. In other words, whereas a White American may have attached substantial meaning and identity to his or her profession, such an attachment may not be true for African-Americans or Latinos. As always, when considering ethnic differences, it is important to remember that typically there is more difference *within groups* than there is *between groups*. The scarcity of research shows that much study is needed to promote greater understanding in this area.

Leisure and Volunteer Activities

Retirement can be a time when older adults pursue recreational activities, enjoy spending time with partners and extended family, devote more time to friends, and participate in lifelong learning activities. Certainly, health concerns may limit some of the "hoped-for" leisure activities, particularly in regard to travel, which tends to decline after the age of 75 (Berk, 2010). Nonetheless, Baby Boomers are taking better care of themselves than any generation before them; they have lower rates of disability and fewer are living in poverty (Maples & Abney, 2006).

During the past few decades, many organizations, such as the American Association for Retired Persons (now simply AARP), have provided older adults with opportunities to learn about other retirees' activities through publications and through the Internet. Other groups, such as senior centers, clubs, and retirement villages, promote lifelong learning through book clubs and other venues (Kail & Cavanaugh, 2010). Many seniors recognize the need to remain cognitively active and choose to participate in these and other activities.

Volunteering is another way that many retired adults choose to structure their time. Older adults contribute significantly to society through volunteer work, and this trend continues to grow (Berk, 2010). Volunteering gives people a chance to make valuable contributions to society. The degree to which older adults volunteer depends on a host of factors, including earlier patterns of civic involvement, the meaningfulness associated with volunteering, and general attitudes. In other words, if an older adult sees no need to volunteer, is limited by health conditions, or does not find the act of volunteering rewarding, he or she is less likely to engage in that activity. However, approximately one-third of people in their 60s and 70s in industrialized nations report volunteering (Berk, 2010). Volunteering not only fulfills multiple societal needs; it can also give older adults a sense of purpose—a sense of mattering (Dixon, 2007). It enables people to contribute to the well-being of current and future generations.

Volunteering can take many forms. Some retirees develop and run their own programs at senior centers. Others choose to volunteer in hospitals, assist with programs like Meals on Wheels, and find niches where their skills can be used to enrich society. For example, the Peace Corps is actively recruiting older volunteers, such as Francine Connolly, a 67-year-old former social worker, along with her husband, who also a retired social worker, to help in Africa. Like other retirees, Mr. and Mrs. Connolly, now freed from the responsibilities of full-time work and child-rearing, may choose to participate in service teams or mission trips, which may be local, national, or international in scope. Often, these retirees use the skills honed during their working years to help people in need. Service teams often consist of volunteers who are skilled in medicine, dentistry, construction, mental health provision, and foreign-language interpretation, to name just a few.

Environmental volunteerism is one way older adults can participate in civic engagement (Bushway, Dickinson, Stedman, Wagenet, & Weinstein, 2011). Although environmental volunteerism among older adults is not as well documented as other types of volunteerism, it offers benefits for volunteers on multiple levels. Retirees who are environmental activists and have the physical capability to work outside are less likely to engage in sedentary behavior, which is a risk factor for chronic disease, morbidity, and premature mortality. Bushway et al. suggested that aging environmental volunteers bring many positives to the table, including "wisdom, experience, technical expertise, and enthusiasm for creating meaning through socio-emotional activities" (p. 193). As with many volunteer

---

REFLECTION 18.3 ROBERT AND POLLY

After retiring, Robert and Polly joined a bridge club at their local senior center. Avid bridge players, they had enjoyed the game for many years, although the time they could devote to this shared activity was limited. They decided to take a refresher course in bridge at a local community college, after which they felt ready to join a bridge club that met twice a week. At the center, they met new people, enjoyed friendly competition, and found that playing bridge helped keep them "mentally sharp." They also invited neighbors to their home for bridge parties. The card game they learned to play when they were younger now became a primary leisure activity that served multiple purposes: It helped them remain cognitively active, it provided them with a new social network, and it was an impetus for getting together with neighbors on a regular basis. [~DWN]

activities, environmental volunteerism is a way to express altruism by giving back to the community and environment.

In summing up ways older adults integrate leisure activities and volunteer work into their retirement paths, Schlossberg (2011) emphasizes that *retirement* does not mean *retreating*. It involves changing gears—leaving one set of activities and moving toward new paths. Older adults, who identify their expectations for retirement, while also preparing for unexpected twists and turns, typically are involved, productive, and engaged. Schlossberg recommends that older adults who are discovering their retirement paths consider asking themselves, "Which do you want to be?"

- A *Continuer*—someone who does more of the same but in a different way,
- An *Adventurer*—someone who engages in something entirely new,
- A *Searcher*—someone who is looking for a niche,
- An *Easy Glider*—someone who "goes with the flow,"
- An *Involved Spectator*—someone who cares and continues learning, but is no longer a key player in what is going on in his or her world, or
- A *Retreater*—someone who has given up.

Schlossberg highlights the need for older adults to get involved. She suggests that if something is troubling retirees, encourage them to check in with themselves. "Can I change what is going on?" If the answer is no, then ask, "Can I change the way I look at the situation?" "Can my stress be reduced through meditation, exercise, counseling, or some combination of the three?" As with people at all stages of life, the importance of *attitude* and the ability to use multiple coping strategies cannot be overemphasized. Involvement, buffered by a positive attitude, can help make retirement activities meaningful and worthwhile.

➤ CASE EXAMPLE **18.4** ACTIVE AT 92.

When I first met Pearl, I was astounded to learn that this 70ish-looking, vibrant, keenly intelligent woman was almost 90 years old. Now, at age 92, she has not slowed down a bit. I recently interviewed her to find out more about this active nonagenarian.

Pearl worked over 30 years as a nurse. For 25 of those years she was a nurse anesthetist. She retired in 1980, at the age of 60. Pearl said that she missed work initially—she missed her connections and attachments associated with the hospital. But she felt it was time to retire. Her energy level had lessened over the years, and she wanted to spend more time doing things she enjoyed, like gardening, sewing, and participating in lifelong learning classes.

One of the first things Pearl did after retiring was to enroll in a course, Learning in Retirement, that was offered at a local community college center. She remained in the course for three years, where she met retired people from all walks of life. They read and discussed classic literature, studied areas of interest that they had not pursued earlier, and formed selective deep friendships.

In 2001, Pearl and her husband separated. She moved across the country to be closer to her daughters and siblings. She now has lived in the southeastern United States for 11 years. Her life is rich—she participates in book clubs, volunteers, and attends classes at a community center called Adventures in Learning. She also spends time with family and recently moved to a retirement village to be close to her brother, whose health is failing. Although she misses living in her own home, she is very involved in the activities at the village, where she exercises, attends arts events, participates in singing groups, and attends Sunday vespers.

What does Pearl find most meaningful at this point in her life? She stated that spending time with friends, participating in a variety of activities, and visiting with her siblings and children are especially rewarding. I then asked her about challenges. She said that losing the freedom of living in her own home was a big challenge initially, but that she has adjusted. She recognizes the need to adapt to having less energy and is careful to avoid falls because her balance "isn't what it used to be." For Pearl, the joy of living far outweighs any challenges. "How life changes!" she said to me. "I am not bored. I choose to keep busy all the time. And I have a wonderful support system of friends and family. I feel blessed."

1. Who do you know that is currently retired? Interview one of these persons to find out his or her views about adjusting to retirement.
2. Does the government do enough to support its aging population? What will happen to people if Social Security funding runs out within the next two decades?
3. How do you envision yourself at the age of 65? Do you intend to continue working? If not, what plans are you making now to ensure that retirement will be feasible?
4. Use the Internet or other resources to discover the percentage of people who have sufficient financial means to retire at the age of 65. What percentage of individuals is dependent on Social Security, friends, relatives, or charity after they stop working? Discuss your findings and reactions.
5. What is age discrimination in the workplace? What regulations were put into place in 2006 to protect employees from age discrimination? Do you think these regulations are sufficient?

SECTION IV: Socioemotional Development in Later Life

Socioemotional Theories Related to Aging

Selective optimization with compensation theory (SOC) has been researched extensively by Margret Baltes (1996), Paul Baltes (1997), and their colleagues (e.g., Baltes & Dickson, 2001). The theory has generated much interest and has applications throughout the lifespan. In this section, the focus will be on the theory's application to later adulthood.

According to SOC, successful aging is linked with three primary factors: selection, optimization, and compensation. For many older adults, losses in certain areas, such as dexterity, certain memory functions, and other areas make it necessary for older adults to adapt. Adaptation may include searching for new goals, reconstructing goal hierarchies, and focusing on goals that are most meaningful (Baltes, 1997, p. 372). When performance is reduced in specific areas, older adults select what is most important to them, which may mean changing priorities. **Optimization** refers to the ways older adults optimize positive changes, thus finding ways to adapt toward a set of desirable outcomes (Baltes, 1997). **Compensation** takes place when life tasks require a level of ability beyond the individual's current level of ability. Older adults, in particular, may need to compensate in areas that may require sustained energy or focus, high physical demands, or quick reaction time (Santrock, 2012).

An oft-cited example of a well-known classical pianist who used *selection, optimization,* and *compensation* to maintain a high level of expert piano playing is Artur Rubinstein. This famous pianist (1897–1982) was asked how, at the age of 80, he was able to continue doing what he loved at such a high performance level. Rubinstein responded that he played fewer pieces (selection) and practiced those pieces more frequently (optimization). As a result of aging, Rubinstein no longer had the mechanical speed that had impressed audiences for so many years. To counteract the loss of speed, Rubinstein slowed his pace before playing fast sections, which made the latter sound faster to the audience (compensation) (Baltes, 1997).

Another well-known older adult who has successfully used selection, optimization, and compensation is Madonna Buder, a Roman Catholic religious sister who is also known as the Iron Nun (Buder & Evans, 2010). Buder began training for Ironman competitions at the age of 48, an age at which most people have already stopped competing in athletic events. She ran her first Ironman event when she was 55 years old and has been competing ever since. She was the oldest woman to complete the prestigious Ironman Triathlon in Hawaii, at the age of 75. A year later she again competed, finishing the grueling event a minute before the cut-off time of 17 hours.

In what way has the Iron Nun implemented SOC theory? At first glance, it appears that she began training at a later age, experienced the benefits of training, and was blessed with a body not afflicted by many of the physical challenges of aging. However, Sister Madonna exemplified *selection* by choosing to focus on exercise and training. She utilized *optimization* by training in a way that adapted for an aging body. She exhibited *compensation* by slowing down her pace, while still choosing to compete.

Certainly not every older adult (or younger adult!) is able to participate in the grueling training required to complete an Ironman triathlon. However, older adults who recognize the benefits of exercise may choose to walk or swim rather than run, participate in water aerobics, and partake in activities that are less strenuous, such as chair exercises or stretching exercises (U.S. Department of Health and Human Services, 2002).

There are many social and socioemotional theories of aging with varying degrees of empirical support. Rather than describe these theories in detail, they are presented in table format. When reviewing Table 18.1, examine the basic premises of the theory, think about which components of the theory have merit, and be prepared to discuss some of the weaknesses associated with each theory.

Think About It   18.3

1. Think of an older adult who has experienced cognitive decline. In what way has that individual used selection, optimization, and compensation in his or her life?
2. In what ways might SOC be used by someone with a chronic illness?
3. Which of the three socioemotional theories described in Table 18.1 seem most applicable to the development of older adults in today's society?

TABLE 18.1 ✦ ADDITIONAL EXAMPLES OF SOCIOEMOTIONAL THEORIES OF AGING

Name of Theory	General Premises	Weaknesses	Theorists and Dates
Disengagement theory	Views aging as a process of gradual withdrawal from society and relationships. Seniors become preoccupied with their inner lives and mortality.	No research support. Many older adults desire to remain occupied and involved with society. Theory largely discounted by gerontologists.	Cumming & Henry (1961)
Activity theory	Remaining active and engaged is paramount to successful aging. Activity may be physical or intellectual. Activity improves health and prosperity.	Not all aging persons can maintain active roles in society. Some elders may persist in continuing activities that pose danger to themselves or others, thus denying their limitations and engaging in unsafe behavior.	Havighurst et al. (1953)
Continuity theory	In making adaptive choices, older adults prefer to use strategies tied to past experiences and their social worlds. Older adults will usually maintain the same activities, behaviors, personalities, and relationships that defined their earlier experiences.	Definition of "normal aging" based on males, not females. Older adults with chronic illnesses are not addressed. The theory does not demonstrate how social institutions affect individuals as they age.	Maddox (1968); Atchley (1989)

Stability and Change of Personality

To what degree does aging influence individual personality traits? In general, personality traits are relatively stable in adults (Roberts, Wood, & Caspi, 2008). However, defining the term *personality* is not a simple task. External and internal events can shape certain personality traits across the life course. Developmental researchers and gerontologists have researched the effects of aging, life events, stress, physical health, and other factors on personality (e.g., Costa, Terraciano, & McCrae, 2001; Roberts & DelVecchio, 2000; Specht, Egloff, & Schmukle, 2011). In this section, personality research is summarized and influences are discussed that may contribute to overall life satisfaction and well-being.

The Big Five personality domains—extraversion, agreeableness, conscientiousness, neuroticism, and openness to experience—have been the focus of recent research on personality. Noftle and Fleeson (2010) found that several of the Big Five factors continued to change in late adulthood. In particular, aspects of conscientiousness and agreeableness tend to increase as adults age (Santrock, 2011). The constructs (or facets) of conscientiousness most likely to change include impulse control, reliability, and conventionality. Furthermore, older adults tend to score lower on measures of neuroticism than their younger counterparts. Finally, some (but not all) adults become more extraverted as they age.

Are there gender differences in the **Five Factor Model (FFM)** for older adults? Costa et al. (2001) reported that women in general score higher than men on the traits of neuroticism and agreeableness, but there were few differences in aggregate measures of extraversion, openness, and conscientiousness. Biological and sociocultural influences may explain some of these differences.

Chapman, Duberstein, Sörensen, and Lyness (2007) assessed differences between genders in a sample of older adults ranging in age from 65 to 98. They also found that women scored higher on measures of neuroticism and agreeableness, indicating that these latent traits increased more for older women than for older men.

Although these findings are important, perhaps even more important is the stability and multifaceted nature of older adults' self-concept (Berk, 2010). Adults whose autobiographical selves emphasize consistency and coherence in spite of physical, cognitive, and occupational changes tend to possess a higher level of psychological well-being and life satisfaction. Seniors who continue to set goals and take steps to attain them also tend to be more satisfied with life.

Adversity, Resilience, and Aging

How do adults weather adversity as they age? To an extent, the manner in which they have managed adverse circumstances in the past is a predictor of the way they handle hardships in later adulthood. In the previous section, personality traits were described; some traits tend to remain stable, whereas other traits are susceptible to change. Other factors, including coping skills, managing stress, the nature and number of negative life events faced during older adulthood, health, social networks, and community resources also play large roles in the various ways aging individuals respond to adversity. In this section, adversity is discussed as it relates to later adulthood, and factors are described that seem to make some adults more resilient and others more vulnerable to adverse events.

➤ CASE EXAMPLE **18.5**   THE CASE OF JANICE.

Janice, an 85-year-old widow, has dealt with numerous challenging life events. Her husband of 40 years died of pancreatic cancer 10 years ago. Macular degeneration has made it difficult for her to read and to get around the way she did in the past. Two years ago, she realized that it was no longer safe to drive. With the encouragement of her three children, she sold the family car and quit driving. She has arthritis in her hips and lower back, which make it difficult to walk and sit pain-free.

For many aging adults, these situations are not unusual. Negative life events often accumulate, age-related health concerns become issues, and family changes are more the norm than not. The ways older adults respond to the life challenges that come with aging differ. Resilience, which we discuss later in this section, is a key factor in adapting to adversity.

For Janice, although faced with many challenges, resilience has enabled her to continue aging successfully. Some of the factors that helped attenuate the negative impact of adversity included an adaptive and solution-driven coping system, an integrated sense of self, her faith, and her social support system, which included family, friends, and her church community.

Adversity

Adversity, as it applies to aging adults, includes limitations imposed by health conditions, both acute and chronic. It also includes daily and chronic stressors, changing life circumstances, financial difficulties, and the loss of a life partner, friend, or loved one. Being forced to retire, no longer being able to drive, and cognitive decline also fit into the broad category of adversity (Hildon, Montgomery, Blane, Wiggins, & Netuveli, 2009). Adversity represents change and risk, and while everyone experiences adversity in some form, by the time one reaches later adulthood, the number of adverse experiences tends to increase. According to Hildon, Smith, Netuveli, and Blane (2008), adversity can be understood "either in terms of disruptions to expected life trajectories or changes in the structure of people's lives" (p. 737).

Resilience

Traditionally, research on resilience has focused on children and adolescents who are able to succeed in spite of facing adverse circumstances (Masten, 2001). More recently, however, attention has been directed toward resilience as it relates to older adults (Hildon et al., 2008; Ong & Bergeman, 2004). **Resilience** has been defined as an ability to "bounce back" (Ong & Bergeman, 2004). It is multidimensional in that it is both a trait and a process. Furthermore, resilience may be demonstrated in one domain in an adult's life but not in another (Hildon et al., 2009). Some of the dimensions associated with resilience include:

- Personality factors, including openness to change, agreeableness, and extraversion
- Optimism
- Adaptive and solution-focused coping skills (as opposed to avoidance)
- Religiosity/spirituality
- A sense of personal control
- Quantity and quality of social relationships, including family and friends
- Community resources
- Acceptance of change
- Cultural influences
- Humor

Older adults who are more resilient than their counterparts tend to experience higher levels of personal health, subjective well-being, and life satisfaction (Hildon et al., 2009; Mathieu, 2008; Ong & Bergeman, 2004).

In contrast, some older adults are more vulnerable and thus may be less likely to experience life satisfaction. Complicated (pathological) grief, compounded adverse events, a perceived loss of control, financial distress, and loneliness can result in a host of problematic psychological difficulties. In particular, a cascade of negative events and/or insufficient social capital can lead to a sense of isolation and despair (Hildon et al., 2008; Shallcross, 2009). Counselors need to be aware of the factors related to resilience and vulnerability and be knowledgeable about ways to work effectively to help older adults who are experiencing adversity. Interventions that provide elders with a safe space to focus on the full range of emotions and interventions that contribute to feelings of mastery and control are particularly important (Ong & Bergeman, 2004).

One of the most devastating events an adult can experience is the loss of a partner or spouse (Bonanno, 2004). Finding ways to restructure one's life after such a loss can be especially challenging. Although people respond in different ways, resilience can help older adults who have experienced the death of their loved one attenuate their ongoing grief as the individual adapts to a new way of living.

REFLECTION 18.4 ONE RESILIENT MOTHER!

My 80-year-old mother was widowed two days before her 65th birthday. My father, who was a 64-year-old Baptist minister at the time, was diagnosed with cancer in February of 1996. In three months, after undergoing chemotherapy and radiation, my father died. I was heartbroken. My mother was devastated, angry, and lost. Her soul mate of almost 40 years had been taken from her unexpectedly, and within a short two-month period her world was forever changed. My sister and I, both in our mid-30s, wondered how on Earth we would be able to meet the needs of my mother, who had depended on my father for a myriad of things.

Early on, my mother realized that she didn't know how to pump gas into her car. That was something "J.L. had always done." Full-service gas stations were becoming a thing of the past and learning to put gas into her vehicle was a necessity. Such an act seems trivial, but it was of vital importance to her ability to function independently.

One of my mother's strongest qualities is her determination. The gas-pumping issue was resolved quickly. Less quickly resolved were issues related to caring for a relatively large home, handling yard work, and developing a new social network when her "couple friends" drifted away. Although it took time, she learned to live independently, hire people to handle the yard work, and reestablish friendships with others who were single.

One of Mother's greatest regrets—outside the obvious, which was losing her husband— was the fact that she and my father never got to enjoy the plans they had made for retirement. My mother had been forced to retire early due to health issues. However, my father had planned to continue pastoring our church for a few more years. After retirement, he and Mother had many plans: go to Hawaii, lead marriage workshops, visit friends in other states, and enjoy leisure time together.

When I talked to my mother recently—some 15 years since my father's untimely death— she indicated that she still missed what they never had the opportunity to do. Men and women plan, but God's plans don't always comply. I can say that my children, my mother's new set of friends, her volunteer work with those who are sick or grieving, and her willingness to figure out new ways of living have all contributed to her overall sense of well-being, in spite of needing to help my sister financially after she was diagnosed with multiple sclerosis. Would life be better had my father lived? Undoubtedly so! However, Mother's resilience has contributed to a life that is meaningful and complete—a life that matters. No one knows what the future holds, but her belief in who holds the future is a constant source of sustenance. [~DWN]

Think About It 18.4

1. Do you think the Big Five Factor theory of personality sufficiently covers the aspects of personality that are most salient in older adults? Explain.
2. Is having a positive attitude always the best way to deal with adversity? Explain.
3. Can resilience be learned, or is a person born with a "hardy" or "vulnerable" personality? In what way does an older adult's environment influence what is perceived as resilience?
4. Think of an older adult you know who appears to be especially resilient. What do you think contributes to that resilience?

REFLECTION 18.5 PATSY'S FAITH AND STRENGTH

Patsy, aged 75, has been affiliated with a local Protestant church all of her life. Even though she has emphysema, carries an oxygen tank, and has battled cancer for several years, she is an active member of her congregation. She spends a significant amount of time working in her church's nursery, a role she has embraced for over two decades. Her devotion to God and her commitment to people in need have become even more evident as she ages. In spite of diminishing physical capacities, she continues to dedicate herself to service and draws strength from her spiritual beliefs and religious participation. [~DWN]

Spirituality, Religion, and Aging

How do spirituality and religiosity affect the well-being of seniors? As adults age, many develop a more mature sense of spirituality (Berk, 2010; Fowler, 1981). According to Fowler (1981), some adults who have achieved midlife and beyond are in the universalizing faith stage. Fowler suggests that people in this stage are more altruistic, with many elders being devoted to overcoming division, oppression, and violence. During this final development of faith, individuals may focus on connecting with others, finding meaning and purpose in life, and using personal power to influence outcomes [Navigating the Aging Process (NAP), 2012]. Fowler gives examples of Mother Teresa, Gandhi, and others who exemplified this type of spiritual commitment. Although it would be inaccurate to state that all (or even most) older adults commit themselves to causes like those mentioned above, many older adults do find a sense of meaning and purpose through spiritual and religious involvement.

Terminology

Distinguishing between **spirituality** and **religion** (or religiosity) is not an easy task. The Association for Spiritual, Ethical, and Religious Values in Counseling (ASERVIC), a division of the American Counseling Association, conducted a Summit on Spirituality in 1995. During the Summit, a description of spiritualty was generated:

> [Spirituality is a] capacity and tendency that is innate and unique to all persons. The spiritual tendency moves the individual toward knowledge, love, meaning, peace, hope, transcendence, connectedness, compassion, wellness, and wholeness. Spirituality includes one's capacity for creativity, growth, and the development of a values system. (ASERVIC, 1995, p. 30)

Religion has been defined in multiple ways as well. It can be referred to as the social or organized means by which a person expresses spirituality (Burke, Chauvin, & Miranti, 2005). Religiosity is often conceptualized as having more organizational and behavioral components, whereas spirituality is considered to be oriented around personal experiences that may be transcendent in nature (Jackson & Bergeman, 2011). For many people, both older and younger, religious organizations, rituals, and collective worship provide a means through which spirituality can be outwardly expressed.

Positive Effects of Spirituality and Religious Involvement

In general, adults who are committed to their religious faith and spiritual convictions tend to be happier, healthier, have more coping resources, and experience more perceived control than those for whom religion and spirituality are less important (e.g., Ellison & Fan, 2008; Fiori, Brown, Cortina, & Antonucci, 2006; Jackson & Bergeman, 2011). In later

REFLECTION 18.6 LOUISE'S RELIGIOUS CONVOY!

Louise, an elderly African-American woman, had been an active member of the Willow Creek Baptist Church for over 65 years. She led Bible studies, sang in the choir, cooked meals for Wednesday night suppers, and volunteered in the after-school program her church hosted. When Louise turned 85, she realized that she could no longer drive to services. Worship and church involvement were central to her life. Fortunately, the church provided a transportation service, and Louise was able to remain an engaged, vital member of her congregation until she died at the age of 90. Her faith and her "religious convoy" of support contributed greatly to her overall well-being and ego integrity during the final stage of her life. [~DWN]

adulthood, it is possible that connections with a religious community contribute to involvement in social and community activity as well as to increased generativity. Formal and informal religious involvement is especially high among ethnic minority elders. For example, in African-American communities, churches often are centers for education, social welfare, and social justice, and elders typically are held in high esteem (Berk, 2010).

Well-being related to spirituality expresses itself in personal growth, involvement in creative life tasks, and wisdom (Wink & Dillon, 2003). Other positive effects associated with religious and spiritual beliefs include lower levels of stress and loneliness, less depression, higher self-esteem, and greater psychosocial competence (Hill & Pargament, 2003). For many older adults, spiritual well-being can provide a buffer against end-of-life despair, suicidal ideation, and hopelessness in the face of a terminal illness (Okon, 2005).

> Even when a person can no longer be cured in his body, he can be healed in his soul. (Bogins, 2000, p. 55)

Do Religious and Spiritual Beliefs Change with Age?

The role of religious and spiritual beliefs and practices in later adulthood does not present a uniform picture. However, many people are able to draw on their spiritual beliefs as a way of maintaining a sense of ego integrity and purpose (Lyon, 2004). Spirituality and religiosity do not necessarily increase with age. Research results on the topic are mixed (Moberg & Binstock, 2001). Even so, many adults do mature spiritually as they age. There are many possible explanations for this phenomenon. One is associated with the fact that older adults are almost always somewhere in the grief process. Their experiences are dominated by losses: loss of loved ones, loss of physical abilities, and often loss of income. The accumulation of these losses, combined with an awareness of their own mortality, may lead to a greater exploration of spiritual issues (NAP, 2012).

Earlier in the chapter, Erikson and Erikson's theory of gerotranscendence was introduced. Gerotranscendence is a process that occurs when older adults shift their focus to a more cosmic and transcendent view of the world (Thornstam, 1997). Through this process, seniors are more likely to consider the spiritual dimension of their lives and the mysteries of life and death. Gerotranscendence, which is spiritual in nature and occurs later in life, is marked by a decrease in self-centeredness and an increase in life satisfaction (Lyon, 2004).

Whereas spirituality may become a stronger factor for many adults as they age, religiousness remains relatively stable throughout the adult years (Wink & Dillon, 2003). Religious practices established in early adulthood tend to carry on through later adulthood, although health and transportation difficulties may impede some older adults' participation in organized religious activities (Berk, 2010). In a study carried out by the Pew Forum (2010), researchers compared religious practices of young people (i.e., the Millennial generation) with those of older adults. Older adults were more likely to affiliate with religious tradition and to engage in religious services, scripture reading, prayer, and meditation. In making this observation, it is important to remember that different generations were compared (i.e., a cross-sectional design), which differs greatly from researching the religious practices of a single generation longitudinally. In another study by the Pew Research Center Organization (2009), which focused on older adults only, 34% of seniors said that religion had grown more important to them over the course of their lives. Four percent stated that it had become less important, and the majority of older adults (60%) said that it had remained the same.

Although the effects of spirituality and religiosity clearly differ from individual to individual, adults appear to mature spiritually as they age. While they are different terms that have overlapping meanings, both religiosity and spirituality contribute to general well-being and life satisfaction. There is still much to be learned about the beneficial effects of spirituality and religiosity in later life (Jackson & Bergeman, 2011); even so, the positive effects of resilience, continued personal growth, altruism, and social connectivity serve as buffers against the cascade of losses that accompany increased aging.

Think About It   18.5

- In what ways are spirituality and religiosity similar? How are they different?
- What are some of the positive effects associated with religiosity and spirituality?
- Think of some of the older adults you know well. Do they talk much about their faith? Do you see differences between older adults who do not consider themselves religious or spiritual and older adults who do?
- Why do you think that the statistics contrasting a sample of the Millennial generation with older adults differ so much?
- Ask someone from your parents' and grandparents' generations about their definition of "old." How do those definitions differ from your own ideas about aging?
- At what age should a person be eligible to receive Social Security or Medicare? Explain.
- If you could live to be as old as you wanted, how old would that be? Under what conditions?
- Imagine that you are asked to interview a supercentenarian. What are the first three questions you would ask?
- Do you think there should be an age limit on aggressive medical treatment—for example, undergoing major surgery?
- Visit http://www.kaiseredu.org/Issue-Modules/US-Health-Care-Costs/Background-Brief.aspx. Health care costs have increased substantially, making up almost 18% of the nation's gross domestic product (GDP) in 2010. Medicare costs contributed significantly to the ever-increasing bill. What would you do to make this massive bill more equitable?
- Do you think that you will live to be 100 years or older? Go to http://www.bumc.bu.edu/centenarian/the-living-to-100-life-expectancy-calculator/ and check it out. What factors do you think centenarians have in common?

Summary

The degree to which people are involved in social relationships in later adulthood is largely dependent on their social networks and support systems. Topics such as sexual relations (yes, older adults do engage in sexual activity), marriage, divorce, remarriage, widowhood, and relations with children, grandchildren, and siblings were discussed. Other important social relationships include friendships, which may be particularly poignant during older adulthood, particularly when friends outlive one another. LGBT relationships are not always viewed positively by society. However, older adults are as diverse in their sexual orientations, attitudes, and behaviors as younger individuals. Counselors can be instrumental in advocating for the rights and privileges deserved by this population. They also can be instrumental in taking action to reduce ageism and elder abuse.

Psychosocial theories of development help explain some of the ways older adults develop and change as they age, but not all adults experience these developmental changes in the same way. Also, it is important to keep in mind that later adulthood can encompass a span of almost four decades. Attempting to generalize across decades would be both inaccurate and unhelpful. With that in mind, some of the key developmental theorists who have addressed later adulthood include Erikson, Peck, Fisher, and Labouvie-Vief. Knowledge about key concepts associated with the related theories is essential for counselors working with older adults.

Retirement is a topic that has particular pertinence for older adults. Many factors figure into the decision about when an adult retires from paid work. Some of those factors are voluntary and others are involuntary (e.g., being laid off). The circumstances surrounding retirement strongly affect the manner in which men and women adjust to retirement. According to many gerontologists, older adults who adjust best to retirement are healthy, active, educated, and financially stable. They have strong support networks and were satisfied with their lives before retirement. Adults who are financially stressed, have health issues, and have poor support systems are less likely to adjust well. Schlossberg's transition theory helps explain the various facets of adjustment that face people going through any major change. Understanding transition theory as it relates to older adults can help you work more effectively with adults approaching retirement. Many adults find that retirement provides new opportunities to participate in leisure and volunteer activities that are meaningful and fulfilling.

Other topics covered in this chapter included socioemotional theories related to aging, personality stability and change, adversity and resilience, and spirituality and religion. As you review those topics, consider how the information included in each section will affect your interactions with the increasingly growing population of older adults. Working with older adults can be both challenging and rewarding, and counselors must continue to stay abreast of developing topics related to later adulthood.

Glossary

abnormality Behavior that is deviant from the norm, distressing, dysfunctional, or potentially dangerous to the individual or others.

abusive head trauma Updated term for *shaken baby syndrome*, including other abusive head injuries inflicted on an infant or toddler, such as with a blunt object.

accommodation Addition of new information that may require that more sophisticated cognitive structures be formed and organized.

acquiring a taste for food In infancy, the early experiences with flavors shape which foods will later be preferred.

active development The view that children actively construct their own worlds and initiate their own growth.

active genotype–environment correlations The view that the child seeks out environments consistent with his genetic makeup and thereby creates his own environment, which then strengthens his inherent qualities.

acute illness Conditions that develop quickly but are usually temporary.

adaptation Process by which the human mind constructs knowledge (Piaget, 1970).

adaptation of life theory Vaillant's theory of development, in which developmental stages do not follow a strict age-related sequence; according to Vaillant, adult development follows this sequence: intimacy, career consolidation (early adulthood), generativity, keeper of meaning (middle adulthood), and ego integrity (late adulthood).

adjustment disorder A disorder in which children's reactions to change are more extreme than might be expected in a normal child.

adolescence The period from about 12 to 19 years of age, during which children experience substantial changes, including puberty, the capacity to think abstractly, and the search for identity.

adult attachment styles Unique patterns of thinking, feeling, and behaving in intimate relationships; influenced by early attachment experiences with caregivers.

affect complexity Complex and cognitively demanding strategy that helps individuals gain insight from emotions, maintain relative objectivity, form a distinct and historically situated sense of self, and realistically blend positive and negative emotions.

affect optimization Process through which older adults cognitively maximize positive emotions and dampen negative emotions, enabling them to maintain positive emotions and psychological well-being in the face of major stressors.

affectionate love The type of love you feel for a close friend or family member (also referred to as companionate love).

age cohort Group of people born within a certain period of time, set apart from earlier or later generations.

ageism Prejudice and discrimination directed against older adults.

amblyopia "Lazy eye," a visual disorder that only children can develop, but that is preventable and treatable.

American Sign Language An organized system for communicating with gestures, widely used among the hearing impaired.

amniocentesis Extraction of amniotic fluid from the mother during the second trimester to examine the cells of the fetus.

amniotic sac Tissue that encloses the embryo, except where the *umbilical cord* passes through to the placenta; contains amniotic fluid, which protects the embryo from being injured by internal pressures and bumps.

amodal information Sensory information that is not tied to a specific sensory system.

amygdala Two almond-sized and -shaped structures, one on each side of the brain near the side of the head; receives information from the senses directly and activates a response before the neocortex has a chance to fully recognize the sensory input.

anabolism The process by which one's body builds up to peak biological performance.

anal stage According to Freud, the stage from 18 months to 3 years, centered on pleasure received from controlling one's excretory functions.

anemia Lack of sufficient iron in the bloodstream.

anger Emotion in which the brain directs more blood flow to the hands, preparing the person to defend against the strike of an opponent.

animism The tendency of children to believe that inanimate objects have the characteristics and feelings of living things.

anoxia Condition in which a fetus is cut off from oxygen supply.

anorexia nervosa Self-starvation, potentially life-threatening; more prevalent in girls than in boys, but increasing in males.

anxious-ambivalent attachment Condition in which a child is preoccupied with the parent throughout the strange situation procedure; the child demonstrates little exploration and is wary of the stranger.

anxious-avoidant attachment Condition in which a child does not cry at separation from the parent but rather continues to play; when the parent returns, the infant actively avoids and ignores the parent but does not resist the mother's efforts at contact.

Apgar test Test given to an infant one minute after they are born and again five minutes later to assess how well the infant is adapting to their environment.

approach Behavior in which one moves toward an object or person.

approach-approach conflict Situations where one has to choose between two desirable things.

approach-avoidance conflict Occurs when the same behavior produces feelings of approach and avoidance.

acquaintance rape Includes rapes in which the victim and perpetrator have been in some sort of relationship, for example, as coworkers or neighbors. See *date rape.*

artificial insemination (AI) Procedure in which sperm is injected into the uterus.

artificialism The belief that natural phenomena such as rain or sunrise are caused by people.

asphyxia Choking; in newborns, asphyxia may result from an entangled umbilical cord, maternal medicine interfering with breathing, or the baby being in a *breech presentation.*

assimilate To take in new information, fitting it into the already existing cognitive structures.

assistive reproductive technology (ART) Technological means of achieving fertilization, including *artificial insemination* and *in vitro* fertilization.

atherosclerosis A buildup of plaque inside the coronary arteries, which supply blood to the heart muscle.

attachment Emotional connection with important people in one's life.

attention-deficit/hyperactivity disorder A disorder characterized by executive functioning deficits affecting inhibition, paying attention, rule following, self-directed speech, motivation, and self-awareness.

attention-seeking Actions of a child who believes she matters only if she is being noticed, and therefore engages in behavior that will draw the attention of the adult.

attention switching The ability to switch between two tasks simultaneously, such as reading a book and listening to the radio (*divided attention*).

attribute substitution Process in peer relations in which children imitate behaviors and other characteristics they see in others.

attribution styles How individuals cognitively appraise an event.

attrition (mortality) A potential problem with longitudinal studies; the possibility that researchers may lose participants due to death, relocation, or a loss of interest in a long-term undertaking.

attunement The process cultivated by a nurturing, responsive parent in the journey toward building an attachment bond with the infant (Stern, 1987).

authoritarian parents Parents who are demanding, actively attempting to shape and control a child's behavior.

authoritative parents Parents who provide structure and direction to the child while still allowing a significant amount of freedom and room for exploration and self-expression.

automatization The process whereby, as patterns of thought and behavior are repeated, the neural connections involved are strengthened and less effort is required.

autonomous morality According to Piaget, the period from around 8 to 12 years of age when children learn that the rules are set by society, including their peers, in a cooperative fashion.

autonomy The ability of research participants to make their own well-informed decisions.

autonomy vs. shame and doubt Erikson's second stage of development; from about ages 1 to 3 years, children need to explore the world and experiment.

autosomal disorders Chromosomal disorders that involve anomalies on any of the chromosomal pairs other than the sex-determining chromosome.

average life expectancy Statistical measure of the average number of years a person born in a given country and of a given age would be expected to live.

avoidance-avoidance conflict Occurs when one is forced to choose between two equally undesirable options.

axon Tube-like part of a neuron that allows signals to be passed from one neuron to another.

Babinski reflex Extension and/or flexion of a newborn's toes when the bottom of the foot is stroked.

Baby Boomers Age cohort of Americans who were born between 1944 and 1964.

baby teeth First set of teeth that erupt in an infant; also called primary teeth or deciduous teeth.

Back to Sleep Campaign AAP program to help parents adopt practices that have correlated with a reduction in SIDS.

Bayley-III Most recent version of the Bayley Scales of Infant Development, consisting of three sections for the infant: Cognitive Scale, Language Scale, and Motor Scale.

behaviorist One who adheres to the theory psychology can be accurately studied through examination of objectively observable and quantifiable behavioral events.

beneficence Ethical principle of promoting the welfare of those involved.

bereavement Sadness resulting from the recent death of a family member or friend.

binge drinking Defined as having five or more drinks in a row on at least one day in the past month.

biological aging Changes in how the human body functions across the lifespan.

biological essentialism Concept used by Bem to describe the tendency to ground gender differences in biology, thus becoming natural, normal, and necessary.

biracial Descriptor of a person conceived by people of different races.

biracial identity development model Model that attempts to address some of the complexities associated with being biracial (Poston, 1990).

birth order A major facet of the family constellation; research reveals support for the existence of distinctive birth order characteristics.

Black racial identity development Model of development toward social and political commitment against singular or multiple forms of oppression (Cross, 1971, 1995).

blink reflex In infants, an automatic response used in situations that warrant protection for the eyes.

Bobo doll An experiment that examined the effects of models of aggression on preschool children's aggressive behavior (Bandura, Ross, and Ross, 1961).

body fat Percentage of fat tissue in the body; in infants, roughly 13% body fat at birth, increasing to 20–25% body fat by the first birthday.

body transcendence vs. body preoccupation According to Peck, the second developmental task in older people, who must learn to cope with and move beyond changes in physical capabilities that accompany the aging process.

brain lateralization Refers to the fact that the two halves of the human brain house different functions.

breech presentation Condition in which a newborn presents feet first.

bridge job Job serving as a transition between full-time work and retirement following a full-time career.

caloric restriction effect The idea that limiting calories extends lifespan (also known as the dietary restriction theory).

canalization The process by which, for some traits, humans are restricted to a small number of outcomes simply as a function of their genes.

cardiovascular system Body system involving organs that provide the body with blood, oxygen, and nutrients.

care perspective Having concern for those in need, being mindful of relationships.

career interests Preferences that individuals have for particular life activities (e.g., writing, working on cars, solving math problems).

case study An open-ended, in-depth examination of a "unit," such as a single individual, family, or small group.

catabolism Following the attainment of peak potential, the process by which the human body inevitably begins to slowly deteriorate.

cataracts Condition in which the normally clear optic lens becomes progressively cloudier, affecting the quality of light filtering into the retina; can be surgically corrected or repaired with a laser.

cathexis A term that psychoanalysts have used to mean attachment.

centenarians People who are alive and at least 100 years of age.

cesarean section (C-section) Cutting an opening in the mother's stomach to remove the newborn.

chemosensory Relating to taste and smell.

choice theory Glasser's (1998) theory that all humans are born with five basic needs that they continually seek to fulfill: survival, love/belonging, power, fun/learning, and freedom.

chronic illness A condition that has developed over time, and is typically persistent and not completely cured.

chronosystem The changes experienced by a child throughout development and the historical and social events of the time.

chunking In information processing, grouping associated items, thereby making one item out of several.

class inclusion The ability to perceive part-to-whole relationships and to distinguish categories and subcategories.

classical conditioning Process of behavior modification in which an innate response to a biological stimulus is expressed in response to a previously neutral stimulus.

climacteric The end of the ability of the *reproductive system* to function, generally occurring in middle adulthood.

clique Peer group (perhaps 6–10) whose members adopt the mannerisms of the group and socialize more or less exclusively with its members.

cluster Randomly positioned neurons in the brain that have physically moved to a distinct place in the brain.

coaching Intervention technique involving three-step process: (1) providing the child with specific instruction in how to perform certain social skills, (2) giving the opportunity to rehearse the skills, and (3) providing with feedback regarding success in using those skills.

cognitive-affective complexity The capacity to integrate one's emotions and pragmatic reasoning when solving problems and making decisions.

cohabitation Living with a sexual partner outside of marriage

cohesion How close or distant family members feel themselves to be.

cohort effects In research studies, effects that occur when observed differences may be due to shared experiences rather than maturation.

cohort-sequential studies See *time-lag designs*.

collectivistic worldview Cultural values that emphasize the centrality of the family and broader groupings, as opposed to individualism and independence.

commitment in relativism developed Third phase of Perry's (1970) theory of development, in which one commits to a set of chosen values and beliefs without knowing, definitively, if they are *right* or *true*.

compensation Adaptation when life tasks require a level of ability beyond the individual's current level of ability; older adults, in particular, may need to compensate in areas that may require sustained energy or focus, high physical demands, or quick reaction time.

comprehension The ability to understand language.

compression of morbidity The way chronic illness seems to be highly concentrated in the last years of life.

conception The merger of two haploid cells (i.e., sperm and egg) to become a single zygote cell with the full complement of 23 pairs of chromosomes.

conceptual knowledge Knowing why—understanding why something is the way it is.

concrete operations As described by Piaget, the stage from approximately age 7 through 11, during which children become able to reason and to use logic to solve problems about the concrete elements of the world around them.

conditioned response (CR) Learned response to a previously neutral stimulus.

conditioned stimulus (CS) Previously neutral stimulus that, after becoming associated with an unconditioned stimulus, eventually comes to trigger a conditioned response.

conduct disorder A disorder in hildren characterized by a general disregard for the basic rules and norms of society and, more specifically, aggression against people and animals, destruction of property, deceitfulness and theft, and serious violations of rules.

conjunctive faith Stage of faith in which one has developed personal beliefs about spirituality that are not based solely on what one has been told throughout life.

connectedness Having relationships of quality with other people in a social circle of family, friends, and acquaintances.

consonance See *goodness of fit.*

conservation The understanding that an object maintains its basic properties even if some attribute of the object changes.

consummate love According to Sternberg, the most complete form of love; occurs when all three dimensions of love—passion, intimacy, and commitment—exist in a relationship.

continuous In terms of development, the view that developmental change is continually occurring at a gradual, steady pace.

conventional level Stage of moral development in which children see rules and expectations as good; focus is on social relationships as well as compliance with social norms.

convergent production Deriving a single, correct answer to an objective question.

coping Any way in which one handles stress.

coping strategies Strategies and postures people use to protect themselves and provide safety from anxiety.

co-sleeping The practice of children and parents sharing a bed.

critical periods Certain limited periods of time when humans have the maximum opportunity for optimal development given appropriate environmental inputs.

cross-cultural research Studies conducted in order to illuminate differences and similarities among various people of diverse cultures.

cross-sectional designs Studies in which researchers measure individuals of different ages at a single point in time.

crowd Influential peer groups larger than cliques; may carry various labels, such as popular, jock, dirt head, druggie.

crystallization Process in which adolescents begin to develop ideas about careers based on their ideas about their interests and talents.

crystallized intelligence The breadth of knowledge acquired through formal education and life experiences in a particular culture; the ability to use the specific skills, knowledge, and experiences gained throughout a lifetime.

culture The entire worldview of a group of people, including their beliefs, values, attitudes, language, and knowledge.

cultural differences Variations across cultures with respect to, e.g., country of origin, race, ethnicity, sexual orientation, religion, gender identity, socioeconomic status, and disability status.

cyclical/repetitive Used to describe the normal human developmental process, with loss and gain inextricably linked, loss always bringing some sort of gain and gain always bringing some sort of loss.

cytoplasm Cellular fluid.

date rape A form of *acquaintance rape* in which there has been some sort of potentially romantic or sexual relationship between the two parties.

day care Institutionalized, fee-based child care outside the home, as when parents are working.

debriefing Explanation of the purpose of a study purpose at the end of the study; necessary in all studies, but especially important in studies where deception is used.

decentration The ability to focus on more than one dimension at a time.

deception Sometimes required when the potential benefits of a study outweigh the risks and there is no alternative way to achieve the desired results.

declarative knowledge Factual knowledge that the individual has learned, such as when the Civil War ended.

defense mechanisms Strategies people employ to protect themselves from unwanted anxiety, experiences, or pain.

deferred imitation The ability to remember an action performed by someone else and later reenact it.

deoxyribonucleic acid (DNA) Molecules that are the carrier of genetic information, made up of four bases: adenine (A), thymine (T), guanine (G), and cytosine (C).

depression Intense sadness, that may include multiple cognitive, emotive, and behavioral symptoms including pessimism, hopelessness, loss of interest in usual activities, lack of motivation, loss of concentration, difficulty making decisions, apathy, changes in eating and sleeping patterns, lethargy or listlessness, diminished self-esteem, and feelings of worthlessness.

despair Reaction to parental separation characterized by increasing hopelessness that the parent would return.

detachment Reaction to parental separation characterized by withdrawal from interacting with the environment.

developmental niche model The Super and Harkness (1994) model, which places increased emphasis on the overarching effects of culture on all of the systems influencing child development.

developmental quotient (DQ) Score yielded by development tests given to infants and toddlers.

developmental tasks Problems and life adjustments that individuals must accomplish; successful resolution of these tasks results in happiness and success, while unsuccessful resolution can lead to unhappiness and difficulty with future tasks.

differentiation of self A process that includes separating oneself from one's family of origin and distinguishing one's emotions from one's cognitions.

diploid state Having the full complement of 23 pairs of chromosomes.

discontinuous In terms of development, the view that children go through relatively stable periods of development that culminate in abrupt transformations as they transition to the next stage of functioning.

discriminative touch Sensations of touch, pressure, and vibration; allows one to perceive a stuffed animal in the dark that he can feel but not see.

disequilibrium Feeling of unbalance signaling the need to accommodate something new into existing schemas.

disgust Emotion that produces a curling of the upper lip to the side while wrinkling the nose simultaneously, which closes the nostrils against an offensive odor and allows the person to spit out a poisonous food.

disorganized-disoriented attachment Condition in which a child appears confused and displays contradictory behaviors in the presence of the parent.

dissonance "Poorness of fit," a mismatch between an organism's capabilities and characteristics and the environment's opportunities and demands.

divergent production The ability to generate multiple solutions to a question or problem, to draw on ideas from multiple disciplines and sources of knowledge to create one's own solutions to open-ended problems.

divided attention See *attention switching*.

diving reflex Demonstrated by an infant immersed in a pool of water holding his breath and opening his eyes, allowing him to block off his airway and protect himself from inhaling water or other noxious substances.

dizygotic twins Twins who began as two eggs, each fertilized separately by different sperm cells (*fraternal twins*).

dominant genes Genes that are generally expressed in a phenotype and thus can be observed.

double approach-avoidance conflict Occurs when one is faced with two choices that have both desirable and undesirable aspects.

double-track career pattern Career track, particularly among women, who may establish a career and take on a second career as a homemaker, raising children while working full time (also called double career).

Down syndrome Chromosomal disorder caused by an extra 21st chromosome, which results in cognitive delays and physical abnormalities seen in the facial region.

dual-career household One in which both partners have individual careers that are not sacrificed by the other or by the family.

dualism Polarized thinking (e.g., good or bad, right or wrong) and the existence of absolute truth.

dualism modified The first phase of Perry's (1970) theory of development, also called dualism and multiplicity; involves recognition that there are differences of opinion and uncertainties among authority figures.

dynamic systems perspective Viewpoint in which each new motor skill that the baby masters is influenced by both the baby and her environment.

dysfunctional Abnormal thoughts, behaviors, or emotions that are so distracting that the individual can no longer go about everyday activities appropriately or productively.

dysthymic disorder A disorder characterized by people having little or no joy in their lives, but instead being rather gloomy most of the time.

early childhood The period from 3 to about 6 years of age, during which children further refine their gross and fine motor skills and make gains in independence, self-control, language, and memory.

Early Head Start Offshoot of Head Start program that provides interventions in the form of child development and family support services.

Early Intervention Program For infants and toddlers through age 2 who have special needs, program available to help children be ready to attend preschool and kindergarten.

early-onset antisocial behavior Deviant behavior beginning by age 11, a serious manifestation that generally leads to chronic delinquency.

ecological model of child development The view that the developing child is continually influenced by the systems within which the child is embedded.

ego According to Freud, that part of a person's unconscious mind that is governed by reality and logic (the *reality principle*).

ego development Loevinger's term for development through stage she labeled (1) presocial, (2) impulsive, (3) self-protective, (4) conformist, (5) self-aware, (6) conscientious, (7) individualistic, (8) autonomous, and (9) integrated.

ego differentiation vs. work-role preoccupation According to Peck, the first developmental task in older people, who must redefine themselves in ways that do not relate to their work roles or occupations.

ego transcendence vs. ego preoccupation According to Peck, the third developmental task in older people, who must learn to cope with the reality of their coming death in the wake of the loss of significant others, siblings, friends, and loved ones.

elaboration Information processing strategy involving reasoning, logic, and sometimes imagination.

elder abuse "[P]sychological, physical, and sexual abuse; neglect (caregiver neglect and self-neglect), and financial exploitation" (Dong, 2014) (also called elder mistreatment or elder maltreatment).

elimination communication (EC) Infant potty training and natural infant hygiene, based on the belief that the infant is not only aware of the elimination function from birth, but that the infant also has some measure of ability to control sphincter muscles from infancy.

embryonic period Period of development from the 14th day (uterine implantation) to the end of the second month, a time of rapid cell division and specialization.

emerging adulthood period from late adolescence through the 20s as a distinctive developmental phase, characterized as a time when individuals have moved out of adolescence, but have not quite reached full adulthood (also called young adulthood).

emic Culture-specific approach to understanding the cultural meaning behind different practices and behaviors.

emotion schemas Framework for how to conceptualize and show emotion.

emotional competence Awareness of one's own and others' emotions and ability to regulate one's emotional responses.

emotional intelligence The ability to navigate the emotional brain/thinking brain system and develop "self-control, zeal and persistence, and the ability to motivate oneself" (Goleman, 1995, p. xii).

emotional regulation The capacity to manage one's own emotions, thoughts, and behavior.

emotions Brain-based impulses that motivate a person to act in a particular way.

empathy The ability to understand the feelings of others by interpreting signals of distress or pleasure (adj. form: empathic).

emphysema Disease involving damage to the elastic tissues of the, thus making it more difficult to exhale; typically caused by smoking.

encoding The process of making an experience relevant to one's life in order to access the information later.

encouragement Feedback during an activity that focuses on the child's effort and ingenuity.

endogenous stimulation Stimulation from internal sources.

environmental mastery The ability to control various external activities.

environmental volunteerism One way older adults can participate in civic engagement; retirees who are environmentalists and have the physical capability to work outside are less likely to engage in sedentary behavior, a risk factor for chronic disease, morbidity, and premature mortality.

epigenesis The idea that environments shape our genetic expressions, which in turn further shape our environments.

epiphyses The active growing areas at the end of each growing bone.

episodic memory Remembering information or events one has experienced from a specific time or event; includes things such as remembering where you are going or where you put something.

erectile dysfunction Impotence, the inability to obtain and maintain an erection firm enough for sex.

esteem needs The fourth level of Maslow's hierarchy of needs, the need for self-esteem, personal worth, and social recognition.

ethology The study of the adaptive and evolutionary basis of animal behavior.

etic Universalistic approach to understanding the cultural meaning behind different practices and behaviors.

evocative genotype–environment correlations The view that the features of the child, which are influenced by his genes, evoke reactions from others toward him, and these responses then further shape the child's development.

exosystem The connections and relationships between two or more settings, at least one of which the developing child does not experience directly.

explicit memory The conscious recollection of previous experiences or information.

explicit self-awareness By 18 months, the infant can now symbolically represent self-recognition of the infant's own body.

extended self See *self-continuity*.

external validity The applicability and generalizability of a study to the real world.

exogenous stimulation Stimulation from external sources.

faith development theory "[A] framework for understanding the evolution of how human beings conceptualize God, or a Higher Being, and how the influence of that Higher Being has an impact on core values, beliefs, and meanings in their personal lives and in their relationships with others" (Fowler & Dell, 2006, p. 34).

family atmosphere The climate that exists within and between people in a family system.

family constellation Structure of the family system and how each person defines his or her place within the family system.

family lifecycle The patterned stages of family composition and changes that affect family members' behavior over time.

fear Emotion that causes blood to be directed to the legs, preparing the body to make a quick getaway from whatever danger is causing the fear response.

fine motor skills Smaller bodily muscle movements, such as reaching and grasping, and those that often require eye-hand coordination.

Five Factor Model (FFM) Model of personality development focused on characteristics of extraversion, agreeableness, conscientiousness, neuroticism, and openness to experience.

fixed interval Applying a reinforcement after a specific amount of time.

fixed ratio Applying a reinforcement after a specific number of behaviors.

flexibility The amount of structure in a family.

fluid intelligence The ability to think logically, demonstrate mental flexibility, and solve problems in new and unfamiliar situations.

focused attention Ability to restrict awareness to a specific stimulus while ignoring other distractions.

food insecurity Condition in which, at some time during the year, a household is either uncertain of having enough food to meet the needs of all the members or is unable to acquire enough food because of insufficient money or other resources for food.

food secure Having continuous access to enough food for all household members to live healthily.

foreclosure State in which adolescents may have committed themselves to certain choices, but haven't explored all alternatives; may adopt their parents' values and choose something others want for them as opposed to exploring options and making a personal commitment.

four-phase model for the development of infant-parent attachments Bowlby's (1969) categorization of the course of development of parent–infant attachment.

frameworklessness Seltzer's (1982) model of how the changes during puberty result in anxiety and instability; the adolescent flounders, caught between the familiarity of childhood and the unfamiliarity of adolescence.

fraternal twins See *dizygotic twins.*

fully functioning person The outcome of successful personality development and self-actualization (Rogers, 1961).

gang A group of teens or young adults who spend time together, engaging in activities that typically involve violence.

gender identity Recognition of one's own gender and ability to identify others of the same gender.

gender polarization Tendency to dichotomize the world of gender; things are either male or female and there is no room for ambiguity.

gender stereotypes Expectations that boys and girls are different and will behave and interact in ways that are predictable on that basis.

Generation X Age cohort of Americans born from 1964 to about 1984.

generativity The concept of giving back through caring for others and the production of something that contributes to the betterment of society.

generativity vs. stagnation Erikson's seventh stage of development; for adults ages 35 to 60, the focus is on transcending self and family and focusing on the next generation.

genital stage According to Freud, the stage that begins at puberty and lasts through the remainder of the person's life.

genograms Pictorial, symbolic representations that elucidate the structure and processes of multiple generations within a family system.

genotype The genetic makeup which comprises the inheritance from both parents.

germ cells Sex cells, which are the cells used to procreate new organisms, and which divide through a process called *meiosis.*

gerotranscendence Developmental task associated with Peck's task of ego transcendence in which adults shift from a connection with the material world to a more transcendent, cosmically directed sense of connection.

gestures Intentional motor actions used to request and direct another's attention.

glaucoma A rise in pressure leading to optic nerve damage; treatable with varying degrees of success if caught early enough.

goals of misbehavior According to Dreikurs and Soltz (1991), if a child is not able to belong in a positive way, he will try to find significance and belonging through mistaken goals: attention seeking, power, revenge, and inadequacy.

goodness of fit In developmental research, a "two-way street, in which a child's temperament and other characteristics could influence the parent's attitude and behavior, as much as the parent's functioning could influence the child's behavior" (Chess & Thomas, 1996, p. 52).

grasping reflex In an infant, when pressure is put on the palm, he clenches his fingers around whatever is pressing on them.

gross motor skills Skills involving the large muscles of the body, enabling such functions as walking, kicking, sitting upright, lifting, and throwing a ball.

grouping A child's ability to sort objects by various dimensions such as color or shape (also called categorization).

growth charts Charts published by WHO and CDC outlining parameters of normal growth patterns in children.

guilt A feeling of responsibility or remorse for some offense, crime, wrong, etc., real or otherwise.

habituation Process that occurs in infants and toddlers when they are shown a stimulus enough times that in each subsequent viewing the child looks at it for a shorter period of time.

handedness Refers to the preference for using the right or left hand.

haploid state Property of germ (sex) cells, which have only one copy of each chromosome.

happiness Emotion that quiets the areas of the brain that generate troubling thoughts, by activating the part of the brain that inhibits negative feelings.

heritability The extent to which the outward expression of a trait is genetically determined.

heteronomous morality According to Piaget, the period from around 5 to 8 years of age when children adopt rules from authorities without question.

hierarchy of needs Maslow's theory that human beings have basic needs that must be met before they can meet other developmental needs.

horizontal stressors The expected and unexpected developmental events that occur across time.

humanistic theories Theories rooted in the philosophies of existentialism and phenomenology, embracing a holistic, positive approach to human existence, and focusing on the individual's potential for growth and self-actualization.

Huntington's disease Chromosomal disease caused by the gene huntingtin (HTT), in which the protein is abnormally expanded and misfolded, resulting in a terminal, progressive neurodegenerative disorder.

hyperphonated cries Children's cries of exceptionally high wavelength, between 1000 and 2000 Hz. resulting in high arousal in adults.

hypothetical-deductive reasoning The ability to develop a hypothesis and test it out, reasoning from general ideas to specific implications.

hypoxia Condition in which a fetus receive an insufficient supply of oxygen.

hysterectomy Surgical removal of the uterus.

id According to Freud, that part of a person's unconscious mind that is governed by pleasure and instinct (the *pleasure principle*).

identical twins See *monozygotic twins.*

identity achievement The desired goal in identity construction; occurs when adolescents have explored options and thought about what they want in life.

identity diffusion Condition in which adolescents are unsure of themselves and have not actively explored many options relative to what they want to do with their lives.

identity vs. role confusion Erikson's fifth stage of development; during adolescence and puberty, individuals need to explore limits, boundaries, meaning, identity, and goals.

ignoring See *neglecting-uninvolved style.*

imaginary audience Adolescent self-consciousness, the belief that one is the focus of everyone's attention; as a result, adolescents may become supersensitive and overly concerned about their appearance or their performance.

imitation Behavior in which an individual observes and replicates another's behavior.

immanent justice An innate belief in children in a just world that makes causal connections between their own misdeeds and later adversity.

implementation Phase beginning in the early 20s when young adults get a job and move into the workforce.

implicit Implied, unspoken; characteristics that may not be openly revealed, but can be implied from behavior.

implicit memory The unconscious recollection of information learned at a given point in time.

imprinting The process by which a newly hatched duck will bond with the first moving object they see, even if it is a human instead of another duck.

inadequacy The final goal of misbehavior; the child displaying inadequacy has given up and displays hopelessness.

incremental theories Developmental theories that see development progressing along a gradual, continuous path, constantly building upon itself little by little.

individual differences Experiences that individuals seek out, coupled with their genetic predispositions, interacting to produce unique developmental trajectories.

individualistic values Cultural values centered around individualism and independence.

individualized family development plan Working document produced by program staff and family members, containomg the agreed-upon early intervention services for a child and family.

inductive reasoning Process of making broad generalizations from specific observations.

industry vs. inferiority Erikson's fourth stage of development; for children ages 6–12, the focus is on goal-setting and achievement.

infancy The period from birth to about two years, encompassing great gains in sensorimotor and cognitive development.

infant-directed speech Also referred to as child-directed speech, motherese, and parentese; distinguished by its elongated, exaggerated vowels, use of high pitches, simple, repeated phrases, and its sing-song, lilting quality.

infant–parent play Important because infants who played with their mothers, as opposed to playing with the same objects by themselves, had more complex and more sustained sensorimotor play than infants who did not have play interactions with adults.

infertility The inability to conceive a child after one year of sexual intercourse without the use of contraception.

information processing Theory encompassing an infant's ability to categorize situations, create memories, and become familiar with recurring stimuli.

informed consent Ethical principle that research participants must have full knowledge of the potential risks, benefits, procedures, and purpose of the study.

inheritance The transmission of (genetic) characteristics from parents to offspring.

inhibited Temperament that involves being socially withdrawn, anxious, and fearful.

interpersonal attraction The attraction between two people that leads to the development of an intimate relationship.

initiative vs. guilt Erikson's third stage of development; between ages 3 and 6, the focus is on developing a basic sense of competence.

inner continuity Preservation and maintenance of existing internal and external structures in the context of changes in middle-aged and older adults.

insecure attachment Various forms of *avoidant attachment* and *ambivalent (resistant) attachment.*

integrity vs. despair Erikson's eighth stage of development; those over age 60 must deal with coming to terms with their life.

intellectual disability Refers to children who have significant limitations in intellectual functioning and adaptive behavior, with IQ scores below 70 (formerly called mental retardation).

intermodal perception The ability to perceive stimulation from events or objects by using multiple senses simultaneously.

internal validity The soundness of a study, meaning that a researcher can confidently determine that the change in the dependent variable (outcome) is due to the conditions the researcher introduced in the independent variable.

interpretivist approaches Models that emphasize the collectivist (vs. individualistic) nature of socialization.

intersectionality The disadvantages (particularly within the context of power and social status) of belonging to multiple categories of social group membership.

intersensory redundancy When identical amodal information—the texture of a stuffed animal—perceived in synchrony by more than one sense modality.

interviews Research designs involving a series of questions asked of subjects either in person or over the telephone to elicit opinions or facts.

intimacy vs. isolation Erikson's sixth stage of development; for individuals ages 18 to 35, the major task is development of and security within intimate relationships.

invincibility fable Belief that bad things might happen to others who take risks, but not to oneself; often seen in adolescents.

justice perspective Having concern for fairness and focusing on what is right.

Klinefelter's syndrome A chromosomal abnormality in males involving one or more extra X chromosomes, resulting in physical features such as long legs, above average height, small and firm testes, and sterility, as well as deficits in language and executive functioning.

Lamaze method Approach to natural birth that stresses that women should be educated and prepared for a safe, natural birth without medical intervention through support, relaxation, and optimal birth positions.

language Communication system consisting of the four basic components: phonology, semantics, pragmatics, and syntax.

lanugo Downy growth of hair covering the entire body of the fetus.

late adulthood The period of life from about 60 to 75 years, when most individuals are nearing the end of their career and are launching children.

late-onset antisocial behavior Deviant behavior that begins after puberty; generally involves only minor offenses.

late-onset babbling Delay in beginning of babbling until after 10 months; in the absence of any significant medical problems, such children are at extreme risk for hearing impairment.

latent stage According to Freud, the stage from age 5 until puberty begins, marked by calm after the torment of the earlier years.

law of effect Thorndike's (1932) theory that learning results from associating stimuli and responses.

learning acquisition device (LAD) According to Chomsky, an inborn system containing a *universal grammar.*

learning disability Refers to children who have difficulties in specific cognitive processes involving perception, memory, language, or metacognition, leading to difficulty in scholastic performance, despite being within the normal or above normal range of measured intelligence.

learning theories Theories that stress the role of external influences on behavior.

Level 1 self-awareness (self-world differentiation) According to Rochat, the newborn comes into the world predisposed to make a distinction between the world outside the infant and the infant's own body and actions.

Level 2 self-awareness (situated self) The infant's ability to map her own bodily space to the bodily space of the adult shows that she is able to situate herself in relation to the other person.

Level 3 self-awareness (identification) The toddler demonstrates identification of the entity in the mirror as standing in for a representation of self, manifesting recognition of self.

life accidents Events that people are powerless to prevent (e.g., war, economic decline, death of a family member) and that may influence how we resolve our life passage.

life review The process of reflecting on and reevaluating one's life.

lifespan The average length of time that members of a population or species will live.

life structure the underlying pattern of a person's life, shaped primarily through your interactions with individuals, groups, and institutions.

lifestyle The way in which a person interfaces with social context.

locomotion Moving one's body from place to place, such as by rolling over, crawling, standing, and walking.

logical consequences Occurs when a child's behavior results in unpleasant effects; allowing children to experience such consequences teaches responsibility and helps them make the connection between their decisions and outcomes.

longitudinal designs Studies in which researchers follow one group, or cohort, of participants over an extended period of time in order to repeatedly measure different aspects of development.

long-term memory In information processing, data is transferred here from *working memory;* has a large capacity and long, perhaps unlimited, duration.

macrosystem The overarching cultural context in which the other systems (micro-, meso-, exosystems) are embedded.

major depressive disorder A condition characterized by serious depressive episodes that are out of character with previous behavior.

malnutrition In infants, diagnosed by comparing weight-for-height score with a healthy reference group's score.

"Man as Hunter" hypothesis Ardrey's (1976) theory that men have always been hunters, and as a result have characteristics such as aggression, ambition, leadership, and interest in technological innovation.

marker events Concrete events in our lives (e.g., graduation, marriage, childbirth), which do not define our developmental stages but may accentuate our need to change.

maturation theory Theories that focus on the idea that human development is biological and that development happens automatically and in predictable, sequential stages with few individual differences.

meiosis Process by which the sex cells (germ cells) are divided into a *haploid state*.

memory Process by which information is encoded, stored, and retrieved.

menopausal hormone therapy Treatment of women with estrogen and progesterone to deal with the symptoms of menopause.

menopause Period in which a woman's monthly menstrual flow discontinues, she no longer releases monthly eggs from her ovaries, and her production of estrogen and progesterone declines.

mental combinations Means through which toddlers use physical experimentation to gain insight.

mentoring programs Enhancement of the school experience by giving adolescents access to relationships with successful community members who provide career and educational support, advice, and encouragement.

mesosystem The connections and relationships between two or more microsystems.

messenger ribonucleic acid (messenger RNA) Molecules within cells that carry instructions from the DNA.

metabolic syndrome Syndrome X; term given to a set of characteristics that increase a person's risk of heart attack and premature death.

metacognition Knowledge about cognitive states or processes; thinking about thinking.

microsystem A pattern of activities, social roles, and interpersonal relations experienced by the developing person in a given face-to-face setting with particular physical, social, and symbolic features that invite, permit, or inhibit engagement in sustained, progressively more complex interaction with, and activity in, the immediate environment (Bronfenbrenner, 1994).

middle adulthood The longest lifespan period, lasting from about 30 to 60 years of age, when many adults either experience career success or reevaluate and change their careers.

middle childhood The period from about 6 to 12 years, during which children begin to think more logically and concretely in the structured educational environment they now inhabit.

midlife crisis A difficult transition period occurring around the age of 40.

mirror neurons Specialized cells in the brain that imitate the behaviors of what children see before they can actually perform the behavior themselves.

miscarriage Spontaneous death of a fetus.

mitosis Process by which a somatic cell divides and duplicates itself into two new cells with replicated genetic information.

modalities of sensation Unique pathways in the spinal cord, reaching distinct targets in the brain: *discriminative touch, pain and temperature,* and *proprioception.*

mode In Beck's (1996) theory of the development of cognitive function, the integration of *systems* and the many *schemas* that make up each system that is being integrated.

monozygotic twins Twins who began as one egg, which was fertilized by one sperm and that split into two separate eggs that developed independently in the mother's womb (*identical twins*).

moral development The process through which children adopt principles and guidelines that allow them to judge whether behavior is right or wrong.

moral intuition Instantaneous emotional reaction of approval or disapproval of a person's actions or behavior.

moral judgment The process of reasoning through and reaching a decision about moral issues.

moral relativism Recognition that differences in moral judgments (i.e., what is right vs. wrong) exist across diverse cultures, that no universal moral standard can be applied to all individuals.

morality principle See *superego.*

moratorium period Crisis period in which adolescents struggle with decisions, are actively exploring relationships and career options, and experimenting with different identities.

Moro reflex Reaction that causes an infant to stretch out his arms, legs, and fingers while elongating the neck muscles simultaneously when the infant is moved suddenly or hears a loud sound.

morpheme The smallest unit of a language that has meaning.

multidimensional theories Developmental theories that integrate stage and incremental theories, acknowledging the importance of both.

multigenerational family systems Developmental theories that focus on how previous generations greatly affect the development of future generations' egos.

multiplicity In Perry's model, the transition from dualistic to more relativistic thinking; individuals realize the legitimacy of multiple viewpoints and no longer believe authorities hold absolute truth.

muscle growth In a normally developing infant, muscle increases gradually throughout the first year and continues slowly and steadily until adolescence.

myelin Fatty substance coating axons, facilitating "the rapid and synchronized information transfer required for coordinated movement, decision-making, and other higher order cognitive, behavioral, and emotive functions" (Deoni et al., 2011, p. 784).

myelination Process of coating the neural fibers, crucial to the development of the infant brain.

nativist Chomsky's perspective focusing on the active role that the infant's brain plays in developing language.

naturalistic observation Unobtrusive observation of people going about their usual business in everyday settings.

natural selection The process whereby certain traits or characteristics of a species that are more adaptable to the environment survive.

nature The biological characteristics and predispositions that an individual inherits.

need for belonging The third level of Maslow's hierarchy of needs, accomplished through relationships with family and friends and involvement in social groups.

negative punishment Removal or withholding of a pleasant event.

negative reactivity Temperamental trait involving negative reactions to parental attention.

negative reinforcement Removal of an unfavorable event or outcome (i.e., relief) after a behavior with the goal of increasing the frequency of that behavior.

neglecting-uninvolved style Parental style characterized by a lack of communication or expressions of affection.

neocortex The large area of the brain responsible for rational thoughts such as strategizing and long-term planning.

neophobia Fear of something new.

neurons Nerve cells.

nine categories of temperament Thomas and Chess's (1977) categorization of temperamental styles along nine parameters.

nonmaleficence Doing no harm, a primary principle of ethical research.

nonnormative or highly individualized life events Those unusual occurrences that greatly affect an individual's life.

non-rapid eye movement (NREM) A quieter type of sleep characterized by slower breathing, lower heart rate, and less brain activity.

normative age-graded influences The predictable changes that every individual will encounter throughout his or her lifespan.

normative history-graded influences The historical circumstances that affect people of common generations similarly.

nosological classification system Any system that provides descriptions of symptoms and guidelines for determining if an individual meets the clinical diagnosis for specifically described disorders.

nucleoplasm The fluid within the cellular nucleus.

nucleus In eukaryotic cells, the command or activity control center, which houses the chromosomes.

numeracy Understanding of numbers and ability to do mathematical operations; number sense.

nurture Environmental influences and experiences as they relate to human development.

nutrition "[T]he intake of food, considered in relation to the body's dietary needs. Good nutrition—an adequate, well balanced diet combined with regular physical activity—is a cornerstone of good health. Poor nutrition can lead to reduced immunity, increased susceptibility to disease, impaired physical and mental development, and reduced productivity" (WHO, 2013).

object categorization Process enabling infants and toddlers to think in categories (e.g., animals, colors, food).

object-directed vocalizations (ODVs) Infants' vocalizations when looking at an object that is either being held or within reach.

object permanence The understanding that when a previously seen object is no longer visible, it still exists.

old age Includes individuals over the age of about 75, who face challenges such as retirement and loss of a spouse.

onlooker play Where the child observes other children playing but does not participate.

open marriages Marriages in which both partners agree that the other may engage in sexual relationships with other individuals.

operant conditioning Process of learning by associating a consequence with a behavior.

oppositional defiant disorder A disorder in children characterized by hostile, negative behavior, particularly directed toward adults.

optimal level of development The highest level of cognitive performance (i.e., information processing) that a person is capable of achieving.

optimization Ways older adults optimize positive changes, finding ways to adapt toward a set of desirable outcomes.

oral stage According to Freud, the stage from birth to 18 months, centered on the pleasure of sucking and eating.

organization Strategy of looking for associations and combining information into groups or categories to make it easier to recall.

original sin Christian doctrine that all infants are born with the hereditary stain left behind from Adam's sin.

ossification In fetal development, the process by which bones form and harden.

overextension Speech error in which the toddler applies a word to a wider range of objects than is accurate.

pain and temperature *Modality of sensation* that includes the sensations of tickle and itch.

parallel play Where children are engaged in the same activity at the same time, but they are playing separately.

parataxic distortions The patterns of skewed or irrational perceptions people have regarding others' perceptions of them.

parent guidance treatment program Treatment program focusing on changing parents' behavior and overtly expressed attitudes toward their child.

parental warmth Conveyed through hugs, kisses, praise, encouragement, terms of endearment, and by telling children they are loved.

passive development The view that children are passively shaped by their environments.

passive genotype–environment correlations The view that parents provide both genes and environment, which influence the child's development.

Peer pressure Influence exerted by one's peers, particularly strong during early adolescence; may be positive or negative.

perception The act of apprehending by means of the senses or of the mind; cognition.

period of the ovum The first 14 days after *conception,* during which the developing organism travels down the fallopian tube and implants onto the blood- and nutrient-rich uterine wall.

permissive parents Parents who are accepting, affirmative, and tolerant of their children's behavior, the goal being to create an environment in which the child exercises significant amounts of discretion with respect to their own behaviors.

person-praise Feedback that includes statements about stable, global traits.

personal fable Typically adolescent belief that they are unlike everyone else—that no one experiences things in the same way as they do, and, consequently, that nobody will understand what they are going through.

perspective taking Children's understanding of how they and their actions are viewed by others.

phallic stage According to Freud, the stage from 3 to 5 years, centered on children's fascination with their genitalia and other bodily functions.

phenotype The expression of genotypes given an individual's environment.

phenylketonuria (PKU) Condition caused by a gene mutation in which the enzyme phenylalanine hydroxylase (PAH) is not properly metabolized into the amino acid tyrosine.

phoneme A speech sound, the smallest unit of language.

phonology The study of a language's sounds.

physiological needs The first level of Maslow's hierarchy of needs, namely basic needs for survival—water, air, food, and sleep.

physiological responses Reactions to stimuli measured to assess activity of the amygdale, including heart rate, pupillary dilation, norepinephrine , muscle tension, and cortisol level.

pincer grasp A precise movement that brings together the thumb and index finger, enabling an infant to pick up objects such as small pieces of cereal.

planned happenstance Theory that recognizes the importance of unplanned, chance events in people's vocational lives.

plasticity Flexibility, an important characteristic of much of human development.

play A range of activities associated with recreational pleasure and enjoyment.

play with objects Play involving an infant intentionally manipulating objects to observe the results.

pleasure principle See *id.*

point of view Individual position or perspective from which something is considered or evaluated.

polygenic inheritance The concept that individual differences in biological characteristics are not traceable to one single gene.

positive psychology Psychology focusing on the mental health of individuals rather than mental disease.

positive parent–child relationships Relationships that promote self-regulation; they positively affect children's ability to learn at school and simultaneously lower the child's risk of developing deviant behaviors or other adjustment problems.

positive punishment Presentation of an adverse event.

positive reinforcements Favorable events or outcomes (rewards) that follow a behavior with the goal of increasing the frequency of that behavior.

postauricular reflex (PAR) Reflex involving pinning the ears against the head, used to signal infants are ready to feed, as well as to make themselves more comfortable during the process of nursing.

postconventional level Stage of moral development not often not attained, in which morality is defined by self-chosen principles seen as having validity.

postformal thought Advanced adult cognition characterized by relativistic thinking, flexibility and pragmatics, tolerance for ambiguity and contradictions, and cognitive-affective complexity.

power Second goal of misbehavior; a child with this goal is trying to achieve significance by being in control and by proving no one can have power over them.

pragmatics The way in which we use language to communicate with a specific listener.

praise Feedback focused on the outcome or completion of a task.

preconventional level Stage of moral development in whichchildren conceptualize things as good or bad as related to the consequences of their behavior, which may result in punishment or rewards.

premoral According to Piaget, the period from birth to around 4 years of age when children are not concerned with rules and have little to no sense of morality.

prenatal period The entire period from conception to birth.

preoperational period The second stage in Piaget's (1983) theory of cognitive development, characterized by changes in how children think.

prereaching Action involving an infant swiping at an object but rarely reaching it.

presbyopia Inability to focus on objects at a close distance.

pretend play Where not only can objects be used to symbolize or represent other objects, but also children can take on dramatic roles as well.

primary circular reactions Substage of *sensorimotor* stage involving coordination of internal sensations and new schemas.

primary emotions The emotions of *happiness, joy, anger, sadness, fear, surprise,* interest, and *disgust.*

primary sex characteristics Organs needed for reproduction: prostate gland, seminal vesicles, testes, scrotum, and penis in males; ovaries, fallopian tubes, uterus, clitoris, and vagina in females.

private logic A person's internal logic, consisting of the person's core assumptions, beliefs, and philosophies about life

private speech The idea that one talks aloud to oneself and not to others for the purposes of self-guidance.

proactive aggression Aggressive behavior aimed at attempting to obtain a desired goal through coercion.

procedural knowledge Skills that have been learned, such as how to play a musical instrument.

process-praise Feedback that focuses on effort rather than a fixed ability.

processing speed As mental activities are repeated, the neural pathways used become myelinated and automatization occurs, and children become quicker at responding and performing mental activities.

production The ability to actually speak language.

professional nonparental caregiver Professionals such as day care providers who function as caregivers.

progeroid Conditions such as progeria or Werner's syndrome, characterized by premature and accelerated aging, accompanied by increased risk for cardiovascular disease and cancer.

proprioception Sensations that happen beneath the surface of the body, such as muscle stretch, joint position.

protest Reaction to parental separation characterized by distress, fear, angry protests, desperate efforts to find the missing parent, and hopefulness that the parent would return.

protoplasm General term for cytoplasm and nucleoplasm.

Proustian memories Memories involuntarily retrieved as a result of stimuli associated with the memories.

proximal processes The reciprocal, enduring interactions between the developing child and his environment.

pruning The process by which the brain rids itself of unnecessary or redundant cells or cell connections.

psychoanalytic learning theory Theory focused on the concept that drive, cue, response, and reinforcement combine to form the foundation of learning.

psychological aging Processes involving an individual's perception of his or her age.

psychosexual stages According to Freud, the phases of human development: *oral, anal, phallic, latent,* and *genital stages.*

psychosocial stages According the Erikson, the eight stages people encounter over the course of their lives, each presenting a unique challenge or crisis that must be met for healthy development.

punishments Adverse events that decrease the frequency of the behavior they follow.

quality world Picture album each person holds in mind, made up or remembered pictures of "the people we most want to be with; the things we most want to own or experience; and the ideas or systems of belief that govern much of our behavior" (Glasser, 1998, p. 45).

questionnaires Research designs involving a written set of questions that administered to people in order to collect facts or opinions about something.

rapid eye movement (REM) Sleep typified by breathing and heart rates similar to waking states, eye movement, and increased brain activity.

reactive aggression Reactive aggression based on misinterpretations of the intentions of others; seeing accidental behavior as purposeful, suggesting a hostile attribution bias.

reactivity When people being observed act differently than they usually would simply because they know that they are being observed.

reality principle See *ego.*

recall Generating a mental image of a previously experienced object without the benefit of having something in the present moment to stimulate recognition of it.

recessive genes Genes that are usually not expressed in a phenotype and thus are not observed.

reciprocal determinism The idea that there is a mutual relationship between an individual and the environment.

recognition Noticing when a new object or event is the same as or similar to one that was previously encountered.

reflexes Acts performed involuntarily in response to a stimulus. ftg

reflexive judgment The way adults analyze and reason through a dilemma, as well as justify the solutions they develop.

rehearsal The conscious repetition of one or more pieces of information as a way of holding the information in the working memory temporarily.

reinforcement schedules How and when reinforcements are applied; may be continuous or variable.

reinforcements Consequences that strengthen or increase the frequency of the behavior they follow.

relational-cultural theory Theory developed by Miller (1976), which posits that people grow through and toward relationships throughout the lifespan, and that culture powerfully impacts relationships.

relativism discovered The second phase of Perry's (1970) theory of development, involving an understanding that most knowledge is contextual, the world is complex, and Truth is not always clearly available.

religion Social or organized means by which a person expresses spirituality.

religious judgment Refers to the human "reasoning that relates reality as experienced to something beyond reality and that serves to provide meaning and direction beyond learned content" (Oser, 1994, p. 376).

reminiscence Recall of memories; in later life, a means by which people recall, assess, and evaluate past events.

reproductive system Body system made up of the organs responsible for reproduction.

resilience An ability to "bounce back" (Ong & Bergeman, 2004).

respiratory system System involving the organs that deliver oxygen to the body.

response Behavior in reaction to a stimulus.

retrieval Gaining access to stored information.

revenge The third goal of misbehavior; the revenge-seeking child has been hurt in some way and is lashing out at those around her.

reversibility In its simplest form, the child's ability to mentally undo or reverse an action.

ribosomes Small particles in the cytoplasm that help produce products necessary for cellular functions, such as cellular replication.

role overload Having more family and work demands than time needed to fulfill them, as well as conflicts between work and family responsibilities.

romantic love Often associated with being "in love" with someone; involves complex emotions, such as passion, anger, joy, jealousy, and fear; also linked to sensual feelings, infatuation, and sexual desire (also referred to as passionate love).

rooting reflex Demonstrated when something is rubbed against an infant's cheek and he turns his mouth toward the object.

sadness Emotion that produces a decrease in energy or enthusiasm.

sandwich generation In general, those, usually middle-aged, who are "stuck" between responsibilities of caring for their parents and their children.

sarcopenia Deterioration of muscle mass as one ages.

scaffolding The process helpful others facilitating children's move from a position of inability to complete challenging tasks to a position where they can eventually complete the tasks independently.

schema Frameworks or basic building blocks of the mind.

schizophrenia A chronic and severe mental disorder characterized by a breakdown in thought processes and perceptions.

school phobia Dread related to going to school; as the thought or reality of school attendance becomes more imminent, children may experience physiological symptoms of anxiety.

school-to-work programs Programs in high schools combining classroom-based education with practical work experience.

scrupulosity Form of obsessive-compulsive disorder seen in individuals who take religious activities to extremes, such as constant worry over sin or rituals like prayer that are taken to an unhealthy level.

secondary circular reactions Substage of *sensorimotor* period during which the child becomes more focused on the world and begins to intentionally repeat actions in order to trigger a response in the environment.

secondary emotions Emotions that include both *self-conscious* and *self-evaluative emotions.*

secondary sex characteristics Physical signs of maturation not associated with the sex organs: breast development and pubic hair in girls; facial, pubic, and body hair in boys.

secular trend Population trend in the onset of puberty, which appears to be occurring at an earlier age than in previous generations, along with increases in weight and height.

secure attachment Condition in which, although the child demonstrates signs of missing a parent, the child easily separates from the mother and becomes engaged in exploration.

security needs The second level of Maslow's hierarchy of needs, the need for safety and security.

selective attention The ability to focus on relevant information and screen out irrelevant information, a skill essential to learning.

self-actualization The highest level of Maslow's hierarchy of needs, the need for fulfillment of one's potential.

self-awareness Recognizing that one's identity is separate and distinct from everyone and everything else.

self-concept The way in which children view themselves as well as how they assess that content.

self-conscious emotions Seen between 15 and 24 months; include embarrassment (the type that results from being the object of attention), envy, and empathy.

self-continuity A type of self-knowledge in which the toddler is self-aware of existing as a continuous being outside of the present moment, that the infant existed in the past, and that the infant will continue to exist into the future.

self-efficacy Beliefs children develop about their capabilities and their ability to influence events that affect their lives.

self-evaluative emotions Emotions such as pride, guilt, shame, and embarrassment.

self-regulation Ability to sooth oneself or control one's behavior to avoid negative stimuli.

self-report The use of questionnaires, checklists, or interviews to get participants to report various data about themselves.

semantic memory Memory involving the basic information learned in school, such as historical facts and concepts.

semantics The meaning of words.

senescence Decline to death, usually with normal aging.

sensation Physically experiencing sensory stimulation.

sensitive period A timeframe when responses to development in certain areas will be optimal.

sensorimotor According to Piaget, the stage from birth to 2 years, during which the infant experiences the surrounding environment, learning information through the senses.

sensory register Part of the information processing system; takes in data through the senses, essentially all the environmental stimuli that the senses pick up (also called sensory memory).

separation protest Distressed behavior when an infant's parent leaves, involving crying and other distressed behaviors, designed to signal a parent to return (also called separation anxiety).

sequential methods Studies that measure multiple age cohorts at multiple intervals over time, allowing researchers to pinpoint which observed differences are due to maturation and which are due to shared historical or generational experiences.

seriation The ability to arrange items in order along some quantitative dimension such as height.

service learning Method of engaging students by having adolescents volunteer in various community agencies.

seven vectors Chickering's term for areas that people navigate as they grow and develop, not necessarily sequentially; people may negotiate multiple vectors simultaneously or revisit vectors over time.

sex chromosomal disorders chromosomal disorders that are caused by missing or extra chromosomes on the 23rd chromosomal pair, which is the sex-determining chromosome.

sexual dysfunction A multidimensional health issue resulting from biological, psychological, and interpersonal factors that inhibit normal sexual function.

sexually transmitted diseases (STDs) Serious infections that are primarily transmitted by unprotected sexual contact [also known as sexually transmitted infections (STIs)].

shaken baby syndrome (SBS) Head injuries resulting from abuse, which occurs when a parent becomes so frustrated with an infant's cries that the parent shakes the baby.

short-term memory See *working memory.*

simple social play Play in which the child makes active attempts to mimic the behaviors of others and are more active at responding to others as well as encouraging responses from others to themselves.

skeletal age The most accurate estimate of an infant's or toddler's physical maturity, obtained by taking an X-ray of the child's hand and wrist and comparing the bones in this area of the body to standards of bone growth on X-rays in an assessment atlas.

skill acquisition The gradual process of learning new cognitive abilities.

sleep disorders Problems involving difficulty falling asleep and frequent waking during the night with subsequent difficulties falling back asleep.

social aging The way individuals view aging within their own culture or society.

social cognition The way children think about people and relationships.

social cognitive theory Updated version of social learning theory reflecting a greater emphasis on cognitive processes as a part of one's development.

social interest View that people endeavor to belong.

social intervention program Intervention that might be employed when working with parents of toddlers who are demonstrating destructive and disruptive behaviors during social play.

social learning theory Theories focusing on the idea that learning occurs through observation, imitation, or modeling.

social phobia Dread characterized by anxiety symptoms that are similar to those of school phobia and separation anxiety, but occurring in most social situations, in and out of school.

social referencing Using the emotional expressions of others to decipher unfamiliar events.

social roles Set of rights and obligations associated with each social status, guiding social interactions as they correspond to social status.

Social Security Federal retirement program enacted in 1935; allows people to retire in their 60s; also provides survivors' and disability benefits.

social status Social positions within the social structures, organized in hierarchies of relative status based on influence and power.

social structures The basic organizational concepts about how society works.

socialization Lifelong process whereby individuals learn social norms, customs, practices, values and beliefs, and, most importantly, role expectations.

socioeconomic status (SES) Social status based on parental income level as well as such markers of "cultural capital" as educational attainment.

solitary play Where the child plays alone even in the presence of other children.

somatic cells Virtually all of the cells which make up the human body, divide through a process called *mitosis.*

somatosensory System that responds to stimulation by creating specialized receptors, linking the body site to the spinal column and brain.

specification Phase in which adolescents begin to limit their options by learning about specific jobs.

spirituality A "capacity and tendency that . . . moves the individual toward knowledge, love, meaning, peace, hope, transcendence, connectedness, compassion, wellness, and wholeness" (ASERVIC, 1995, p. 30).

spontaneous recurrent abortions (SRAs) Repeated miscarriages.

stage theories Class of developmental theories that propose that human development across the lifespan changes abruptly via rapid transformations that propel individuals from one stage of functioning to the next, where they remain quite stable for long periods of time.

standardized testing Tests that are given and scored using uniform procedures for all test takers and normed on large populations.

stepping reflex When held above the floor, infants kick their legs in ways that simulate walking (*walking reflex*).

strange situation Experimental procedure that assesses the security of attachment in children 10–24 months old (Ainsworth & Bell, 1970; Ainsworth, Blehar, Waters, and Wall, 1978).

stranger wariness (stranger anxiety) Distressed behavior toward people an infant does not know.

strategies More deliberate, less automatic mental activities that are involved in learning and moving information to long-term memory.

stress Any internal or external force in the world that affects the individual.

structured observation Tests in which researchers design situations or stimuli to elicit behaviors of interest.

sucking reflex In infants, the natural reaction when something is placed inside their mouths such as a nipple.

sudden infant death syndrome (SIDS) Spontaneous death of an infant 1–12 months old.

supercentenarians People who have reached 115 years of age.

superego According to Freud, that part of a person's unconscious mind that is governed by society and morality (the *morality principle*).

supine Recumbent position of lying on one's back.

surveys Research designs asking a series of questions in order to gather information about what people do or think about something.

surprise Emotion that producesa lifting of the eyebrows, lettin the person increase their visual field so that they can better appraise the surprising event and make a plan of action.

sustained attention Ability to focus attention over an extended period of time.

swingers Partners in a committed relationship who mutually agree to engage in sexual activities with other like-minded couples as a social activity.

symbolic Make-believe play, when an infant uses one object to represent another, usually appearing around 12 or 13 months.

syntax Grammatical component of language, how words are ordered and word forms changed, as in changing a verb from present to future tense.

systems In Beck's (1996) theory of the development of cognitive function, the five basic building blocks of the mind: cognitive (or information processing), affective (or emotional), behavioral, motivational, and physiological.

tabula rasa Literally, blank slate; the idea that we are born without innate ideas and that knowledge is determined by experience and perception.

tasting exposures In infancy, necessary for the brain to accept the taste of a particular food.

teething process Typically begins at 5–9 months, with the eruption of the first *baby teeth*.

telegraphic speech Speech that is pared down to the basic elements, with nonessential words eliminated.

teleological Goal-directed.

telomeres Minute structures capping the chromosomes, containing long repetitive sequences of noncoding genetic material.

temper tantrum An explosive external presentation of an inner emotional state, usually a mixture of both anger and distress.

temperament Unique behavioral dispositions that are stable over time.

teratogens Substances that may cause abnormalities in newborns.

teratology Study of structural malformations in newborns.

tertiary circular reactions Substage of *sensorimotor* period, during which children begin a period of trial-and-error experimentation.

testosterone A steroid hormone found in humans and other vertebrates, secreted primarily by the testicles of males and, to a lesser extent, the ovaries of females.

theory of evolution Darwin's theory that all living species have descended over time from common ancestors through *natural selection.*

theory of multiple intelligences "[A] pluralistic view of mind, recognizing many different and discrete facets of cognition, acknowledging that people have different cognitive strengths and contrasting cognitive styles" (Gardner, 1996, p. 6).

time-lag designs Replications of previous studies using the same age groups and parameters as researchers from a previous era, allowing researchers from the current era to determine if dated findings still apply today or have changed in some way.

toddlerhood The period from about 2 to 3 years, during which children further develop their language skills and begin mastering such tasks as potty training and feeding and dressing themselves.

toilet training Method endorsed by the AAP to teach a toddler to transition from eliminating in a diaper to using the toilet independently, usually beginning about 18–24 months.

transition theory Developmental theory focusing on positive and negative changes that cause discomfort as roles, routines, relationships, and assumptions change.

transivity A more sophisticated variation of *seriation;* the ability to understand the relationship between items in a series and be able to draw conclusions based on that understanding.

traumatic stress disorders Disorders characterized by symptoms of anxiety and arousal, avoidance, and psychological reexperiencing of trauma that may be triggered by anything that remotely reminds a child of the traumatic event.

trust vs. mistrust Erikson's first stage of development; infants must develop trust with secure caregiver relationships as their basic needs are met.

Turner's syndrome Disorder in which a female loses an X from the 23rd chromosomal pair, resulting in shortened height, webbed neck, heart disease, and infertility.

Type A personality Personality style characterized by extreme competitiveness, intense anger, hostile tendencies, restlessness, being overly aggressive, and frequent impatience.

Type B personality Personality style that tends to be calm, easygoing, relaxed, and not often hurried.

ulnar grasp Closing the fingers against the palm to grasp an object.

umbilical cord Carries oxygenated blood from the placenta to the fetus and carries away deoxygenated blood and waste products from the embryo or fetus.

unconditioned response (UCR) Unlearned response that occurs naturally in reaction to an unconditioned stimulus.

unconditioned stimulus (UCS) Stimulus that unconditionally, naturally, and automatically triggers a response.

unintentional injuries Injuries not deliberately inflicted, such as burns and scalds, poisoning, head injuries, and pedestrian and street safety.

universal grammar According to Chomsky, a set of grammatical rules shared by all languages and hardwired into an infant's brain before the infant even hears a word spoken.

vaccines Substances that work to immunize the body against a particular disease by introducing a small-scale version of the pathogen into the body, usually by injection, causing the body to respond by producing antibodies as if it is really under attack.

variable interval Giving reinforcements following variable amounts of time.

variable ratio Giving reinforcements following a variable number of responses.

vasectomy Surgical procedure in which the vas is sealed by either clamping or cutting, thus preventing sperm from mixing with semen and ejaculating through the penis.

vernix caseosa Waxy substance covering the skin to protect a fetus's skin from constant exposure to amniotic fluid.

vertical stressors Patterns such as familial behavioral and communication styles passed down through generations, as well as long-term poverty and oppression across generations.

videotaped playroom observations Research designs involving videotaped sessions in which particular, often novel, situations are presented, and observations are later analyzed for content and meaning.

vision impairment Damage to the eye, incorrect eye shape, or difficulties with brain processing of visual stimuli.

visual cliff Experiments in which infants who can already crawl look to their mothers' expressions for guidance as to whether or not to crawl over the visual cliff with a transparent covering.

vital capacity The amount of air the lungs can inhale and expel.

vocational education Instruction that prepares young adults for nonacademic careers related to a specific trade (e.g., plumbing, masonry) [also known as career and technical education (CTE)].

vocational self-concept A part of one's broader sense of identity, including ideas about which characteristics of the self are congruent with the requirements of an occupation.

walking reflex See *stepping reflex.*

White racial identity development A model that includes statuses that demonstrate an evolution in abandoning racism and developing a positive identity (Helms, 1990).

work values Values reflecting what a person needs to have present in the work environment in order to find satisfaction on the job.

working memory In the information processing system, where we reason, comprehend, and problem solve; has a limited capacity and a short duration, about 20 seconds.

young adulthood The period from about 19 to 30 years, during which individuals face the challenges of establishing a career and seeking out intimate relationships.

zone of proximal development Vygotsky's term for the difference or distance between what children can achieve individually versus what they can achieve with adult guidance and support.

zygote The single-celled product of *conception,* which immediately undergoes mitosis.

zygotic period The period of development following immediately after *conception.*

References

Abjullah, B., Nasreen, R., & Ravichandran, N. (2012). A comprehensive review of consumption pattern and strategies in cosmeceutical market with a focus on dermaceuticals in Indian market. *International Journal of Scientific and Research Publications, 2,* 171–180.

Acredolo, L., & Goodwyn, S. (1988). Symbolic gesturing in normal infants. *Child Development, 59,* 450–466. doi: 10.2307/1130324

Actis-Grosso, R., & Zavagno, D. (2008). The representation of time course events in visual arts and the development of the concept of time in children: A preliminary study. *Spatial Vision, 21,* 313–336. doi: 10.1163/156856808784532590

Adam, B. D. (2006). Relationship innovation in male couples. *Sexualities, 9,* 5–26. doi: 10.1177/1363460706060685

Adams, G., & Rau, B. (2011). Putting off tomorrow to do what you want today: Planning for retirement. *American Psychologist, 66,* 180–192. doi: 10.1037/a0022131

Adler, A. (1970). Fundamentals of individual psychology. *Journal of Individual Psychology, 26*(1), 36–49.

Administration on Aging (AoA). (2011). *A profile of older Americans: 2011.* Retrieved from http://www.aoa.gov/AoARoot/Aging _Statistics/Profile/index.aspx

Ahnert, L., Pinquart, M., & Lamb, M. E. (2006). Security of children's relationships with nonparental care providers: A meta-analysis. *Child Development, 74,* 664–679. doi: 10.1111/j.1467-8624.2006 .00896.x

Ainsworth, M. D. S., & Bell, S. M. (1970). Attachment, exploration, and separation: Illustrated by the behavior of one-year-olds in a strange situation. *Child Development, 41,* 49–67. doi: 10.2307/1127388

Ainsworth, M. D. S., Blehar, M. C., Waters, E., & Wall, S. (1978). *Patterns of attachment: A psychological study of the strange situation.* Hillsdale, NJ: Erlbaum.

Ainsworth, M. D. S., & Bowlby, J. (1989). An ethological approach to personality development. *American Psychologist, 46,* 333–341. doi: 10.1037/0003-066X.46.4.333

Akos, P., Niles, S. G., & Erford, B. T. (2015). Fostering educational and career planning in students. In B. T. Erford (Ed.), *Transforming the school counseling profession* (4th ed., pp. 202–221). Upper Saddle River, NJ: Pearson Merrill.

Akos, P., Niles, S. G., Miller, E. M., & Erford, B. T. (2011). Promoting educational and career planning in schools. In B. T. Erford (Ed.), *Transforming the school counseling profession* (3rd ed., pp. 202–221). Columbus, OH: Pearson Merrill Prentice Hall.

Albers, C. A., & Grieve, A. J. (2007). Test review: Bayley Scales of Infant and Toddler Development—Third Edition. *Journal of Psychoeducational Assessment, 25,* 180–190.

Albers, L. L., Migliaccio, L., Bedrick, E. J., Teaf, D., & Peralta, P. (2007). Does epidural analgesia affect the rate of spontaneous obstetric lacerations in normal births? *Journal of Midwifery & Women's Health, 52,* 31–33. doi: 10.1016/j.jmwh.2006.08.016

Aldwin, C. M., & Levenson, M. R. (2001). Stress, coping, and health at mid-life: A developmental perspective. In M. E. Lachman (Ed.), *The handbook of midlife development* (pp. 118–124). New York, NY: Wiley.

Aldwin, C. M., Spiro, A., & Levenson, M. R. (1989). Longitudinal findings from the normative aging study: Does mental health change with age? *Psychology and Aging, 4,* 295–306. doi: 10.1037/0882-7974.16.3.450

Allen, B. (2009). Are researchers ethically obligated to report suspected child maltreatment? A critical analysis of opposing perspectives. *Ethics & Behavior, 19,* 15–24. doi: 10.1080/10508420802623641

Allen, E. S., & Baucom, D. H. (2006). Dating, marital, and hypothetical extradyadic involvements: How do they compare? *The Journal of Sex Research, 43,* 307–317. doi: 10.1080/00224490609552330

Alley, D. E., Putney, N. M., Rice, M., & Bengtson, V. L. (2010). The increasing use of theory in social gerontology: 1990–2004. *The Journals of Gerontology Series B: Psychological Sciences and Social Science, 65B,* 583–590. doi: 10.1093/geronb/gbq053

Allport, G. W. (1961). *Pattern and growth in personality.* New York, NY: Holt, Rinehart & Winston.

Almeida, D. M., Neupert, S. D., Banks, S. R., & Serido, J. (2005). Do daily stress processes account for socioeconomic health disparities? *Journals of Gerontology: Social Sciences, 60B* (Special Issue II), 34–39. doi: 10.1093/geronb/60.Special_Issue_2

Alspaugh, P., & Birren, J. E. (1977). Variables affecting creative contributions across the life span. *Human Development, 20,* 240–248. doi: 10.1159/000271559

Alvarez, G., & Cavanagh, P. (2004). The capacity of visual short-term memory is set both by visual information load and by number of objects. *Psychological Science, 15,* 106–111. doi: 10.1111/j.0963 -7214.2004.01502006.x

Amato, P. R. (2000). The consequences of divorce for adults and children. *Journal of Marriage and Family, 62,* 1269–1287. doi: 10.1111/j.1741-3737.2000.01269.x

Amato, P. R. (2004). Tension between institutional and individual views of marriage. *Journal of Marriage and Family, 66,* 959–965. doi: 10.1111/j.0022-2445.2004.00065.x

Amato, P. R. (2007). Transformative processes in marriage: Some thoughts from a sociologist. *Journal of Marriage and the Family, 69,* 305–309. doi: 10.1111/j.1741-3737.2007.00365.x

Amato, P. R. (2010). Research on divorce: Continuing trends and new developments. *Journal of Marriage and Family, 72,* 650–666. doi: 10.1111/j.1741-3737.2010.00723.x

Amato, P. R., Booth, A., Johnson, D. R., & Rogers, S. J. (2007). *Alone together: How marriage in America is changing,* Cambridge, MA: Harvard University Press.

Amato, P. R., & DeBoer, D. D. (2001). The transmission of marital instability across generations: Relationship skills or commitment to marriage? *Journal of Marriage and Family, 63,* 1038–1051. doi: 10.1111/j.1741-3737.2001.01038.x

American Academy of Pediatrics. (2009a). Media violence. *Pediatrics, 124,* 1495–1503. doi: 10.1542/peds.2009-2146

American Academy of Pediatrics. (2009b). *Toilet training.* Elk Grove Village, IL: American Academy of Pediatrics.

American Academy of Pediatrics. (2011). *AAP expands guidelines for infant sleep safety and SIDS risk reduction.* Retrieved from rhttp:// www.aap.org/en-us/about-the-aap/aap-press-room/pages/AAP

-Expands-Guidelines-for-Infant-Sleep-Safety-and-SIDS-Risk-Reduction.aspx?nfstatus

American Academy of Pediatrics. (2012a). *Where we stand: Breastfeeding*. Retrieved from http://www.healthychildren.org/English/ages-stages/baby/breastfeeding/pages/Where-We-Stand-Breastfeeding.aspx

American Academy of Pediatrics. (2012b). *Benefits of breastfeeding for mom*. Retrieved from http://www.healthychildren.org/English/ages-stages/baby/breastfeeding/pages/Benefits of-Breastfeeding-for-Mom.aspx

American Academy of Pediatrics. (2012c). *Breastfeeding benefits your baby's immune system*. Retrieved from http://www.healthy-children.org/English/ages-stages/baby/breastfeeding/pages/Breastfeeding-Benefits-Your-Baby's-Immune-System.aspx

American Academy of Pediatrics. (2013). *Is vision screening needed in children under three?* Retrieved from http://www.aap.org/en-us/about-the-aap/aap-press-room/Pages/Is-Vision-Screening-Needed-in-Children-Under-Three.aspx

American Association for Pediatric Ophthalmology and Strabismus. (2013). *What is amblyopia?* Retrieved from http://www.aapos.org/terms/conditions/21

American Association on Intellectual and Developmental Disabilities (AAIDD). (2010). *Intellectual disability: Definition, classification, and systems of support* (11th ed.). Annapolis Junction, MD: Author.

American Cancer Society. (2011a). *Breast cancer*. Retrieved from http://www.cancer.org/Cancer/BreastCancer/DetailedGuide/breast-cancer-key-statistics

American Cancer Society. (2011b). *Prostate cancer*. Retrieved from http://www.cancer.org/Cancer/ProstateCancer/DetailedGuide/index

American Cancer Society. (2013). *Cancer figures and facts for African Americans 2013–2014*. Atlanta, GA: American Cancer Society.

American Congress of Obstetricians and Gynecologists. (2011). *2011 women's health: Stats and facts*. Retrieved from http://www.acog.org/~/media/NewsRoom/MediaKit.pdf

American Counseling Association (ACA). (2005). *American Counseling Association code of ethics*. Alexandria, VA: Author.

American Hair Loss Association. (2010a). *Men's hair loss*. Retrieved from http://www.americanhairloss.org/men_hair_loss/

American Hair Loss Association. (2010b). *Women's hair loss*. Retrieved from http://www.americanhairloss.org/women_hair_loss/

American Heart Association. (2007). *Physical activity improves quality of life*. Retrieved from http://www.heart.org/HEARTORG/GettingHealthy/PhysicalActivity/StartWalking/Physical-activity-improves-quality-of-life_UCM_307977_Article.jsp

American Heart Association. (2010). *Binge drinking increases death risk in men with high blood pressure*. Retrieved from http://www.newsroom.heart.org/index.php?s=43&item=1094

American Lung Association. (2011a). *About smoking*. Retrieved from http://www.lungusa.org/stop-smoking/about-smoking/

American Lung Association. (2011b). *Warning signs of lung disease*. Retrieved from http://www.lungusa.org/your-lungs/signs-of-lung-disease/

American Psychiatric Association. (2013). *Diagnostic and statistical manual of mental disorders* (5th ed.). Washington, DC: Author.

American Society for Reproductive Medicine (Producer). (2011). *Understanding fertility*. Retrieved from http://www.asrm.org/search/detail.aspx?id=2356&q=infertility

American Society of Plastic Surgeons. (2011). *2011 plastic surgery procedural statistics*. Retrieved from http://www.plasticsurgery.org/News-and-Resources/2011-Statistics-.html

American Speech-Language-Hearing Association. (2005). *Unsafe usage of portable music players may damage your hearing*. Retrieved from http://www.asha.org/about/news/atitbtot/mp3players.htm

American Speech-Language-Hearing Association. (2006). *ASHA to consumers: Save your hearing by lowering personal stereo system volume*. Retrieved from http://www.asha.org/about/news/atitbtot/stereo-vol-1-12-2006.htm

American Speech-Language-Hearing Association. (2013). *Self-test for hearing loss*. Retrieved from http://www.asha.org/public/hearing/Self-Test-for-Hearing-Loss/

Amsterdam, B. (1972). Mirror self-image reactions before age two. *Developmental Psychobiology, 5*, 297–305. doi: 10.1002/dev.420050403

Anaby, D., Miller, W. C., Eng, J. J., Jarus, T., & Noreau, L. (2011). Participation and well-being among older adults living with chronic conditions. *Social Indicators Research, 100*(1), 171–183. doi: 10.1007/s11205-010-9611-x

Andreoletti, C., Zebrowitz, L. A., & Lachman, M. E. (2001). Physical appearance and control beliefs in young, middle-aged, and older adults. *Personality & Social Psychology Review, 27*, 969–981. doi: 10.1177/0146167201278005

Ängarne-Lindberg, T., Wadsby, M., & Berterö, C. (2009). Young adults with childhood experience of divorce: Disappointment and contentment. *Journal of Divorce and Remarriage, 50*, 172–184. doi: 10.1080/10502550902717749

Antonucci, T. C., Akiyama, H., & Takahashi, K. (2004). Attachment and close relationships across the life span. *Attachment and Human Development, 6*, 353–370. doi: 10.1080/1461673042000303136

Appel, J. (2005). Defining death: When physicians and families differ. *Law, Ethics, and Medicine, 31*, 641–642. doi: 10.1186/1747-5341-2-27

Archambault, I., Eccles, J. S., & Vida, M. N. (2010). Ability self-concepts and subjective value in literacy: Joint trajectories from grades 1 through 12. *Journal of Educational Psychology, 102*, 804–816. doi: 10.1037/a0021075

Ardila, A., Rosselli, M., Matute, E., & Inozemtseva, O. (2011). Gender differences in cognitive development. *Developmental Psychology, 47*, 984–990.

Ardrey, R. (1976). *The hunting hypothesis*. New York, NY: Antheneum Press.

Aries, P. (1962). *Centuries of childhood: A social history of family life*. New York, NY: Vintage Books.

Armstrong, M. J. (2003). Is being a grandmother being old? Cross-ethnic perspectives from New Zealand. *Journal of Cross-Cultural Gerontology, 18*, 185–202. doi: 10.1023/B:JCCG.0000003089.53598.73

Arnett, J. J. (2004). *Emerging adulthood: The winding road from the late teens through the twenties*. New York, NY: Oxford University Press.

Arnett, J. J., & Tanner, J. L. (2006). *Emerging adults in America: Coming of age in the 21st century*. Washington, DC: American Psychological Association.

Aronson, K., Almeida, D. M., Stawski, R., Kline, L., & Kozlowski, L. T. (2008). Smoking is associated with worse mood on stressful days: Results of a national diary study. *Annals of Behavioral Medicine, 36*, 259–269. doi: 10.1007/s12160-008-9068-1

Asher, S. R., & Gottman, J. (Eds.) (1981). *The development of children's friendships*. New York, NY: Cambridge University Press.

Ashtari, M., Cervellione, K. L., Hasan, K. M., Wu, J., McIlree, C., Kester, H., . . . & Kumra, S. (2007). White matter development during late adolescence in healthy males: A cross-sectional diffusion tensor imaging study. *Neuroimage, 35,* 501–510. doi: 10.1016/j.neuroimage.2006.10.047

Association for Play Therapy. (2013). *Play therapy makes a difference.* Retrieved from http://www.a4pt.org/ps.index.cfm

Association for Spiritual, Ethical, and Religious Issues in Counseling (ASERVIC). (1995, December). Summit results in formation of spiritual competencies. *Counseling Today, 30.*

Association for Spiritual, Ethical, and Religious Values in Counseling. (2009). *Competencies for addressing spiritual and religious issues in counseling.* Retrieved from http://www.aservic.org/resources/spiritual-competencies/

Atchley, R. C. (1989). A continuity theory of normal aging. *The Gerontologist, 29*(2), 183–190. doi: 10.1093/geront/29.2.183

Atkins, D. C., & Furrow, J. (2008, November). *Infidelity is on the rise: But for whom and why?* Paper presented at the annual meeting of the Association for Behavioral and Cognitive Therapies, Orlando, FL.

Atwater, E. (1996). *Adolescence* (4th ed.). Upper Saddle River, NJ: Prentice Hall.

Aud, S., Kewal-Ramani, A., & Frohlich, L. (2011). *America's youth: Transition to adulthood.* Retrieved from http://nces.ed.gov/pubs2012/2012026.pdf

August, K. J., & Sorkin, D. H. (2011). Racial/Ethnic disparities in exercise and dietary behaviors of middle-aged and older adults. *Journal of General Internal Medicine, 26,* 245–250. doi: 10.1007/s11606-010-1514-7

Avolio, B. J., & Sosik, J. J. (1999). A life-span framework for assessing the impact of work on white-collar workers. In S. L. Willis & J. D. Reid (Eds.), *Life in the middle* (pp. 249–274). San Diego, CA: Academic Press.

Bada, H. S., Bann, C. M., Bauer, C. R., Shankaran, S., Lester, B., LaGasse, L., . . . & Higgins, R. (2011). Preadolescent behavior problems after prenatal cocaine exposure: Relationship between teacher and caretaker ratings (Maternal Lifestyle Study). *Neurotoxicology and Teratology, 33,* 77–87. doi: 10.1542/peds.2011-2209

Bahrick, L. E., & Lickliter, R. (2009). Perceptual development: Intermodal perception. In B. Goldstein (Ed.), *Encyclopedia of perception,* Vol. 2 (pp. 753–756). Newbury Park, CA: Sage Publishers.

Baillargeon, R., & DeVos, J. (1991). Object permanence in young infants: Further evidence. *Child Development, 62,* 1227–1246. doi: 10.2307/1130803

Bair, E. M., & Williams, J. (2007). Management of the third stage of labor. *Journal of Midwifery & Women's Health, 52,* 412–414. doi: 10.1016/j.jmwh.2007.02.019

Bale, R., Robertson, I., Leavitt, S., Loader, N., Harlan, T., Gagen, M., . . . & Froyd, C. A. (2010). Temporal stability in bristlecone pine tree-ring stable oxygen isotope chronologies over the last two centuries. *The Holocene, 20*(1), 3–6. doi: 10.1177/0959683609348867

Ball, T. M., & Wright, A. L. (1999). Health care costs of formula-feeding in the first year of life. *Pediatrics, 103,* 870–877.

Balter, L., & Tamis-LeMonda, C. S. (Eds.). (2006). *Child psychology: A handbook of contemporary issues* (2nd ed.). New York, NY: Taylor & Francis.

Baltes, B. B., & Dickson, M. W. (2001). Using life-span models in industrial-organizational psychology: The theory of selective optimization with compensation. *Applied Developmental Science, 5*(1), 51–62. doi: 10.1207/S1532480XADS0501_5

Baltes, M. M. (1996). *The many faces of dependency in old age.* New York, NY: Cambridge University Press.

Baltes, P. B. (1987). Theoretical propositions of life-span developmental psychology: On the dynamics between growth and decline. *Developmental Psychology, 23,* 611–626. doi: 10.1037/0012-1649.23.5.611

Baltes, P. B. (1997). On the incomplete architecture of human ontogeny: Selection, optimization, and compensation a foundation of developmental theory. *American Psychologist, 52,* 366–380. doi: 10.1037/0003-066X.52.4.366

Baltes, P. B. (2003). On the incomplete architecture of human ontogeny: Selection, optimization and compensation as foundation of developmental theory. In U. M. Staudinger & U. Lindenberger (Eds.), *Understanding human development: Dialogues with lifespan psychology* (pp. 17–43). Dordrecht, Netherlands: Kluwer Academic Publishers.

Bancroft, J., Loftus, J., & Long, J. S. (2003). Distress about sex: A national survey of women in heterosexual relationships. *Archives of Sexual Behavior, 32,* 193–208. doi: 10.1023/A:1023420431760

Bandura, A. (1977). *Social learning theory.* New York, NY: General Learning Press.

Bandura, A. (1986). *Social foundations of thought and action: A social cognitive theory.* Englewood Cliffs, NJ: Prentice-Hall.

Bandura, A. (1989). Social cognitive theory. In R. Vasta (Ed.), *Annals of child development,* Vol. 6: *Six theories of child development* (pp. 1–60). Greenwich, CT: JAI Press.

Bandura, A. (1991). Social cognitive theory of moral thought and action. In W. M. Kurtines & J. L. Gewirtz (Eds.), *Handbook of moral behavior and development,* Vol. 1 (pp. 45–103). Hillsdale, NJ: Erlbaum.

Bandura, A. (1994). Self-efficacy. In V. S. Ramachaudran (Ed.), *Encyclopedia of human behavior,* Vol. 4 (pp. 71–81). New York, NY: Academic Press.

Bandura, A. (2001). Social cognitive theory: An agentic perspective. *Annual Review of Psychology, 52,* 1–26. doi: 10.1146/annurev.psych.52.1.1

Bandura, A., Ross, D., & Ross, S. A. (1961). Transmission of aggression through imitation of aggressive models. *Journal of Abnormal and Social Psychology, 63,* 575–582. doi: 10.1037/h0045925

Bankart, C. P. (1997). *Talking cures: A history of western and eastern psychotherapies.* Pacific Grove, CA: Brooks/Cole.

Barak, Y., Heroman, W., & Tezel, T. (2012). The past, present and future of exudative age-related macular degeneration treatment. *Middle East African Journal of Ophthalmology, 19*(1), 43–51.

Barger, M. K. (2010). Maternal nutrition and perinatal outcomes. *Journal of Midwifery & Women's Health, 55,* 502–511. doi: 10.1016/j.jmwh.2010.02.017

Barkley, R. A. (2006). *Attention deficit hyperactivity disorder: A handbook for diagnosis and treatment.* New York, NY: Guilford.

Barkley, R. A. (2011). *The important role of executive functioning and self-regulation in ADHD.* Retrieved from http:/www.russellbarkley.org

Barnes, T. P., & Austin, A. M. B. (1995). The influence of parents and siblings on the development of a personal premise system in middle childhood. *Journal of Genetic Psychology, 156,* 73–85. doi: 10.1080/00221325.1995.9914807

Barnha, K. T. (2011). Epidemiology of male and female reproductive disorders and impact on fertility regulation and population growth. *Fertility and Sterility, 95,* 2200–2203. doi: 10.1016/j.fertnstert.2011.03.044

Barr, J. J. (2009). Key historical events in human growth and development. In American Counseling Association (Ed.),

The ACA encyclopedia of counseling (pp. 269–270). Alexandria, VA: American Counseling Association.

Barry, C. L., Carlson, M. D., Thompson, J. W., Schlesinger, M., McCorkle, R., Kasl, S., & Bradley, E. H. (2012). Caring for grieving family members: Results from a national hospice survey. *Medical Care, 50,* 578. doi: 10.1097/MLR.0b013e318248661d

Barsky, A. E. (2009). The legal and ethical context for knowing and using the latest child welfare research. *Child Welfare, 88,* 69–92.

Barth, R. (2009). Preventing child abuse and neglect with parent training: Evidence and opportunities. *The Future of Children, 19,* 95–118. doi: 10.1353/foc.0.0031

Bartzokis, G., Beckson, M., Lu, P. H., Nuechterlein, K. H., Edwards, N., & Mintz, J. (2001). Age-related changes in frontal and temporal lobe volumes in men: A magnetic resonance imaging study. *Archives of General Psychiatry, 58,* 461–465. doi: 10.1001/archpsyc.58.5.461

Bauer, I. (2001). *Diaper free! The gentle wisdom of natural infant hygiene.* Saltspring Island, BC, Canada: Natural Wisdom Press.

Baumrind, D. (1971). Current patterns of parental authority. *Developmental Psychology Monographs, 4*(1), 1–102. doi: 10.1037/h0030372

Baumrind, D. (1980). New directions in socialization research. *American Psychologist, 35,* 639–652. doi: 10.1037/0003-066X.35.7.639

Baumrind, D. (1996). The discipline controversy revisited. *Family Relations, 45,* 405–414. doi: 10.2307/585170

Bayley, N. (2005). *Bayley Scales of Infant and Toddler Development* (3rd ed.) [Bayley-III]. San Antonio, TX: Harcourt Assessment.

Bazelon, E. (2011). *Shaken-baby syndrome faces new questions in court.* Retrieved from http://www.nytimes.com/2011/02/06/magazine/06baby-t.html?pagewanted=all&_r=0

Beatty, B. (2009). Transitory connections: The reception and rejection of Jean Piaget's psychology in the nursery school movement in the 1920s and 1930s. *History of Education Quarterly, 49,* 442–464. doi: 10.1111/j.1748-5959.2009.00225.x

Beck, A. T. (1996). Beyond belief: A theory of modes, personality, and psychopathology. In P. Salkovskis (Ed.), *Frontiers of cognitive therapy* (pp. 1–25). New York, NY: Guilford.

Beck, A. T., Steer, R. A., & Brown, G. K. (1996). *Manual for the Beck Depression Inventory—Second Edition.* San Antonio, TX: Psychological Corporation.

Beck, A. T., & Weishaar, M. E. (2000). Cognitive therapy. In R. J. Corsini & D. Wedding (Eds.), *Current psychotherapies* (pp. 241–272). Istasca, IL: F. E. Peacock.

Beck, M. (2012). *Is baby too small? Charts make it hard to tell.* Retrieved from http://online.wsj.com/article/SB10000872396390443437504577544861908329668.html

Bedi, G., & Goddard, C. (2007). Intimate partner violence: What are the impacts on children? *Australian Psychologist, 42,* 66–77. doi: 10.1080/00050060600726296

Beechem, M. H., Anthony, C., & Kurtz, J. (1998). A life review interview guide: A structured systems approach to information gathering. *The International Journal of Aging & Human Development, 46*(1), 25–44. doi: 10.2190/NFNC-UNNL-5N5G-MQNY

Belenky, M. F., Bond, L. A., & Weinstock, J. S. (1997). *A tradition that has no name: Nurturing the development of people, families,* and *communities.* New York, NY: Basic Books.

Belloc, N., & Breslow, L. (1972). Relationship of physical health status and health practices. *Preventative Medicine, 1,* 409–421. doi: 10.1016/0091-7435(72)90014-X

Belsky, J. (1996). Parent, infant and social-contextual antecedents of father-son attachment security. *Developmental Psychology, 32,* 905–913.

Belsky, J. (2005). Attachment theory and research in ecological perspective. In K. E. Grossmann, K. Grossmann, & E. Waters (Eds.), *Attachment from infancy to adulthood: The major longitudinal studies* (pp. 71–97). New York, NY: Guilford.

Bem, S. L. (1993). *The lenses of gender: Transforming the debate on sexual inequality.* New Haven, CT: Yale University Press.

Bemak, F., Chung, R. C.-Y., & Murphy, C. S. (2003). A new perspective in counseling at-risk youth. In B. T. Erford (Ed.), *Transforming the school counseling profession* (pp. 285–296). Columbus, OH: Merrill Prentice Hall.

Bender, A., Spada, H., Rothe-Wulf, A., Traber, S., & Rauss, K. (2012). Anger elicitation in Tonga and Germany: The impact of culture on cognitive determinants of emotions. *Frontiers in Psychology, 3*(435), 1–20. doi: 10.3389

Bender, D. (2011). Bullying at school as a predictor of delinquency, violence and other anti-social behaviour in adulthood. *Criminal Behaviour & Mental Health, 21*(2), 99–106.

Benes, F. M., Turtle, M., Khan, Y., & Farol, P. (1994). Myelination of a key relay zone in the hippocampal formation occurs in the human brain during childhood, adolescence, and adulthood. *Archives of General Psychiatry, 51,* 477–484. doi: 10.1001/archpsyc.1994.03950060041004

Bennett, C. M., & Baird, A. A. (2006). Anatomical changes in the emerging adult brain: A voxel-based morphometry study. *Human Braining Mapping, 27,* 766–777. doi: 10.1002/hbm.20218

Berger, K. S. (2008). The *developing person through childhood and adolescence* (8th ed.). New York, NY: Worth.

Bergin, C. B., & Bergin, D. A. (2012). *Child and adolescent development in your classroom.* Belmont, CA: Wadsworth.

Berk, L. (2008). *Child development* (7th ed.). Boston, MA: Allyn & Bacon.

Berk, L. (2010). *Development through the lifespan* (5th ed.). Boston, MA: Pearson–Allyn & Bacon.

Bernert, R. A., Merrill, K. A., Braithwaite, S. R., Van Orden, K., & Joiner, T. E. (2007). Family life stress and insomnia symptoms in a prospective evaluation of young adults. *Journal of Family Psychology, 21,* 58–66. doi: 10.1037/0893-3200.21.1.58

Berscheid, E. (2010). Love in the fourth dimension. *Annual Review of Psychology, 61,* 1–25. doi: 10.1146/annurev.psych.093008.100318

Bettelheim, B. (2010). The *uses of enchantment: The meaning and importance of fairy tales.* New York, NY: Vintage.

Bhatia, K., Martindale, E. A., Rustamov, O., & Nysenbaum, A. M. (2009). Surrogate pregnancy: An essential guide for clinicians. *The Obstetrician & Gynaecologist, 11*(1), 49–54. doi: 10.1576/toag.11.1.49.27468

Bianchi, S. M., Milkie, M. A., Sayer, L. C., & Robinson, J. P. (2000). Is anyone doing the housework? Trends in the gender division of household labor. *Social Forces, 79,* 191–228. doi: 10.1093/sf/79.1.191

Bianchi, S. M., Robinson, J. P., & Milkie, M. A. (2006). *Changing rhythms of American family life.* New York, NY: Russell Sage.

Biblarz, T. J., & Stacey, J. (2010). How does the gender of parents matter? *Journal of Marriage and Family, 72,* 3–22. doi: 10.1111/j.1741-3737.2009.00678.x

Bifulco, A., Moran, P., Ball, C., & Bernazzoni, O. (2002). Adult attachment style, I: Its relationship to clinical depression. *Social Psychiatry and Psychiatric Epidemiology, 37,* 50–59. doi: 10.1007/s127-002-8215-0

Bigelow, A. E., MacLean, K., & Proctor, J. (2004). The role of joint attention in the development of infants' play with objects. *Developmental Science, 7,* 518–526. doi: 10.1111/j.1467-7687.2004.00375.x

Binet, A., & Simon, T. (1916). *The development of intelligence in children.* Baltimore, MD: Williams & Wilkins.

Bitter, J. R. (2009). *Theory and practice of family therapy and counseling.* Belmont, CA: Brooks/Cole.

Bjorkland, D. F., & Pelligrini, A. D. (2002). *The origins of human nature: Evolutionary developmental psychology.* Washington, DC: American Psychological Association.

Bjorvan, C., Eide, G. E., Hanestad, B. R., & Havik, O. E. (2008). Anxiety and depression among subjects attending genetic counseling for hereditary cancer. *Patient Education and Counseling, 71,* 234–243. doi: 10.1016/j.pec.2008.01.008

Blackwell, P. (2000). The influence of touch on child development: Implications for intervention. *Infants and Young Children, 13*(1), 25–39.

Blake, V., Joffe, S., & Kodish, E. (2011). Harmonization of ethics policies in pediatric research. *Journal of Law, Medicine & Ethics, 39,* 70–78. doi: 10.1111/j.1748-720X.2011.00551.x

Bleeker, M. M., & Jacobs, J. E. (2004). Achievement in math and science: Do mothers' beliefs matter 12 years later? *Journal of Educational Psychology, 96*(1), 97–109. doi: 10.1037/0022-0663.96.1.97

Blekesaune, M. (2008). Partnership traditions and mental distress: Investigating temporal order. *Journal of Marriage and Family, 70,* 879–890.

Bleyer, A., O'Leary, M., Barr, R., & Ries, L. A. G. (2006). *Cancer epidemiology in older adolescents and young adults 15 to 29 years of age, including SEER incidence and survival: 1975–2000.* National Cancer Institute, NIH Pub. No. 06-5767. Bethesda, MD: National Institutes of Health.

Blieszner, R. (2009). Who are the aging families? Aging families and caregiving. In S. H. Qualls & S. H. Zarit (Eds.), *Aging families and caregiving* (pp. 1–18). Hoboken, NJ: John Wiley & Sons Inc.

Blume, J. (1970). *Hello God, it's me Margaret.* Scarsdale, NY: Bradbury Press.

Blume, J. (1971). *Then again, maybe I won't.* Scarsdale, NY: Bradbury Press.

Boden, J. S., Fischer, J. L., & Niehuis, S. (2009). Predicting marital adjustment from young adults' initial levels and changes in emotional intimacy over time: A 25-year longitudinal study. *Journal of Adult Development, 17,* 121–134. doi: 10.1007/s10804-009-9078-7

Boersma, B., & Wit, J. M. (1997). Catch-up growth. *Endocrine Reviews, 18,* 646–661.

Bogins, S. (2000, December 1). Spiritual issues of palliative care. *Nursing Homes: Long Term Care Management 49,* 1–55.

Bohlmeijer, E., Roemer, M., Cuijpers, P., & Smit, F. (2007). The effects of reminiscence on psychological well-being in order adults: A meta-analysis. *Aging and Mental Health, 11,* 291–300. doi: 10.1080/13607860600963547

Bonanno, G. (2004). Loss, trauma, and human resilience: Have we underestimated the human capacity to thrive after extremely aversive events? *American Psychologist, 59,* 20–28. doi: 10.1037/0003-066X.59.1.20

Bonnel, S., Mohand-Said, S., & Sahel, J. A. (2003). The aging of the retina. *Experimental Gerontology, 38,* 825–831. doi: 10.1016/S0531-5565(03)00093-7

Borba, M. (2003). *No more misbehavin': 38 difficult behaviors and how to stop them.* San Francisco, CA: Jossey-Bass.

Borella, E., Carretti, B., & De Beni, R. (2007). Working memory training in older adults: Evidence of transfer and maintenance effects. *Psychology and Aging, 25,* 767–778. doi: 10.1037/a0020683

Bornstein, M. H., & Arterberry, M. E. (2010). The development of object categorization in young children: Hierarchical inclusiveness, age, perceptual attribute, and group versus individual analyses. *Developmental Psychology, 46,* 350–365. doi: 10.1037/a0018411

Bos, H. M. W., van Balen, F., & van den Boom, D. C. (2007). Child adjustment and parenting in planned lesbian-parent families. *American Journal of Orthopsychiatry, 77,* 38–48. doi: 10.1037/0002-9432.77.1.38

Bouchard, T. J., Jr., Lykken, D. T., McGue, M., Segal, N. L., & Tellegen, A. (1990). Sources of human psychological differences: The Minnesota study of twins reared apart. *Science, 250*(4978), 223–228. doi: 10.1126/science.2218526

Bowen, M. (1978). *Family therapy in clinical practice.* New York, NY: Aronson.

Bowker, J. C. W., Rubin, K. H., Burgess, K. B., Booth-LaForce, C., & Rose-Krasnor, L. (2006). Behavioral characteristics associated with stable and fluid best friendship patterns in middle childhood. *Merrill-Palmer Quarterly, 52,* 671–693. doi: 10.1353/mpq.2006.0000

Bowlby, J. (1969). *Attachment and loss: Attachment.* New York, NY: Basic Books.

Bowlby, J. (1973). *Attachment and loss,* Vol. 2: *Separation: Anxiety and anger.* New York, NY: Basic Books.

Bowlby, R. (2007). Babies and toddlers in non-parental daycare can avoid stress and anxiety if they develop a lasting secondary attachment bond with one carer who is consistently accessible to them. *Attachment & Human Development, 9,* 307–319. doi: 10.1080/14616730701711516

Boyer, W. (2009). Crossing the glass wall: Using preschool educators' knowledge to enhance parental understanding of children's self-regulation. *Early Childhood Education Journal, 37,* 175–182. doi: 10.1007/s10643-009-0343-y

Bradley, R. H. (2002). Environment and parenting. In M. H. Bornstein (Ed.), *Handbook of parenting,* Vol. 2: *Biology and ecology of parenting* (2nd ed., pp. 281–314). Mahwah, NJ: Erlbaum.

Bradshaw, Z., & Slade, P. (2003). The effects of induced abortion on emotional experiences and relationships: A critical review of the literature. *Clinical Psychology Review, 23,* 929–958. doi: 10.1016/j.cpr.2003.09.001

Bramlett, M. D., & Mosher, W. D. (2002). Cohabitation, marriage, divorce, and remarriage in the United States. *Vital Health Statistics,* Series 23, No. 22.

Brandl, B., Dyer, C., Heisler, C., Otto, J., Stiegel, L., & Thomas, R. (2007). *Elder abuse detection and intervention: A collaborative approach.* New York, NY: Springer Publishing.

Brant, A. M., Haberstick, B. C., Corley, R. P., Wadsworth, S. J., DeFries, J. C., & Hewitt, J. K. (2009). The developmental etiology of high IQ. *Behavior Genetics, 39,* 393–405. doi: 10.1007/s10519-009-9268-x

Brassard, M. R., & Boehm, A. E. (2007). *Preschool assessment: Principles and practices.* New York, NY: Guilford.

Braten, A. L., & Hulme, C. (2009). The cognitive and linguistic foundations of early reading development: A Norwegian latent variable longitudinal study. *Developmental Psychology, 45,* 764–781. doi: 10.1037/a0014132

Brazelton, T. B., & Nugent, J. K. (1995). *The Neonatal Behavioral Assessment Scale.* Cambridge, UK: Mac Keith Press.

Bridgett, D. J., Gartstein, M. A., Putnam, S. P., Oddi Lance, K., Iddins, E., Waits, R., VanVleet, J., & Lee, L. (2010). Emerging effortful control in toddlerhood: The role of infant orienting/regulation, maternal effortful control, and maternal time spent in caregiving activities. *Infant Behavior and Development, 34*(1), 189–199. doi: 10.1016/j.infbeh.2010.12.008

Broderick, P. C., & Blewitt, P. (2014). *The life span: Human development for helping professionals* (4th ed.). Upper Saddle River, NJ: Pearson.

Bronfenbrenner, U. (1977). Toward an experimental ecology of human development. *American Psychologist, 32,* 513–531. doi: 10.1037/0003-066X.32.7.513

Bronfenbrenner, U. (1978). *The ecology of human development.* Cambridge, MA: Harvard University Press.

Bronfenbrenner, U. (1994). Ecological models of human development. In M. Gauvain & M. Cole (Eds.), *Readings on the development of children* (2nd ed., pp. 37–43). New York, NY: Freeman.

Bronstein, P. (1988). Father-child interaction. In P. Bronstein & C. P. Cowan (Eds.), *Fatherhood today: Men's changing role in the family* (pp. 107–124). New York, NY: John Wiley.

Broude, G. J. (1995). *Growing up: A cross-cultural encyclopedia.* Santa Barbara, CA: ABC-CLIO.

Brown, S. L. (2010). Marriage and child well-being: Research and policy perspectives. *Journal of Marriage and Family, 72,* 1059–1077. doi: 10.111/j.1741-3737.2010.00750.x

Brown, W., Pfeiffer, K. A., McIver, K. L., Dowda, M., Addy, C. L., & Pate, R. R. (2009). Social and environmental factors associated with preschoolers non-sedentary physical activity. *Child Development, 80,* 45–58.

Browne, J. V. (2008). Chemosensory development in the fetus and newborn. *Newborn & Infant Nursing Reviews, 8*(4), 180–186. doi: 10.1053/j.nainr.2008.10.009

Brownridge, D. A. (2009). *Violence against women: Vulnerable populations.* New York, NY: Routledge.

Bruer, J. T. (2001). A critical and sensitive period primer. In D. B. Bailey, J. T. Bruer, F. J. Symons, & J. W. Lichtman (Eds.), *Critical thinking about critical periods: A series from the National Center for Early Development and Learning* (pp. 289–292). Baltimore, MD: Paul Brooks Publishing.

Bryson, K., & Casper, L. M. (1999). *Current population reports: Coresident grandparents* and grandchildren. U.S. Census Bureau, 23–198.

Bucciol, A., & Piovesan, M. (2011). Luck or cheating? A field experiment on honesty with children. *Journal of Economic Psychology, 32,* 73–78. doi: 10.1016/j.joep.2010.12.001

Buckley, T., Sunari, D., Marshall, A., Bartrop, R., McKinley, S., & Tofler, G. (2012). Physiological correlates of bereavement and the impact of bereavement interventions. *Dialogues in Clinical Neuroscience, 14*(2), 129.

Buder, M., & Evans, K. (2010). *The grace to race: The wisdom of the 80-year-old world champion triathlete known as the Iron Nun.* New York, NY: Simon and Shuster.

Budney, A. J., Hughes, J. R., Moore, B. A., & Vandrey, R. (2004). Review of the validity and significance of cannabis withdrawal syndrome. *American Journal of Psychiatry, 161,* 1967–1977. doi: 10.1016/j.jsat.2008.01.002

Budney, A. J., Vandrey, R. G., Hughes, J. R., Thostenson, J. D., & Bursac, Z. (2008). Comparison of cannabis and tobacco withdrawal: Severity and contribution to relapse. *Journal of Substance Abuse Treatment, 35,* 362–368. doi: 10.1016/j.drugalcdep.2011.06.003

Bühler, C. (1929). Jugendpsychologie und Schule. *Suddeneutscher Monatshefte, 27,* 186.

Bühler, C., & Allen, M. (1972). *Introduction to humanistic psychology.* Monterey, CA: Brooks/Cole Publishing Co.

Bulanda, J. R. (2011). Doing family, doing gender, doing religion: Structured ambivalence and the religion-family connection. *Journal of Family Theory and Review, 3,* 179–197.

Bumpass, L., & Lu, H. H. (2000). Trends in cohabitation and implications for children's family contexts in the United States. *Population Studies, 54,* 29–41. doi: 10.1080/713779060

Burchinal, M. R., Roberts, J. E., Riggins, R., Jr., & Zeisel, S. A. (2000). Relating quality of center-based child care to early cognitive and language development longitudinally. *Child Development, 71,* 339–357. doi: 10.1111/1467-8624.00149

Burgess, A., & Hanrahan, N. (2006). *Identifying forensic markers in elderly sexual abuse.* Washington, DC: National Institute of Justice.

Burke, M. T., Chauvin, J. C., & Miranti, J. G. (2005). *Religious and spiritual issues in counseling: Applications across diverse populations.* New York, NY: Brunner-Routledge.

Burne, A., & Carr, D. (2005). Caught in the cultural lag: The stigma of singlehood. *Psychological Inquiry, 16,* 84–141. doi: 10.1080/1047840X.2005.9682919

Burnham, S., & Arnold, M. (2000). I am somebody: Gang membership. In D. Capuzzi & D. Gross (Eds.), *Youth at risk: A prevention resource for counselors, teachers, and parents* (pp. 353–384). Alexandria, VA: American Counseling Association.

Bushway, L. J., Dickinson, J. L., Stedman, R. C., Wagenet, L. P., & Weinstein, D. A. (2011). Benefits, motivations, and barriers related to environmental volunteerism for older adults: Developing a research agenda. *International Journal of Aging and Human Development, 72,* 189–206. doi: 10.2190/AG.72.3.b

Butler, R. N. (1968). The life review: An interpretation of reminiscence in the aged. In B. L. Neugarten (Ed.), *Middle age and aging* (pp. 486–496). Chicago, IL: University of Chicago Press.

Buunk, B. (1980). Sexually open marriages: Ground rules for countering potential threats to marriage. *Journal of Family and Economic Issues, 3,* 312–328. doi: 10.1007/BF01083061

Buunk, B. (1981). Jealousy in sexually open marriages. *Journal of Family and Economic Issues, 4,* 357–372. doi: 10.1007/BF01257944

Byers, A., Levy, B., Allore, H., Bruce, M., & Kasl, S. (2008). When parents matter to their adult children: Filial reliance associated with parents' depressive symptoms. *Journal of Gerontology Series B, 63B,* 33–40.

Byock, I. (1997). *Dying well: The prospect for growth at the end of life.* New York, NY: Riverhead Books.

Cadwell, K. (2007). Latching-on and suckling of the healthy term neonate: Breastfeeding assessment. *Journal of Midwifery & Women's Health, 52,* 638–642. doi: 10.1016/j.jmwh.2007.08.004

Callahan, S. T., & Cooper, W. O. (2005). Uninsurance and health care access among young adults in the United States. *Pediatrics, 116,* 88–95. doi: 10.1542/peds.2004-1449

Calvete, E., Camara, M., Estevez, A., & Villardón, L. (2011). The role of coping with social stressors in the development of depressive symptoms: Gender differences. *Anxiety Stress Coping, 42*(4), 387–406. doi: 10.1080/10615806.2010.515982

Campos, J. J., & Stenberg, C. (1981). Perception, appraisal, and emotion: The onset of social referencing. In M. E. Lamb, & L. R. Sherrod (Eds.), *Infant social cognition: Empirical and theoretical considerations* (pp. 273–314). Hillsdale, NJ: Erlbaum.

Camras, L. A., Oster, H., Campos, J. J., & Bakeman, R. (2003). Emotional facial expressions in European-American, Japanese, and Chinese infants. *Annals of the New York Academy of Sciences, 1000*, 1–17. doi: 10.1196/annals.1280.007

Cansino, S., Guzzon, D., Martinelli, M., Barollo, M., & Casco, C. (2011). Effects of aging on interference control in selective attention and working memory. *Memory and Cognition, 39*, 1409–1422. doi: 10.3758/s13421-011-0109-9

Capone, N. C., & McGregor, K. K. (2005). The effect of semantic representation on toddlers' word retrieval. *Journal of Speech, Language, and Hearing Research, 48*, 1468–1480. doi: 10.1044/1092-4388(2005/102)

Capuzzi, D., & Gross, D. R. (Eds). (2004). *Youth at risk*. Alexandria, VA: American Counseling Association.

Carbery, J., & Buhrmester, D. (1998). Friendship and need fulfilment during three phases of young adulthood. *Journal of Social and Personal Relationships, 15*, 393–409. doi: 10.1177/0265407598153005

Career Vision. (2005). *Job satisfaction statistics*. Retrieved from http://www.careervision.org/about/pdfs/mr_jobsatisfaction.pdf

Carpenter, C., & Gates, G. J. (2008). Gay and lesbian partnership: Evidence from California. *Demography, 45*, 573–590.

Carter, B., & McGoldrick, M. (Eds.). (2005). *The expanded family life cycle: Individual, family, and social perspectives* (3rd ed.). Boston, MA: Allyn & Bacon.

Carver, P. R., Egan, S. K., & Perry, D. G. (2004). Children who question there heterosexuality. *Developmental Psychology, 40*(1), 43–53. doi: 10.1037/0012-1649.40.1.43

Caspi, A., Sugden, K., Moffitt, T. E., Taylor, A., Craig, I. W., Harrington, H., . . . & Poulton, R. (2003). Influence of life stress on depression: Moderation by a polymorphism in the 5-HTT gene. *Science, 301*, 386–389. doi: 10.1126/science.1083968

Cass, V. C. (1979). Homosexual identity formation: A theoretical model. *Journal of Homosexuality, 4*, 219–235. doi: 10.1080/00224498409551214

Cassidy, J. (1999). The nature of the child's ties. In J. Cassidy & P. Shaver (Eds.), *Handbook of attachment: Theory, research and clinical aspirations* (pp. 3–20). New York, NY: Guilford Press.

Cautilli, J. D., & Dziewolska, H. (2006). Brief report: The use of opportunity to respond and practice to increase efficiency of the stepping reflex in a five-month-old infant. *The Behavior Analyst Today, 7*, 538–547.

Centers for Disease Control and Prevention. (2004). *Smoking and tobacco use: Within 20 minutes of quitting*. Retrieved from http://www.cdc.gov/tobacco/data_statistics/sgr/2004/posters/20mins/index.htm

Centers for Disease Control and Prevention. (2008). *Use of mental health services in the past twelve months by children ages 4–17 years: United States, 2005–2006*. NCHS Data Brief No. 8. Retrieved from http://www.cdc.gov-nchs-data-databriefs.db08.pdf

Centers for Disease Control and Prevention. (2009). *Women's reproductive health: Hysterectomy*. Retrieved from http://www.cdc.gov/reproductivehealth/womensrh/hysterectomy.htm

Centers for Disease Control and Prevention. (2010a). *Cancer statistics by cancer type*. Retrieved from http://www.cdc.gov/cancer/dcpc/data/types.htm

Centers for Disease Control and Prevention. (2010b). *Child maltreatment*. Retrieved from http://www.cdc.gov/violenceprevention/pdf/CM-DataSheet-a.pdf

Centers for Disease Control and Prevention. (2010c). Vital signs: Current cigarette smoking among adults aged ≥ 18 years—United States, 2009. *Morbidity and Mortality Weekly Report, 59*(35), 1135–1140.

Centers for Disease Control and Prevention. (2010d). *WHO growth standards are recommended for use in the U.S. for infants and children 0 to 2 years of age*. Retrieved from http://www.cdc.gov/growthcharts/who_charts.htm

Centers for Disease Control and Prevention. (2011a). *Alcohol and public health: Fact sheets*. Retrieved from www.cdc.gov/alcohol/fact-sheets/alcohol-use.htm

Centers for Disease Control and Prevention. (2011b). *Health effects of cigarette smoking*. Retrieved from http://www.cdc.gov/tobacco/data_statistics/fact_sheets/health_effects/effects_cig_smoking/

Centers for Disease Control and Prevention. (2011c). *Heart disease fact sheet*. Retrieved from http://www.cdc.gov/heartdisease/

Centers for Disease Control and Prevention. (2011d). *Overweight and obesity: Data and statistics*. Retrieved from www.cdc.gov/obesity/data/index.html

Centers for Disease Control and Prevention. (2011e). *Smoking cessation*. Retrieved from http://www.cdc.gov/tobacco/data_statistics/fact_sheets/cessation/quitting/index.htm

Centers for Disease Control and Prevention. (2011f). *Workplace safety and health topics: Noise and hearing loss prevention*. Retrieved from http://www.cdc.gov/niosh/topics/noise/

Centers for Diseases Control and Prevention. (2011g). Contraceptive methods available to patients of office-based physicians and Title X clinics—United States, 2009–2010. *Morbidity and Mortality Weekly Report, 60*(1), 1–4.

Centers for Disease Control and Prevention. (2011h). *Addressing obesity in the childcare setting: Program highlights*. Retrieved from http://www.cdc.gov/obesity/downloads/obesity_program_highlights.pdf

Centers for Disease Control and Prevention. (2011i). *Recommended immunization schedule for persons age 0–6 years—United States 2011*. Retrieved from http://www.cdc.gov/vaccines/recs/schedules/downloads/child/0-6yrs-schedule-bw.pdf

Centers for Disease Control and Prevention. (2011j). *Vision impairment*. Retrieved from http://www.cdc.gov/ncbddd/dd/ddvi.htm

Centers for Disease Control and Prevention. (2011k). *HIV among youth*. Retrieved from http://www.cdc.gov/hiv/youth/pdf/youth.pdf

Centers for Disease Control and Prevention. (2012a). *Prostate cancer screening: A decision guide*. Retrieved from http://www.cdc.gov/cancer/prostate/informed_decision_making.htm

Centers for Disease Control and Prevention. (2012b). Estimated HIV incidence in the United States, 2007–2010. *HIV Surveillance Supplemental Report, 17*(4), 1–25. doi: 10.1056/NEJMsa042088

Centers for Disease Control and Prevention. (2012c). *Sudden unexpected infant death (SUID)*. Retrieved from http://www.cdc.gov/sids/

Centers for Disease Control and Prevention. (2014). *Depression in the U.S. household population, 2009–2012*. Retrieved from http://www.cdc.gov/nchs/data/databriefs/

Cevenini, E., Bellavista, E., Tieri, P., Castellani, G., Lescai, F., France!sconi, M., . . . & Franceschi, C. (2010). Systems biology and longevity: An emerging approach to identify innovative anti-aging targets and strategies. *Current Pharmaceutical Design, 16*, 802–813. doi: 10.2174/138161210790883660

Chairney, J., Boyle, M., Offord, D. R., & Racine, Y. (2003). Stress, social support, and depression in single and married mothers.

Social Psychiatry and Psychiatric Epidemiology, 38, 442–449. doi: 10.1007/s00127-003-0661-0

Chalmers, B., Kaczorowski, J., Darling, E., Heaman, M., Fell, D. B., O'Brien, B., & Lee, L. (2010). Cesarean and vaginal birth in Canadian women: A comparison of experiences. *Birth Issues in Prenatal Care, 37,* 44–49. doi: 10.1111/j.1523-536X.2009.00377.x

Chancey, L. (2006). Voluntary childlessness in the United States: Recent trends by cohort and period. Unpublished thesis, Louisiana State University, Baton Rouge, LA.

Chang, R. S., & Thompson, N. S. (2010). The attention-getting capacity of whines and child-directed speech. *Evolutionary Psychology, 8,* 260–274.

Chang, R. S., & Thompson, N. S. (2011). Whines, cries and motherese: Their relative power to distract. *Journal of Social, Evolutionary, and Cultural Psychology, 5*(2), 10–20. doi: 10.1037/h0099270

Chanrachakul, B., & Herabuya, Y. (2003). Postterm with favorable cervix: Is induction necessary? *European Journal of Obstetrics & Gynecology and Reproductive Biology, 106,* 154–157. doi: 10.1016/S0301-2115(02)00243-9

Chao, R. (1994). Beyond parental control: Authoritarian parenting styles: Understanding Chinese parenting through the cultural notion of training. *Child Development, 45,* 1111–1119. doi: 10.1111/j.1467-8624.1994.tb00806.x

Chao, R. (2001). Extending research on the consequences of parenting style for Chinese-Americans and European-Americans. *Child Development, 72,* 1832–1843. doi: 10.1111/1467-8624.00381

Chapin, L. A., & Yang, R. K. (2009). Perceptions of social support in urban at-risk boys and girls. *Journal of At-Risk Issues, 15,* 1–7.

Chapman, B. P., Duberstein, P. R., Sörensen, S., & Lyness, J. M. (2007). Gender differences in Five Factor Model personality traits in an elderly cohort. *Personality and Individual Differences, 43,* 1594–1603. doi: 10.1016/j.paid.2007.04.028

Charlesworth, W. R. (1992). Darwin and developmental psychology: Past and present. *Developmental Psychology, 28,* 5–16. doi: 10.1037/0012-1649.28.1.5

Charness, N., & Bosman, E. A. (1990). Expertise and aging: Life in the lab. In T. H. Hess (Ed.), *Aging and cognition: Knowledge organization and utilization* (pp. 343–385). Amsterdam, Netherlands: Elsevier.

Charny, I. W., & Parnass, S. (1995). The impact of extramarital relationships on the continuation of marriages. *Journal of Sex & Marital Therapy, 21,* 100–115. doi: 10.1080/00926239508404389

Chaves, A. P., Diemer, M. A., Blustein, D. L., Gallagher, L. A., DeVoy, J. E., Casares, M. T., & Perry, J. C. (2004). Conceptions of work: The view from urban youth. *Journal of Counseling Psychology, 51,* 275–286. doi: 10.1037/0022-0167.51.3.275

Chen, K., Kandel, D. B., & Davies, M. (1997). Relationships between frequency and quantity of marijuana use and last year proxy dependence among adolescents and adults in the United States. *Drug and Alcohol Dependency, 46,* 53–67. doi: 10.1016/S0376-8716(97)00047-1

Chess, S., & Thomas, A. (1996). *Temperament: Theory and practice.* New York, NY: Brunner/Mazel.

Chickering, A. W. (1969). *Education and identity.* San Francisco, CA: Jossey-Bass.

Chickering, A. W., & Reisser, L. (1993). *Education and identity* (2nd ed.). San Francisco, CA: Jossey-Bass.

Child Welfare Information Gateway. (2007). *Recognizing child abuse and neglect: Signs and symptoms.* Retrieved from http://www.childwelfare.gov/pubs/factsheets/signs.cfm

Children of Alcoholic Families. (2011). *How many COAs are there?* Retrieved from http://www.coaf.org/researchlinks/numbers.htm

Ching-Yun, Y., Chich-Hsiu, H., Te-Fu, C., Ching-Hsueh, Y., & Chien-Yu, L. (2012). Prenatal predictors for father-infant attachment after childbirth. *Journal of Clinical Nursing, 21,* 1577–1583. doi: 10.1111/j.1365-2702.2011.04003.x

Chodorow, N. (1978). *The reproduction of mothering.* Berkeley, CA: University of California Press.

Chodorow, N. (1994). *Femininities, masculinities, sexualities: Freud and beyond.* Lexington, KY: University of Kentucky Press.

Choi, S., & Gopnik, A. (1995). Early acquisition of verbs in Korean: A cross-linguistic study. *Journal of Child Language, 22,* 497–529. doi: 10.1017/S0305000900009934

Chomsky, N. (1968). *Language and mind.* New York, NY: Harcourt, Brace & World.

Christensen, K., Doblhammer, G., Rau, R., & Vaupel, J. (2009). Ageing populations: The challenges ahead. *Lancet, 374*(9696), 1196–1208. doi: 10.1016/S0140-6736(09)61460-4

Chu, S. Y., Barber, L. E., & Smith, P. J. (2004). Racial/ethnic disparities in preschool immunizations. United States—1996–2001. *American Journal of Public Health, 94,* 973–977. doi: 10.2105/AJPH.94.6.973

Ciaramelli, E., Muccioli, M., Ladavas, E., & di Pellegrino, G. (2007). Selective deficit in personal moral judgment following damage to ventromedial prefrontal cortex. *Social Cognitive and Affective Neuroscience, 2,* 84–92. doi: 10.1093/scan/nsm001

Ciarocchi, J. (2009). *The doubting disease: Help for scrupulosity and religious compulsions.* Mahwah, NJ: Paulist Press.

Cicourel, A. V. (1974). *Theory and method in a study of Argentine fertility.* New York, NY: Wiley.

Clarke-Steart, A., & Allhusen, V. (2005). *What we know about childcare.* Cambridge, MA: Harvard University Press

Clasien De Schipper, J., Tavecchio, L. W. C., & Van IJzendoorn, M. H. (2008). Children's attachment relationships with day care caregivers: Associations with positive caregiving and the child's temperament. *Social Development, 17,* 454–470. doi: 10.1111/j.1467-9507.2007.00448.x

Clay, A. R. (2006). Battling the self-blame of infertility: The frustration of infertility. *Monitor on Psychology, 37*(8), 44–45.

Clay, O., Edwards, J., Ross, L. Okonkwo, O., Wadley, V., Roth, D., & Ball, K. (2009). Visual function and cognitive speed of processing mediate age-related decline in memory span and fluid intelligence. *Journal of Aging & Health, 21,* 547–566. doi: 10.1177/0898264309333326

Cleland, J., Bernstein, S., Ezeh, A., Faundes, A., Glasier, A., & Inni, J. (2006). Family planning: The unfinished agenda. *The Lancet, 368,* 1810–1827. doi: 10.1016/S0140-6736(06)69480-4

Clements, M. L., Stanley, S. M., & Markman, H. J. (2004). Before they said "I do": Discriminating among marital outcomes over 13 years based on premarital data. *Journal of Marriage and Family, 66,* 613–626. doi: 10.1111/j.0022-2445.2004.00041.x

Cobb, N. J. (2001). *The child: Infants, children, and adolescents.* Mountain View, CA: Mayfield.

Cocke, A. (2002). *Brain may also pump up from workout.* Retrieved from http://www.neurosurgery.medsch.ucla.edu/whastnew/societyforneuroscience.htm

Cohany, S. R., & Sok, E. (2007). Trends in labor force participation of married mothers of infants. *Monthly Labor Review, 130,* 9–16.

Cohen, C. (2012). Bioethicists must rethink the concept of death: The idea of brain death is not appropriate for cryopreservation. *Clinics, 67*(2), 93–94. doi: http://dx.doi.org/10.6061/clinics/2012(02)01

Colby, A., & Kohlberg, L. (1987). *The measurement of moral judgment: Theoretical foundations and research validation,* Vol. 1. Cambridge, MA: Cambridge University Press.

Coleman, M., Ganong, L., & Rothrauff, T. (2006). Racial and ethnic similarities and differences in beliefs about intergenerational assistance to older adults after divorce and remarriage. *Family Relation, 55,* 576–587. doi: 10.1111/j.1741-3729.2006.00427.x

Coles, R. (1977). *Children of crisis.* Boston, MA: Little, Brown.

Collins, W. A., & van Dulmen, M. (2006). Friendships and romance in emerging adulthood: Assessing distinctiveness in close relationships. In J. J. Arnett & J. L. Tanner (Eds.), *Emerging adults in America: Coming of age in the 21st century* (pp. 219–234). Washington, DC: American Psychological Association.

Connor, S. (2006). Grandparents raising grandchildren: Formation, disruption and intergenerational transmission of attachment. *Australian Social Work, 59,* 172–184. doi: 10.1080/03124070600651887

Consedine, N. S., & Fiori, K. L. (2009). Gender moderates the associations between attachment and discrete emotions in middle age and later life. *Aging and Mental Health, 13,* 847–862.

Considine, J., & Miller, K. (2010). The dialectics of care: Communicative choices at the end of life. *Health Communications, 25,* 165–174. doi: 10.1080/10410230903544951

Cooney, C., Howard, R., & Lawlor, B. (2006). Abuse of vulnerable people with dementia by their caregivers: Can we identify those most at risk? *International Journal of Geriatric Psychiatry, 21,* 564–571. doi: 10.1002/gps.1525

Coontz, S. (2006). *Marriage, a history: From obedience to intimacy, or how love conquered marriage.* New York, NY: Viking.

Cooper, C., Dere, W., Evans, W., Kanis, J. A., Rizzoli, R., Sayer, A. A., . . . & Reginster, J. Y. (2012). Frailty and sarcopenia: Definitions and outcome parameters. *Osteoporosis International, 23,* 1839–1848.

Cooper, C., Selwood, A., & Livingston, G. (2008). The prevalence of elder abuse and neglect: A systematic review. *Age and Ageing, 37,* 151–160. doi: 10.1093/ageing/afm194

Cooper, M. J. (2002). Alcohol use and risky sexual behavior among college students and youth: Evaluating the evidence. *Journal of Studies on Alcohol, 14,* 101–117.

Corey, G. (2012). *Theory and practice of counseling and psychotherapy* (9th ed.). Belmont, CA: Brooks/Cole.

Corrigan, P. W. (2007). How clinical diagnosis might exacerbate the stigma of mental illness. *Social Work, 52,* 31–39. doi: 10.1093/sw/52.1.31

Corsaro, W. A. (1979). "We're friends, right?": Children's use of access rituals in a nursery school. *Language in Society, 8,* 315–336. doi: 10.1017/S0047404500007570

Corsaro, W. A. (1981). Friendship in the nursery school: Social organization in a peer environment. In S. R. Asher & J. Gottman (Eds.), *The development of children's friendships* (pp. 207–241). New York, NY: Cambridge University Press.

Corsaro, W. A. (1985). *Friendship and peer culture in the early years.* Norwood, NJ: Ablex.

Corsaro, W. A., & Eder, D. (1990). Children's peer cultures. *Annual Review of Sociology, 16,* 197–220. doi: 10.1146/annurev.so.16.080190.001213

Costa, P., Jr., & McCrae, R. R. (2006). Age changes in personality and their origins: Comment on Roberts, Walton, and Viechtbauer (2006). *Psychological Bulletin, 132,* 26–28. doi: 10.1037/0033-2909.132.1.26

Costa, P., Terracciano, A., & McCrae, R. R. (2001). Gender differences in personality traits across cultures: Robust and surprising findings. *Journal of Personality and Social Psychology, 81,* 322–331. doi: 10.1037/0022-3514.81.2.322

Couchenour, D., & Chrisman, K. (2011). *Families, schools, and communities: Together for young children* (4th ed.). Belmont, CA: Cengage.

Cowan, N., Morey, C. C., AuBuchon, A. M., Zwilling, C. E., & Gilchrist, A. L. (2010). Seven-year-olds allocate attention like adults unless working memory is overloaded. *Developmental Science, 13*(1), 120–133. doi: 10.1111/j.1467-7687.2009.00864.x

Cozier, Y. C., Yu, J., Coogan, P. F., Bethea, T. N., Rosenberg, L., & Palmer, J. R. (2014). Racism, segregation, and risk of obesity in the Black women's health study. *American Journal of Epidemiology.* doi: 10.1093/aje/kwu004

Cozolino, L. (2006). *The neuroscience of human relationships: Attachment and the developing social brain.* New York, NY: Norton.

Crandell, T. L., Crandell, C. H., & VanderZanden, J. W. (2009). *Human development* (9th ed.). Boston, MA: McGraw-Hill.

Cree, L. M., Samuels, D. C., & Chinnery, P. F. (2009). The inheritance of pathogenic mitochondrial DNA mutations. *Biochimica et Biophysica Acta, 1792,* 1097–1102. doi: 10.1016/j.bbadis.2009.03.002

Crenshaw, K. W. (1989). Demarginalizing the intersection of race and sex: A Black feminist critique of antidiscrimination doctrine, feminist theory and antiracist politics. *University of Chicago Legal Forum, 1989,* 139–167.

Criss, M. M., Shaw, D. S., Moilanen, K. L., Hitchings, J. E., & Ingoldsby, E. M. (2009). Family, neighborhood, and peer characteristics as predictors of child adjustment: A longitudinal analysis of additive and mediation models. *Social Development, 18,* 511–535. doi: 10.1111/j.1467-9507.2008.00520.x

Cross, W. E. (1971). The Negro-to-Black conversion experience. *Black World, 20,* 13–27.

Cross, W. E. (1995). The psychology of Nigrescence. In J. G. Ponterotto, J. M Casas, L. A. Suzuki, & C. M. Alexander (Eds.) *Handbook of multicultural counseling* (pp. 93–122). Thousand Oaks, CA: Sage.

Cross, W. E., Parham, T. A., & Helms, J. E. (1991). The stages of Black identity development: Nigrescence models. In R. L. Jones (Ed.), *Black psychology* (3rd ed., pp. 319–338). Hampton, VA: Cobb & Henry.

Crowe, H. P., & Zeskind, P. S. (1992). Psychophysiological and perceptual responses to infant cries varying in pitch: Comparison of adults with low and high scores on the Child Abuse Potential Inventory. *Child Abuse and Neglect, 16,* 16–29.

Crowne, D. P., & Marlowe, D. (1960). A new scale of social desirability independent of psychopathology. *Journal of Consulting Psychology, 24,* 349–354. doi: 10.1037/h0047358

Csikszentmihalyi, M. (2000). *Beyond boredom and anxiety.* San Francisco, CA: Jossey-Bass.

Cumming, E., & Henry, W. E. (1961). *Growing old.* New York, NY: Basic Books.

Cummings, J., Lee, J., & Kraut, R. (2006). Communication technology and friendship during the transition from high school to college. In R. E. Kraut, M. Brynin, & S. Kiesler (Eds.), *Computers, phones, and the Internet: Domesticating information technology* (pp. 265–278). New York, NY: Oxford University Press.

Cunningham, H. (1995). *Children and childhood in Western society since 1500.* London, UK: Longman.

Cwikel, J., Gramotnev, H., & Lee, C. (2006). Never married childless women in Australia: Health and social circumstances in older age. *Social Science & Medicine, 62,* 1991–2001. doi: 10.1016/j.socscimed.2005.09.006

Dacey, J. S., & Travers, J. F. (2006). *Human development over the lifespan* (6th ed.). New York, NY: McGraw-Hill.

Dacey, J., Travers, J., & Fiore, L. (2009). *Human development across the lifespan* (7th ed.). Boston, MA: McGraw-Hill.

Daniels, J. (1995). Homeless students: Recommendations to school counselors based on semistructured interviews. *School Counselor, 42,* 346–352. doi: 10.1016/S0190-7409(01)00176-1

Darwin, C. (1869). *On the origin of species by means of natural selection or the preservation of favoured races in the struggle for life* (5th ed). Retrieved from http://darwin-online.org.uk/content/frameset?itemID=F387&viewtype=text&pageseq=1

Davanzo, R. (2004). Newborns in adverse conditions: Issues, challenges, and interventions. *Journal of Midwifery & Women's Health, 49,* 29–35. doi: 10.1016/j.jmwh.2004.05.002

David, A., & Zimmerman, M. (2010). Cancer: An old disease, a new disease or something in between? *Nature Reviews Cancer, 10,* 728–733. doi: 10.1038/nrc2914

Daviglus, M. L., Bell, C. C., Berrettini, W., Bowen, P. E., Connolly, E. S., Cox, N. J., . . . & Trevisan, M. (2010). National Institutes of Health State-of-the-Science Conference statement: Preventing Alzheimer disease and cognitive decline. *Annals of Internal Medicine, 153,* 176–181. doi: 10.7326/0003-4819-153-3-201008030-0026

Davis, C. G., & Asliturk, E. (2011). Toward a positive psychology of coping with anticipated events. *Canadian Psychology, 52,* 101–110. doi: 10.1037/a0020177

Davis, E. P., & Sandman, C. A. (2010). The timing of prenatal exposure to maternal cortisol and psychosocial stress is associated with human infant cognitive development. *Child Development, 81,* 131–148. doi: 10.1111/j.1467-8624.2009.01385.x

Deary, I. J., Spinath, F. M., & Bates, T. C. (2006). Genetics of intelligence. *European Journal of Human Genetics, 14,* 690–700. doi: 10.1038/sj.ejhg.5201588

Deary, I. J., Whiteman, M. C., Starr, J. M., Whalley, L. J., & Fox, H. C. (2004). The impact of childhood intelligence on later life: Following up the Scottish mental surveys of 1932 and 1947. *Journal of Personality and Social Psychology, 86,* 130–147. doi: 10.1037/0022-3514.86.1.130

DeBeauvoir, S. (1972). *The second sex.* New York, NY: Penguin Books.

DeBoulay, S. (1984). *Cicely Saunders: Founder of the modern hospice movement.* London, UK: Hodder and Stoughton.

DeCasper, A. J., Lecanuet, J., Busnel, M., & Granier-Deferre, C. (1994). Fetal reactions to recurrent maternal speech. *Infant Behavior and Development, 17,* 159–164. doi: 10.1016/0163-6383(94)90051-5

Degges-White, S. (2005). Understanding gerotranscendence in older adults: A new perspective for counselors. *Adultspan, 4*(1), 36–48. doi: 10.1002/j.2161-0029.2005.tb00116.x

DeKlyen, M., Brooks-Gunn, J., McLanahan, S., & Knab, J. (2006). The mental health of married, cohabiting, and non-coresident parents with infants. *American Journal of Public Health, 96,* 1836–1841. doi: 10.2105/AJPH.2004.049296

Delany, S., Delany, E., & Hearth, A. (1993). *Having our say: The Delany sisters' first 100 years.* New York, NY: Kodansha International.

Deleire, T., & Kalil, A. (2003). Good things come in threes: Single-parent multigenerational family structure and adolescent adjustment. *Demography, 39,* 393–413. doi: 10.1353/dem.2002.0016

Dell'Antonia, K. J. (2013). *The A.A.P. has a new vaccine schedule. Will you follow it?* Retrieved from http://parenting.blogs.nytimes.com/2013/01/29/theres-a-new-vaccine-schedule-will-you-follow-it/

Demerath, E., Jones, L., Hawley, N., Norris, S., Pettifor, J., Duren, D., Chumlea, W. C., & Towne, B. (2009). Rapid infant weight gain and advanced skeletal maturation in childhood. The *Journal of Pediatrics, 155,* 355–361. doi: 10.1016/j.jpeds.2009.03.016

Demo, D. H., & Fine, M. A. (2010). *Beyond the average divorce.* Thousand Oaks, CA: Sage.

Dempsey, A. G., & Storch, E. A. (2010). Psychopathology and health problems affecting involvement in bullying. In E. M. Vernberg, & B. K. Biggs (Eds.). *Preventing and treating bullying and victimization* (pp. 107–131). New York, NY: Oxford University Press.

Denham, S. A., Blair, K. A., DeMulder, E., Levitas, J., Sawyer, K. Auerbach-Major, S., & Queenan, P. (2003). Preschool emotional competence: Pathway to social competence. *Child Development, 74,* 238–256. doi: 10.1111/1467-8624.00533

Deoni, S. L., Mercure, E., Blasi, A., Gasston, D., Thomson, A., Johnson, M., & Murphy, D. M. (2011). Mapping infant brain myelination with magnetic resonance imaging. *The Journal of Neuroscience, 31,* 784–791. doi: 10.1523/JNEUROSCI.2106-10.2011

DePaulo, B. (2006). *Singled out: How singles are stereotyped, stigmatized, and ignored, and still live happily ever after.* New York, NY: St. Martin's Press.

De Raad, B., & Doddema-Winsemius, M. (1992). Factors in the assortment of human mates: Differential preferences in Germany and the Netherlands. *Personality and Individual Differences, 13,* 103–114. doi: 10.1016/0191-8869(92)90226-F

Dermody, S. S., Marshal, M. P., Cheong, J. W., Burton, C., Hughes, T., Aranda, F., & Friedman, M. S. (2013). Longitudinal disparities of hazardous drinking between sexual minority and heterosexual individuals from adolescence to young adulthood. *Journal of Youth and Adolescence, 43,* 30–39. doi: 10.1007/s10964-013-9905-9

Derobertis, E. M. (2006). Charlotte Buhler's existential-humanistic contributions to child and adolescent psychology. *Journal of Humanistic Psychology, 46,* 48–76. doi: 10.1177/0022167805277116

Derryberry, D., & Reed, M. A. (1996). Regulatory processes and the development of cognitive representations. *Development and Psychopathology, 8,* 215–234. doi: 10.1017/S0954579400007057

Dias, M. S., Smith, K., deGuehery, K., Mazur, P., Li, V., & Shaffer, M. L. (2005). Preventing abusive head trauma among infants and young children: A hospital-based, parent education program. *Pediatrics, 115,* 470–477. doi: 10.1542/peds.2004-1896

DiFranza, J. R., Rigotti, N. A., McNeill, A. D., Ockene, J. K., Savageau, J. A., Cyr, D. S., & Coleman, M. (2000). Initial symptoms of nicotine dependence in adolescents. *Tobacco Control, 9,* 313–319. doi: 10.1136/tc.9.3.313

DiFranza, J. R., Savageau, J. A., Fletcher, K., O'Loughlin, J., Pbert, L., Ockene, J. K., . . . & Wellman, R. J. (2007). Symptoms of tobacco dependence after brief intermittent use: The development and assessment of nicotine dependence in youth-2 study. *Archives of Pediatrics & Adolescent Medicine, 16,* 704–710. doi:10.1001/archpedi.161.7.704

DiLeo, H. A., Reiter, R. J., & Taliaferro, D. H. (2002). Chronobiology, melatonin, and sleep in infants and children. *Pediatric Nursing, 28*(1), 35–39. doi: 35400010030667.0040

Dilworth-Bart, J. E., & Moore, C. F. (2006). Mercy mercy me: Social injustice and the prevention of environmental pollutant exposures among ethnic minority and poor children. *Child Development, 77,* 247–265. doi: 10.1111/j.1467-8624.2006.00868.x

Dinkmeyer, D., Jr., & Carlson, J. (2001). *Consultation creating school based interventions* (2nd ed.). Philadelphia, PA: Brunner-Routledge.

Dinkmeyer, D. C., & McKay, G. D. (1989). *STEP: The parent's handbook.* Circle Pines, MN: American Guidance Service.

DiPietro, J. A., Costigan, K. A., & Pressman, E. K. (2002). Fetal state concordance predicts infant state regulation. *Early Human Development, 68,* 1–13. doi: 10.1016/S0378-3782(02)00006-3

Dixon, A. L. (2007). Mattering in the later years: Older adults' experiences of mattering to others, purpose in life, depression, and wellness. *Adultspan: Theory Research & Practice, 6*(2), 83–95. doi: 10.1002/j.2161-0029.2007.tb00034.x

Dixon, R. A., De Frias, C. M., & Maitland, S. B. (2001). Memory in midlife. In M. E. Lachman (Ed.), *Handbook of midlife development* (pp. 248–278). New York, NY: Wiley.

Dobbs, D., Emmett, C. P., Hammarth, A., & Daaleman, T. P. (2012). Religiosity and death attitudes and engagement of advance care planning among chronically ill older adults. *Research on Aging, 34*(2), 113–130. doi: 10.1177/0164027511423259

Dodge, K. A. (1983). Behavioral antecedents of peer social status. *Child Development, 54,* 1386–1399. doi: 10.1177/0164027511423259

Dohm, A. (2000). Gauging the labor force effects of retiring baby-boomers. *Monthly Labor Review, 17,* 17–25.

Dolan, M. A., & Hoffman, C. D. (1998). Determinants of divorce among women: A reexamination of critical influences. *Journal of Divorce and Remarriage, 28,* 97–106. doi: 10.1300/J087v28n03_05

Dolbin-MacNab, M. L., & Keiley, M. K. (2006). A systemic examination of grandparents' emotional closeness with their custodial grandchildren. *Research in Human Development, 3*(1), 59–71. doi:10.1207/s15427617rhd0301_6

Dollard, J., & Miller, N. (1950). *Personality and psychotherapy: An analysis in terms of learning, thinking, and culture.* New York, NY: McGraw-Hill.

Dong, X. (2014). Elder abuse: Research, practice, and health policy. The 2012 GSA Maxwell Pollack award lecture. *The Gerontologist, 44*(2), 153–162. doi: 10.1093/geront/gnt 139

Donley, M. G., & Likins, L. (2010). The multigenerational impact of sibling relationships. *The American Journal of Family Therapy, 38,* 383–396. doi: 10.1080/01926187.2010.513905

Dooley, C. M. (2010). Young children's approaches to books: The emergence of comprehension. *Reading Teacher, 64,* 120–130. doi: 10.1598/RT.64.2.4

Dooley, E. (2014). *George H. W. Bush marks 90th birthday by skydiving.* ABC News, June 12. Retrieved from http://abcnews.go.com/Politics/george-bush-marks-90th-birthday-skydiving/story?id=24103264

Downing, N. E., & Roush, K. L. (1985). From passive acceptance to active commitment: A model of feminist identity development for women. *The Counseling Psychologist, 13,* 695–709. doi: 10.1177/0011000085134013

Downing, P. (2000). Interactions between visual working memory and selective attention. *Psychological Science, 11,* 467–473. doi: 10.1111/1467-9280.00290

Doyle, D. A. (2009). *Physical growth of infants and toddlers.* Retrieved from http://www.merckmanuals.com/professional/pediatrics/physical_growth_and_development/physical_growth_of_infants_and_children.html

Drag, L., & Bieliauskas, L. (2010). Contemporary review 2009: Cognitive aging. *Journal of Geriatric Psychiatry and Neurology, 23*(2), 75–93. doi: 10.1177/0891988709358590

Dreikurs, R., & Soltz, V. (1991). *Children the challenge: The classic work on improving parent-child relations: Intelligent, humane and eminently practical.* New York, NY: Plume.

Duffy, M., Gillig, S. E., Tureen, R. M., & Ybarra, M. A. (2002). A critical look at the DSM-IV. *The Journal of Individual Psychology, 58,* 363–373.

Duggan, M. B. (2010). Anthropometry as a tool for measuring malnutrition: Impact of the new WHO growth standards and reference. *Annals of Tropical Paediatrics, 30,* 1–17. doi: 10.1179/146532810X12637745451834

Dunn, J. (1988). Sibling influences on child development. *Child Psychology, Psychiatry and Allied Disciplines, 29*(2), 118–127. doi: 10.1111/j.1469-7610.1988.tb00697.x

Durkheim, E. (1897/1951). *Suicide: A study in sociology.* (Translated by J. A. Spaulding & G. Simpson.) Glencoe, IL: The Free Press.

Duvall, E. M. (1957). *Family development.* New York, NY: Lippincott.

Duvall, E. M. (1967). *Family development.* Philadelphia, PA: Lippincott.

Duvall, E. M. (1977). *Marriage and family development* (5th ed.) New York, NY: Lippincott.

Dweck, C. S. (2006). *Mindset.* New York, NY: Random House.

Dwyer, J. B., McQuown, S. C., & Leslie, F. M. (2009). The dynamic effects of nicotine on the developing brain. *Pharmacology & Therapeutic, 122,* 125–139. doi: 10.1016/j.pharmthera.2009.02.003

Eckstein, D., Aycock, K. J., Sperber, M. A., McDonald, J., Van Wiesner, W., Watts, R. E., & Ginsburg, P. (2010). A review of 200 birth order studies: Lifestyle characteristics. *Journal of Individual Psychology, 66,* 408–434.

Economic Research Service. (2012). *Household food security in the United States in 2011: Key statistics and graphics.* Retrieved from http://www.ers.usda.gov/topics/food-nutrition-assistance/food-security-in-the-us/key-statistics-graphics.aspx#children

Eggebeen, D. J. (2005). Cohabitation and exchanges of support. *Social Forces, 83,* 1097–1110. doi: 10.1353/sof.2005.0027

Egger, H. C., & Emde, R. N. (2011). Developmentally sensitive diagnostic criteria for mental health disorders in early childhood. *American Psychologist, 66,* 95–106. doi: 10.1037/a0021026

Egger, H. L., & Angold, A. (2006). Common emotional and behavioral disorders in preschool children: Presentation, nosology, and epidemiology. *Journal of Child Psychology and Psychiatry, 47,* 313–337. doi: 10.1111/j.1469-7610.2006.01618.x

Eiden, R. D., Schuetze, P., & Coles, C. D. (2011). Maternal cocaine use and mother–infant interactions: Direct and moderated associations. *Neurotoxicology and Teratology, 33,* 120–128. doi: 10.1016/j.ntt.2010.08.005

Eisenberg, N. (2012). Temperamental effortful control (self-regulation). Retrieved from http://www.child-encyclopedia.com/documents/EisenbergANGxp2-Temperament.pdf

Elagouz, M., Jyothi, S., Gupta, B., & Sivaprasa, S. (2010). Sickle cell disease and the eye: Old and new concepts. *Survey of Opthalmology, 55,* 359–377. doi: 10.1016/j.survophthal.2009.11.004

Elder, G. H., Jr. (1974). *Children of the Great Depression: Social change in the life experience.* Chicago, IL: University of Chicago Press.

Elkind, D. (1984). *All grown up and no place to go: Teenagers in crisis.* Reading, MA: Addison-Wesley.

Elkind, D. (1988). *The hurried child: Growing up too fast too soon.* Reading, MA: Addison-Wesley.

Ellfolk, M., & Malm, H. (2010). Risks associated with in utero and lactation exposure to selective serotoninreuptake inhibitors (SSRIs). *Reproductive Toxicology, 30,* 249–260. doi: 10.1016/j.reprotox.2010.04.01

Elliot, E., & Gonzalez-Mena, J. (2011). Babies' self-regulation: Taking a broad perspective. Part of a special section: Emotional intelligence: A 21st century skill for children and adults. *Young Children, 66*(1), 28–32.

Ellis, A. (1980). Rational-emotive therapy and cognitive behavior therapy: Similarities and differences. *Cognitive Therapy and Research, 4,* 325–340. doi: 10.1007/BF01178210

Ellis, A. (1991). The revised ABC's of rational-emotive therapy (RET). *Journal of Rational-Emotive and Cognitive-Behavior Therapy, 9,* 139–172. doi: 10.1007/BF01061227

Ellis, A. (2003). Early theories and practices of rational emotive behavior therapy and how they have been augmented and revised during the last three decades. *Journal of Rational—Emotive and Cognitive-Behavior Therapy, 21,* 219–243. doi: 10.1023/A:1025890112319

Ellison, C. G., & Fan, D. (2008). *Daily spiritual experiences and psychological well-being.* New York, NY: Guilford Press.

Ellison, N. B., Steinfield, C., & Lampe, C. (2007). The benefits of Facebook "friends": Social capital and college students' use of online social network sites. *Journal of Computer-Mediated Communication, 12,* 1143–1168. doi: 10.1111/j.1083-6101.2007.00367.x

El-Sakka, A., Morsey, A. M., & Fagih, B. I. (2011). Severity of erectile dysfunction could predict left ventricular diastolic dysfunction in patients without overt cardiac complaint. *Journal of Sexual Medicine, 8,* 2590–2597. doi: 10.1111/j.1743-6109.2011.02350.x

Endresen, I. M., & Olweus, D. (2005). Participation in power sports and antisocial involvement in preadolescent and adolescent boys. *Journal of Child Psychology and Psychiatry, 46,* 468–478. doi: 10.1111/j.1469-7610.2005.00414.x

Erford, B. T. (2013). *Assessment for counselors* (2nd ed.). Belmont, CA: Cengage.

Erford, B. T. (2015). *Research and evaluation in counseling* (2nd ed.). Boston, MA: Cengage.

Erford, B. T., Erford, B. M., Lattanzi, G., Weller, J., Schein, H., Wolf, E., . . . & Peacock, E. (2011). Counseling outcomes from 1990–2008 for school-aged youth with depression: A meta-analysis. *Journal of Counseling & Development, 89,* 439–458.

Erford, B. T., Lee, V. V., Newsome, D. W., & Rock, E. (2011). Systemic approaches to counseling students experiencing complex and specialized problems. In B. T. Erford (Ed.), *Transforming the school counseling profession* (3rd ed., pp. 288–313). Upper Saddle River, NJ: Pearson Merrill.

Erford, B. T., Richards, T., Peacock, E. R., Voith, K., McGair, H., Muller, B., Duncan, K., & Chang, C. Y. (2013). Counseling and guided self-help outcomes for clients with bulimia nervosa: A meta-analysis of clinical trials from 1980–2010. *Journal of Counseling & Development, 91,* 152–172. doi: 10.1002/j.1556-6676.2013.00083.x

Erikson, E. H. (1950). *Childhood and society.* New York, NY: Norton

Erikson, E. (1959). Identity and the life cycle. *Psychological Issues, 1,* 1–171.

Erikson, E. H. (1963). *Childhood and society* (2nd ed.). New York, NY: Norton.

Erikson, E. H. (1982). *The life cycle completed: Review.* New York, NY: Norton.

Erikson, E. H., with Erikson, J. M. (1997). *The life cycle completed: Extended version.* New York, NY: W. W. Norton.

Erlangsen, A., Nordentoft, M., Conwell, Y., Waern, M., De Leo, D., Lindner, R., . . . & Lapierre, S. (2011). Key considerations for preventing suicide in older adults: Consensus opinions of an expert panel. *Crisis: The Journal of Crisis Intervention and Suicide Prevention, 32*(2), 106. doi: 10.1027/0227-5910/a000053

Escalona, S. (1968). *The roots of individuality.* Chicago, IL: Aldine.

Evans, W. N., & Lien, D. S. (2005). The benefits of prenatal care: Evidence from the PAT bus strike. *Journal of Econometrics, 125,* 207–239. doi: 10.1016/j.jeconom.2004.04.007

Evenson, R. J., & Simon, R. W. (2005). Clarifying the relationship between parenthood and depression. *Journal of Health and Social Behavior, 46,* 341–358. doi: 10.1177/002214650504600403

Eyberg, S. M., Nelson, M. M., & Boggs, S. R. (2008). Evidence-based psychosocial treatments for children and adolescents with disruptive behavior. *Journal of Clinical Child and Adolescent Psychology, 37*(1), 215–237. doi: 10.1080/15374410701820117

Familyfacts.org. (2006). *Top ten findings: The benefits of marriage.* Retrieved from http://www.familyfacts.org/topten/topten_0606.cfm

Familyfacts.org. (2012). *The benefits of marriage.* Retrieved from http://www.familyfacts.org/briefs/1/the-benefits-of-marriage

Family Watch. (2011). *Trends that affect parents and children in our present world.* Retrieved from http://www.un.org/esa/socdev/family/docs/egm11/Doha%20Statement%20TFW%20ENGLISH.pdf

Fasig, L. G. (2000). Toddlers' understanding of ownership: Implications for self-concept development. *Social Development, 9,* 370–382. doi: 10.1111/1467-9507.00131

Fässberg, M. M., Orden, K. A. V., Duberstein, P., Erlangsen, A., Lapierre, S., Bodner, E., . . . & Waern, M. (2012). A systematic review of social factors and suicidal behavior in older adulthood. *International Journal of Environmental Research and Public Health, 9,* 722–745. doi: 10.3390/ijerph9030722

Fausto-Sterling, A. (1985). *The myths of gender.* New York, NY: Basic Books.

Fein, J. A., Zempsky, W. T., Cravero, J. P., & The Committee on Pediatric Emergency Medicine and Section on Anesthesiology and Pain Medicine. (2012). Relief of pain and anxiety in pediatric patients in emergency medical systems. *Pediatrics, 130,* 1391–1405.

Ferber, R. (2006). *Solve your child's sleep problems: New, revised, and expanded edition.* New York, NY: Fireside.

Ferdous, T., Cederholm, T., Kabir, Z., Hamadani, J., & Wahlin, A. (2010). Nutritional status and cognitive function inn community-living rural Bangladeshi older adults: Data from the Poverty and Health in Ageing Project. *Journal of the American Geriatrics Society, 58,* 919–924.

Fernald, A., & Morikawa, H. (1993). Common themes and cultural variations in Japanese and American mothers' speech to infants. *Child Development, 64,* 637–656. doi: 10.1111/j.1467-8624.1993.tb02933.x

Fester, C. B., & Skinner, B. F. (1957). *Schedules of reinforcement.* New York, NY: Appleton-Century-Crofts.

Festinger, L., Schachter, S., & Black, I. (1950). *Social pressure in informal groups: A study of human factors in housing.* Stanford, CA: Stanford University Press.

Fielding, R., Rejeski, W. J., Blair, S., Church, T., Espeland, M. A., Gill, T. M., . . . & Pahor, M. for the LIFE Research Group. (2011). The Lifestyle Interventions and Independence for Elders Study: Design and methods. *Journal of Gerontology (A): Biological Sciences and Medical Sciences, 66A*(11), 1226–1237. doi: 10.1093/gerona/glr123

Fifer, W. P., & Moon, C. M. (1995). The effects of fetal experience with sound. In J. Lecanuet, W. P. Fifer, N. A. Krasnegor, & W. P.

Smotherman (Eds.), *Fetal development: A psychobiological perspective* (pp. 351–366). Hillsdale, NJ: Erlbaum.

Fine, G.A. (1987). *With the boys: Little league baseball and pre-adolescent culture.* Chicago, IL: University of Chicago Press.

Finkelstein, E. A., Trogdon, J. G., Cohen, J. W., & Dietz, W. (2009). Annual medical spending attributable to obesity: Payer- and service-specific estimates. *Health Affairs, 28,* 822–831. doi: 10.1377/hlthaff.28.5.w822

Fiore, F. (2011, October). "Will I ever work again?" *AARP Bulletin, 52*(8), 18–19.

Fiore, M. C., Jaén, C. R., Baker, T. B., Bailey W. C., Benowitz, N. L., & Curry, S. J. (2008). *Treating tobacco use and dependence: 2008 update.* Rockville, MD: U.S. Department of Health and Human Services.

Fiori, K. L., Brown, E. E., Cortina, K. S., & Antonucci, T. C. (2006). Locus of control as a mediator of the relationship between religiosity and life satisfaction: Age, race, and gender differences. *Mental Health, Religion, and Culture, 9,* 239–263. doi: 10.1080/13694670600615482

Fischer, H. (1994). *Anatomy of love: The natural history of mating, marriage and why we stray.* New York, NY: Random House.

Fischer, K. W., & Pruyne, E. (2003). Reflective thinking in adulthood: Emergence, development and variation. In J. Demick & C. Andreoletti (Eds.), *Handbook of adult development* (pp. 169–198). New York, NY: Kluwer Academic/Plenum Publishers.

Fish, M. (2004). Attachment in infancy and preschool in low socioeconomic status rural Appalachian children: Stability and change and relations to preschool and kindergarten competence. *Development and Psychopathology, 16,* 293–312. doi: 10.1017/S0954579404044529

Fisher, J. C. (1993). A framework for describing developmental change among older adults. *Adult Education Quarterly, 43*(2), 76–89. doi: 10.1177/0741713693043002002

Fitzgerald, H. E., McKelvey, L. M., Schiffman, R. F., & Montanez, M. (2006). Exposure of low-income families and their children to neighborhood violence and paternal antisocial behavior. *Parenting: Science and Practice, 6,* 243–258. doi: 10.1080/15295192.2006.9681308

Fitzgerald, K., Henriksen, R. C., & Garza, Y. (2013). Perceptions of counselors regarding the effectiveness of interventions for traumatized children. *International Journal of Play Therapy, 21,* 45–56. doi: 10.1037/a0026737

Fivush, R. (2008). Remembering and reminiscing: How individual lives are constructed in family narratives. *Memory Studies, 1*(1), 49–58. doi: 10.1177/1750698007083888

Foley, D. (2010). *Learning capitalist culture: Deep in the heart of Tejas* (2nd ed.). Philadelphia, PA: University of Pennsylvania Press.

Fonagy, P., & Target, M. (2002). Early intervention and the development of self-regulation. *Psychoanalytic Quarterly, 22,* 307–335. doi: 10.1080/07351692209348990

Foos, P. W., & Boone, D. (2008). Adult age differences in divergent thinking: It's just a matter of time. *Educational Gerontology, 34,* 587–594. doi: 10.1080/03601270801949393

Foot, P. (1978). *The problem of abortion and the doctrine of the double effect in virtues and vices.* Oxford, UK: Basil Blackwell.

Fouad, N. A. (2002). Cross-cultural differences in vocational interests: Between-groups differences on the Strong Interest Inventory. *Journal of Counseling Psychology, 49,* 283–289. doi: 10.1037/0022-0167.49.3.282

Fowler, J. W. (1974). Agenda toward a developmental perspective on faith. *Religious Education, 69,* 209–219.

Fowler, J. W. (1981). *Stages of faith: The psychology of human development and the quest for meaning.* San Francisco, CA: Harper & Row.

Fowler, J. W. (1995). *Stages of faith: The psychology of human development and the quest for meaning.* New York, NY: HarperCollins.

Fowler, J. W., & Dell, M. L. (2006). Stages of faith from infancy through adolescence: Reflections on three decades of faith development theory. In E. C. Roehlkepartain , P. E. King, L. M. Wagener, & P. L. Benson (Eds.), *The handbook of spiritual development in childhood and adolescence* (pp. 34–45). Newbury Park, CA: Sage.

Fox News. (2010). *World's oldest new mom dying after IVF pregnancy at age 72.* Retrieved from http://www.foxnews.com/story/0,2933,594684,00.html

Fozard, J. L., & Gordon-Salant, S. (2001). Sensory and perceptual changes with aging. In J. E. Birren & K. W. Schaie (Eds.), *Handbook of the psychology of aging* (5th ed., pp. 241–266). San Diego, CA: Academic Press, Inc.

Fraley, R. C., & Shaver, P. R. (2000). Adult romantic attachment: Theoretical developments, emerging controversies, and unanswered questions. *Review of General Psychology, 4,* 132–154. doi: 10.1037/1089-2680.4.2.132

Franco-Borges, G., Vaz-Rebelo, P., & Kourkoutas, E. (2010). The identity function of parenthood: A systemic and developmental approach. *Procedia Social and Behavioral Sciences, 5,* 1721–1725. doi: 10.1016/j.sbspro.2010.07.354

Frank, A. (1963). *The diary of a young girl.* New York, NY: Washington Square Press.

Franklyn, N., & Tate, C. (2008). Lifestyle and successful aging: An overview. *American Journal of Lifestyle Medicine, 3,* 6–11. doi: 10.1177/1559827608326125

Freud, S. (1971). The ego and the id (1923). Part II: The ego and the id. *Abstracts of the Standard Edition of Freud, volume. 127.*

Freud, S. (1938/1973). *An outline of psychoanalysis.* London, UK: Hogarth.

Freund, A. (2008). Successful aging as management of resources: The role of selection, optimization, and compensation. *Research in Development, 5*(2), 94–108. doi: 10.1080/15427600802034827

Frías, V. D., Varela, O., Oropeza, J. J., Bisiacchi, B., & Álvarez, A. (2010). Effects of prenatal protein malnutrition on the electrical cerebral activity during development. *Neuroscience Letters, 482,* 203–207. doi: 10.1016/j.neulet.2010.07.033

Friedberg, R. D., & McClure, J. M. (2002). *Clinical practice of cognitive therapy with children and adolescents.* New York, NY: Guilford Press.

Friedman, H. S., Martin, L. R., Tucker, J. S., Criqui, M. H., Kern, M. L., & Reynolds, C. A. (2008). Stability of physical activity across the lifespan. *Journal of Health Psychology, 13,* 1092–1104. doi: 10.1177/1359105308095963

Friedman, M., & Rosenman, R. H. (1974). *Type A behavior and your heart.* New York, NY: Knopf.

Friedman, R., & Downey, J. (2008). Sexual differentiation of behavior: The foundation of a developmental model of psychosexuality. *Journal of the American Psychoanalytic Association, 56,* 147–175. doi: 10.1177/0003065108315690

Fries, J. (1980). Aging, natural death, and the compression of morbidity. *New England Journal of Medicine, 303*(3), 130–135. doi: 10.1590/S0042-96862002000300012

Fries, J., Bruce, B., & Chakravarty, E. (2011). Compression of morbidity 1980–2011: A focused review of paradigms and progress. *Journal of Aging Research, 32,* 2109–2120. doi: 10.4061/2011/261702

Fromkin, V. (1974). The development of language in Genie: A case of language acquisition beyond the critical period. *Brain and Language, 1,* 81–107. doi: 10.1016/0093-934X(74)90027-3

Frost, D. (2011). Similarities and difference in the pursit of intimacy among sexual minority and heterosexual individuals: A personal projects analysis. *Journal of Social Issues, 67,* 282–301.

Frye, D. P. (2005). Rough-and-tumble social play in humans. In A. D. Pelligrini & P. K. Smith (Eds.). *The nature of play: Great apes and humans* (pp. 50–85). New York, NY: Guilford.

Fuchs, C. S., Stampfer, M. J., Colditz, G. A., Civannucci, E. L., Manson, J. E., Kawachi, I., . . . & Rosener, B. (1995). Alcohol consumption and mortality among women. *New England Journal of Medicine, 332*(19), 245–250. doi: 35400005690483.0010

Fussell, E., & Furstenberg, F. F. (2005). The transition to adulthood during the twentieth century: Race, nativity, and gender. In R. A. Settersten, F. F. Furstenberg, & R. G. Rumbaut (Eds.), *On the frontier of adulthood* (pp. 29–75). Chicago, IL: University of Chicago Press.

Gagne, D. A., Von Holle, A., Brownley, K. A., Runfola, C. D., Hofmeier, S., Branch, K. E., & Bulik, C. M. (2012). Eating disorder symptoms and weight and shape concerns in a large Web-based convenience sample of women ages 50 and above: Results of the gender and body image (GABI) study. *International Journal of Eating Disorders, 45,* 832–844. doi: 10.1002/eat.22030

Galinsky, E., Aumann, K., & Bond, J. T. (2011). *2008 national study of the changing workforce: Times are changing: Gender and generation at work and at home.* New York, NY: Families and Work Institute.

Gallant, M., Spitz, G., & Grove, J. (2010). Chronic illness self-care and the family lives of older adults: A synthetic review across four ethnic groups. *Journal of Cross Cultural Gerontology, 25*(1), 21–43. doi: 10.1007/s10823-010-9112-z

Gallicchio, L., Miller, S. R., Visvanathan, K., Lewis, L. M., Babus, J., Zacur, H., & Flaws, J. A. (2006). Cigarette smoking, estrogen levels, and hot flashes in midlife woman. *Maturitas, 53,* 133–143. doi: 10.1016/j.maturitas.2005.03.007

Ganger, J., & Brent, M. R. (2004). Reexamining the vocabulary spurt. *Developmental Psychology, 40,* 621–632. doi: 10.1037/0012-1649.40.4.621

Gano-Overway, L. A., Newton, M., Magyar, T. M., Fry, M. D., Kim, M., & Guivernau, M. R. (2009). Influence of caring youth sport contexts on efficacy related beliefs and social behaviors. *Developmental Psychology, 45,* 329–340. doi: 10.1037/a0014067

Garber, K. B., Visootsak, J., & Warren, S. T. (2008). Fragile X syndrome. *European Journal of Human Genetics, 16,* 666–672. doi: 10.1038/ejhg.2008.61

Gardner, H. (1983/2003). *Frames of mind: The theory of multiple intelligences.* New York, NY: Basic Books.

Gardner, H. E. (1996). *Multiple Intelligences: The theory in practice.* New York, NY: Basic Books.

Gardner, H. E. (1999). *Intelligences reframed: Multiple intelligences for the 21st century.* New York, NY: Basic Books.

Garstka, T. A., Schmitt, M. T., Branscombe, N. R., & Hummert, M. L. (2004). How young and older adults differ in their responses to perceived age discrimination. *Psychology and Aging, 19,* 326–335. doi: 10.1037/0882-7974.19.2.326

Gartstein, M., Gonzalez, C., Carranza, J., Ahadi, S., Ye, R., Rothbart, M., & Wen Yang, S. (2006). Studying cross-cultural differences in the development of infant temperament: People's Republic of China, the United States of America, and Spain. *Child Psychiatry Human Development, 37,* 145–161. doi: 10.1007/s10578-006-0025-6

Gartstein, M. A., & Rothbart, M. K. (2003). Studying infant temperament via a revision of the infant behavior questionnaire. *Infant Behavior and Development, 26,* 64–86. doi: 10.1016/S0163-6383(02)00169-8

Gartstein, M. A., Slobodskaya, H. R., & Kinsht, I. A. (2003). Cross-cultural differences in the first year of life: United States of America (U.S.) and Russian. *International Journal of Behavioral Development, 27,* 316–328. doi: 10.1080/01650250244000344

Gartstein, M. A., Slobodskaya, H. R., Zylicz, P. O., Gosztyla, D., & Nakagawa, A. (2010). A cross-cultural evaluation of temperament: Japan, USA, Poland and Russia. *International Journal of Psychology and Psychological Therapy, 10*(1), 55–75.

Gaskins, S., Miller, P., & Corsaro, W. A. (1992). Theoretical and methodological perspectives in the interpretive study of children. *New Directions For Child Development, 58,* 5–23. doi: 10.1002/cd.23219925803

Gavin, N. I., Gaynes, B. N., Lohr, K. N., Meltzer-Brody, S., Gartlehner, G., & Swinson, T. (2005). Perinatal depression: A systematic review of prevalence and incidence. *Obstetrics & Gynecology, 106,* 1071–1083. doi: 10.1097/01.AOG.0000183597.31630.db

Geangu, E. (2008). Notes on self awareness development in early infancy. *Cognition, Brain, Behavior, 11*(1), 103–113.

Geertz, C. (1973a). *The interpretation of cultures.* New York, NY: Basic Books.

Geertz, C. (1973b). Thick description: Toward an interpretive theory of culture. In C. Geertz (Ed.), *The interpretation of culture: Selected essays* (pp. 3–30). New York, NY: Basic Books.

Gesell, A. (1929). Maturation and infant behavior pattern. *Psychological Review, 36,* 307–319. doi: 10.1037/h0075379

Gesell, A., Ilg, F. L., & Ames, L. B. (1974). *Infant and child in the culture of today: The guidance of development in home and nursery school.* New York, NY: Harper & Row.

Gewirtz, A. H., & Edleson, J. L. (2007). Young children's exposure to intimate partner violence: Towards a developmental risk and resilience framework for research and intervention. *Journal of Family Violence, 22,* 151–163. doi: 10.1007/s10896-007-9065-3

Gibbons, W. E., Cedars, M., & Ness, R. B. (2011). Toward understanding obstetrical outcome in advanced assisted reproduction: Varying sperm, oocyte, and uterine source and diagnosis. *Fertility and Sterility, 95,* 1645–1649. doi: 10.1016/j.fertnstert.2010.11.029

Giedd, J. N. (2003). The anatomy of mentalization: A view from developmental neuroimaging. *Bulletin of the Menninger Clinic, 67,* 132–142. doi: 10.1521/bumc.67.2.132.23445

Giedd, J. N., Blumenthal, J., Jeffries, N. O., Castellanos, F. X., Liu, H., Zijdenbos, T. P., . . . & Rapoport, J. L. (1999). Brain development during childhood and adolescence: A longitudinal MRI study. *Nature Neuroscience, 2,* 861–863. doi:10.1038/13158

Giesbrecht, G. F., Miller, M. R., & Muller, U. (2010). The anger distress model of temper tantrums: Associations with emotional reactivity and emotional competence. *Infant and Child Development, 19,* 478–497. doi: 10.1002/icd.677

Gillanders, C. (2007). An English speaking prekindergarten teacher for young Latino children: Implications of teacher-child relationship on second language learning. *Early Childhood Education Journal, 35*(1), 47–54. doi: 10.1007/s10643-007-0163-x

Gilligan, C. (1982). *In a different voice: Psychological theory and women's development.* Cambridge, MA: Harvard University Press.

Gilligan, C. (1993). *In a different voice: Psychological theory and women's development.* Cambridge, MA: Harvard University Press.

Gilligan, C., & Attanucci, J. (1988). Two moral orientations: Gender differences and similarities. *Merrill-Palmer Quarterly, 34,* 223–237.

Ginsburg, H. P., & Opper, S. (1987). *Piaget's theory of intellectual development* (3rd ed.). Englewood Cliffs, NJ: Prentice Hall.

Gladding, S. T. (2011), *Family therapy history theory and practice* (5th ed.). Upper Saddle River, NJ: Pearson Merrill.

Glasser, W. (1998). *Choice theory: A new psychology of personal freedom.* New York, NY: Harper Collins.

Gleason, J. B. (2005). The development of language: An overview and a preview. In J. B. Gleason (Ed.), *The development of language* (6th ed., pp. 1–38). Boston, MA: Pearson.

Glenn, E. N. (1985). Racial ethnic women's labor: The intersection of race, gender and class oppression. *Review of Radical Political Economics, 7*(3), 86–108. doi: 10.1177/048661348501700306

Gloria, A. M., & Hird, J. S. (1999). Influences of ethnic and nonethnic variables on the career decision-making self-efficacy of college students. *The Career Development Quarterly, 48,* 157–174. doi: 10.1002/j.2161-0045.1999.tb00282.x

Gogate, L. J., & Bahrick, L. E. (2001). Intersensory redundancy and 7-month-old infants' memory for arbitrary syllable-object relations. *Infancy, 2,* 219–231. doi: 10.1207/S15327078IN0202_7

Goh, J. O., & Park, D. C. (2009). Neuroplasticity and cognitive aging: The scaffolding theory of aging and cognition. *Restorative Neurology and Neuroscience, 27,* 391–403. doi: 10.3233/RNN -2009-0493

Goldberg, H., & Goldberg, I. (2013). *Family therapy: An overview* (8th ed.). Belmont, CA: Cengage.

Goldsmith, H. H., Buss, A. H., Plomin, R., Rothbart, M. K., Thomas, A., Chess, S., Hinde, R. A., & McCall, R. B. (1987). Roundtable: What is temperament? Four approaches. *Child Development, 58,* 505–529. doi: 10.2307/1130527

Goldstein, M. H., & Schwade, J. A. (2010). From birds to words: Perception of structure in social interactions guides vocal development and language learning. In M. S. Blumberg, J. H. Freeman, & S. R. Robinson (Eds.), *The Oxford handbook of developmental behavioral neuroscience* (pp. 708–729). Oxford, UK: Oxford University Press.

Goldstein, M. H., Schwade, J., Briesch, J., & Syal, S. (2010). Learning while babbling: Prelinguistic object-directed vocalizations indicate a readiness to learn. *Infancy, 15,* 362–391. doi: 10.1111/j.1532-7078.2009.00020.x

Goleman, D. (1995). *Emotional intelligence: Why it can matter more than IQ.* New York, NY: Bantam.

Goleman, D. J. (2001). Emotional intelligence: Issues in paradigm building. In C. Cherniss & D. J. Goleman (Eds.), *The emotionally intelligent workplace: How to select for, measure, and improve emotional intelligence in individuals, groups, and organizations* (pp. 13–26). San Francisco, CA: Jossey-Bass.

Gonyea, J. G., & Hooyman, N. R. (2005). Reducing poverty among older women: Social Security reform and gender equity. *Families in Society, 86,* 338–346. doi: 10.1606/1044-3894.3431

Goodman, J. H. (2004). Paternal postpartum depression, its relationship to maternal postpartum depression, and implications for family health. *Journal of Advanced Nursing, 45,* 26–35. doi: 10.1046/j.1365-2648.2003.02857.x

Goodnough, G. E., Perusse, R., & Erford, B. T. (2011). Developmental classroom guidance. In B. T. Erford (Ed.), *Transforming the school counseling profession* (3rd ed., pp. 154–177). Columbus, OH: Pearson Merrill.

Goodwin, P., McGill, B., & Chandra, A. (2009). *Who marries and when? Age at first marriage in the United States, 2002.* NCHS Data Brief No. 19. Hyattsville, MD: National Center for Health Statistics.

Goodwyn, S. W., Acredolo, L. P., & Brown, C. A. (2000). Impact of symbolic gesturing on early language development. *Journal of Nonverbal Behavior, 24*(2), 81–103. doi: 10.1023 /A:1006653828895

Goossens, F. A., & van IJzendoom, M. H. (1990). Quality of infants' attachments to professional caregivers: Relation to infant-parent attachment and day-care characteristics. *Child Development, 61,* 832–837. doi: 10.1111/j.1467-8624.1990.tb02825.x

Gordon-Salant, S. (2005). Hearing loss and aging: New research findings and clinical implications. *Journal of Rehabilitation Research and Development, 42,* 9–23. doi: 10.1682 /JRRD.2005.01.0006

Gottesman, I. I., & Hanson, D. R. (2005). Human development: Biological and genetic processes. *Annual Review of Psychology, 6,* 263–286. doi: 10.1146/annurev.psych.56.091103.070208

Gottfredson, L. S. (1996). Gottfredson's theory of circumscription and compromise. In D. Brown & L. Brooks (Eds.), *Career choice and development* (3rd ed., pp. 179–232). San Francisco, CA: Jossey-Bass.

Gottlieb, G. (1991). Experiential canalization of behavioral development: Theory. *Developmental Psychology, 27,* 4–13. doi: 10.1037/0012-1649.27.1.4

Gottman, J., & Levenson, R. (2003). *Gay and lesbian couples research: A case of similarities of same-sex and cross-sex couples*, differences between gay and lesbian couples. Retrieved from http://www .gottman.com/SubPage.aspx?spdt_id=2&sp_id =100842&spt_id=1

Gould, R. (1972). The phases of adult life: A study in developmental psychology. *The American Journal of Psychiatry, 129,* 521–531.

Gould, R. L. (1978). *Transformations: Growth and change in adult life.* New York, NY: Simon and Schuster.

Gow, A., Johnson, W., Pattie, A., Brett, R., Roberts, B., Starr, J., & Deary, I. (2011). Stability and change in intelligence from age 11 to ages 70, 79, and 87: The Lothian Birth Cohorts of 1921 and 1936. *Psychology and Aging, 26*(1), 232–240. doi: 10.1037 /a0021072

Gralinski-Bakker, J. H., Hauser, S., Billings, R., Allen, J., Lyons, P., & Melton, G. (2005, July). *Transitioning to adulthood for young adults with mental health issues.* Issue Brief No. 21. Retrieved from http://www.nhchc.org/transitiontoadulthood.pdf

Gralinski-Bakker, J. H., Hauser, S. T., Stott, C., Billings, R. L., & Allen, J. P. (2004). Markers of resilience and risk: Adult lives in a vulnerable population. *Research in Human Development, 1,* 291–326. doi: 10.1207/s15427617rhd0104_4

Grall, T. S. (2009). *Custodial mothers and fathers and their child support: 2007.* Current Population Reports No. P60-237. Retrieved from http://www.census.gov/prod/2009pubs/p60-237 .pdf

Grant, B. F., Dawson, D. A., Stinson, F. S., Chou, S. P., Dufour, M. C., & Pickering, R. P. (2004). The 12-month prevalence and trends in DSM-IV alcohol abuse and dependence: United States, 1991–1992 and 2001–2002. *Drug and Alcohol Dependence, 74,* 223–234. doi: 10.1016/j.drugalcdep.2004.02.004

Grant, L. (1984). Black females' "place" in desegregated classrooms. *Sociology of Education, 57,* 58–76. doi: 10.2307/2112632

Grant, N., Wardle, J., & Steptoe, A. (2009). The relationship between life satisfaction and health behaviour: A cross-cultural analysis of young adults. *International Journal of Behavioral Medicine, 16,* 259–268. doi: 10.1007/s12529-009-9032-x

Graven, S. N., & Browne, J. V. (2008). Sleep and brain development: The critical role of sleep in fetal and early neonatal brain development. *Newborn & Infant Nursing Reviews, 8*(4), 173–179. doi: 10.1053/j.nainr.2008.10.008

Gray, A. (2011). *Midlife adults: Lifestyle, leisure and health.* Retrieved from http://www.TeAra.govt.nz/en/midlife-adults/4

Green, R. F., Devine, O., Crider, K. S., Olney, R. S., Archer, N., Olshan, A. F., & Shapira, S. K. (2010). Association of paternal age and risk for major congenital anomalies from the national birth defects prevention study, 1997 to 2004. *Annals of Epidemiology, 20,* 241–249. doi: 10.1016/j.annepidem.2009.10.009

Greene, A. G. (2009). *Feeding baby green: The earth-friendly program for healthy, safe nutrition during pregnancy, childhood, and beyond.* San Francisco, CA: Jossey-Bass.

Greene, J. D., Sommerville, R. B., Nystrom, L. E., Darley, J. M., & Cohen, J. D. (2001). An fMRI investigation of emotional engagement in moral judgment. *Science, 293,* 2105–2108. doi: 10.1126/science.1062872

Greene, J. P., & Winters, M. (2005). *Public high school graduation and college readiness: 1991–2002.* New York, NY: Manhattan Institute for Policy Research.

Greenfield, E., & Marks, N. (2006). Linked lives: Adult children's problems and their parents' psychological and relational well-being. *Journal of Marriage and Family, 68,* 442–454. doi: 10.1111/j.1741-3737.2006.00263.x

Greenfield, E. A., Vaillant, G. E., & Marks, N. F. (2009). Do formal religious participation and spiritual perceptions have independent linkages with diverse dimensions of psychological well-being? *Journal of Health and Social Behavior, 50,* 196–212. doi: 10.1177/002214650905000206

Greer, F. R. (2010). Vitamin K the basics—What's new? *Early Human Development, 86,* S43–S47. doi: 10.1016/j.earlhumdev.2010.01.015

Greven, C. U., Rijsdijk, F. V., & Plomin, R. (2011). A twin study of ADHD symptoms in early adolescence: Hyperactivity-impulsivity and inattentiveness show substantial genetic overlap but also genetic specificity. *Journal of Abnormal Child Psychology, 39,* 265–275. doi: 10.1007/s10802-010-9451-9

Griffin, K. W., Botvin, G. J., Scheier, L. M., Diaz, T., & Miller, N. L. (2000). Parenting practices as predictors of substance use, delinquency, and aggression among urban minority youth: Moderating effects of family structure and gender. *Psychology of Addictive Behaviors, 14,* 174–184. doi: 10.1037/0893-164X.14.2.174

Griffiths, P. E., & Taberyb, J. (2008). Behavioral genetics and development: Historical and conceptual causes of controversy. *New Ideas in Psychology, 26,* 332–352. doi: 10.1016/j.newideapsych.2007.07.016

Grobman, W. A., & Simon, C. (2007). Factors associated with e length of the latent phase during labor induction. *European Journal of Obstetrics & Gynecology and Reproductive Biology, 132,* 163–166. doi: 10.1016/j.ejogrb.2006.09.002

Grohol, J. (2006). *Study: Brain continues development in early adulthood.* Retrieved from http://psychcentral.com/blog/archives/2006/02/07/study-brain-continues-development-in-early-adulthood/

Grossmann, K., Grossmann, K. E., Spangler, G., Suess, G., & Unzer, L. (1985). Maternal sensitivity and newborns' orientation responses as related to quality of attachment in northern Germany. In I. Bretherton & E. Waters (Eds.), *Growing points of attachment theory and research. Monographs of the Society for Research in Child Development, 50*(1–2, Serial No. 209).

Grote, N. K., & Frieze, I. H. (2005). The measurement of friendship-based love in intimate relationships. *Personal Relationships, 1,* 275–300. doi: 10.1111/j.1475-6811.1994.tb00066.x

Gruber, A. J., Pope, H. G., Hudson, J. I., & Yurgelun-Todd, D. (2003). Attributes of long-term heavy cannabis users: A case-control study. *Psychological Medicine, 33,* 1415–1422. doi: 10.1017/S0033291703008560

Grundy, E. (2005). Reciprocity in relationships: Socio-economic and health influences on intergenerational exchanges between third age parents and their adult children in Great Britain. *British Journal of Sociology, 56,* 233–255. doi: 10.1111/j.1468-4446.2005.00057.x

Grundy, E., & Tomassini, C. (2010). Marital history, health and mortality among older men and women in England and Wales. *BMC Public Health, 10,* 554. doi: 10.1186/1471-2458-10-554

Guilford, J. P. (1967). *The nature of human intelligence.* New York, NY: McGraw-Hill.

Guilford, J. P. (1975). Creativity: A quarter century of progress. In I. A. Taylor & J. W. Getzels (Eds.), *Perspectives in creativity* (pp. 37–59). Chicago, IL: Aldine.

Guilford, J. P., & Hoepfner, R. (1971). *The analysis of intelligence.* New York, NY: McGraw-Hill.

Guinness Book of Records. (2014). *Oldest living humans.* Retrieved from http://www.guinnessworldrecords.com/records-5000/oldest-person/

Gunnar, M. R. (1998). Quality of early care and buffering of neuroendocrine stress reactions: Potential effects on the developing human brain. *Preventive Medicine, 27,* 208–211. doi: 10.1006/pmed.1998.0276

Gunnar, M. R. (2000, July). *Brain-behavior interface: Studies of early experiences and the physiology of stress.* Presentation at the World Association for Infant Mental Health, Montreal, Quebec, Canada.

Gunnar, M. R. (2006). Social regulation of stress in early childhood development. In K. McCartney & D. Phillips (Eds.), *Handbook of early childhood development* (pp. 106–125). Malden, MA: Blackwell.

Gunnar, M. R., & Cheatham, C. L. (2003). Brain and behavior interface: Stress and the developing brain. *Infant Mental Health Journal, 24,* 195–211. doi: 10.1002/imhj.10052

Guo, J., Chung, I., Hill, K., Hawkins, D., Catalano, R., & Abbott, R. (2002). Developmental relationships between adolescent substance use and risky sexual behaviour in young adulthood. *Journal of Adolescent Health, 31,* 354–362. doi: S1054-139X(02)00402-0

Gurian, M., & Stevens, K. (2005). *The minds of boys: Saving our sons from falling behind in school and life.* San Francisco, CA: Jossey-Bass.

Gutmann, D. (1994). *Reclaimed power: Men and women in later life* (2nd ed.). Evanston, IL: Northwestern University Press.

Guyuron, B., Rowe, D., Weinfield, A., Eshraghi, Y., Fathi, A., & Iamphongsai, S. (2009). Factors contributing to the facial aging of identical twins. *Plastic & Reconstructive Surgery, 123,* 1321–1331. doi: 10.1097/PRS.0b013e31819c4d42

Gysbers, N. C., Heppner, M. J., & Johnson, J. A. (2009). *Career counseling: Contexts, processes, and techniques.* Alexandria, VA: American Counseling Association.

Haber, D. (2006). Life review: Implementation, theory, research, and therapy. *The International Journal of Aging and Human Development, 63*(2), 153–171. doi: 10.2190/DA9G-RHK5-N9JP-T6CC

Hafen, L. B., Hulinsky, R. S., Simonssen, S. E., Wilder, S., & Rose, N. C. (2009). The utility of genetic counseling prior to offering first trimester screening options. *Journal of Genetics Counseling, 18,* 395–400. doi: 10.1007/s10897-009-9230-3

Haidt, J. (2001). The emotional dog and its rational tail: A social intuitionist approach to moral judgment. *Psychological Review, 108,* 814–834. doi: 10.1037/0033-295X.108.4.814

Haidt, J. (2007). The new synthesis in moral psychology. *Science, 316,* 998–1002. doi: 10.1126/science.1137651

Haight, B. K., & Haight, B. S. (2007). *The handbook of structured life review.* Baltimore, MD: Health Professions Press.

Hall, C. T. (2002, April 30). Study speeds up biological clock: Fertility rates dip after women hit 27. *San Francisco Chronicle.* Retrieved from http://www.sfgate.com/cgi-bin/article.cgi?file=/chronicle/archive/2002/04/30/MN182697.DTL

Hamilton, S. F., & Hamilton, M. A. (2006). School, work, and emerging adulthood. In J. J. Arnett & J. L. Tanner (Eds.), *Coming of age in the 21st century: The lives and contexts of emerging adults.* Washington, DC: American Psychological Association.

Hansen, C. C., & Zambo, D. (2006). Loving and learning with Wemberly and David: Fostering emotional development in early childhood education. *Early Childhood Education Journal, 34,* 273–278. doi: 10.1007/s10643-006-0124-9

Haque, F. N., Gottesman, I. I., & Wong, A. H. C. (2009). Not really identical: Epigenetic differences in monozygotic twins and implications for twin studies in psychiatry. *American Journal of Medical Genetics, 151C*(2), 136–141. doi: 10.1002/ajmg.c.30206

Hariri, A. R. (2010). The neurobiology of individual differences in complex behavioral traits. *Annual Review of Neuroscience, 32,* 225–247. doi: 10.1146/annurev.neuro.051508.135335

Harlow, H. F. (1958). The nature of love. *American Psychologist, 13,* 673–685. doi: 10.1037/h0029383

Harman, D. (1955). *Aging: A theory based on free radical and radiation chemistry.* Berkeley, CA: University of California Radiation Laboratory Press.

Harris, K. M., Gordon-Larson, P., Chantala, K., & Udry, J. R. (2006). Longitudinal trends in race/ethnic disparities in leading health indicators from adolescence to young adulthood. *Archives of Pediatrics & Adolescent Medicine, 160*(1), 74–81. doi: 10.1001/archpedi.160.1.74.

Hart, B. (2004). What toddlers talk about. *First Language, 24,* 91–106. doi: 10.1177/0142723704044634

Hart, B., & Risley, T. R. (1995). *Meaningful differences in the everyday experiences of young American children.* Baltimore, MD: Paul H. Brookes.

Hart, S., Field, T., & Roitfarb, M. (1999). Depressed mothers' assessments of their neonates' behavior. *Infant Mental Health Journal, 20,* 200–210. doi: 10.1002/(SICI)1097-0355(199922)20:2<200::AID-IMHJ7>3.0.CO;2-8

Harter, S. (2006). The development of self-esteem. In M. H. Kernis (Ed.), *Self-esteem issues and answers: A sourcebook of current perspectives* (pp. 144–150). New York, NY: Psychology Press.

Harvey, J. H. & Fine, M. A. (2010). *Children of divorce: Stories of loss and growth.* New York, NY: Taylor & Francis.

Haskett, M. E., Ahern, L. S., Sabourin Ward, C., & Allaire, J. C. (2006). Factor structure and validity of the Parenting Stress Index/Short Form. *Journal of Clinical Child and Adolescent Psychology, 35,* 302–312. doi: 10.1207/s15374424jccp3502_14

Hatch, S. L., Feinstein, L., Link, B. G., Wadsworth, M. E., & Richards, M. (2007). The continuing benefits of education: Adult education and midlife cognitive ability in the British 1946 birth cohort. *The Journal of Gerontology Series B: Psychological Sciences and Social Sciences November, 62*(6), S404–S414. doi: 10.1093/geronb/62.6.S404

Hautvast, J. G. (1997). Adequate nutrition in pregnancy does matter. *European Journal of Obstetrics & Gynecology and Reproductive Biology, 75,* 33–35. doi: 10.1016/S0301-2115(97)00198-X

Havighurst, R. J. (1952). *Human development and education.* New York, NY: Longman.

Havighurst, R. J. (1956). Research on the developmental task concept. *The School Review, 64,* 215–223.

Havighurst, R. J. (1973). *Developmental tasks and education.* New York, NY: McKay.

Hayashi, A., Karasawa, M., & Tobin, J. (2009). The Japanese preschool's pedagogy of feeling: Cultural strategies for supporting young children's emotional development. *Ethos, 37,* 32–49. doi: 10.1111/j.1548-1352.2009.01030.x

Hayden, K., Reed, B., Manly, J., Tommet, D., Pietrzak, R., Chelune, G., . . . & Jones, R. (2011). Cognitive decline in the elderly: An analysis of population heterogeneity. *Age and Aging, 40,* 684–689. doi: 10.1093/ageing/afr101

Hayes, M. J., Fukumizu, M., Troese, M., Sallinen, B. A., & Gilles, A. A. (2007). Social experiences in infancy and early childhood co-sleeping. *Infant and Child Development, 16,* 403–416. doi: 10.1002/icd.524

Hayflick, L., & Moody, H. R. (2003). *Has anyone ever died of old age?* New York, NY: International Longevity Center.

Hays, D. G., & Erford, B. T. (Eds.). (2014). *Developing multicultural counseling competence* (2nd ed.). Columbus, OH: Pearson.

Haywood, K. M., & Getchell, N. (2009). *Life span motor development* (5th ed.). Champaign, IL: Human Kinetics.

Hazen, A. L., Connelly, C. D., Kelleher, K., Landsverk, J., & Barth, R. (2004). Intimate partner violence among female caregivers of children reported for child maltreatment. *Child Abuse & Neglect, 28,* 301–319. doi: 10.1016/j.chiabu.2003.09.016

Hazen, C., & Shaver, P. R. (1987). Romantic love conceptualized as an attachment process. *Journal of Personality and Social Psychology, 52,* 511–524. doi: 10.1037/0022-3514.52.3.511

Hazen, N. L., & Black, B. (1989). Preschool peer communication skills: The role of social status and interaction context. *Child Development, 60,* 867–876. doi: 10.2307/1131028

Heath, S., & Cleaver, E. (2003). *Young, free and single? Twenty-somethings and household change.* Basingstoke, UK: Palgrave Macmillan.

Heath, S. B. (1983). *Ways with words: Language, life and work in communities and classrooms.* Cambridge, MA: Cambridge University Press.

Heaven, B., Brown, L. J. E., White, M., Errington, L., Mathers, J. C., & Moffatt, S. (2013). Supporting well-being in retirement through meaningful social roles: Systematic review of intervention studies. *The Milbank Quarterly, 91,* 222–287.

Hediger, M. L., Overpeck, M. D., Kuczmarski, R. J., McGlynn, A., Maurer, K. R., & Davis, W. W. (1998). *Muscularity and fatness of infants and young children born small- or large-for-gestational-age.* Retrieved from http://pediatrics.aappublications.org/content/102/5/e60.full.html

Heidrich, S. M., & Denney, N. W. (1994). Does social problem solving differ from other types of problem solving during the adult years? *Experimental Aging Research, 20,* 105–126. doi: 10.1080/03610739408253957

Hellemans, K. G., Sliwowska, J. H., Verma, P., & Weinberg, J. (2010). Prenatal alcohol exposure: Fetal programming and later life vulnerability to stress, depression and anxiety disorders. *Neuroscience and Biobehavioral Reviews, 34,* 791–807. doi: 10.1016/j.neubiorev.2009.06.004

Helms, J. E. (1984). Toward a theoretical explanation of the effects of race on counseling: A Black and White model. *The Counseling Psychologist, 12*(4), 153–165. doi: 10.1177/0011000084124013

Helms, J. E. (Ed.). (1990). *Black and White racial identity: Theory, research, and practice.* Westport, CT: Greenwood Press.

Hemphill, S., & Sanson, A. (2001). Matching parenting to child temperament. *Family Matters, 59,* 42–47.

Henderson, H. A., & Wachs, T. D. (2007). Temperament theory and the study of cognition–emotion interactions across development. *Developmental Review, 27,* 396–427. doi: 10.1016/j.dr.2007.06.004

Henning, A., Striano, T., & Lieven, E. V. M. (2005). Maternal speech to infants at 1 and 3 months of age. *Infant Behavior & Development, 28,* 519–536. doi: 10.1016/j.infbeh.2005.06.001

Henriksen, R. C., Jr., & Paladino, D. A. (2009). *Counseling multiple heritage individuals, couples, and families.* Alexandria, VA: American Counseling Association.

Herlihy, B., & Corey, G. (2006). *ACA ethical standards casebook* (6th ed.). Alexandria, VA: American Counseling Association.

Herman, K. C., Reinke, W. M., Parkin, J., Traylor, K. B., & Agarwal, G. (2009). Childhood depression: Rethinking the role of the school. *Psychology in the Schools, 46,* 433–446. doi: 10.1002/pits.20388

Hermus, M. A., Verhoeven, C. J., Mol, B. W., de Wolf, G. S., & Fiedeldeij, C. A. (2009). Comparison of induction of labour and expectant management in post term pregnancy: A matched cohort study. *Journal of Midwifery & Women's Health, 54,* 351–356.

Herr, E. L., Cramer, & Niles, S. G. (2003). *Career guidance and counseling through the lifespan: Systematic approaches* (6th ed.). Boston, MA: Allyn & Bacon.

Herrnstein, R. J., & Murray, C. A. (1994). *The bell curve: Intelligence and class structure in American life.* New York, NY: Free Press.

Hertzog, C., Kramer, A., Wilson, R., & Lindenberger, U. (2008). Enrichment effects on adult cognitive development: Can the functional capacity of older adults be preserved and enhanced? *Psychology Science in the Public Interest, 9*(1), 1–65. doi: 10.1111/j.1539-6053.2009.01034.x

Hetherington, E. M. (2006). The influence of conflict, marital problem solving, and parenting on children's adjustment in nondivorced, divorced and remarried families. In A. Clarke-Stewart & J. Dunn (Eds.). *Families count: Effects on child and adolescent development.* (pp. 203–237). New York, NY: Cambridge University Press.

Hildon, Z., Montgomery, S. M., Blane, D., Wiggins, R. D., & Netuveli, G. (2009). Examining resilience of quality of life in the face of health-related and psychosocial adversity at older ages: What is "right" about the way we age? *The Gerontologist, 5*(1), 36–47. doi: 10.1093/geront/gn067

Hildon, Z., Smith, G., Netuveli, G., & Blane, D. (2008). Understanding adversity and resilience at older ages. *Sociology of Health and Illness, 30,* 726–740. doi: 10.1111/j.1467-9566.2008.01087.x

Hill, P. C., & Pargament, K. I. (2003). Advances in the conceptualization and measurement of religion and spirituality: Implications for physical and mental health research. *American Psychologist, 58,* 64–74. doi: 10.1037/1941-1022.S.1.3

Hillman, C. H., Buck, S. M., Themanson, J. R., Pontifex, M. B., & Castelli, D. M. (2009). Aerobic fitness and cognitive development: Event-related brain potential and task performance indices of executive control in preadolescent children. *Developmental Psychology, 45*(1), 114–129. doi: 10.1037/a0014437

Hinde, R. A. (1989). Ethological and relationship approaches. In R. Vatsa (Ed.), *Annals of child development,* Vol. 6 (pp. 251–285). Greenwich, CT: JAI Press.

Hinnant, J. B., & O'Brien, M. (2007). Cognitive and emotional control and perspective taking and their relationship to empathy in five year old children. *The Journal of Genetic Psychology, 168,* 301–322. doi: 10.3200/GNTP.168.3.301-322

Hinshaw, S. P., & Lee, S. S. (2003). Conduct and oppositional defiant disorders. In E. J. Mash & R. A. Barkley (Eds.), *Child psychopathology* (2nd ed., pp. 144–198). New York, NY: Guilford Press.

Hoeksta, R. A., Bartels, M., & Boomsma, D. I. (2007). Longitudinal genetic study of verbal and nonverbal IQ from childhood to young adulthood. *Learning and Individual Differences, 17,* 97–114. doi: 10.1016/j.lindif.2007.05.005

Hoel, S., Wiese, L., & Striano, T. (2008). Young infants' neural processing of objects is affected by eye gaze direction and emotional expression. *PLoS ONE, 3*(6), e2389. doi: 10.1371/journal.pone.0002389

Hoff, E. (2006). How social contexts support and shape language development. *Developmental Review, 26,* 55–88. doi: 10.1016/j.dr.2005.11.002

Hofferth, S. L. (2010). Home media and children's achievement and behavior. *Child Development, 81,* 1598–1619. doi: 10.1111/j.1467-8624.2010.01494.x

Hohmann-Marriott, B. (2009). The couple context of pregnancy and its effects on prenatal care and birth outcomes. *Maternal and Child Health Journal, 13,* 745–754. doi: 10.1007/s10995-009-0467-0

Holcomb-McCoy, C. C. (2005). Ethnic identity development in early adolescence: Implications and recommendations for middle school counselors. *Professional School Counseling, 9,* 120–127.

Holland, J. L. (1973). *Making vocational choices: A theory of careers.* Upper Saddle River, NJ: Prentice Hall.

Holland, J. L. (1985). *Making vocational choices: A theory of vocational personalities and work environments* (2nd ed.). Upper Saddle River, NJ: Prentice Hall.

Holland, J. L. (1997). Making vocational choices: A theory of vocational personalities and work environments (3rd ed.). Englewood Cliffs, NJ: Prentice-Hall.

Holland, J. L., Gottfredson, G. D., & Baker, H. G. (1990). The validity of vocational aspirations and interest inventories: Extended, replicated, and reinterpreted. *Journal of Counseling Psychology, 37,* 337–342. doi: 10.1037/0022-0167.37.3.337

Hollich, G., Hirsh-Pasek, K., & Golinkoff, R. M. (2000). Breaking the language barrier: An emergentist coalition model of word learning. *Monographs of the Society for Research in Child Development, 65*(3, Serial No. 262).

Hollier, L. M., Leveno, K. J., Kelly, M. A., McIntire, D. D., & Cunningham, F. G. (2000). Maternal age and malformations in singleton births. *Obstetrics & Gynecology, 96,* 701–706. doi: 10.1016/S0029-7844(00)01019-X

Hollist, C. S., & Miller, R. B. (2005). Perceptions of attachment style and marital quality in midlife marriage. *Family Relations, 54,* 46–57. doi: 10.1111/j.0197-6664.2005.00005.x

Hood, R. W., Jr., Hill, P. C., & Spilka, B. (2009). *The psychology of religion: An empirical approach.* New York, NY: Guilford Press.

Hooyman, N., & Kiyak, H. (2011). *Social gerontology* (9th ed.). New York, NY: Pearson.

Horm, L., & Nevill, S. (2006). *Profile of undergraduates in U.S. postsecondary education institutions: 2003–04: With a special analysis of community college students*. NCES 2006-184. U.S. Department of Education. Washington, DC: National Center for Education Statistics.

Horn, J. L. (1968). Organization of abilities and the development of intelligence. *Psychological Review, 75,* 242–259. doi: 10.1037/h0025662

Horn, J. L. (1982). The theory of fluid and crystallized intelligence in relation to concepts of cognitive psychology and aging in adulthood. In F. I. M. Craik & S. E. Trehub (Eds.), *Aging and cognitive processes* (pp. 847–870). New York, NY: Plenum Press.

Horn, J. L., & Cattell, R. B. (1963). Age differences in fluid and crystallized intelligence. *Acta Psychologica, 26,* 107–129. doi: 10.1016/0001-6918(67)90011-X

Horn, J. L., & Hofer, S. M. (1992). Major abilities and development in the adult period. In R. I. Sternberg & C. A. Berg (Eds.), *Intellectual development* (pp. 44–99). Cambridge, UK: Cambridge University Press.

Horn, L., & Berger, R. (2004). *College persistence on the rise? Changes in 5-year degree completion and postsecondary persistence rates between 1994 and 2000*. NCES 2005-156. Washington, DC: U.S. Department of Education, National Center for Education Statistics.

Horney, K. (1950). *Neurosis and human growth*. New York, NY: W. W. Norton.

Hornik, R., Risenhoover, N., & Gunnar, M. (1987). The effects of maternal positive, neutral, and negative affective communications on infant responses to new toys. *Child Development, 58,* 937–944. doi: 10.2307/1130534

Howes, C., & Matheson, C. C. (1993). Contextual constraints on the constraints of the concordance of mother-child and teacher-child relationships. In R. Pianta (Ed.), *"Beyond parents": The role of alternative adults* (pp. 23–40). San Francisco, CA: Jossey-Bass.

Hsu, C., Soong, W., Stigler, J. W., Hong, C., & Liang, C. (1981). The temperamental characteristics of Chinese babies. *Child Development, 53,* 1337–1340. doi: 10.1111/j.1467-8624.1981.tb03188.x

Hughes, F. P. (2010). *Children, play, and development* (4th ed.). Thousand Oaks, CA: Sage.

Hultsch, D. F., Hertzog, C., Small, B. J., & Dixon, R. A. (1999). Use it or lose it: Engaged lifestyle as a buffer of cognitive decline in aging? *Psychology and Aging, 14,* 245–263.

Hummert, M. L., Garstka, T. A., & Shaner, J. L. (1997). Stereotyping of older adults: The role of target facial cues and perceiver characteristics. *Psychology and Aging, 12,* 107–114. doi: 10.1037/0882-7974.12.1.107

Hunt, S. A., & Kraus, S. W. (2009). Exploring the relationship between erotic disruption during the latency period and the use of sexually explicit material, online sexual behaviors, and sexual dysfunctions in young adulthood. *Sexual Addiction & Compulsivity, 16,* 79–100. doi: 10.1080/10720160902724228

Hunt, W. A., & Landis, C. C. (1938). A note on the difference between the Moro reflex and the startle pattern. *Psychological Review, 45,* 267–269. doi: 10.1037/h0059938

Hunter, M. (2011). Mid-life crisis, transition and the propensity to embark upon entrepreneurship. *International Journal of Business and Technopreneurship, 1*(2), 237–244.

Hurley, B. F. (1995) Age, gender, and muscular strength. *Journals of Gerontology, 50A,* 41–44. doi: 10.1093/gerona/50A.Special_Issue.41

Hurtado, S., Cuellar, M., & Guillermo-Wann, C. (2011). Quantitative measures of students' sense of validation: Advancing the study of diverse learning environments. *Enrollment Management Journal, 4,* 53–71.

Huttenlocher, J., Duffy, S., & Levine, S. (2002). Infants and toddlers discriminate amount: Are they measuring? *Psychological Science, 13,* 244–249. doi: 10.1111/1467-9280.00445

Iles, J., Slade, P., & Spiby, H. (2011). Posttraumatic stress symptoms and postpartum depression in couples after childbirth: The role of partner support and attachment. *Journal of Anxiety Disorders, 25,* 520–530. doi: 10.1016/j.janxdis.2010.12.006

Impett, E. A., & Peplau, L. A. (2006). "His" and "her" relationships? A review of the empirical evidence. In A. L. Vangelisti & D. Perlman (Eds.), *The Cambridge handbook of personal relationships* (pp. 273–291). New York, NY: Cambridge University Press.

International Rett Syndrome Foundation. (2008). *About Rett syndrome*. Retrieved from http://www.rettsyndrome.org/content/blogsection/4/1000/

Ivey, A. E., D'Andrea, M., Ivey, M. B., & Simek-Morgan, L. (2007). *Theories of counseling and psychotherapy: A multicultural perspective* (6th ed.). Boston, MA: Allyn & Bacon.

Ivey, A. E., & Ivey, M. B. (1998). Reframing DSM-IV: Positive strategies from developmental counseling and therapy. *Journal of Counseling & Development, 76,* 334–350. doi: 10.1002/j.1556-6676.1998.tb02550.x

Izard, C. E. (2007). Basic emotions, natural kinds, emotion schemas and a new paradigm. *Perspectives on Psychological Science, 2,* 260–280. doi: 10.1111/j.1745-6916.2007.00044.x

Jackson, B. R., & Bergeman, C. S. (2011). How does religiosity enhance well-being? The role of perceived control. *Psychology of Religion and Spirituality, 3*(2), 149–161. doi: 10.1037/a0021597

Jacobs, M. (2004). The perils of latency. *Psychodynamic practice: Individuals, groups, and organisations, 10,* 500–514. doi: 10.1080/14753630412331313721

Jacobson, P. F., & Schwartz, R. J. (2005). Past tense use in bilingual children with language impairment. *American Journal of Speech Language Pathology, 14,* 213–223.

Jacobzone, S. (2000). Coping with aging: International challenges. *Health Affairs, 19,* 213–225. doi: 10.1377/hlthaff.19.3.213

Jaffe, M. L. (1998). *Adolescence*. New York, NY: John Wiley & Sons.

Jaffee, S. R., & Maikovich-Fong, A. K. (2011). Effects of chronic maltreatment and maltreatment timing on children's behavior and cognitive abilities. *The Journal of Child Psychology and Psychiatry, 52,* 184–194. doi: 10.1111/j.1469-7610.2010.02304.x

Jahoda, M. (1958). *Current concepts of positive mental health*. New York, NY: Basic Books.

Jain, S., Arya, V. K., Gopalan, S., & Jain, V. (2003). Analgesic efficacy of intramuscular opioids versus epidural analgesia in labor. *International Journal of Gynecology and Obstetrics, 83,* 19–27. doi: 10.1016/S0020-7292(03)00201-7

Jarrett, M. A., & Ollendick, T. H. (2012). Treatment of comorbid attention-deficit/hyperactivity disorder and anxiety in children. *Journal of Consulting and Clinical Psychology, 80,* 239–244. doi: 10.1037/a0027123

Jarvis, R. M., Thompson, M., & Wadsworth, N. (2003). Cigarette smoking and cognitive decline in midlife: Longitudinal population based study. *American Journal of Public Health, 93,* 994–998. doi: 10.2105/AJPH.93.6.994

Jennings, N. S., Hooker, S. D., & Linebarger, D. L. (2009). Educational television as mediated literacy environments for preschoolers. *Learning, Media and Technology, 34,* 229–242. doi: 10.1080/17439880903141513

Jensen, A. R. (1969). How much can we boost IQ and scholastic achievement? *Harvard Educational Review, 39,* 1–123.

Jensen, J. P., & Bergin, A. E. (1988). Mental health values of professional therapists: A national interdisciplinary survey. *Professional Psychology: Research and Practice, 19,* 290–297. doi: 10.1037/0735-7028.19.3.290

Jepsen, L., & Jepsen, C. (2002). An empirical analysis of the matching patterns of same-sex and opposite-sex couples. *Demography, 39,* 435–453.

Jeune, B., Ronine, J., Young, R., Dejarines, B., Skytthe, A., & Vaupel, J. (2010). Jeanne Calment and her successors: Biological notes on the longest living humans. In H. Maier, J. Gampe, B. Jeune, J. Robine, & J. Vaupel (Eds.), *Supercentenarians* (pp. 285–322). Heidelberg, Germany: Springer-Verlag.

John J. Heldrich Center for Workforce Development. (2009). *The anguish of unemployment.* Retrieved from http://www.heldrich .rutgers.edu/sites/default/files/content/Heldrich_Work_Trends _Anguish_Unemployment.pdf

Johnson, D. E. (2002). Adoption and the effect on children's development. *Early Human Development, 68,* 39–54. doi: 10.1016 /S0378-3782(02)00017-8

Johnson, D. W., Nicholls, M. E. R., Shah, M., & Shields, M. (2009). Nature's experiment? Handedness and early childhood development. *Demography, 46,* 281–301. doi: 10.1353/dem.0.0053

Johnson, G. M., Valle-Inclán, F., Geary, D. C., & Hackley, S. A. (2012). The nursing hypothesis: An evolutionary account of emotional modulation of the postauricular reflex. *Psychophysiology, 49,* 178–185. doi: 10.1111/j.1469-8986.2011.01297.x

Johnston, L. D., O'Malley, P. M., Bachman, J. G., & Schulenberg, J. E. (2012). *Monitoring the future national results on adolescent drug use: Overview of key findings.* NIH Publication No. 08-6418. Bethesda, MD: National Institute on Drug Abuse.

Jones, D., Macias, R. L., Gold, P. B., Barreira, P., & Fisher, W. (2008). When parents with severe mental illness lose contact with their children: Are psychiatric symptoms or substance use to blame? *Journal of Loss & Trauma, 13,* 261–287. doi: 10.1080/15325020701741849

Jones, E. H., & Herbert, J. S. (2006). Exploring memory in infancy: Deferred imitation and the development of declarative memory. *Infant and Child Development, 15,* 195–205. doi: 10.1002/icd.436

Jose, A., O'Leary, K. D., & Moyer, A. (2010). Does premarital cohabitation predict subsequent marital stability and marital quality? A meta-analysis. *Journal of Marriage and the Family, 72,* 105–116. doi: 10.1111/j.1741-3737.2009.00686.x

Jose, P. E. (1990). Just world reasoning in children's immanent justice judgments. *Child Development, 61,* 1024–1033. doi: 10.1111/j .1467-8624.1990.tb02839.x

Josefen, J. (2011). The impact of pregnancy nutrition on offspring obesity. *Journal of the American Dietetic Association, 111,* 50–52. doi: 10.1016/j.jada.2010.10.015

Jourard, S. M., & Landsman, T. (1980). Healthy personality. An approach from the viewpoint of humanistic psychology (4th ed.). New York, NY: Macmillan.

Jung, C. G. (1961). *Memories dreams reflections.* New York, NY: Vintage.

Jung, C. G. (1965). *Memories dreams reflections.* (Edited by A. Jaffe, Translated by R. Winston & C. Winston) (p. 358). New York, NY: Vintage Books. (Original work published in 1961.)

Kagan, J., Arcus, D., Snidman, N., Yu Feng, W., Hendler, J., & Greene, S. (1994). Reactivity in infants: A cross-national comparison. *Developmental Psychology, 30,* 342–345. doi: 10.1037/0012 -1649.30.3.342

Kagan, J., Reznick, S., & Snidman, N. (1987). The physiology and psychology of behavioral inhibition in children. *Child Development, 58,* 1459–1473. doi: 10.1111/j.1467-8624.1987.tb03858.x

Kail, R. V., & Cavanaugh J. C. (2010). *Human development: A lifespan view* (5th ed.). Belmont, CA: Wadsworth.

Kaiser Family Foundation. (2002). *Substance use and risky sexual behavior: Attitudes and practices among adolescents and young adults.* Retrieved from http://www.kff.org/youthhivstds/upload /KFF-CASASurveySnapshot.pdf

Kaiser Family Foundation. (2006). *Sexual health statistics for teenagers and young adults in the United States.* Retrieved from http://www .kff.org/womenshealth/upload/3040-03.pdf

Kalter, H. (2003). Teratology in the 20th century: Environmental causes of congenital malformations in humans and how they were established. *Neurotoxicology and Teratology, 25,* 131–282. doi: 10.1016/S0892-0362(03)00010-2

Kandel, D. B., & Chen, K. (2000). Extent of smoking and nicotine dependence in the United States: 1991–1993. *Nicotine and Tobacco Research, 2,* 263–274. doi: 10.1080/14622200050147538

Kandiah, J., & Amend, V. (2010). An exploratory study on perceived relationship of alcohol, caffeine, and physical activity on hot flashes in menopausal women. *Health, 2,* 989–996. doi: 10.4236 /health.2010.29146

Kaplan, L. A., Evans, L., & Monk, C. (2008). Effects of mothers' prenatal psychiatric status and postnatal caregiving on infant biobehavioral regulation: Can prenatal programming be modified? *Early Human Development, 84,* 249–256. doi: 10.1016/j .earlhumdev.2007.06.004

Kaplan, P. S. (2000). *A child's odyssey: Child and adolescent development* (3rd ed.). Belmont, CA: Wadsworth.

Karon, J. M., Fleming, P. L., Steketee, R. W., & De Cock, K. M. (2001). HIV in the United States at the turn of the century: An epidemic in transition. *American Journal of Public Health, 91,* 1060–1068. doi: 10.2105/AJPH.91.7.1060

Karpowitz, D. H. (2000). American families in the 1990's and beyond. In M. J. Fine & S. W. Lee (Eds.), *Handbook of diversity in parent education: The changing faces of parenting and parent education* (pp. 3–12). San Diego, CA: Academic Press.

Kawada. T., & Otsuka, T. (2010). Framingham hypertension risk score: The prevalence estimation of hypertension after 1 year in the population. *The Journal of Clinical Hypertension, 12,* 814–815. doi: 10.1111/j.1751-7176.2010.00345.x

Kegan, R. (1980). Making meaning: The constructive-developmental approach to persons and practice. *Personnel & Guidance Journal, 58,* 373–380. doi: 10.1002/j.2164-4918.1980.tb00416.x

Kegan, R. (1982). *The evolving self: Problem and process in human development.* Cambridge, MA: Harvard University Press.

Kehily, M. J. (Ed.). (2004). *An introduction to childhood studies.* Maidenhead, MA: Open University Press/McGraw Hill.

Kelcourse, F. B. (Ed.). (2004). Human development and faith: Life-cycle stages of body, mind, and soul. St. Louis, MO: Chalice Press.

Kellehear, A. (2009). On dying and human suffering. *Palliative Medicine, 23,* 388–397.

Kelleher, C. (2009). Minority stress and health: Implications for lesbian, gay, bisexual, transgender, and questioning (LGBTQ) young people. *Counselling Psychology Quarterly, 22,* 373–379. doi: 10.1080/09515070903334995

Keller, M. A., & Goldberg, W. A. (2004). Co-sleeping: Help or hindrance for young children's independence? *Infant and Child Development, 13*, 369–388. doi: 10.1002/icd.365

Keller, M. C. (2008). The evolutionary persistence of genes that increase mental disorders risk. *Current Directions in Psychological Science, 17*, 395–399. doi: 10.1111/j.1467-8721.2008.00613.x

Kendrick, C. M. (2004). Engagement in safety practices to prevent home injuries in preschool children among White and non-White ethnic minority families. *Injury Prevention, 10*, 375–378. doi: 10.1136/ip.2004.005397

Kerr, M. E., & Bowen, M. (1988). *Family evaluation.* New York, NY: W. W. Norton & Company.

Killen, M., Mulvey, K. L., & Hitti, A. (2013). Social exclusion in childhood: A developmental intergroup perspective. *Child Development, 84*, 772–790. doi: 10.1111/cdev.12012

Kim, J., & Cicchetti, D. (2010). Longitudinal pathways linking child maltreatment, emotion regulation, peer relationships and psychopathology. *The Journal of Child Psychology and Psychiatry, 51*, 706–716. doi: 10.1111/j.1469-7610.2009.02202.x

Kim, M. J., Catalano, R. F., Haggerty, K. P., & Abbott, R. D. (2011). Bullying at elementary school and problem behaviour in young adulthood: A study of bullying, violence and substance use from age 11 to age 21. *Criminal Behaviour & Mental Health, 21*, 136–144. doi: 10.1002/cbm.804

Kim-Cohen, J., Caspi, A., Moffitt, T. E., Harrington, H., Milne, B. J., & Poulton, R. (2003). Prior juvenile diagnoses in adults with mental disorder: Developmental follow-back of a prospective-longitudinal cohort. *Archives of General Psychiatry, 60*, 709–717. doi: 10.1001/archpsyc.60.7.709

Kim-Cohen, J., & Gold, A. L. (2009). Measured gene-environment interactions and mechanisms promoting resilient development. *Current Directions in Psychological Science, 18*, 138–142. doi: 10.1111/j.1467-8721.2009.01624.x

King, P. M., & Kitchener, K. S. (1994). *Developing reflective judgment.* San Francisco, CA: Jossey-Bass.

King, V., & Scott, M. (2005), A comparison of cohabiting relationships among older and younger adults. *Journal of Marriage and Family, 67*, 271–285. doi: 10.1111/j.0022-2445.2005.00115.x

Kinnaert, P. (2009). Some historical notes on the diagnosis of death: The emergence of the brain death concept. *Acta Chrurgica Belgica, 109*, 421–428.

Kirkwood, T. (2011). Systems biology of ageing and longevity. *Philosophical Transactions of the Royal Society of Biological Sciences, 366*, 64–70. doi: 10.1098/rstb.2010.0275

Kitchener, K. (1983). Cognition, metacognition, and epistemic cognition. *Human Development, 26*, 222–232. doi: 10.1159/000272885

Kitchener, K. S., & Fischer, K. W. (1990). A skill approach to the development of reflective thinking. *Contributions to Human Development, 21*, 48–62.

Kitchener, K. S., & King, P. M. (1990). The reflective judgment model: Transforming assumptions about knowing. In J. Mezirow (Ed.), *Fostering critical reflection in adulthood* (pp. 159–176). San Francisco, CA: Jossey-Bass.

Kitchener, K., King, P., & DeLuca, S. (2006). Development of reflective judgment in adulthood. In C. Hoare (Ed.), *Handbook of adult development and learning* (pp. 73–98). New York, NY: Oxford University Press.

Kitchener, K., Lynch, C., Fischer, K., & Wood, P. (1993). Developmental range of reflective judgment: The effect of contextual support and practice on developmental stage.

Developmental Psychology, 29, 893–906. doi: 10.1037/0012-1649.29.5.893

Kitchener, R. F. (1986). *Piaget's theory of knowledge: Genetic epistemology and scientific reason.* New Haven, CT: Yale University Press.

Kloss, R. J. (1994). A nudge is best: Helping students through the Perry scheme of intellectual development. *College Teaching, 42*(4), 151–158. doi: 10.1080/87567555.1994.9926847

Knauer, N. J. (2009). LGBT elder law: Towards equity in aging. *Harvard Journal of Law and Gender, 32*, 308–358.

Knudsen, B., & Liszkowski, U. (2012). Eighteen- and 24-month-old infants correct others in anticipation of action mistakes. *Developmental Science, 15*(1), 113–122. doi: 10.1111/j.1467-7687.2011.01098.x

Kochanek, K. D., Xu J. Q., Murphy S. L., Minino, A. M., & Kung, H. (2011). *Deaths: Preliminary data for 2009. National vital statistics reports, 59*(4), Hyattsville, MD: National Center for Health Statistics.

Kochanska, G., Murray, K., & Coy, K. C. (1997). Inhibitory control as a contributor to conscience in childhood: From toddler to early school age. *Child Development, 68*, 263–277. doi: 10.2307/1131849

Kochanska, G., Murray, K. T., & Harlan, E. T. (2000). Effortful control in early childhood: Continuity and change, antecedents, and implications for social development. *Developmental Psychology, 36*, 220–232. doi: 10.1037/0012-1649.36.2.220

Kochanska, G., Murray, K., Jacques, T. Y., Koenig, A. L., & Vandegeest, K. A. (1996). Inhibitory control in young children and its role in emerging internationalization. *Child Development, 67*, 490–507.

Kohlberg, L. (1963). Development of children's orientation towards a moral order, Part I: Sequencing in the development of moral thought. *Vita Humana, 6*, 11–36. doi: 10.1159/000269667

Kohlberg, L. (1969). Stage and sequence: The cognitive-developmental approach to socialization. In D. A. Goslin (Ed.), *Handbook of socialization theory and research* (pp. 348–480). Chicago, IL: Rand McNally.

Kohlberg, L. (1971). Stages of moral development. In C. M. Beck, B. S. Crittenden, & E. V. Sullivan (Eds.), *Moral education* (pp. 23–92). Toronto, ON, Canada: University of Toronto Press.

Kohlberg, L. (1975). The cognitive-developmental approach to moral education. *Phi Delta Kappan, 56*, 670–677.

Kohlberg, L. (1981). *Essays on moral development: The philosophy of moral development*, Vol. 1. San Francisco, CA: Harper & Row.

Kohlberg, L. (1984). *Essays on moral development: The psychology of moral development: The nature and validity of moral stages*, Vol. II. San Francisco, CA: Harper & Row.

Kohlberg, L., & Hersh, R. H. (1977). Moral development: A review of the theory. *Theory into Practice, 16*(2), 53–59. doi: 10.1080/00405847709542675

Kolb, P. J. (2008). Developmental theories of aging. In S. G. Austrian (Ed.), *Developmental theories through the life cycle* (pp. 285–364). New York, NY: Columbia.

Kompanje, E. (2010). The worst is yet to come: Many elderly patients with chronic terminal illness will eventually die in the emergency department. *Intensive Care Medicine, 36*, 732–734. doi: 10.1007/s00134-010-1803-y

Koplewicz, H. S. (2002). *More than moody: Recognizing and treating adolescent depression.* New York, NY: Berkley Publishing.

Kotlowitz, A. (1991). *There are no children here: The story of two boys growing up in the other America.* New York, NY: Knopf Doubleday Publishing Group.

Kraut, R., Patterson, M., Lundmark, V., Kiesler, S., Mukophadhyay, T., & Scherlis, W. (1998). Internet paradox: A social technology that reduces social involvement and psychological well-being? *American Psychologist, 53,* 1017–1031. doi: 10.1037/0003 -066X.53.9.1017

Kreider, R. M. (2005). *Number, timing, and duration of marriages and divorces: 2001.* Current Population Reports, P70-97. Washington, DC: U.S. Census Bureau.

Kreider, R. M. (2007). *Living arrangements of children: 2004.* Current Population Reports, P70-114. Washington, DC: U.S. Census Bureau.

Kreider, R. M., & Elliott, D. B. (2009). *America's families and living arrangements: 2007.* Current Population Reports, P20-561. Washington, DC: U.S. Census Bureau.

Kroger, J. (2003). Identity development during adolescence. In G. R. Adams & M. D. Berzonsky (Eds.), *Blackwell handbook of adolescence* (pp. 205–226). Malden, MA: Blackwell.

Kruger, J., & Kohl, H. W. (2007). Prevalence of regular physical activity among adults: United States, 2001–2005. *Journal of Morbidity and Mortality Weekly Report, 56*(46), 1209–1212.

Krumboltz, J. D. (1979). A social learning theory of career decision making. In A. M. Mitchell, G. B. Jones, & J. D. Krumboltz (Eds.), *Social learning and career decision making* (pp. 19–49). Cranston, RI: Carroll Press.

Kübler-Ross, E. (1969). *On death and dying.* New York, NY: Macmillan.

Kuczmarski, R. J., Ogden, C. L., Grummer-Strawn, L. M., Flegal, K. M., Guo, S. S., Wei, R., & Johnson, C. L. (2000). *CDC growth charts: United States.* Advance Data No. 314. Washington, DC: Centers for Disease Control and Prevention, U.S. Department of Health and Human Services.

Kuehner, C., & Huffziger, S. (2012). Response styles to depressed mood affect the long-term course of psychosocial functioning in depressed patients. *Journal of Affective Disorders, 136,* 627–633.

Kuhl, D., Stanbrook, M. B., & Hébert, P. C. (2010). What people want at the end of life. *Canadian Medical Association Journal, 182,* 1707.

Kuhl, P. (2004). Early language acquisition: Cracking the speech code. *Nature Reviews Neuroscience, 5,* 831–843. doi: 10.1038/nrn1533

Kuhl, P., & Rivera-Gaxiola, M. (2008). Neural substrates of language acquisition. *Annual Review of Neuroscience, 31,* 511–534. doi: 10.1146/annurev.neuro.30.051606.094321

Kuhn, D. (2006). Do cognitive changes accompany developments in the adolescent brain? *Perspectives on Psychological Science, 1,* 59–67. doi: 10.1111/j.1745-6924.2006.t01-2-.x

Kurdek, L. A. (1991). Sexuality in homosexual and heterosexual couples. In K. McKinney & S. Sprecher (Eds), *Sexuality in close relationships* (pp. 177–191). Hillsdale, NJ: Erlbaum.

Kurdek, L. A. (1998). Relationship outcomes and their predictors: Longitudinal evidence from heterosexual married, gay cohabiting, and lesbian cohabiting couples. *Journal of Marriage and Family, 60,* 553–568. doi: 10.2307/353528

Kurdek, L. A. (2001). Differences between heterosexual-nonparent couples and gay, lesbian, and heterosexual-parent couples. *Journal of Family Issues, 22,* 727–754. doi: 10.1177/019251301022006004

Kurdek, L. A. (2006). Differences between partners from heterosexual, gay, and lesbian cohabiting couples. *Journal of Marriage and Family, 68,* 509–528. doi: 10.1111/j.1741-3737.2006.00268.x

Kurdek, L. A., & Schmidt, J. P. (1987). Perceived emotional support from family and friends in members of homosexual, married, and heterosexual cohabiting couples. *Journal of Homosexuality, 14,* 57–68. doi: 10.1300/J082v14n03_04

Kuwabara, S. A., Van Voorhees, B. W., Gollan, J. K., & Alexander, G. C. (2007). A qualitative exploration of depression in emerging adulthood: Disorder, development, and social context. *General Hospital Psychiatry, 29,* 317–324. doi: 10.1016/j.genhosppsych .2007.04.001

Labouvie-Vief, G. (1990). Wisdom as integrated thought: Historical and developmental perspectives. In R. J. Sternberg (Ed.), *Wisdom: Its nature, origins, and development* (pp. 52–83). New York, NY: Cambridge University Press.

Labouvie-Vief, G. (2003). Dynamic integration: Affect, cognition, and the self in adulthood. *Current Directions in Psychological Science, 12*(6), 201–206. doi: 10.1046/j.0963-7214.2003.01262.x

Labouvie-Vief, G. (2006). Emerging structures of adult thought. In J. Arnett (Ed.), *Psychological development during emerging adulthood* (pp. 60–84). Washington, DC: American Psychological Association.

Labouvie-Vief, G., Chiodo, L. M., Goguen, L. A., Diehl, M., & Orwoll, L. (1995). Representations of self across the life span. *Psychology and Aging, 10,* 404–415. doi: 10.1037/0882-7974.10.3.404

Labouvie-Vief, G., & DeVoe, M. (1991). Emotional regulation in adulthood and later life: A developmental view. In K. W. Schaie (Ed.), *Annual review of gerontology and geriatrics* (pp. 172–194). New York, NY: Springer.

Labouvie-Vief, G., Diehl, M., Jain, E., & Zhang, F. (2007). Six-year change in affect optimization and affect complexity across the adult life span: A further examination. *Psychology and Aging, 22,* 738–751. doi: 10.1037/0882-7974.22.4.738

Labouvie-Vief, G., Grühn, D., & Studer, J. (2010). Dynamic integration of emotion and cognition: Equilibrium regulation in development and aging. In R. M. Lerner, M. E. Lamb, & A. M. Freund (Eds.), *The handbook of life-span development,* Vol. 2: *Social and emotional development* (pp. 79–115). Hoboken, NJ: Wiley.

Ladd, G. W. (2005). Children's peer relations and social competence: A century of progress. New Haven, CT: Yale University Press.

Laidlaw, K., & Pachana, N. A. (2009). Aging, mental health, and demographic change: Challenges for psychotherapists. *Professional Psychology: Research and Practice, 40,* 601–608. doi: 10.1037/a0017215

Lamanna, M. A., Riedmann, A. C., & Riedmann, A. (2006). *Marriage and families.* Boston, MA: Cengage Learning.

Lamaze.org. (2013). About us. Retrieved from http://www.lamaze.org/

La Merrill, M., Stein, C. R., Landrigan, P., Engel, S. M., & Savitz, D. A. (2011). Prepregnancy body mass index, smoking during pregnancy, and infant birth weight. *Annals of Epidemiology, 21,* 413–420. doi: 10.1016/j.annepidem.2010.11.012

Landivar, L. C. (2013). *Disparities in STEM employment by sex, race, and Hispanic origin.* American Community Survey Reports. Retrieved from http://www.census.gov/prod/2013pubs/acs-24.pdf

Landreth, G. L., Ray, D. C., & Bratton, S. C. (2009). Play therapy in elementary schools. *Psychology in the Schools, 46,* 281–289. doi: 10.1002/pits.20374

Lanfranco, F., Kamischke, A., Zitzmann, M., & Nieschlag, E. (2004). Klinefelter's syndrome. *Lancet, 64,* 273–283. doi: 10.1016/S0140 -6736(04)16678-6

Lang, I. A., Llwellyn, D. J., Hubbard, R. E., Langa, K. M., & Melzer, M. (2011). Income and the midlife peak in common mental disorder prevalence. *Psychological Medicine, 41,* 1365–1372. doi: 10.1017 /S0033291710002060

Langa, K., Llewellyn, D., Lang, I., Weir, D., Wallace, R., Kabeto, M., & Huppert, F. A. (2009). Cognitive health among older adults in the United States and in England. *BMC Geriatrics, 9,* 23. PMCID: PMC2709651

Langer, S. (2009). *Counter clockwise: Mindful health and the power of possibility.* New York, NY: Ballantine Books.

Lannutti, P. J. (2013). Same-sex marriage and privacy management: Examining couples communication with family members. *Journal of Family Communications, 13,* 60–75.

Lansford, J. E., Chang, L. Dodge, K. A., Malone, P. S., Oburu, P., Palmerus, K., . . . & Quinn, N. (2005). Physical discipline and children's adjustment: Cultural normativeness as a moderator. *Child Development, 76,* 1234–1246. doi: 10.1111/j.1467 -8624.2005.00847.x

Lansford, J. E., Deater-Deckard, K., Dodge, K. A., Bates, J. E., & Pettit, G. S. (2004). Ethnic differences in the link between physical discipline and later adolescent externalizing behaviors. *Journal of Child Psychology and Psychiatry, 45,* 801–812. doi: 10.1111/j.1469 -7610.2004.00273.x

Lapkin, S., Swain, M., & Psyllakis, P. (2010). The role of languaging in creating zones of proximal development (ZPDs): A long-term care resident interacts with a researcher. *Canadian Journal on Aging, 29,* 477–490. doi: http://dx.doi.org/10.1017 /S0714980810000644

Lapointe, J., & Hekimi, S. (2010). When a theory of aging goes badly. *Cellular Molecular Life Sciences, 67,* 1–8.

Latane, B., & Darley, J. M. (1968). Group inhibition of bystander intervention in emergencies. *Journal of Personality and Social Psychology, 10,* 215–221. doi: 10.1037/h0026570

Lau, J. Y., Burt, M., Leibenluft, E., Pine, D. S., Rijsdijk, F., Shiffrin, N., & Eley, T. C. (2009). Individual differences in children's facial expression recognition ability: The role of nature and nurture. *Developmental Neuropsychology, 34*(1), 37–51. doi: 10.1080/87565640802564424

Laumann, E. O., & Michael, R. T. (2001). *Sex, love and health in America.* Chicago, IL: University of Chicago Press.

Laumann, E. O., Paik, A., Glasser, D. Kang, J., Wang, T., Levinson, B., . . . & Gingell, C. (2006). A cross-national study of subjective sexual well-being among older women and men: Findings from the Global Study of Sexual Attitudes and Behaviors. *Archives of Sexual Behavior, 35,* 145–161. doi: 10.1007/s10508-005-9005-3

Laumann, E. O., Paik, A., & Rosen, R. C. (1999). Sexual dysfunction in the United States: Prevalence and predictors. *Journal of the American Medical Association, 281,* 537–544. doi: 10.1001 /jama.281.6.537

Laureys, S. (2005, November). Death, unconsciousness and the brain. *Nature Reviews, 6,* 899–909. doi: 10.1038/nrn1789

Lawn, J. E., Lee, A. C., Kinney, M., Sibley, L., Carlo, W. A., Paul, V. K., Pattinson, R., & Darmstadt, G. L. (2009). Two million intrapartum-related stillbirths and neonatal deaths: Where, why, and what can be done? *International Journal of Gynecology and Obstetrics, 107,* S5–S19. doi: 10.1016/j.ijgo.2009.07.016

Leach, R., Phillipson, C., Biggs, S., & Money, A. (2008). Sociological perspectives on the baby boomers. *Quality in Aging and Older Adults, 9*(4), 19–26.

Lebel, C., & Beaulieu, C. (2011). Longitudinal development of human brain wiring continues from childhood into adulthood. *Journal of Neuroscience, 31,* 10937–10947. doi: 10.1523/JNEUROSCI .5302-10

Lebel, C., Walker, L., Leemans, A., Phillips, L., & Beaulieu, C. (2008). Microstructural maturation of the human brain from childhood to adulthood. *Neuroimage, 40,* 1044–1050. doi: 10.1016/j .neuroimage.2007.12.053

Ledger, W. (2009). Demographics of infertility. *Reproductive BioMedicine Online, 18,* 11–14. doi: 10.1016/S1472 -6483(10)60442-7

Lee, H.-M., & Galloway, J. C. (2012). Early intensive postural and movement training advances head control in very young infants. *Physical Therapy, 92,* 935–947. doi: 10.2522/ ptj.20110196

Lee, S. (2009). East Asian attitudes towards death: A search for the ways to help East Asian elderly dying in contemporary America. *The Permanente Journal, 13*(3), 55–60.

Lee, S. M., & Kushner, J. (2008). Single-parent families: The role of parent's and child's gender on academic achievement. *Gender and Education, 20,* 607–621. doi: 10.1080/09540250802415132

Lefkowitz, E. S., & Gillen, M. M. (2006). Sex is just a normal part of life: Sexuality in emerging adulthood. In J. J. Arnett & J. L. Tanner (Eds.), *Emerging adults in America: Coming of age in the 21st century* (pp. 235–255). Washington, DC: American Psychological Association.

Lehman, H. C. (1960). The age decrement in outstanding scientific creativity. *American Psychologist, 15,* 128–134. doi: 10.1037 /h0041844

Leigh, B. C., Ames, S. L., & Stacy, A. W. (2008). Alcohol, drugs, and condom use among drug offenders: An event-based analysis. *Drug and Alcohol Dependence, 9,* 38–42. doi: 10.1016/j .drugalcdep.2007.08.012

Lengua, L. J., Wolchick, S. A., Sandler, I. N., & West, S. G. (2000). The additive and interactive effects of parenting and temperament in predicting adjustment problems of children of divorce. *Journal of Clinical Child Psychology, 29,* 232–244. doi: 10.1207 /S15374424jccp2902_9

Lenters, K. (2004). No half measures: Reading instruction for young second language learners. *Reading Teacher, 58,* 313–333.

Lerman, S. E., & Liao, J. C. (2001). Neonatal circumcision. *Pediatric Clinics of North America, 48,* 1539–1557.

Lerner, H. (1989). *The dance of intimacy.* New York, NY: Harper & Row.

Levasseur, M., Desrosiers, J., & Whiteneck, G. (2010). Accomplishment level and satisfaction with social participation of older adults: association with quality of life and best correlates. *Quality of Life Research, 19,* 665–675. doi: 10.1007/s11136-010 -9633-5

Levine, E. S., & Anshel, D. J. (2011). "Nothing works!" A case study using cognitive-behavioral interventions to engage parents, educators, and children in the management of attention-deficit/ hyperactivity disorder. *Psychology in the Schools, 48,* 297–306. doi: 10.1002/pits.20554

Levine, M. H. (2005). Take a giant step: Investing in preschool education in emerging nations. *Phi Delta Kappan, 87,* 196–200.

Levinson, D. J. (1986). A conception of adult development. *American Psychologist, 41,* 3–13. doi: 10.1037/0003-066X.41.1.3

Levinson, D., Darrow, C. N., Klein, E. B., Levinson, M. H., & McKee, B. (1978). *The seasons of a man's life.* New York, NY: Knopf.

Lewis, B. A., Minnes, S., Short, E. J., Weishampel, P., Satayathum, S., Min, M. O., Nelson, S., & Singer, L. T. (2011). The effects of prenatal cocaine on language development at 10 years of age. *Neurotoxicology and Teratology, 33,* 17–24. doi: 10.1016/j .ntt.2010.06.006

Lewis, M. (1997). The self in self-conscious emotions. In S. G. Snodgrass & R. L. Thompson (Eds.), *The self across psychology: Self-recognition, self-awareness, and the self-concept,* Vol. 818. New York, NY: New York Academy of Sciences.

Lewis, M. (2000). Self-conscious emotions: Emotional self-organization at three time scales. In M. D. Lewis & I. Granic

(Eds.), *Emotion, development, and self-organization: Dynamic systems approaches to emotional development* (pp. 37–69). New York, NY: Cambridge University Press.

Lewis, O. (1961). *The children of Sanchez: Autobiography of a Mexican family.* New York, NY: Random House.

LGBT Movement Advancement Project (MAP). (2010). *Improving the lives of LGBT older adults.* Denver, CO: Author.

Lightfoot, C., Cole, M., & Cole, S. R. (2008). *The development of children* (6th ed.). New York, NY: Macmillan.

Lin, I. (2008). Consequences of parental divorce for adult children's support of their frail parents. *Journal of Marriage & Family, 70*(1), 113–128. doi: 10.1111/j.1741-3737.2007.00465.x

Lindau, S. T., Schumm, P. L., Laumann, E. O., Levinson, W., O'Muircheartaigh, C. A., & Waite, L. J. (2007). A study of sexuality among older adults in the United States. *New England Journal of Medicine, 357,* 762–774. doi: 10.1056/NEJMoa067423

Lino, M. (2011). *Expenditures on children by families, 2010.* Retrieved from http://www.cnpp.usda.gov/Publications/CRC/crc2010.pdf

Livesey, D., Lum Mow, M., Toshack, T., & Zheng, Y. (2011). The relationship between motor performance and peer relations in 9- to 12-year old children. *Child: Care, Health, and Development, 37,* 581–588. doi: 10.1111/j.1365-2214.2010.01183.x

Ljunger, E., Stavreus-Evers, A., Cnattingius, S., Ekbom, A., Lundin, C., Annaren, G., & Sundstrum-Poromaa, I. (2011). Ultrasonographic findings in spontaneous miscarriage: Relation to euploidy and aneuploidy. *Fertility & Sterility, 95,* 221–224. doi: 10.1016/j.fertnstert.2010.06.018

Lloyd-Jones, D. M., Nam, B., D'Agostino, R. B., Levy, D., Murabito, J. M., Wang, T. J., Wilson, P. W. F., & O'Donnell, C. J. (2004). Parental cardiovascular disease as a risk factor for cardiovascular disease in middle-aged adults. T*he Journal of the American Medical Association, 291,* 2204–2211. doi: 10.1001/jama.291.18.2204

Locke, J. (1689/1996). An essay concerning human understanding. In K. P. Winkler (Ed.), *An essay concerning human understanding: Abridged and edited with an introduction and notes* (pp. 4–357). Indianapolis, IN: Hackett.

Lockhart, T. E., & Shi, W. (2010). Effects of age on dynamic accommodation. *Ergonomics, 53,* 892–903. doi: 10.1080/00140139.2010.489968

Loeckenhoff, C., Fruyt, F., Terracciano, A., McCrae, R., DeBolle, M., & Costa, P., Jr. (2009). Perceptions of aging across 26 cultures and their culture-level associates. *Psychology and Aging, 24,* 941–954. doi: 10.1037/a0016901

Loevinger, J. (1976). *Ego development.* San Francisco, CA: Jossey-Bass

Lohaus, A., Keller, H., Lamm, B., Teubert, M., Fassbender, I., Freitag, C., . . . & Schwarzer, G. (2011). Infant development in two cultural contexts: Cameroonian Nso farmer and German middle-class infants. *Journal of Reproductive and Infant Psychology, 29,* 148–161. doi: 10.1080/02646838.2011.558074

Lopez, B. (1999). About this life: Journeys on the threshold of memory. New York, NY: Random House.

Losse, A., Henderson, S., Elliman, D., Hall, D., Knight, E., & Jongmans, M. (1991). Clumsiness in children. Do they grow out of it? A 10-year follow up study. *Developmental Medicine and Child Neurology, 33,* 55–68. doi: 10.1111/j.1469-8749.1991.tb14785.x

Lövdén, M., Bäckman, L., Lindenberger, U., Schaefer, S., & Schmiedek, F. (2011). A theoretical framework for the study of adult cognitive plasticity. *Psychological Bulletin, 136,* 659–676. doi: 10.1037/a0020080

Lowenstein, T., Shubert, B., & Timofeeff, M. (2011). Microbial communities in fluid inclusions and long-term survival in halite. *GSA Today, 21*(1), 4–9. doi: 10.1130/GSATG81A.1

Lu, L. (2010). Leisure and depression in midlife: A Taiwanese national survey of middle-aged adults. *Journal of Health Psychology, 16,* 137–147. doi: 10.1177/1359105310370501

Luby, J., Heffelfinger, A., Mrakotsky, C., Hessler, M., Brown, K., & Hildebrand, T. (2002). Preschool major depressive disorder: Preliminary validation for developmentally modified DSM-IV criteria. *Journal of the American Academy of Child and Adolescent Psychiatry, 41,* 928–937. doi: 10.1097/00004583-200208000-00011

Ludwig, J., & Phillips, D. (2007). *The benefits and costs of Head Start.* SRCD Social Policy Report. Retrieved from home.uchicago.edu/~ludwigj/papers/SRCD_Headstart_2007.pdf

Luepker, E. T. (2010). Videotaped life review: Its personal and intergenerational impact. *Clinical Social Work Journal, 38*(2), 183–192. doi: 10.1007/s10615-008-0175-z

Lumeng, J. C., Cabral, H. J., Gannon, K., Heeren, T., & Frank, D. A. (2007). Pre-natal exposures to cocaine and alcohol and physical growth patterns to age 8 years. *Neurotoxicology and Teratology, 29,* 446–457. doi: 10.1016/j.ntt.2007.02.004

Luppa, M., Sikorski, C., Luck, T., Ehreke, L., Konnopka, A., Wiese, B., . . . & Riedel-Heller, S. G. (2010). Age- and gender-specific prevalence of depression in latest-life: Systematic review and meta-analysis. *Journal of Affective Disorders, 136,* 212–221.

Lurie, S., Rotmench, S., & Glezerman, M. (2001). Prenatal management of women who have partial Rh (D) antigen. *British Journal of Obstetrics and Gynecology, 108,* 895–897. doi: 10.1111/j.1471-0528.2001.00232.x

Luszki, M., & Luszki, W. (1985). Advantages of growing older. *Journal of the American Geriatric Society, 33,* 216–217.

Luthar, S. S., & Latendresse, S. J. (2005). Children of the affluent: Challenges to well-being. *Current Directions in Psychological Science, 14,* 49–53. doi: 10.1111/j.0963-7214.2005.00333.x

Lutz-Zois, C. J., Bradley, A. C., Mihalik, J. L., & Moorman-Eavers, E. R. (2006). Perceived similarity and relationship success among dating couples: An idiographic approach. *Journal of Social and Personal Relationships, 23,* 865–880. doi: 10.1177/0265407506068267

Lynch, A., Mcduffie, R., Murphy, J., Faber, K., Leff, M., & Orleans, M. (2001). Assisted reproductive interventions and multiple birth. *Obstetrics & Gynecology, 97,* 195–200. doi: 10.1016/S0029-7844(00)01145-5

Lyon, K. B. (2004). Faith and development in late adulthood. In F. B. Kelcourse (Ed.), *Human development and faith: Life-cycle stages of body, mind, and soul* (pp. 269–284). St. Louis, MO: Chalice Press.

Lyons, M. J., York, T. P., Franz, C. E., Grant, M. D., Eaves, L. J., Jacobson, K. C., . . . & Kremen, W. S. (2009). Genes determine stability and the environment determines change in cognitive ability during 35 years of adulthood. *Psychological Science, 20,* 1146–1152. doi: 10.1111/j.1467-9280.2009.02425.x

Maccoby, E. E., & Martin, J. A. (1983). Socialization in the context of the family: Parent-child interaction. In P. H. Mussen & E. M. Hetherington (Eds.), *Handbook of child psychology: Socialization, personality and social development* (4th ed., pp. 1–101). New York, NY: Wiley.

MacDonald, W. L., & DeMaris, A. (1996). Parenting stepchildren and biological children: The effects of stepparent's gender and new biological children. *Journal of Family Issues, 17,* 5–25. doi: 10.1177/019251396017001002

MacDorman, M. F., Declercq, E., & Zhang, J. (2010). Obstetrical intervention and the singleton preterm birth rate in the United States from 1991–2006. *American Journal of Public Health, 100,* 2241–2247. doi: 10.2105/AJPH.2009.180570

MacKinlay, E., & Trevitt, C. (2010). Living in aged care: Using spiritual reminiscence to enhance meaning in life for those with dementia. *International Journal of Mental Health Nursing, 19,* 394–401. doi: 10.1111/j.1447-0349.2010.00684.x

Macmillan, M. (2000). Restoring Phineas Gage: A 150th retrospective. *Journal of the History of the Neurosciences, 9,* 46–66. doi: 10.1076/0964-704X(200004)9:1;1-2;FT046

MacWhitney, B. (2005). Language development. In M. H. Bornstein & M. E. Lamb (Eds.), *Developmental science: An advanced textbook* (5th ed., pp.359–387). Mahwah, NJ: Erlbaum.

Maddox, G. L. (1968). Persistence in life style among the elderly: A longitudinal study of patterns of social activity in relation to life satisfaction. In B. L. Neugarten (Ed.), *Middle age and aging: A reader in social psychology* (pp. 181–183). Chicago, IL: University of Chicago Press.

Maguire, E. A., Spiers, H. J., Good, C. D., Hartley, T., Frackowiak, R. S. J., & Burgess, N. (2003). Navigation expertise and the human hippocampus: A structural brain imaging analysis. *Hippocampus, 13,* 250–259. doi: 10.1002/hipo.10087

Magyar-Moe, J. L. (2009). *Therapist's guide to positive psychological interventions.* Burlington, MA: Academic Press.

Maier, A., Chabanet, C., Schaal, B., Issanchou, S., & Leathwood, P. (2007). Effects of repeated exposure on acceptance of initially disliked vegetables in 7-month old infants. *Food Quality and Preference, 18,* 1023–1032. doi: 10.1016/j.foodqual.2007.04.005

Maier, H., Gampe, J., Jeune, B., Robine, J., & Vaupel, J. (Eds.). (2010). *Supercentenarians.* Heidelberg, Germany: Springer-Verlag.

Main, M., & Solomon, J. (1986). Discovery of an insecure, disorganized/disoriented attachment pattern: Procedures, findings, and implications for the classification of behavior. In M. Yogman & T. B. Brazelton (Eds.), *Affective development in infancy* (pp. 94–124). Norwood, NJ: Ablex.

Main, M., & Solomon, J. (1990). Procedures for identifying disorganized/disoriented infants during the Ainsworth strange situation. In M. T. Greenberg, D. Cicchetti, & E. M. Cummings (Eds.), *Attachment in the preschool years* (pp. 121–160). Chicago, IL: University of Chicago Press.

Maiques, V., García-Tejedor, A., Perales, A. Cordoba, J., & Esteban, R. J. (2003). HIV detection in amniotic fluid samples: Amniocentesis can be performed in HIV pregnant women? *European Journal of Obstetrics & Gynecology and Reproductive Biology, 108,* 137–141. doi: 10.1016/S0301-2115(02)00405-0

Maisel, N. C., & Fingerhut, A. W. (2011). California's ban on same-sex marriage: The campaign and its effects on gay, lesbian, and bisexual individuals. *Journal of Social issues, 67,* 242–263.

Maitland, S. B., Intrieri, R. C., Schaie, K. W., & Willis, S. L. (2000). Gender differences and changes in cognitive abilities across the adult life span. *Aging, Neuropsychology, and Cognition, 7,* 32–53. doi: 10.1076/anec.7.1.32.807

Maldonado-Carreno, C., & Votruba-Drzal, E. (2011). Teacher–child relationships and the development of academic and behavioral skills during elementary school: A within- and between-child analysis. *Child Development, 82,* 601–616. doi: 10.1111/j.1467-8624.2010.01533.x

Mallak, J. (2009). Natural birth vs. birthing naturally. *International Journal of Childbirth Education, 24*(3), 35–38.

Manly, J. T., Kim, J. E., Rogosch, F. A., & Cicchetti, D. (2001). Dimensions of child maltreatment and children's adjustment: Contributions of developmental timing and subtype. *Development and Psychopathology, 13,* 759–782.

Manning, M. A., Bear, G. G., & Minke, K. M. (2006). Self concept and self-esteem. In G. G. Bear & K. M Minke (Eds.), *Children's needs III: Development, prevention, and intervention* (pp. 341–356). Washington, DC: National Association of School Psychologists.

Mansfield, B. (2008). The social nature of natural childbirth. *Social Science & Medicine, 66,* 1084–1094. doi: 10.1016/j.socscimed.2007.11.025

Maples, M. F. (2009). The "transition experience": Group counseling for baby boomers. In L. B. Golden (Ed.), *Case studies in counseling older adults* (pp. 29–37). Upper Saddle River, NJ: Pearson Merrill Prentice Hall.

Maples, M. F., & Abney, P. C. (2006). Baby boomers mature and gerontological counseling comes of age. *Journal of Counseling & Development, 84,* 3–9. doi: 10.1002/j.1556-6678.2006.tb00374.x

Markos, P. A., & Lima, N. R. (2003). Homelessness in the United States and its effect on children. *Guidance & Counseling, 18,* 118–124.

Marrs, J., Trumbley, S., & Malik, G. (2011). Early childhood caries: Determining the risk factors and assessing prevention strategies for nursing intervention. *Pediatric Nursing, 37,* 9–15.

Marshall, J. (2011). Infant neurosensory development: Considerations for infant child care. *Early Childhood Education Journal, 39,* 175–181. doi: 10.1007/s10643-011-0460-2

Martin, D. G. (2003). *Clinical practice with adolescents.* Pacific Grove, CA: Brooks/Cole.

Martin, J. A., Hamilton, B. E., Sutton, P. D., Ventura, S. J., Menacker, F., Kirmeyer, S., & Matthews, T. J. (2009). *Births: Final data for 2006.* National Vital Statistics Reports. Retrieved from http://www.cdc.gov/nchs/data/nvsr/nvsr57/nvsr57_07.pdf

Martin, M., Jäncke, L., & Röcke, C. (2012). Functional approaches to lifespan development: Toward aging research as the science of stabilization. *The Journal of Gerontopsychology and Geriatric Psychiatry, 25,* 185–188. doi: 10.1024/1662-9647/a000069

Martin, P. P., & Weaver, D. A. (2005). Social Security: A program and policy history. *Social Security Bulletin, 66*(1). Retrieved from http://www.ssa.gov/policy/docs/ssb/vv66n1p1.html

Martin, S. P., & Parashar, S. (2006). Women's changing attitudes toward divorce, 1974–2002: Evidence for an educational crossover. *Journal of Marriage and Family, 68*(1), 29–40. doi: 10.1111/j.1741-3737.2006.00231.x

Martinez-Biarge, M., Diez-Sebastian, J., Kapellou, O., Gindner, D., Allsop, J. M., Rutherford, M. A., & Cowan, F. M. (2011). Predicting motor outcome and death in term hypoxic-ischemic encephalopathy. *Neurology, 76,* 2055–2061. doi: 10.1212/WNL.0b013e31821f442d

Maslow, A. H. (1943). A theory of human motivation. *Psychological Review, 50,* 370–396. doi: 10.1037/h0054346

Maslow, A. H. (1954/1987). *Motivation and personality.* New York, NY: Harper and Row.

Maslow, A. H. (1962). *Towards a psychology of being.* Princeton, NJ: D. van Nostrand.

Maslow, A. H. (1965). *Self-actualization and beyond.* Brookline, MA: Center for the Study of Liberal Education for Adults; Winchester, MA: New England Board of Higher Education.

Maslow, A. H. (1968). *Toward a psychology of being* (2nd ed.). Princeton, NJ: Van Norstrand.

Masten, A. S. (2001). Ordinary magic: Resilience in development. *American Psychologist, 56,* 227–238. doi: 10.1037/0003-066X.56.3.227

Masters, W. H., & Johnson, V. E. (1966). *Human sexual response.* New York, NY: Bantam Books.

Mather, K. (1943). Polygenic inheritance and natural selection. *Biological Reviews, 18,* 32–64. doi: 10.1111/j.1469-185X.1943.tb00287.x

Mathews, T. J., & MacDorman, M. F. (2010). Infant mortality statistics from the 2006 period linked birth/infant death data set. *National Vital Statistics Reports, 58*(17), 1–31.

Mathieu, S. I. (2008). Happiness and humor group promotes life satisfaction for senior center participants. *Adaptation and Aging, 32*(2), 134–144. doi: 10.1080/01924780802143089

Matlin, M. (2004). *The psychology of women.* New York, NY: Holt, Rinehart, & Winston.

Mattick, J. S. (2007). A new paradigm for developmental biology. *Journal of Experimental Biology, 210,* 1526–1547. doi: 10.1242/jeb.005017

Mattison, J., Roth, G. S., Beasley, T. M., Tilmont, E. M., Handy, A. M., Herbert, R. L., . . . & de Cabo, R. (2012, August). Impact of caloric restriction on the health and survival of rhesus monkeys from the NIA study. *Nature 489,* 317–321. doi: 10.1038/nature11432

Matud, M. (2004). Gender differences in stress & coping styles. *Personality and Individual Differences, 37,* 1401–1415. doi: 10.1016/j.paid.2004.01.010

Maunder, R. G., & Hunter, J. J. (2001). Attachment and psychosomatic medicine: Developmental contributions to stress and disease. *Psychosomatic Medicine, 63,* 556–567. doi: 10.1097/00006842-200107000-00006

Mayer, J. D., Salovey, P., & Caruso, D. R. (2008). Emotional intelligence: New ability or eclectic traits? *American Psychologist, 63,* 503–517. doi: 10.1037/0003-066X.63.6.503

Mayo Clinic. (2012). *Childhood disintegrative disorder.* Retrieved from http://www.mayoclinic.com/health/childhood-disintegrative-disorder/DS00801

McCabe, S. E., Schulenberg, J. E., Johnston, L. D., O'Malley, P. M., Bachman, J. G., & Kloska, D. D. (2004). Selection and socialization effects of fraternities and sororities on U.S. college substance use: A multi-cohort national longitudinal study. *Society for the Study of Addiction, 100,* 512–524. doi: 10.1111/j.1360-0443.2005.01038.x

McClatchey, I. S., & Wimmer, J. S. (2014). Coping with parental death as seen from the perspective of children who attended a grief camp. *Qualitative Social Work, 13,* 221–236. doi: 10.1177/1473325012465104

McConatha, J. T., Hayta, V., Rieser-Danner, L., McConatha, D., & Polat, T. S. (2004). Turkish and U.S. attitudes towards aging. *Educational Gerontology, 30,* 169–183. doi: 10.1080/03601270490272106

McCrae, R. R., Arenberg, D., & Costa, P. T. (1987). Declines in divergent thinking with age: Cross-sectional, longitudinal, and cross-sequential analyses. *Psychology & Aging, 2,* 130–137. doi: 10.1037/0882-7974.2.2.130

McDevitt, T. M., & Ormrod, J. E. (2012). *Child development and education* (5th ed). Upper Saddle River, NJ: Pearson.

McDonald, S. D., Han, Z., Mulla, S., Murphy, K. E., Beyene, J., & Ohlsson, A. (2009). Preterm birth and low birth weight among in vitro fertilization singletons: A systematic review and meta-analyses. *European Journal of Obstetrics & Gynecology and Reproductive Biology, 146,* 138–148. doi: 10.1016/j.ejogrb.2009.05.03

McDowell, M. A., Fryar, C. D., Ogden, C. L., & Flegal, K. M. (2008). *Anthropometric reference data for children and adults: United States, 2003–2006.* National Health Statistics Reports, No. 10. Hyattsville, MD: National Center for Health Statistics.

McFarland, M., Uecker, J., & Regnerus, M. (2011). The role of religion in shaping sexual frequency and satisfaction: Evidence from married and unmarried older adults. *Journal of Sex Research, 48*(2–3), 297–308. doi: 10.1080/00224491003739993

McFarland, W. P., & Tollerud, T. (2009). Counseling children and adolescents with special needs. In A. Vernon (Ed.), *Counseling children and adolescents* (4th ed., pp. 287–334). Denver, CO: Love Publishing.

McGinty, K., Knox, D., & Zusman, M. (2007). Friends with benefits: Women want friends and men want benefits. *College Student Journal, 41,* 1128–1131.

McGoldrick, M., & Carter, B. (Ed.). (1999). *The expanded family life cycle: Individual, family, and social perspectives* (3rd ed., pp. 27–46). Boston, MA: Allyn & Bacon.

McIntosh, P. (1989, July/August). White privilege: Unpacking the invisible knapsack. *Peace and Freedom,* 10–12.

McKee, P., & Barber, C. (1999). On defining wisdom. *The International Journal of Aging and Human Development, 49,* 149–164. doi: 10.2190/8G32-BNV0-NVP9-7V6G

McLaughlin, S., Connell, C., Herringa, S., Li, L., & Roberts, S. (2010). Successful aging in the United States: Prevalence estimates from a national sample of older adults. *Journal of Gerontology: Social Sciences, 65B*(2), 216–226. doi: 10.1093/geronb/gbp101

McLoyd, V. C., Aikens, N. L., & Burton, L. M. (2006). Childhood poverty, policy, and practice. In K. A. Renninger & I. E. Sigel (Eds.), *Handbook of child psychology,* Vol. 4: *Child psychology in practice* (6th ed., pp. 700–778). Hoboken, NJ: Wiley.

McWhirter, E. H. (1997). Perceived barriers to education and career: Ethnic and gender differences. *Journal of Vocational Behavior, 50,* 124–140. doi: 0001-8791/97

McWhirter, E. H., & Burrow-Sanchez, J. J. (2009). Counseling at-risk children and adolescents. In A. Vernon (Ed.), *Counseling children and adolescents* (4th ed., pp. 335–358). Denver, CO: Love Publishing.

McWhirter, J. J., McWhirter, B. T., McWhirter, A. M., & McWhirter, E. H. (2007). *At-risk youth: A comprehensive response* (3rd ed.). Pacific Grove, CA: Brooks/Cole.

McWilliams, L. A., & Bailey, S. J. (2010). Associations between adult attachment ratings and health conditions: Evidence from the National Comorbidity Survey Replication. *Health Psychology, 29,* 446–453. doi: 10.1037/a0020061

Mead, G. H. (1934). *Mind, self and society.* Chicago IL: University of Chicago Press.

Medda, E., Donati, S., Spinelli, A., & Di Renzo, G. C. (2003). Genetic amniocentesis: A risk factor for preterm delivery? *European Journal of Obstetrics & Gynecology and Reproductive Biology, 110,* 153–158. doi: 10.1016/S0301-2115(03)00106-4

Meece, J. L. (2002). *Child and adolescent development for educators* (2nd ed.). New York, NY: McGraw Hill.

Mehdizadeh, S. (2010). Self-presentation 2.0: Narcissism and self-esteem on Facebook. *Cyberpsychology, Behavior, and Social Networking, 13,* 357–364. doi: 10.1089=cyber.2009.0257

Meier, A., Hull, K. E., & Ortyl, T. A. (2009). Young adult relationship values at the intersection of gender and sexuality. *Journal of Marriage and Family, 71,* 510–525. doi: 10.1111/j.1741-3737.2009.00616.x

Mangweth-Matzek, B., Rupp, C. I., Hausmann, A., Assmayr K, Mariacher, E., & Kemmler, G. (2006). Never too old for eating disorders or body dissatisfaction: A community study of elderly women. *International Journal of Eating Disorders, 39*(7), 583–586.

Meier, M. H., Slutske, W. S., Heath, A. C., & Martin, N. G. (2011). Sex differences in the genetic and environmental influences on childhood conduct disorder and adult antisocial behavior. *Journal of Abnormal Psychology, 120,* 377–388. doi: 10.1037/a0022303

Meltzer, H., Vostanis, P., Doger, N., Doos, L., Ford, T. & Goodman, R. (2008). Children's specific fears. *Child Care Health and Development, 35,* 781–789. doi: 10.1111/j.1365-2214.2008.00908.x

Meltzoff, A. N., & Moore, M. K. (1992). Early imitation within a functional framework: The importance of person identity, movement, and development. *Infant Behavior and Development, 15,* 479–505. doi: 10.1016/0163-6383(92)80015-M

Menn, L., & Stoel-Gammon, C. (2005). Phonological development: Learning sounds and sound patterns. In J. B. Gleason (Ed.), *The development of language* (6th ed., pp. 39–61). Boston, MA: Pearson.

Menyuk, P., Liebergott, J. W., & Schultz, M. C. (1995). *Early language development in full-term and premature infants.* Hillsdale, NJ: Erlbaum.

Mercer, J. S., Erickson-Owens, D. A., Graves, B., & Haley, M. M. (2007). Evidence-based practices for the fetal to newborn transition. *Journal of Midwifery & Women's Health, 52,* 262–272. doi: 10.1016/j.jmwh.2007.01.005

Mercer, R. T., & Ferketich, S. L. (1990). Predictors of parental attachment during early parenthood. *Journal of Advanced Nursing, 15,* 268–280. doi: 10.1111/j.1365-2648.1990.tb01813.x

Meydani, M., Das, S., Band, M., Epstein, S., & Roberts, S. (2011). The effect of caloric restriction and glycemic load on measures of oxidative stress and antioxidants in humans: Results from the CALERIE Trial of Human Caloric Restriction. *Journal of Nutritional Health and Aging, 15,* 456–460. doi: 10.1007/s12603-011-0002-z

Mickelson, K. D., Kessler, R. C., & Shaver, P. R. (1997). Adult attachment in a nationally representative sample. *Journal of Personality and Social Psychology, 73,* 1092–1106. doi: 10.1037/0022-3514.73.5.1092

Midlarsky, E., & Nitzburg, G. (2008). Eating disorders in middle-aged women. *The Journal of General Psychology, 135,* 393–407.

MIDMAC. (2006). The John D. and Catherine T. Macarthur Foundation Research Network on Successful Midlife Development (MIDMAC). Retrieved from http://midmac.med .harvard.edu/

Mikkelson, A., Myers, S., & Hannawa, A. (2011). The differential use of relational maintenance behaviors in adult sibling relationships. *Communication Studies, 62,* 258–270. doi: 10.1080/10510974.2011.555490

Milan, S. E., & Pinderhughes, E. E. (2000). Factors influencing maltreated children's early adjustment in foster care. *Development and Psychopathology, 12,* 63–81. doi: 10.1017/S0954579400001048

Milkie, M., Bierman, A., & Schieman, S. (2008). How adult children influence older parents' mental health: Integrating stress-process and life-course perspectives. *Social Psychology Quarterly, 71*(1), 86–105. doi: 10.1177/019027250807100109

Miller, C. H., & Hedges, D. W. (2008). Scrupulosity disorder: An overview and introductory analysis. *Journal of Anxiety Disorders, 22,* 1042–1058. doi: 10.1016/j.janxdis.2007.11.004

Miller, J. B. (1976). *Toward a new psychology of women.* Boston, MA: Beacon.

Miller, M. D. (2012). Complicated grief in later life. *Dialogues Clinical Neuroscience, 14,* 195–202.

Miller, R. B. (2002). Misconceptions about the U-shaped curve of marital satisfaction over the life course. *Family Science Review, 13,* 60–73.

Miller, S. (1986). Parents' beliefs about their children's cognitive abilities. *Developmental Psychology, 22,* 276–284. doi: 10.2307/1130311

Mindell, J. A., Kuhn, B., Lewin, D. S., Meltzer, L. J., & Sadeh, A. (2006). Behavioral treatment of bedtime problems and night wakings in infants and young children: An American Academy of Sleep Medicine review. *Sleep, 29,* 1263–1276.

Miščević, N. (2012). Learning about wisdom from Lehrer. *Philosophical Studies, 161*(1), 59–68.

Mitchell, B. A. (1998). Too close for comfort? Parental assessments of "boomerang kids" living arrangements. *The Canadian Journal of Sociology, 23,* 21–46.

Mitchell, K. E., Levin, A. S., & Krumboltz, J. D. (1999). Planned happenstance: Constructing unexpected career opportunities. *Journal of Counseling and Development, 77,* 115–124. doi: 10.1002/j.1556-6676.1999.tb02431.x

Mitteldorf, J. (2010). Aging is not a process of wear and tear. *Rejuvenation Research, 13*(2–3), 322–326. doi: 10.1089/rej.2009.0967

Miyake, Y., Keiko, T., Sasaki, S., & Hirota, Y. (2011). Employment, income, and education and risk of postpartum depression: The Osaka Maternal and Child Health Study. *Journal of Affective Disorders, 130,* 133–137. doi: 10.1016/j.jad.2010.10.024

Moberg, D. O., & Binstock, R. H. (2001). Book reviews. *Gerontologist, 41,* 698.

Moehler, E., Kagan, J., Oelkers-Ax, R., Brunner, R., Poustka, L., Haffner, J., & Resch, F. (2008). Infant predictors of behavioural inhibition. *British Journal of Developmental Psychology, 26,* 145–150. doi: 10.1348/026151007X206767

Mojtabai, R., & Olfson, M. (2008). National patterns in antidepressant treatment by psychiatrists and general medical providers: Results from the National Comorbidity Survey Replication. *Journal of Clinical Psychiatry, 69,* 1064–1074. doi: 10.4088/JCP.v69n0704

Mokdad, A. H., Marks, J. S., Stroup, D. F., & Gerberding, J. L. (2004). Actual causes of death in the United States. *The Journal of the American Medical Association, 291,* 1238–1245. doi: 10.1001/jama.291.10.1238

Molavi, D. W. (2013). *Basic somatosensory pathway.* Neuroscience tutorial: An illustrated guide to the essential basics of clinical neuroscience created in conjunction with the first-year course for medical students. Retrieved from http://www.bioon.com/bioline/neurosci/course/bassens.html

Moldrich, R. X., Dauphinot, L., Laffaire, J., Rossier, J., & Potier, M. C. (2007). Down syndrome gene dosage imbalance on cerebellum development. *Progress in Neurobiology, 82,* 87–94. doi: 10.1016/j.pneurobio.2007.02.006

Monroe, S. M., & Simons, A. D. (1991). Beyond diathesis-stress: Differential susceptibility to environmental influences. *Psychological Bulletin, 135,* 885–908. doi: 10.1037/a0017376

Moody, E. J. (2001). Internet use and its relationship to loneliness. *Cyber Psychology and Behavior, 4,* 393–401. doi: 10.1089/109493101300210303

Moody, H. R. (2010). *Aging: Concepts and controversies* (6th ed.). Thousand Oaks, CA: Pine Forge Press.

Mooney, S. M., & Varlinskaya, E. I. (2011). Acute prenatal exposure to ethanol and social behavior: Effects of age, sex, and timing of exposure. *Behavioural Brain Research, 216,* 358–364. doi: 10.1016/j.bbr.2010.08.014

Morelli, G. A., Rogoff, B., Oppenheimer, D., & Goldsmith, D. (1992). Cultural variations in infants' sleeping arrangements: Question of independence. *Developmental Psychology, 28,* 604–613. doi: 10.1037/0012-1649.28.4.604

Moreno, A. J., & Klute, M. M. (2008). Relational and individual resources as predictors of empathy in early childhood. *Social Development, 17,* 613–637. doi: 10.1111/j.1467-9507.2007.00441.x

Morgenthaler, T. I., Owens, J., Alessi, C., Boehlecke, B., Brown, T. M., Coleman, J., . . . & Swick, T. J. (2006). Practice parameters for behavioral treatment of bedtime problems and night waking infants and young children: An American Academy of Sleep Medicine report. *Sleep, 29,* 1277–1281.

Morikawa, M., Yamada, H., Kato, E. H., Shimada, S., Sakuragi, N., Fujimoto, S., & Minakami, H. (2003). Live birth rate varies with gestational history and etiology in women experiencing recurrent spontaneous abortion. *European Journal of Obstetrics & Gynecology and Reproductive Biology, 109,* 21–26. doi: 10.1016/S0301-2115(02)00464-5

Morry, M. M., & Gaines, S. O. (2005). Relationship satisfaction as a predictor of similarity ratings: A test of the attraction-similarity hypothesis. *Journal of Social and Personal Relationships, 22,* 561–584. doi: 10.1177/0265407505054524

Moscardino, U., Nwobu, O., & Axia, G. (2006). Cultural beliefs and practices related to infant health and development among Nigerian immigrant mothers in Italy. *Journal of Reproductive and Infant Psychology, 24,* 241–255. doi: 10.1080/02646830600821280

Mosher, W., Chandra, A., & Jones, J. (2005). *Sexual behavior and selected health measures: Men and women 15–44 years of age.* Advance Data No. 362. Washington, DC: National Center for Health Statistics.

Mott, V. W. (1998). Women's career development. New Directions for Adult and Continuing Education, 80, 25–33. doi: 10.1002/ace.8003

Moutquin, J. M. (2003). Classification and heterogeneity of preterm birth. *International Journal of Obstetrics and Gynecology, 110,* 30–33. doi: 10.1016/S1470-0328(03)00021-1

Mullen, J. D. (2006). Nature, nurture, and individual change. *Behavior and Philosophy, 34,* 1–17.

Munakata, Y., McClelland, J. L., Johnson, M. H., & Siegler, R. S. (1997). Rethinking infant knowledge: Toward an adaptive process account of successes and failures in object permanence tasks. *Psychological Review, 104,* 686–713. doi: 10.1037/0033-295X.104.4.686

Murphy, A. A., Halamek, L. P., Lyell, D. J., & Druzin, M. L. (2003). Training and competency assessment in electronic fetal monitoring: A national survey. *Obstetrics & Gynecology, 101,* 1243–1248. doi: 10.1016/S0029-7844(03)00351

Murphy, P. E., & Fitchett, G. (2009). Belief in a concerned God predicts response to treatment for adults with clinical depression. *Journal of Clinical Psychology, 65,* 1000–1008. doi: 10.1002/jclp.20598

Murray, A. D. (1985). Aversiveness is in the mind of the beholder: Perception of infant crying by adults. In B. M. Lester & C. F. Z. Boukydis (Eds.), *Infant crying: Theoretical and research perspectives* (pp. 217–240). New York, NY: Plenum Press.

Mussen, P., Honzik, M. P., & Eichorn, D. H. (1982). Early adult antecedents of life satisfaction at age 70. *Journal of Gerontology, 37,* 16–32. doi: 10.1093/geronj/37.3.316

Myers, J. E., & Shannonhouse, L. (2013). Combating ageism: Advocacy for older persons. In C. Lee & G. Walz (Eds.), *Multicultural issues in counseling: New approaches to diversity* (4th ed., pp. 151–170). Alexandria, VA: American Counseling Association.

Myers, S., & Goodboy, A. (2010). Relational maintenance behaviors and communication channel use among adult siblings. *North American Journal of Psychology, 12*(1), 103–116.

Nadler, J. T., & Clark, M. H. (2011). Stereotype threat: A meta-analysis comparing African Americans to Hispanic Americans. *Journal of Applied Social Psychology, 41,* 872–890. doi: 10.1111/j.1559-1816.2011.00739.x

Najman, J. M., Hayatbakhsh, M. R., Clavarino, A., Bor, W., O'Callaghan, M. J., & Williams, G. M. (2010). Family poverty over the early life course and recurrent adolescent and young adult anxiety and depression: A longitudinal study. *American Journal of Public Health, 100,* 1719–1723. doi: 10.2105/AJPH.2009.180943

Naqvi, R., Liberman, D., Rosenberg, J., Alston, J., & Straus, S. (2013). Preventing cognitive decline in healthy older adults. *Canadian Medical Association Journal, 85,* 881–885. doi: 10.1503/cmaj.121448

National Cancer Institute. (2011). *General information about male breast cancer.* Retrieved from http://www.cancer.gov/cancertopics/pdq/treatment/malebreast/patient

National Center for Chronic Disease Prevention and Health Promotion. (2010). *Chronic diseases and health promotion.* Retrieved from http://www.cdc.gov/chronicdisease/overview/index.htm

National Center for Chronic Disease Prevention and Health Promotion. (2011). *Chronic disease prevention and health promotion.* Retrieved from http://www.cdc.gov/chronicdisease/

National Center for Education Statistics. (2007). *The condition of education 2007.* Retrieved from http://nces.ed.gov/pubs2007/2007064.pdf

National Center for Education Statistics. (2011). *Fast facts.* Retrieved from http://nces.ed.gov/fastfacts/display.asp?id=4

National Center for Education Statistics. (2013). *Fast facts.* Retrieved from http://www.nces.ed.gov/fastfacts/display.asp?id=16

National Center for Elder Abuse (NCEA). (2005). *Fact sheet: Older adults abuse prevalence and incidence.* Retrieved from http://www.ncea.aoa.gov/main_site/pdf/publication/FinalStatistics050331.pdf

National Center for Family and Marriage Research. (2010). *Rate of first marriage in the U.S., 2008.* Retrieved from http://ncfmr.bgsu.edu/pdf/family_profiles/file84386.pdf

National Center for Health Statistics. (2004). *NHANES analytic guidelines.* Retrieved from http://www.cdc.gov/nchs/nhanes.htm

National Center for Health Statistics. (2010). *Health, United States, 2010: Special feature on death and dying.* DHHS Publication No. 2010-1232. Retrieved from http://www.cdc.gov/nchs/hus/special.htm

National Center on Elder Abuse (NCEA). (2014). *Frequently asked questions.* Retrieved from http://www.ncca.aoa.gov/faq/index.aspx

National Child Advocacy Center. (2012). *Forensic interviews.* Retrieved from http://www.nationalcac.org/

National Education Association. (2011). *Long term benefits of early childhood education.* Retrieved from http://www.nea.org/home/18163.htm

National Heart, Lung, and Blood Institute. (2000). *The practice guide: Identification, evaluation, and treatment of overweight and obesity in adults.* Retrieved from http://www.nhlbi.nih.gov/guidelines/obesity/practgde.htm

National Highway Traffic Safety Administration (NHTSA). (2010). *Traffic safety facts 2008: Speeding.* Washington, DC: Author.

National Human Genome Research Institute. (2010a). *A brief guide to genomics.* Retrieved from http://www.genome.gov/18016863

National Human Genome Research Institute. (2010b). *Chromosome abnormalities.* Retrieved from http://www.genome.gov/11508982

National Human Genome Research Institute. (2010c). *Chromosomes.* Retrieved from http://www.genome.gov/26524120

National Institute of Child Health and Development (NICHD) Early Child Care Research Network. (1997). The effects of infant child care on infant-mother attachment security: Results of the NICHD study of early child care. *Child Development, 68,* 860–879.

National Institute of Diabetes and Digestive and Kidney Diseases, National Institute of Health. (2010). *Prostate enlargement: Benign prostatic hyperplasia.* Retrieved from http://kidney.niddk.nih.gov /kudiseases/pubs/prostateenlargement/

National Institute of Neurological Disorders and Stroke. (2009a). *Autism fact sheet.* Retrieved from http://www.ninds.nih.gov /disorders/autism/detail_autism.htm

National Institute of Neurological Disorders and Stroke. (2009b). *Pervasive developmental disorders information page.* Retrieved from http://www.ninds.nih.gov/disorders/pdd/pdd.htm

National Institute on Aging. (2011). *Growing older in America: The health and retirement study.* Retrieved from http://www.nia.nih. gov/health/publication/growing-older-america-health-and -retirement-study

National Institute on Alcohol Abuse and Alcoholism. (2006). *Alcohol alert: National epidemiologic survey on alcohol and related conditions.* Retrieved from http://pubs.niaaa.nih.gov /publications/AA70/AA70.htm

National Institute on Alcohol Abuse and Alcoholism. (2013). *Alcohol use disorders.* Retrieved from http://www.niaaa.nih.gov/alcoho l-health/overview-alcohol-consumption/alcohol-use-disorders

National Institute on Drug Abuse. (2012). *Commonly abused drugs: Heath effects chart.* Retrieved from http://www.drugabuse.gov /drugs-abuse/commonly-abused-drugs/health-effects

National Osteoporosis Foundation. (2011). *About osteoporosis.* Retrieved from http://www.nof.org/aboutosteoporosis

National Prevention Council. (2011). *2011 annual status report.* Retrieved from http://www.healthcare.gov/prevention/nphpphc /index.html

National Science Foundation. (2002). *Science and engineering indicators: 2002.* Retrieved from http://www.nsf.gov/statistics /seind02/c3/c3s1.htm#c3s1l7

National Science Foundation. (2011). *Sleep deprived kids.* Retrieved from http://www.nsf.gov/news/special_reports/science_nation /sleepdeprivedkids.jsp

National Senior Citizens Law Center. (2011). *LGBT older adults in long-term care facilities.* Washington, DC: Author.

National Sleep Foundation. (2011). *How much sleep do we really need?* Retrieved from http://www.sleepfoundation.org/article/how -sleep-works/how-much-sleep-do-we-really-need

National Survey of Children's Health. (2007). Data query from the Child and Adolescent Health Measurement Initiative, Data Resource Center for Child and Adolescent Health website. Retrieved from www.childhealthdata.org

National Survey of Sexual Health and Behavior. (2010). Findings from the National Survey of Sexual Health and Behavior. *Journal of Sexual Medicine, 7,* 5.

National Survey on Drug Use and Health (NSDUH). (2005). *College enrollment status and past year illicit drug use among young adults: 2002, 2003, and 2004.* Retrieved from http://oas.samhsa.gov/2k5 /College/college.pdf

Navigating the Aging Process (NAP). (2012). *Spirituality and aging.* Retrieved from http://www.nap411.com/Spirituality-Aging /spirituality-and-aging.html

Neal, J. L., Lowe, N. K., Ahijevych, K. L., Patrick, T. E., Cabbage, L. A., & Corwin, E. J. (2010). "Active labor" duration and dilation rates among low-risk, nulliparous women with spontaneous labor onset: A systematic review. *Journal of Midwifery & Women's Health, 55,* 308–318. doi: 10.1016/j.jmwh.2009.08.004

Neal, M. (2011, February 24). Betty White: Dreading aging is a waste of a wonderful life. *Huffpost Health Living.* Retrieved from http:// www.huffintonpost.com/2011/05/24/betty-white-on -aging_n_865814.html

Neugarten, B. L., Moore, J. W., & Lowe, J. C. (1965). Age norms, age constraints, and adult socialization. *The American Journal of Sociology, 70,* 710–717.

Neuman, M. J. (2005). Global early care and education: Challenges responses and lessons. *Phi Delta Kappan, 87,* 188–192.

Newsome, D. W., & Gladding, S. T. (2014). *Clinical mental health counseling in community and agency settings* (4th ed.). Upper Saddle River, NJ: Pearson Merrill.

New York Post. (2010). *Geez whiz! A dad at 94.* Retrieved from http:// www.nypost.com/p/news/international/geez_whiz_dad_at _W3QyhFSZ1AbLGeDy5tQQaN

Niles, S. G., & Harris-Bowlsbey, J. (2013). *Career development interventions in the 21st century* (4th ed.). Upper Saddle River, NJ: Pearson Merrill.

Noftle, E. E., & Fleeson, W. (2010). Age differences in Big Five behavior averages and variabilities across the adult life span: Moving beyond retrospective, global summary accounts of personality. *Psychology and Aging, 25*(1), 95–107. doi: 10.1037/a0018199

Nolan, R. E., & Kadavil, N. K. (2003, October 8–11). Vaillant's contribution to research and theory of adult development. *Midwest Research-to-Practice Conference in Adult, Continuing, and Community Education.* Columbus, OH.

Nolen-Hoeksama, S., Larson, T., & Grayson, C. (1999). Explaining the gender difference in depressive symptoms. *Journal of Personality and Social Psychology, 5,* 1061–1072. doi: 10.1037/0022-3514 .77.5.1061

Nolen-Hoeksama, S., Morrow, & Frederickson, B. L. (1993). Response styles and the duration of episodes of depressed mood. *Journal of Abnormal Psychology, 102,* 20–28. doi: 10.1037/0021-843X .102.1.20

Nomaguchi, K. M., & Milkie, M. A. (2003). Costs and rewards of children: The effects of becoming a parent on adults' lives. *Journal of Marriage & the Family, 65,* 356–374. doi: 10.1111/j.1741-3737 .2003.00356.x

Noone, J., Alpass, F., & Stephens, C. (2010). Do men and women differ in their retirement planning? Testing a theoretical model of gendered pathways to retirement preparation. *Research on Aging, 32,* 715–738. doi: 10.1177/0164027510383531

North, M. S., & Fiske, S. T. (2012). An inconvenienced youth? Ageism and its potential intergenerational roots. *Psychological Bulletin, 138,* 982–997. doi: 10.1037/a0027843

O'Connell, M. E., Boat, T., & Warner, K. E. (2009). Preventing mental, emotional, and behavioral disorders among young people: Progress and possibilities. Washington, DC: National Academies Press.

Office of Minority Health. (2000). *Assessment of state minority health infrastructure and capacity to address issues of health disparity: Final report.* Retrieved from http://minorityhealth.hhs.gov /templates/content.aspx?lvl=1&lvlID=44&ID=7895

Office of Minority Health. (2011a). *African American profile.* Retrieved from http://minorityhealth.hhs.gov/templates/browse .aspx?lvl=2&lvlID=51

Office of Minority Health. (2011b). *American Indians/Alaska Natives profile.* Retrieved from http://minorityhealth.hhs.gov/templates /browse.aspx?lvl=3&lvlid=26

Office of Minority Health. (2011c). *Hispanics/Latino profile.* Retrieved from http://minorityhealth.hhs.gov/templates/browse .aspx?lvl=3&lvlid=31

Office of the Child Advocate. (2013). *Office of the child advocate: Annual report.* Hartford, CT: Author.

O'Flynn O'Brien, K. L., Varghese, A. C., & Agarwal, A. (2010). The genetic causes of male factor infertility: A review. *Fertility and Sterility, 93,* 1–11. doi: 10.1016/j.fertnstert.2009.10.045

Ogden, C. L., Carroll, M. D., Curtin, L. R., Lamb, M. M., & Flegal, K. M. (2010). Prevalence of high body mass index in US children and adolescents, 2007–2008. *Journal of the American Medical Association, 303,* 242–290. doi: 10.1001 /jama.2009.2012

Ogden, C. L., Carroll, M. D., Curtin, L. R., McDowell, M. A., Tabak, C. J., & Flegal, K. M. (2006). Prevalence of overweight and obesity in the United States, 1999–2004. *The Journal of the American Medical Association, 295,* 1549–1555. doi: 10.1001 /jama.295.13.1549

Ogden, C. L., Carroll, M. D., Kit, B. K., & Flegal K. M. (2014). Prevalence of childhood and adult obesity in the United States, 2011–2012. *Journal of the American Medical Association, 311,* 806–814. doi: 10.1001/jama.2014.732

Ogden, C. L., Kuczmarski, R. J., Flegal, K. M., Mei, Z., Guo, S., Wei, R., . . . & Johnson, C. L. (2002). Centers for Disease Control and Prevention 2000 growth charts: Improvement to the 1977 National Center for Health Statistics version. *Pediatrics, 109*(1), 45–69. doi: 10.1542/peds.109.1.45

Okon, T. R. (2005). Palliative care review: Spiritual, religious, and existential aspects of palliative care. *Journal of Palliative Medicine, 8,* 392–414.

Oliver, M., Schofield, G. M., & Kolt, G. S. (2007). Physical activity in preschoolers: Understanding prevalence and measurement issues. *Sports Medicine, 37,* 1045–1070. doi: 10.2165/00007256 -200737120-00004

Oller, D. K. (2000). *The emergence of the speech capacity.* Mahwah, NJ: Lawrence Erlbaum Associates.

Oller, D. K., Eilers, R. E., & Basinger, D. (2001). Intuitive identification of infant vocal sounds by parents. *Developmental Science, 4*(1), 49–60. doi: 10.1111/1467-7687.00148

Olshansky, J., Passaro, D., Hershow, R., Layden, J., Carnes, B., Brody, J., . . . & Ludwig, D. S. (2005). A potential decline in life expectancy in the United States in the 21st century. *The New England Journal of Medicine, 352,* 1138–1145. doi: 10.1056/NEJMsr043743

Olson, A. (2011). EC simplified: Infant potty training made easy, v. 2.0. EC Simplified LLC and Andrea Olson.

Olson, D. H., & Gorall, D. M. (2003). Circumplex model of marital and family systems. In F. Walsh (Ed), *Normal family processes* (3rd ed., pp. 514–547). New York, NY: Guilford Press.

Oncale, R. M., & King, B. M. (2001). Comparison of men's and women's attempts to dissuade sexual partners from the couple using condoms. *Archives of Sexual Behaviors, 30,* 379–391. doi: 10.1023/A:1010209331697

Ong, A. D., & Bergeman, C. S. (2004). Resilience and adaptation to stress in later life: Empirical perspectives and conceptual implications. *Ageing International, 29,* 219–246.

Opie, I., & Opie, P. (1959). *The lore and language of school children.* Oxford, UK: Oxford University Press.

Opie, I., & Opie, P. (1969). *Children's games in street and playground.* Oxford, UK: Oxford University Press.

O'Reilly, D. (2009). *APGAR.* Retrieved from http://www.nlm.nih.gov /medlineplus/ency/article/003402.htm

Oser, F. K. (1994). The development of religious judgment. In B. Puka (Ed.), *Fundamental research in moral development* (pp. 375–396). New York, NY: Garland.

Ostrov, J. M., & Godleski, S. A. (2010). Toward an integrated gender-linked model of aggression subtypes in early and middle childhood. *Psychological Review, 117,* 233–242. doi: 10.1037 /a0018070

Owens, K. B. (2002). *Child and adolescent development: An integrated approach.* Belmont, CA: Wadsworth.

Pang, Y., & Richey, D. (2007). Preschool education in China and the United States: A preschool perspective. *Early Childhood Development and Care, 177*(1), 1–13. doi: 10.1080 /14797580500252712

Panksepp, J. (2001). The long-term psychobiological consequences of infant emotions: Prescriptions for the twenty first century. *Infant Mental Health Journal, 22,* 132–173. doi: 10.1080/15294145 .2001.10773353

Papadimos, T. J., Gafford, E. F., Stawicki, S. P., & Murray, M. J. (2014). Diagnosing dying. *Anesthesia & Analgesia, 118,* 879–882. doi: 10.1213/ANE.0000000000000043

Papalia, D. E., Olds, S. W., & Feldman, R. D. (2009). *Human development* (11th ed.). Boston, MA: McGraw-Hill.

Park, D. C., & Bischof, G. N. (2013). The aging mind: Neuroplasticity in response to cognitive training. *Dialogues in Clinical Neuroscience, 15,* 109–119.

Park , M. J., Paul, M. T., Adams, S. H., Brindis, C. D., & Irwin, C. E. (2006). The health status of young adults in the United States. *Journal of Adolescent Health, 39,* 305–317. doi: 10.1016/j .jadohealth.2006.04.017

Parten, M. (1932). Social play among preschool children. *Journal of Abnormal and Social Psychology, 28,* 136–147. doi: 10.1037 /h0073939

Pascarella, E. T., & Terenzini, P. T. (2005). *How college affects students,* Vol. 2: *A third decade of research.* San Francisco, CA: Jossey-Bass.

Pastor, P. N., & Reuben, C. A. (2008). *Diagnosed attention deficit hyperactivity disorder and learning disability: United States, 2004–2006.* National Center for Health Statistics. Vital Health Statistics Report 10(237). Hyattsville, MD: National Center for Health Statistics.

Pasupathy, D., Wood, A. M., Pell, J. P., Fleming, M., & Smith, G. C. (2009). Time trend in the risk of delivery-related perinatal and neonatal death associated with breech presentation at term. *International Journal of Epidemiology, 38,* 490–498. doi: 10.1093 /ije/dyn225

Pasupathy, D., Wood, A. M., Pell, J. P., Fleming, M., & Smith, G. C. (2010). Advanced maternal age and the risk of perinatal death due to intrapartum anoxia at term. *Journal of Epidemiology and Community Health, 65*(3), 1–28. doi: 10.1136/jech.2009.097170

Paterson, J. (2011, July). Young and depressed. *Counseling Today, 54,* 32–35.

Patterson, C. J., & Hastings, P. D. (2007). Socialization in the context of family diversity. In J. E. Grusec & P. D. Hastings (Eds.), *Handbook of socialization: Theory and research.* New York, NY: Guilford Press.

Paul, E. L., McManus, B., & Hayes, A. (2000). "Hookups": Characteristics and correlates of college students' spontaneous and anonymous sexual experiences. *The Journal of Sex Research, 37,* 76–88. doi: 10.1080/00224490009552023

Pauli-Pott, U., Mertesacker, B., & Beckmann, D. (2004). Predicting the development of infant emotionality from maternal characteristics.

Development and Psychopathology, 16, 19–42. doi: 10.1017 /S0954579404044396

Pavlov, I. P. (1927). *Conditioned reflexes: An investigation of the physiological activity of the cerebral cortex.* (Translated and edited by G. V. Anrep.) London, UK: Oxford University Press. Retrieved from http://psychclassics.yorku.ca/Pavlov/lecture3.htm

Payne, B. K., Blowers, A., & Jarvis, D. B. (2012). The neglect of elder neglect as a white-collar crime: Distinguishing patient neglect from physical abuse and the criminal justice system's response. *Justice Quarterly, 29,* 448–468. doi: 10.1080/07418825.2011.572559

Payne, B., & Fletcher, L. (2005). Elder abuse in nursing homes: Prevention and resolution strategies and barriers. *Journal of Criminal Justice, 33*(2), 119–125. doi: 10.1016/j .jcrimjus.2004.12.003

Payne, R. (2008). Nine powerful practices. *Educational Leadership, 65*(7), 48–52.

Pearson, J. D., Morrell, C. H., Gordon-Salant, S., Brant, L. J., Meter, E. J., Klein, L. L., & Fozard, J. L. (1995). Gender differences in a longitudinal study of age-associated hearing loss. *Journal of Acoustical Society of America, 97,* 1196–1205. doi: 10.1121/1.412231

Pearson, Q. M. (2008). Role overload, job satisfaction, leisure satisfaction, and psychological health among employed women. *Journal of Counseling & Development, 86,* 57–63. doi: 10.1002 /j.1556-6678.2008.tb00626.x

Peck, R. (1955). Psychological developments in the second half of life. In J. E. Anderson (Ed.), *Psychological aspects of aging* (pp. 42–53). Washington, DC: American Psychological Association.

Peck, R. C. (1968). Psychological developments in the second half of life. In B. L. Neugarten (Ed.), *Middle age and aging* (pp. 88–92). Chicago, IL: University of Chicago Press.

Pedroso, F. S., Riesgo, R. S., Gatiboni, T., & Rotta, N. T. (2012). The diving reflex in healthy infants in the first year of life. *Journal of Child Neurology, 27*(2), 168–171. doi: 10.1177/0883073811415269

Peltz, C., Kim, H., & Kawas, C. (2010). Abnormal EEGs in cognitively and physically health oldest-old: Findings from the 90+ study. *Journal of Clinical Neurophysiology, 27,* 292–295. doi: 10.1097 /WNP.0b013e3181eaad7d

Penhale, B. (2005). Older women, domestic violence, and elder abuse: A review of commonalities, differences, and shared approaches. *Journal of Elder Abuse and Neglect, 15*(3), 163–183. doi: 10.1300 /J084v15n03_10

Penn, A. A., & Shatz, C. J. (2002). Principles of endogenous and sensory activity-dependent brain development: The visual system. In H. Lagercrantz, M. Hanson, P. Evrard, & C. H. Rodeck (Eds.), *The newborn brain: Neuroscience and clinical applications* (pp. 204–255). Cambridge, NY: Cambridge University Press.

Pereira, A. C., Huddleson, D. E., Brickman, A. M., Sosunov, A. A., Hen, R., McKhann, G. M., . . . & Small, S. A. (2007). An *in vivo* correlate of exercise-induced neurogenesis in the adult dentate gyrus. *Proceedings of the National Academy of Sciences of the United States of America, 104,* 5638–5643. doi: 10.1073 /pnas.0611721104

Perls, T., Wilmoth, J., Levenson, R., Drinkwater, M., Cohen, M., Borgan, H., . . . & Puca, A. (2002). Life-long sustained mortality advantage of centenarians. *Proceedings of the National Academy of Sciences, 99*(12). Retrieved from http://www.pnas.org/content /99/12/8442.short

Perry, B. (1997). Incubated in terror: Neurodevelopmental factors in the "cycle of violence." In J. Osofsky (Ed.), *Children, youth, and violence: The search for solutions* (pp. 124–148). New York, NY: Guilford Press.

Perry, B. D. (2009). Examining child maltreatment through a neurodevelopmental lens: Clinical applications of the neurosequential model of therapeutics. *Journal of Loss and Trauma, 14,* 240–255. doi: 10.1080/15325020903004350

Perry, W. G. (1970). Forms of intellectual and ethical development in the college years: A scheme. New York, NY: Holt, Rinehart and Winston.

Perry, W. G. (1981). Cognitive and ethical growth: The making of meaning. In A. Chickering (Ed.), *The modern American college* (pp. 76–116). San Francisco, CA: Jossey-Bass.

Perry, W. G. (1999). Forms of ethical and intellectual development in the college years: A scheme. San Francisco, CA, Jossey-Bass.

Petasnick, W. D. (2011). End-of-life care: The time for a meaningful discussion is now. *Journal of Healthcare Management, 56,* 369–372.

Peterson, C., & Seligman, M. E. P. (2004). *Character strengths and virtues: A handbook and classification.* Oxford, UK: Oxford University Press.

Pew Forum. (2010, February 17). *Religion among the Millennials: Less religiously active than older Americans, but fairly traditional in other ways.* Retrieved from http://www.pewforum.org/Age /Religion-Among-the-Millennials.aspx

Pew Research Center. (2006). *As family forms change, bonds remain strong: Families drawn together by communications revolution.* Washington, DC: Author.

Pew Research Center. (2008). *Baby boomers: The gloomiest generation.* Retrieved from http://pewresearch.org/pubs/880/baby-boomers -the-gloomiest-generation

Pew Research Center. (2009, June 29). *Growing old in America: Expectations vs. reality.* Retrieved from http://pewresearch.org /pubs/1269/agin-survey-expectations-versus-reality

Pew Research Center. (2012). *Young, underemployed, and optimistic: Coming of age, slowly, in a tough economy.* Retrieved from http:// www.pewsocialtrends.org/2012/02/09/young-underemployed -and-optimistic/

Phinney, J. (1990). Ethnic identity in adolescents and adults: Review of research. *Psychological Bulletin, 108*(93), 499–514. doi: 10.1037/0033-2909.108.3.499

Physical Activity Guidelines Advisory Committee. (2008). *Physical Activity Guidelines Advisory Committee report, 2008.* Washington, DC: U.S. Department of Health and Human Services.

Piaget, J. (1932). *The moral judgment of the child.* London, UK: Free Press.

Piaget, J. (1962). *Play, dreams, and imitation in childhood.* New York, NY: Norton.

Piaget, J. (1970). Piaget's theory. In P. H. Mussen (Eds.), *Carmichael's manual of child psychology.* New York, NY: Wiley.

Piaget, J. (1980). *Adaptation and intelligence: Organic selection and phenocopy.* Chicago, IL: University of Chicago Press.

Piaget, J. (1983). Piaget's theory. In P. Mussen (Ed.), *Handbook of child psychology,* Vol. 1 (4th ed.). New York, NY: Wiley.

Pierret, C. (2006). The "sandwich generation": Women caring for parents and children. *Monthly Labor Review, 129*(9), 3–9.

Pinker, S. (1994). *The language instinct.* New York, NY: Morrow.

Pinker, S. (1999). *Words and rules: The ingredients of language.* New York, NY: Basic Books.

Pinquart, M. (2002). Good news about the effects of bad old-age stereotypes. *Experimental Aging Research, 28,* 317–336. doi: 10.1080=03610730290080353

Pinquart, M., & Sorenson, S. (2007). Correlates of physical health of informal caregivers: A meta-analysis. *Journal of Gerontology Series B, 62,* 137–162. doi: 10.1093/geronb/62.2.P126

Piper, M. E., Federman, E. B., Piasecki, T. M., Bolt, D. M., Smith, S. S., Fiore, M. C., & Baker, T. B. (2004). A multiple motives approach to tobacco dependence: The Wisconsin Inventory of Smoking Dependence Motives (WISDM-68). *Journal of Consulting and Clinical Psychology, 72,* 139–154. doi: 10.1037/0022-006X.72.2.139

Platt, O. S., Thorington, B. D., Brambilla, D. J., Milner, P. F., Rosse, W. F., Vichinsky, E., & Kinney, T. R. (1991). Pain in sickle cell disease—Rates and risk factors. *New England Journal of Medicine, 325,* 11–16. doi: 10.1056/NEJM199107043250103

Plude, D. J., & Doussard-Roosevelt, J. A. (1989). Aging, selective attention, and feature integration. *Psychology of Aging, 4*(1), 98–105. doi: 10.1037/0882-7974.7.1.65

Pomerantz, E. M., & Kempner, S. G. (2013). Mothers' daily person and process praise: Implications for children's theory of intelligence and motivation. *Developmental Psychology, 49,* 2040–2046. doi: 10.1037/a0031840

Ponterotto, J. G., Pace, T. M., & Kavan, M. G. (1989). A counselor's guide to the assessment of depression. *Journal of Counseling & Development, 67,* 301–309. doi: 10.1002/j.1556-6676.1989 .tb02608.x

Popkin, D. (1989). *Active parenting.* Atlanta, GA: Active Parenting.

Portrie-Bethke, T. L., Hill, N. R., & Bethke, J. G. (2009). Strength-based mental health counseling for children with ADHD: An integrative model of adventure-based counseling and Adlerian play therapy. *Journal of Mental Health Counseling, 31,* 323–339.

Posada, G., Gao, Y., Fang, W., Posada, R., Tascon, M., Schoelmerich, A., . . . & Synnevaag, B. (1995). The secure base phenomenon across cultures: Children's behavior, mothers' preferences, and experts' concepts. In E. Waters, B. Vaughn, G. Posada, & K. Kondo-Ikemura (Eds.), *Caregiving, cultural and cognitive perspectives on secure-base behaviour and working models: New growing points of attachment theory and research. Monographs of the Society for Research in Child Development, 60*(2–3, Serial No. 244), 27–48. doi: 10.1111/j.1540-5834.1995.tb00202.x

Poston, W. S. C. (1990). The biracial identity development model: A needed addition. *Journal of Counseling and Development, 69,* 152–155. doi: 10.1002/j.1556-6676.1990.tb01477.x

Potegal, M., & Davidson, R. J. (2003). Temper tantrums in young children: Behavioral composition. *Developmental and Behavioral Pediatrics, 24,* 148–154. doi: 10.1097/00004703-200306000-00002

Potter, J. (2010). Aging in America: Essential considerations in shaping senior care policy. *Aging Health, 6,* 289–299. doi: 10.2217 /ahe.10.25

Poulin, F., & Chan, A. (2010). Stability and changes in children and adolescent friendships. *Developmental Review, 30,* 257–252. doi: 10.1037/0012-1649.21.6.1007

Povinelli, D. J. (1995). The unduplicated self. In P. Rochat (Ed.), *The self in infancy: Theory and research* (pp. 161–192). Amsterdam, Netherlands: North-Holland/Elsevier Science.

Powell, K. C., & Kalina, C. J. (2008). Cognitive and social constructivism: Developing tools for effective classrooms. *Education, 130,* 241–250.

Price, T., Langford, J., & Liporace, F. (2012). Essential nutrients for bone health and a review of their availability in the average North American diet. *The Open Orthopedics Journal, 6,* 143–149. doi: 102174/187432500126010143

Prull, M. W., Gabrieli, J. D. E., & Bunge, S. A. (2000). Age related changes in memory: A cognitive neuroscience perspective.

In F. I. Craik & R. Salthouse (Eds.), *Handbook of aging and cognition* (pp. 91–154). Mahwah, NJ: Lawrence Erlbaum Associates.

Quadagno, J. (2011). Aging and the life course: An introduction to social gerontology (5th ed.). New York, NY: McGraw-Hill.

Raley, R. K., & Bumpass, L. (2003). The topography of the divorce plateau: Levels and trends in union stability in the United States after 1980. *Demographic Research, 8,* 245–259.

Rando, T. A., Doka, K. J., Fleming, S., Franco, M. H., Lobb, E. A., Parkes, C. M., & Steele, R. (2012). A call to the field: Complicated grief in the DSM-5. *Omega, 65,* 251–255.

Ranke, M. B., & Saenger, P. (2001). Turner's syndrome. *Lancet, 358,* 309–314. doi: 10.1016/S0140-6736(01)05487-3

Rapee, R., Kennedy, S., Ingram, M., Edwards, S., & Sweeney, L. (2005). Prevention and early intervention of anxiety disorders in inhibited preschool children. *Journal of Consulting and Clinical Psychology, 73,* 488–497. doi: 10.1037/0022-006X.73.3.488

Rathus, S. A. (2012). *HDEV* (2nd ed.). Belmont, CA: Wadsworth.

Rauer, A. J., & Volling, B. L. (2007). Differential parenting and sibling jealousy: Developmental correlates of young adults' romantic relationships. *Personal Relationships, 14,* 495–511. doi: 10.1111/j.1475-6811.2007.00168.x

Ray, D. C., Blanco, P. J., Sullivan, J. M., & Holliman, R. (2009). An exploratory study of child-centered play therapy with aggressive children. *International Journal of Play Therapy, 18,* 162–175. doi: 10.1037/a0014742

Ray, D. C., Schottelkorb, A., & Tsai, M. (2007). Play therapy with children exhibiting symptoms of attention deficit hyperactivity disorder. *International Journal of Play Therapy, 16,* 95–111. doi: 10.1037/1555-6824.16.2.95

Reck, C., Stehle, E., Reinig, K., & Mundt, C. (2009). Maternity blues as a predictor of DSM-IV depression and anxiety disorders in the first three months of postpartum. *Journal of Affective Disorders, 113,* 77–87. doi: 10.1016/.j.jad.2008.05.003

Reed, K. (2009). "It's them faulty genes again": Women, men, and the gendered nature of genetic responsibility in prenatal blood screening. *Sociology of Health & Illness, 31,* 343–359. doi: 10.1111/j.1467-9566.2008.01134.x

Reedy, N. J. (2007). Born too soon: The continuing challenge of preterm labor and birth in the United States. *Journal of Midwifery & Women's Health, 52,* 281–290. doi: 10.1016/j.jmwh.2007.02.022

Reese, H. W., Lee, L. J., Cohen, S. H., & Puckett, J. M. (2001). Effects of intellectual variables, age, and gender on divergent thinking in adulthood. *International Journal of Behavioral Development, 25,* 491–500. doi: 10.1080/01650250042000483

Regan, P. C. (1998). Of lust and love: Beliefs about the role of sexual desire in romantic relationships. *Personal Relationships, 5,* 139–157. doi: 10.1111/j.1475-6811.1998.tb00164.x

Regier, D. A., Narrow, W. E., Rae, D. S., Manderscheid, R. W., Locke, B. Z., & Goodwin, F. K. (1993). The de facto U.S. mental and addictive disorders service system. Epidemiologic catchment area prospective 1-year prevalence rates of disorders and services. *Archives of General Psychiatry, 50*(2), 85–94. doi: 10.1001 /archpsyc.1993.01820140007001

Reichstadt, J., Sengupta, G., Depp,C., Palinkas, L., & Jeste, D. (2010). Older adults' perspectives on successful aging: Qualitative interviews. *American Journal of Geriatric Psychiatry, 18,* 567–575. doi: 10.1097/JGP.0b013e3181e040bb

Remley, R. P., & Herlihy, B. (2010). *Ethical, legal and professional issues in counseling* (3rd ed.). Upper Saddle River, NJ: Pearson Merrill.

Reyna, V., & Farley, F. (2006). Risk and rationality in adolescent decision-making: Implications for theory, practice, and public policy. *Psychological Science in the Public Interest, 7,* 1–44. doi: 10.1111/j.1529-1006.2006.00026.x

Riba, M. B., Wulsin, L., & Rubenfire, M. (Eds.). (2012). *Psychiatry and heart disease: The mind, brain, and heart.* New York, NY: Wiley-Blackwell.

Richards, J. E. (1998). Development of selective attention in young infants: Enhancement and attenuation of startle reflex by attention. *Developmental Science, 1*(1), 45–51. doi: 10.1111/1467-7687.00011

Richards, J., & Deary, I. (2005). A life course approach to cognitive reserve: A model for cognitive aging and development. *Annual Neurology, 58,* 617–622. doi: 10.1002/ana.20637

Richards, M. (2008). Artificial insemination and eugenics: Celibate motherhood, eutelegenesis and germinal choice. *Studies in History and Philosophy of Biological and Biomedical Sciences, 39,* 211–221. doi: 10.1016/j.shpsc.2008.03.005

Riggle, E. D. B., Rotosky, S. S., & Horne, S. G. (2009). Marriage amendments and lesbian, gay, and bisexual individuals in the 2006 election. *Sexuality Research and Social Policy, 6,* 80–89.

Riley, L. D., & Bowen, C. (2005). The sandwich generation: Challenges and coping strategies of multigenerational families. *The Family Journal , 13,* 52–58.

Rimmele, U., Seiler, R., Marti, B., Wirtz, P. H., Ehlert, U., & Heinrichs, M. (2008). The level of physical activity affects adrenal and cardiovascular reactivity to psychosocial stress. *Psychoneuroendocrinology, 34,* 190–198. doi: 10.1016/j.psyneuen.2008.08.023

Ristau, S. (2011). People do need people: Social interaction boosts brain health in older age. *Generations, 35*(2), 70–76.

Rizzoli, R., Åkesson, K., Bouxsein, M., Kanis, J. A., Napoli, N., Papapoulos, S., Reginster, J.-Y., & Cooper, C. (2011). Subtrachanteric fractures after long-term with bisphosphonates: A European Society on Clinical and Economic Aspects of Osteoporosis and Osteoarthritis, and International Osteoporosis Foundation working group report. *Osteoporosis International, 22,* 373–390. doi: 10.1007/s00198-010-1453-5

Roberson, D., Davidoff, J., Davies, I. R. L., & Shapiro, L. R. (2004). The development of color categories in two languages: A longitudinal study. *Journal of Experimental Psychology: General, 133,* 554–571. doi: 10.1037/0096-3445.133.4.554

Roberts, B. W., & DelVecchio, W. F. (2000). The rank-order consistency of personality traits from childhood to old age: A quantitative review of longitudinal studies. *Psychological Bulletin, 126*(1), 3–25. doi: 10.1037/0033-2909.126.1.3

Roberts, B. W., Wood, D., & Caspi, A. (2008). The development of personality traits in adulthood. In O. P. John, R. W. Robins, & L. A. Pervin (Eds.), *Handbook of personality: Theory and research* (3rd ed., pp. 375–398). New York, NY: Guilford Press.

Roberts, J. E. (2002). The "push" for evidence: Management of the second stage. *Journal of Midwifery & Women's Health, 47,* 2–15. doi: 10.1016/S1526-9523(01)00233-1

Roberts, S. T., & Kennedy, B. L. (2006). Why are young college women not using condoms? Their perceived risk, drug use, and developmental vulnerability may provide important clues to sexual risk. *Archives of Psychiatric Nursing, 20,* 32–40. doi: 10.1016/j.apnu.2005.08.008

Robins, L. N., Helzer, J. E., Weissman, M. M., Orvaschel, H., Gruenberg, E., Burke, J. D., & Regier, D. A. (1984). Life-time prevalence of specific psychiatric disorders in three sites. *Archives of General Psychiatry, 41,* 949–958. doi: 10.1001/archpsyc.1984.01790210031005

Robinshaw, H. (2007). Acquisition of hearing, listening and speech skills by and during key stage 1. *Early Childhood Development and Care, 177,* 661–668. doi: 10.1080/03004430701379090

Robinson, E. H., & Rotter J. C. (1991). Children's fears: Toward a preventative model. *School Counselor, 38,* 187–203.

Rochat, P. (2003). Five levels of self-awareness as they unfold early in life. *Consciousness and Cognition, 12,* 717–731. doi: 10.1016/S1053-8100(03)00081-3

Rochat, P., & Hespos, S. (1997). Differential rooting response by neonates: Evidence for an early sense of self. *Early Development and Parenting, 6,* 150–158. doi: 10.1002/(SICI)1099-0917(199709/12)6:3/4<105::AID-EDP150>3.0.CO;2-U

Rodriquez, A., & Waldenstrom, U. (2008). Fetal origins of child non-right handedness and mental health. *Child Psychology and Psychiatry, 49,* 967–976. doi: 10.1111/j.1469-7610.2008.01923.x

Roe, A. (1957). Early determinants of vocational choice. *Journal of Counseling Psychology, 4,* 212–217. doi: 10.1037/h0045950

Roe v. Wade, 410 U.S. 113 (1973).

Rogers, C. R. (1959). A theory of therapy, personality and interpersonal relationships as developed in the client-centered framework. In S. Koch (Ed.), *Psychology: A study of a science,* Vol. 3: *Formulations of the person and the social context.* New York, NY: McGraw Hill.

Rogers, C. R. (1961). On becoming a person: A therapist's view of psychotherapy. Boston, MA: Houghton Mifflin.

Rogers, W. A. (2000). Attention and aging. In D. C. Parks & N. Schwarz (Eds.), *Cognitive aging: A primer* (pp. 57–73). Philadelphia, PA: Psychology Press.

Rohr, M. K., & Lang, F. R. (2009). Aging well together: A mini-review. *Gerontology, 55,* 333–343. doi: 10.1159/000212161

Rolfsnes, E. S., & Idsoe, T. (2011). School-based intervention programs for PTSD symptoms: A review and meta-analysis. *Journal of Traumatic Stress, 24,* 155–165. doi: 10.1002/jts.20622

Roper, A. S. W. (2011). *Baby boomers envision retirement II: Survey of baby boomers' expectations for retirement report.* Retrieved from http://assets.aarp.org/rgcenter/econ/boomers_envision.pdf

Rosen, M. (2010). Anesthesia for ritual circumcision in neonates. *Pediatric Anesthesia, 20,* 1124–1127. doi: 10.1111/j.1460-9592.2010.03445.x

Rosenbaum, J. E., & Becker, K. I. (2011). *The early college challenge: Navigating disadvantaged students' transition to college.* Retrieved from http://www.aft.org/pdfs/americaneducator/fall2011/Rosenbaum.pdf

Rosenbluth, S. C., & Steil, J. M. (1995). Predictors of intimacy for women in heterosexual and homosexual couples. *Journal of Social and Personal Relationships, 12,* 163–175. doi: 10.1177/0265407595122001

Rosenfeld, M. J. (2007). The age of independence: Interracial unions, same-sex unions and the changing American family. Boston, MA: Harvard University Press.

Ross, C. A., & Tabrizi, S. J. (2011). Huntington's disease: From molecular pathogenesis to clinical treatment. *The Lancet Neurology, 10,* 83–98. doi: 10.1016/S1474-4422(10)70245-3

Rothbart, M. K., Ahadi, S. A., & Hershey, K. L. (1994). Temperament and social behavior in childhood. *Merrill-Palmer Quarterly, 40,* 21–39.

Rothbart, M. K., & Bates, J. E. (2006). Temperament. In W. Damon (Series Ed.) & N. Eisenberg (Vol. Ed.), *Handbook of child psychology,* Vol. 3: *Social, emotional, and personality development* (6th ed., pp. 105–176). New York, NY: Wiley.

Rothbart, M. K., & Rueda, M. R. (2005). The development of effortful control. In U. Mayr, E. Awh, & S. Keele (Eds.), *Developing individuality in the human brain: A tribute to Michael I. Posner* (pp. 167–188). Washington, DC: American Psychological Association.

Rothbaum, R., Kakinuma, M., Nagaoka, R., & Azuma, H. (2007). Attachment and amae: Parent-child closeness in the United States and Japan. *Journal of Cross-Cultural Psychology, 38,* 465–486. doi: 10.1177/0022022107302315

Rousseau, J. (1749/1964). Discourse on the arts and sciences. In R. D. Masters (Ed.), *The first and second discourses.* (Translated by R. D. Masters & J. R. Masters.) New York, NY: St. Martins.

Rowe, J., & Kahn, R. (1989). *Successful aging.* New York, NY: Pantheon Books.

Rowe, J., & Kahn, R. (1997). Successful aging. *The Gerontologist, 37,* 433–440. doi: 10.1093/geront/37.4.433

Rowe, J. W., & Kahn, R. L. (1998). *Successful aging.* New York, NY: Dell Publishing.

Rubin, K. H., Bukowsky, W., & Parker, J. G. (2006). Peer interactions, relationships, and groups. In W. Damon, R. M. Lerner, & N. Eisenberg (Eds.), *Handbook of child psychology, Vol. 3: Social, emotional, and personality development* (6th ed., pp. 571–645). New York, NY: Wiley.

Rubin, K. H., Coplan, R. J., Chen, X., Buskirk, A. A., & Wojslawowicz, J. C. (2005). Peer relationships in childhood. In M. H. Bornstein & M. E. Lamb (Eds.), *Developmental science: An advanced textbook* (5th ed., pp. 469–512). London, UK: Taylor & Francis Books.

Rubin, K. H., Fein, G. C., & Vandenberg, B. (1983). Play. In P. H. Mussen (Ed.), *Handbook of child psychology* (4th ed., pp. 693–774). New York, NY: Wiley.

Rucker, J. J., & McGuffi, P. (2010). Polygenic heterogeneity: A complex model of genetic inheritance in psychiatric disorders. *Biological Psychiatry, 68,* 312–313. doi: 10.1016/j.biopsych.2010.06.020

Rule, A. C., & Stewart, R. A. (2002). Effects of practical life materials on kindergarteners' fine motor skills. *Early Childhood Journal, 30*(1), 9–13. doi: 10.1023/A:1016533729704

Ruth, J. E., & Birren, J. E. (1985). Creativity in adulthood and old age: Relations to intelligence, sex, and mode of testing. *International Journal of Behavioral Development, 8,* 99–109. doi: 10.1177/016502548500800107

Saccardi, M. C. (1996). Predictable books: Gateway to a lifetime of reading. *Reading Teacher, 49,* 588–590.

Safdar, S., Matsumoto, D., Kwantes, C. T., Friedlmeier, W., Yoo, S. H., & Kakai, H. (2009). Variations of emotional display rules within and across cultures: A comparison between Canada, USA, and Japan. *Canadian Journal of Behavioral Science, 41,* 1–10. doi: 10.1037/a0014387

Sagi, A., van IJzendoorn, M. H., & Koren-Karie, N. (1991). Primary appraisal of the Strange Situation: A cross-cultural analysis of preseparation episodes. *Developmental Psychology, 27,* 587–596. doi: 10.1037/0012-1649.27.4.587

Saginak, M. A. (2003). Adolescent career development: A holistic perspective. In C. T. Dollarhide & K. A. Saginak (2003). *School counseling in the secondary school: A comprehensive process and program* (pp. 381–390). Boston, MA: Pearson.

St. Clair-Thompson, H., Overton, T., & Botton, C. (2010). Information processing: A review of implications for Johnstone's model for science education. *Research in Science and Technological Education, 28,* 131–148. doi: 10.1080/02635141003750479

St. James-Roberts, I., Alvarez, M., Csipke, E., Abramsky, T., Goodwin, J., & Sorgenfrei, E. (2006). Infant crying and sleeping in London, Copenhagen and when parents adopt a "proximal" form of care. *Pediatrics, 117,* 1146–1155. doi: 10.1542/peds.2005-2387

Saleebey, D. (2001). The diagnostic strengths manual? *Social Work, 46,* 183–187. doi: 10.1093/sw/46.2.183

Salinger, J. D. (1945). *Catcher in the rye.* New York, NY: Bantam.

Salthouse, T. (2000). Aging and measures of processing speed. *Biological Psychology, 54,* 35–54. doi: 10.1016/S0301-0511(00)00052-1

Salzen, E. A. (2010). Whatever happened to ethology? The case for the fixed action pattern in psychology? *History & Philosophy of Psychology, 12*(2), 63–78.

Sameroff, A. (2010). A unified theory of development: A dialectic integration of nature and nurture. *Child Development, 81,* 6–22. doi: 10.1111/j.1467-8624.2009.01378.x

Sander, M., Werkle-Bergner, M., & Lindenberger, U. (2011). Binding and strategic selection on working memory: A lifespan dissociation. *Psychology and Aging, 26,* 612–662.

Sann, L., Durand, M., Picard, J., Lasne, Y., & Bethenod, M. (1988). Arm fat and muscle areas in infancy. *Archives of Disease in Childhood, 63,* 256–260. doi: 10.1136/adc.63.3.256

Santrock, J. W. (2011). *Life-span development* (13th ed.). Boston, MA: McGraw Hill.

Santrock, J. W. (2012). *Essentials of lifespan development* (2nd ed.). Boston, MA: McGraw-Hill.

Saudino, K. J. (2005). Behavioral genetics and child temperament. *Journal of Developmental and Behavioral Pediatrics, 26,* 214–223. doi: 10.1097/00004703-200506000-00010

Saul, R. (2014). ADHD does not exist: The truth about attention deficit hyperactivity disorder. New York, NY: HarperCollins.

Savickas, M. L. (1997). Career adaptability: An integrative construct for life-span, life-space theory. *Career Development Quarterly, 47,* 247–259. doi: 10.1002/j.2161-0045.1997.tb00469.x

Savickas, M. L. (2003). Advancing the career counseling profession: Objectives and strategies for the next decade. *Career Development Quarterly, 52*(1), 87. doi: 10.1002/j.2161-0045.2003.tb00631.x

Savickas, M. L., & Lent, R. W. (Eds.). (1994). Convergence in career development theories: Implications for science and practice. Palo Alto, CA: CPP Books.

Sayfan, L., & Lagattuta, K. H. (2009). Scaring the monster away: What children know about managing fears of real and imaginary creatures. *Child Development, 80,* 1756–1774. doi: 10.1111/j.1467-8624.2009.01366.x

Scarpello, F., & Vandenberg, R. (1992). The importance of occupational and career views to job satisfaction attributes. *Journal of Organizational Behavior, 13*(2), 125–140.

Scarr, S., & McCartney, K. (1983). How people make their own environments: A theory of genotype→environment effects. *Child Development, 54,* 424–435. doi: 10.1111/j.1467-8624.1983.tb03884.x

Schaal, B., Hummel, T., & Soussignan, R. (2004). Olfaction in the fetal and premature infant: Functional status and clinical implications. *Clinics in Perinatology, 31,* 261–285.

Schaefer, C. E. (2011). *Foundations of play therapy.* Hoboken, NJ: John Wiley and Sons.

Schaie, K. W. (1993). The Seattle longitudinal studies of adult intelligence. *Current Directions in Psychological Science, 2,* 171–175. doi: 10.1111/1467-8721.ep10769721

Schaie, K. W., Maitland, S. B., Willis, S. L., & Intrieri, R. C. (1998). Longitudinal invariance of adult psychometric ability factor structures across 7 years. *Psychology and Aging, 13,* 8–20. doi: 10.1037/0882-7974.13.1.8

Scher, A., & Zukerman, S. (2005). Persistent night waking and settling difficulties across the first year: Early precursors of later behavioral problems. *Journal of Reproductive & Infant Psychology, 23*(1), 77–88. doi:10.1080/02646830512331330929

Schermerhorn, A. C., Chow, S.-Y., & Cummings, E. M. (2010). Developmental family processes and interparental conflict: Patterns of microlevel influences. *Developmental Psychology, 46,* 869–885. doi: 10.1037/a0019662

Schiller, N. O., & Costa, A. (2006). Different selection principals of freestanding and bound morphemes in language production. *Journal of Experimental Psychology: Learning Memory and Cognition, 32,* 1201–1207. doi: 10.1037/0278-7393.32.5.1201

Schlossberg, N. K. (2009). *Revitalizing retirement: Reshaping your identity, relationships, and purpose. Washington,* DC: American Psychological Association.

Schlossberg, N. K. (2011, August 17). *Transitions through life: Surviving every stage of life* [Web log post]. Retrieved from http://www.psychologytoday.com/blog/transitions-through-life/201108/what-do-maria-shriver-beef-ranchers-and-medical-faculty-have-in

Schmalz, D. L., Kerstetter, D. L., & Anderson, D. M. (2008). Stigma consciousness as a predictor of children's participation in recreational vs. competitive sports. *Journal of Sport Behavior, 31,* 276–297.

Schmidt, S. W. (2007). The relationship between satisfaction with workplace training and job satisfaction. *Human Resource Development Quarterly, 18,* 481–498. doi: 10.1002/hrdq.1216

Schoen, S., & Schoen, A. (2010). Bullying and harassment in the United States. *The Clearing House, 83*(2), 68–72. doi: 10.1080/00098650903386444

Schoenberg, N., Bardach, S. H., Manchikanti, K., & Goodenow, A. (2011). Appalachian residents' experiences with and management of multiple morbidity. *Qualitative Health Research, 21,* 601–611. doi: 10.1177/1049732310395779

Schonert-Reichl, K. A., Smith, V., Zaidman-Zait, A., & Hertzman, C. (2012). Promoting children's prosocial behaviours in school: Impact of the "Roots of Empathy" program on the social and emotional competence of school-aged children. *School Mental Health, 4*(1), 1–12. doi: 10.1007/s12310-011-9064-7

Schore, A. N. (1994). *Affect regulation and the origin of the self.* Mahwah, NJ: Lawrence Erlbaum Associates.

Schott, J. M., & Rossor, M. N. (2003). The grasp and other primitive reflexes. *Journal of Neurology, Neurosurgery & Psychiatry, 74,* 558–560. doi: 10.1136/jnnp.74.5.558

Schrag, S. J., Arnold, K. E., Mohle-Boetani, J. C., Lynfield, R., Zell, E. R., Stefonek, K...Schuchat, A. (2003). Prenatal screening for infectious diseases and opportunities for prevention. *Obstetrics & Gynecology, 102,* 753–760. doi: 10.1016/S0029-7844(03)00671-9

Schuetze, P., & Eiden, R. D. (2007). The association between prenatal exposure to cigarettes and infant and maternal negative affect. *Infant Behavior & Development, 30,* 387–398. doi: 10.1016/j.infbeh.2006.10.005

Schulenberg, J., Maggs, J. L., Long, S. W., Sher, K. J., Gotham, H. J., Baer, J. S., . . . & Zucker, R. A. (2001). The problem of college drinking: Insights from a developmental perspective. *Alcoholism: Clinical and Experimental Research, 25,* 473–477. doi: 10.1111/j.1530-0277.2001.tb02237.x

Schulenberg. J. E., & Zarrett, N. R. (2006). Mental health during emerging adulthood: Continuity and discontinuity in courses, causes, and functions. In J. J. Arnett, & J. L. Tanner (Eds.), *Emerging adults in America: Coming of age in the 21st century* (pp. 135–172). Washington, DC: APA Books.

Schultz, B. K., Storer, J., Watabe, Y., Sadler, J., & Evans, S. W. (2011). School-based treatment of attention-deficit/hyperactivity disorder. *Psychology in the Schools, 48,* 254–262. doi: 10.1002/pits.20553

Schulz, L. L., & Rubel, D. J. (2011). A phenomenology of alienation in high school: The experiences of five male non-completers. *Professional School Counseling, 14,* 286–298. doi: 10.5330/PSC.n.2011-14.286

Schulz, M. S., Cowan, P. A., & Cowan, C. P. (2006). Promoting healthy beginnings: A randomized controlled trial of a preventive intervention to preserve marital quality during the transition to parenthood. *Journal of Clinical and Consulting Psychology, 74,* 20–31. doi: 10.1037/0022-006X.74.1.20

Schulz, R., & Curnow, C. (1988). Peak performance and age among super-athletes: Track and field, swimming, baseball, tennis, and golf. *Journal of Gerontology: Psychological Sciences, 43,* 113–120. doi: 10.1093/geronj/43.5.P113

Schutz, A. (1970). *On phenomenology and social relations.* Chicago, IL: University of Chicago Press.

Schwartz, C., Wright, C., Shin, L., Kagan, J., & Rauch, S. (2003). Inhibited and uninhibited infants "grown up": Adult amygdalar response to novelty. *Science, 300,* 1952–1953. doi: 10.1126/science.1083703

Sears, W., & Sears M. (1995). The discipline book: How to have a better behaved child from birth to age ten. New York, NY: Little, Brown, & Co.

Seattle.Gov. (2011). *Injury prevention program.* Retrieved from http://www.seattle.gov/fire/pubed/preschool/injuryPrevention.htm

Seeman, T. E., Lusignolo, T. M., Albert, M., & Berkman, L. (2001). Social relationships, social support, and patterns of cognitive aging in healthy, high-functioning older adults: MacArthur Studies of Successful Aging. *Health Psychology, 20,* 243–255. doi: 10.1037//0278-6133.20.4.243

Seftor, N., & Turner, S. (2002). Back to school: Federal student aid policy and adult college age enrollment. *Journal of Human Resources, 37,* 336–352.

Sekuler, R. (1995). Motion perception as a partnership: Endogenous and exogenous contributions. Current Directions in Psychological Science, 4(2), 43–47. doi: 10.1111/1467-8721.ep10771003

Seligman, M. E. P., Rashid, T., & Parks, A. C. (2006). Positive psychotherapy. *American Psychologist, 61,* 774–788. doi: 10.1037/0003-066X.61.8.774

Selman, R. L. (1980). *The growth of interpersonal understanding.* San Diego, CA: Academic Press.

Seltzer, V. C. (1982). Adolescent social development: Dynamic functional interaction. Lexington, MA: Heath.

Selye, H. (1985). History and present status of the stress concept. In A. Monat & R. S. Lazarus (Eds.), *Stress and coping* (2nd ed., pp. 17–29). New York, NY: Columbia University.

Serpanos, Y. C., & Jarmel, F. (2007). Quantitative and qualitative follow-up outcomes from a preschool audio logic screening program: Perspectives over a decade. *American Journal of Audiology, 16,* 4–12. doi: 10.1044/1059-0889(2007/002

Settersen, R. A. (2003). Propositions and controversies in life-course scholarship. In R. A. Settersen, Jr. (Ed.), *Invitation to the life course: Toward new understandings of later life* (pp. 15–45). Amityville, NY: Baywood.

Settersten, R. A. (2006). *Becoming adult: Meanings and markers for young Americans. The Network on Transitions to Adulthood. Research Network.* Working Paper. Retrieved from http://www.transad.pop.upenn.edu/downloads/Settersten%20Becoming%20Adult%20final%203-06%29.pdf

Settersen, R. A., & Hagestad, G. O. (1996). What's the latest? Cultural age deadlines for family transitions. *The Gerontologist, 36,* 178–188. doi: 10.1093/geront/36.2.178

Shaffer, D. R., & Kipp, K. (2010). *Developmental psychology: Childhood and adolescence* (8th ed.). New York, NY: Wadsworth.

Shaffer, D., & Waslick, B. D. (2002). *The many faces of depression in children and adolescents.* Washington, DC: American Psychiatric Publishing.

Shallcross, L. (2009, June). Living live to the full. *Counseling Today,* 1–5.

Shallcross, L. (2012). Retirement, etc.: Making your next move. *Counseling Today, 54*(7), 28–36.

Shapiro, A. F., Gottman, J. M., & Carrere, S. (2000). The baby and the marriage: Identifying factors that buffer against decline in marital satisfaction after the first baby arrives. *Journal of Family Psychology, 14*(1), 59–70. doi: 10.1037/0893-3200.14.1.59

Shapiro, A., & Keyes, C. L. M. (2008). Marital status and social well-being: Are the married always better off? *Social Indicators Research, 88,* 329–346. doi: 10.1007/s11205-007-9194-3

Sharma, G., & Goodwin, J. (2006). Effect of aging on respiratory system physiology and immunology. *Clinical Interventions in Aging, 1,* 253–260. doi: 10.2147/ciia.2006.1.3.253

Shaver, P. R., & Mikulincer, M. (2009). An overview of adult attachment theory. In J. H. Obegi & E. Berant (Eds.), *Attachment theory and research in clinical work* (pp. 17–45). New York, NY: Guilford.

Shealy, K. R., Scanlon, K. S., Labiner-Wolfe, J., Fein, S. B., & Grummer-Strawn, L. M. (2008). Characteristics of breastfeeding practices among US mothers. *Pediatrics, 122,* 50–56. doi: 10.1542/peds.2008-1315f

Shechory, M., & Ziv, R. (2007). Relationships between gender role attitudes, role division, and perception of equity among heterosexual, gay and lesbian couples. *Sex Roles, 56,* 629–638. doi: 10.1007/s11199-007-9207-3

Sheehy, G. (1976). *Passages: Predictable crises of adult life.* New York, NY: Dutton.

Sheehy, G. (1976/2004). *Passages.* New York, NY: Ballantine Books.

Sheehy, G. (1995). *New passages: Mapping your life across time.* New York, NY: Ballantine Books.

Sheppard, S. C., Malatras, J. W., & Israel, A. C. (2010). The impact of deployment on U.S. military families. *American Psychologist, 65,* 599–609. doi: 10.1037/a0020332

Sherman, C. W., Rosenblatt, D. E., & Antonucci, T. C. (2008). Elder abuse and mistreatment: A lifespan and cultural context. *Indian Journal of Gerontology, 22,* 319–339.

Sherman, M. M., & Sherman, I. C. (1925). Sensori-motor responses in infants. *Journal of Comparative Psychology, 5*(1), 53–68. doi: 10.1037/h0074472

Shiha, G., Turokb, D. K., & Parkerc, W. J. (2011). Vasectomy: The other (better) form of sterilization. *Contraception, 83,* 310–315. doi: 10.1016/j.contraception.2010.08.019

Shonkoff, J. P. (2010). Building a new biodevelopmental framework to guide the future of early childhood policy. *Child Development, 81,* 357–367. doi: 10.1111/j.1467-8624.2009.01399.x

Shutts, K. B., Örnkloo, H., von Hofsten, C. Keen, R., & Spelke, E. S. (2009). Young children's representations of spatial and functional relationships between objects. *Child Development, 80,* 1612–1627.

Siegler, R., DeLoache, J., & Eisenberg, N. (2003). *How children develop.* New York, NY: Worth.

Sievert, L. L., Obermeyer, C. M., & Price, K. (2006). Determinants of hot flashes and night sweats. *Animals of Human Biology, 33*(1), 4–16. doi: 10.1080/03014460500421338

Sigelman, C. K., & Rider, E. A. (2012). *Life-span human development* (7th ed.). Belmont, CA: Wadsworth Cengage Learning.

Silverman, W. K., Pina, A. A., & Viswesvaran, C. (2008). Evidence-based psychosocial treatments for phobic and anxiety disorders in children and adolescents. *Journal of clinical child and adolescent psychology, 37,* 105–130. doi: 10.1080/15374410701817907

Simmons, R. K., Singh, G., Maconochic, N., Doyle, P., & Green, J. (2006). Experience of miscarriage in the UK: Qualitative findings from the National Women's Health Study. *Social Science & Medicine, 63,* 1934–1946. doi: 10.1016/j.socscimed.2006.04.024

Simonton, D. K. (1988). Age and outstanding achievement: What do we know after a century of research? *Psychological Bulletin, 104,* 251–267. doi: 10.1037/0033-2909.104.2.251

Singer, D. G., & Revenson, T. A. (1996). *A Piaget primer: How a child thinks.* New York, NY: Plume.

Singer, T., Verhaeghen, P., Ghisletta, P., Lindenberger, U., & Baltes, P. B. (2003). The fate of cognition in very old age: Six-year longitudinal findings in the Berlin Aging Study (BASE). *Psychology of Aging, 18,* 318–331. doi: 10.1037/0882-7974.18.2.318

Sinnott, J. D. (1998). *The development of logic in adulthood: Postformal thought and its applications.* New York, NY: Plenum.

Sisson, M. C., Witcher, P. M., & Stubsten, C. (2004). The role of the maternal-fetal medicine specialist in high-risk obstetric care. *Critical Care Nursing Clinics of North America, 16,* 187–191.

Sisson, S. B., Broyles, S. T., Newton, R. L., Baker, B. L., & Chernausek, S. D. (2011). TVs in the bedrooms of children: Does it impact health and behavior? *Preventive Medicine: An International Journal Devoted to Practice and Theory, 52,* 104–108.

Skalicky, A., Meyers, A. F., Adams, W. G., Yang, Z., Cook, J. T., & Frank, D. A. (2006). Child food insecurity and iron deficiency anemia in low-income infants and toddlers in the United States. *Maternal and Child Health Journal, 10*(2), 177–185. doi: 10.1007/s10995-005-0036-0

Skinner, B. F. (1953). *Science and human behavior.* New York, NY: Macmillan.

Skinner, B. F. (1962). *Walden two.* New York, NY: Macmillan.

Skinner, B. F. (1991). *Verbal behavior.* Acton, MA: Copley. (Original work published in 1957.)

Skwarchak, S. (2009). How do parents support preschoolers numeracy: Learning experiences at home. *Early Childhood Education Journal, 37,* 189–197.

Slevec, J., & Tiggemann, M. (2010). Attitudes towards cosmetic surgery in middle-aged women: Body image, aging anxiety, and the media. *Psychology of Women Quarterly, 34,* 65–74. doi: 10.1111/j.1471-6402.2009.01542.x

Slutsky, C. B., & Simpkins, S. D. (2009). The link between children's sports participation and self-esteem: Exploring the mediating role of sport self-concept. *Psychology of Sport and Exercise, 10,* 381–389. doi: 10.1016/j.psychsport.2008.09.006

Smart, R., & Peterson, C. (1997). Super's career stages and the decision to change careers. *Journal of Vocational Behavior, 51,* 358–374. doi: 10.1006/jvbe.1996.1544

Smith, C., & Lloyd, B. (1978). Maternal behavior and perceived sex of infant: Revisited. *Child Development, 49,* 1263–1265. doi: 10.2307/1128775

Smith, D. K., Johnson, A. B., Pears, K. C., Fisher, P. A., & DeGarmo, D. S. (2007). Child maltreatment and foster care: Unpacking the effects of prenatal and postnatal parental substance use, *Child Maltreatment, 12,* 150–160. doi: 10.1177/1077559507300129

Smith, L. B., Yu, C., & Pereira, A. F. (2011). Not your mother's view: The dynamics of toddler visual experience. *Developmental Science, 14*(1), 9–17. doi: 10.1111/j.1467-7687.2009.00947.x

Smith, T. W. (2006). *American sexual behavior: Trends, sociodemographic differences, and risk behavior.* GSS Topical Report No. 25. Retrieved from http://www.norc.uchicago.edu/NR/rdonlyres/2663F09F-2E74-436E-AC81-6FFBF288E183/0/AmericanSexualBehavior2006.pdf

Snaedal, J. (2011). Person centered medicine for the older patient, with specific reference to the person with dementia. *International Journal of Person Centered Medicine, 1*(1). Retrieved from http://ijpcm.org/index.php/IJPCM/article/view/3/27

Sobralske, M. C., & Gruber, M. E. (2009). Risks and benefits of parent/child bed sharing. *Journal of American Academy of Nurse Practitioners, 21,* 474–479. doi: 10.1111/j.1745-7599.2009.00430.x

Social Security Online. (2012). *Frequently asked questions: Full retirement age.* Retrieved from http://ssa-custhelp.ssa.gov/app/answers/detail/a_id/14

Society for Research in Child Development. (2009). Pragmatic and semantic flexibility in early verb use. *Monographs of the Society for Research in Child Development, 74*(2), 40–48.

Sockol, L. E., Epperson, C. N., & Barber, J. P. (2011). A meta-analysis of treatments for perinatal depression. *Clinical Psychology Review, 31,* 839–849. doi: 10.1016/j.cpr/2011/03/009

Sokol, R. I., Webster, K. L., Thompson, N. S., & Stevens, D. A. (2005). Whining as mother-directed speech. *Infant and Child Development, 14,* 478–490.

Solberg, M. E., Olweus, D., & Endresen, I. M. (2007). Bullies and victims at school: Are they the same pupils? *British Journal of Educational Psychology, 77,* 441–464. doi: 10.1348/000709906X105689

Soons, J. P. M., & Liebroer, A. C. (2008). Together is better? Effects of relationship status and resources on young adults' wellbeing. *Journal of Social and Personal Relationships, 25,* 603–624. doi: 10.1177/0265407508093789

Sorce, J. F., Emde, R. M., Campos, J. J., & Klinnert, M. D. (1985). Maternal emotional signaling: Its effect on the visual cliff behavior of 1-year-olds. *Developmental Psychology, 21,* 195–200. doi: 10.1037/0012-1649.21.1.195

Sousa, N., Mendes, R., Abrantes, C., & Sampaio, J. (2011). Differences in maximum upper and lower limb strength in older adults after a 12 week intense resistance training program. *Journal of Human Kinetics, 30,* 183–188. doi: 10.2478/v10078-011-0086-x

Specht, J., Egloff, B., & Schmukle, S. C. (2011). Stability and change of personality across the life course: The impact of age and major life events on mean-level and rank-order stability of the Big Five. *Journal of Personality and Social Psychology, 101,* 862–882. doi: 10.1037/a0024950

Spector, P. E. (1997). *Job satisfaction: Application, assessment, causes, and consequences.* Thousand Oaks, CA: Sage.

Sperry, L. (2007). *The ethical and professional practice of counseling and psychotherapy.* Boston, MA: Pearson.

Spokane, A. R., & Cruza-Guet, M. C. (2005). Holland's theory of vocational personalities in work environments. In S. D. Brown & R. T. Lent (Eds.), *Career development and counseling: Putting theory and research to work* (pp. 24–41). Hoboken, NJ: Wiley.

Sprecher, S. (1989). Premaritial sexual standards for different categories of individuals. *Journal of Sexual Research, 26,* 232–248. doi: 10.1080/00224498909551508

Sprecher, S., Sullivan, Q., & Hatfield, E. (1994). Mate selection preferences: Gender differences examined in a national sample. *Journal of Personality and Psychology, 66,* 1074–1080. doi: 10.1037/0022-3514.66.6.1074

Sroufe, L. A., Egeland, B., Carlson, E., & Collins, W. A. (2005). *The development of the person: The Minnesota study of risk and adaptation from birth to adulthood.* New York, NY: Guilford.

Stake, R. E. (2010). *Qualitative research.* New York, NY: Guilford Press.

Stanley, S. M., Amato, P. R., Johnson, C. A., & Markman, H. J. (2006). Premarital education, marital quality, and marital stability: Findings from a large, random, household survey. *Journal of Family Psychology, 20,* 117–126. doi: 10.1037/0893-3200.20.1.117

Stapley, J., & Haviland, J. (1989). Beyond depression: Gender differences in normal adolescences' emotional experiences. *Sex Roles, 20,* 295–309. doi: 10.1007/BF00287726

Start ASL. (2012). *Sign language for babies.* Retrieved from http://www.start-american-sign-language.com/sign-language-for-babies.html

Staudinger, U. M., Smith, J., & Baltes, P. B. (1992). Wisdom related knowledge in a life review task: Age differences and the role of professional specialization. *Psychology and Aging, 7,* 271–281. doi: 10.1037/0882-7974.7.2.271

Steele, C. M., & Aronson, J. (1995). Stereotype threat and the intellectual test performance of African Americans. *Journal of Personality and Social Psychology, 69,* 797–811. doi: 10.1037/0022-3514.69.5.797

Steffen, L. M., Kroenke, C. H., Yu, X., Pereira, M. A., Slattery, M. L., Van Horn, L., . . . & Jacobs, D. R. (2005). Associations of plant foods, dairy products, and meat consumption with fifteen-year incidence of elevated blood pressure in young Black and White adults: The CARDIA study. *The American Journal of Clinical Nutrition, 82,* 1169–1177.

Stein, Z., & Dawson-Turnik, T. L. (2004). It's all good: Moral relativism and the millennial mind. Retrieved from https://www.devtestservice.org/PDF/ItsAllGood.pdf

Steinberg, L. (2004). Risk-taking in adolescence: What changes, and why? *Annals of the New York Academy of Sciences, 1021,* 51–58. doi: 10.1196/annals.1308.005

Steinberg, L. (2007). Risk taking in adolescence: New perspectives from brain and behavioral science. *Current Directions in Psychological Science, 16,* 55–59. doi: 10.1111/j.1467-8721.2007.00475.x

Steinberg, L., Bornstein, M. H., Vandell, D. L., & Rook, K. S. (2011). *Lifespan development: Infancy through adulthood.* Belmont, CA: Wadsworth Cengage Learning.

Stern, D. (1987). *The interpersonal world of the infant.* New York, NY: Basic Books.

Sternberg, R. J. (1986). A triangular theory of love. *Psychological Review, 93,* 119–135. doi: 10.1037/0033-295X.93.2.119

Stevens, N., Martina, C., & Westerhof, G. (2006). Meeting the need to belong: Predicting effects of a friendship enrichment program for older women. *The Gerontologist, 46,* 495–502. doi: 10.1093/geront/46.4.495

Stevens-Long, J., & Commons, M. L. (1992). *Adult life: Developmental process* (4th ed.). Mountain View, CA: Mayfield.

Stevenson, M. B., Leavitt, L. A., Thompson, R. H., & Roach, M. A. (1988). A social relations model analysis of parent and child play. *Developmental Psychology, 24,* 101–108. doi: 10.2307/1130782

Stewart, L. M., Holman, C. D., Hart, R., Finn, J., Mai, Q., &, Preen, D. B. (2011). How effective is *in vitro* fertilization, and how can it be improved? *Fertility and Sterility, 95,* 1677–1683. doi: 10.1016/j .fertnstert.2011.01.130

Stickgold, R., & Walker, M. P. (2007). Sleep-dependent memory consolidation and reconsolidation. *Sleep Medicine, 8,* 331–343. doi: 10.1016/j.sleep.2007.03.011

Stimpson, J. P., Yong-Fang, K., Ray, L. A., Rajii, M. A., & Peek, M. K. (2007). Risk of mortality related to widowhood in older Mexican Americans. *Annual Journal of Epidemiology, 17,* 313–319. doi: 10.1016/j.annepidem.2006.10.006

Stine-Morrow, E., Miller, L., & Hertzog, C. (2006). Age and self-regulated language processing. *Psychology Bulletin, 132,* 582–606. doi: 10.1037/0033-2909.132.4.582

Stine-Morrow, E. A. L., Parisi, J. M., Morrow, D. G., & Park, D. C. (2008). The effects of an engaged lifestyle on cognitive vitality: A field experiement. *Psychology and Aging, 23,* 778–786.

Stinson, C. (2009). Structured group reminiscence: An intervention for older adults. *The Journal of Continuing Education in Nursing, 40*(11), 521–528. doi: 10.3928/00220124-20091023-10

Stoner, S. B. (1982). Age differences in crystallized and fluid intellectual abilities. *Journal of Psychology, 110,* 357–383. doi: 10.1080/00223980.1982.9915319

Stormer, V., Passow, S., Biesenack, J., & Li, S. (2011, November 21). Dopaminergic and cholinergic modulations of visual-spatial attention and working memory: Insights from molecular genetic research and implications for adult cognitive development. *Developmental Psychology, 48,* 875–889. doi: 10.1037/a0026198

Strauss, W., & Howe, N. (1992). *Generations: The history of Americans' future, 1584 to 2069.* New York, NY: William Morrow and Company, Inc.

Striano, T., Stahl, D., & Cleveland, A. (2009). Taking a closer look at social and cognitive skills: A weekly longitudinal assessment between 7 and 10 months of age. *European Journal of Developmental Psychology, 1,* 567–591. doi: 10.1080 /17405620701480642

Stroebe, W., Insko, C. A., Thompson, V. D., & Layton, B. D. (1971). Effects of physical attractiveness, attitude similarity, and sex on various aspects of interpersonal attraction. *Journal of Personality and Social Psychology, 18*(1), 79–91. doi: 10.1037/h0030710

Strohschein, L. (2005). Parental divorce and child mental health trajectories. *Journal of Marriage and Family, 67,* 1286–1300. doi: 10.1111/j.1741-3737.2005.00217.x

Su, R., Rounds, J., & Armstrong, P. I. (2009). Men and things, women and people: A meta-analysis of sex differences in interests. *Psychological Bulletin, 135,* 859–884. doi: 10.1037/a0017364

Substance Abuse and Mental Health Services Administration (SAMHSA). (2006). *Results from the 2005 National Survey on Drug Use and Health: National Findings.* Office of Applied Studies, NSDUH Series H-30, DHHS Publication No. SMA 06-4194. Rockville, MD: SAMHSA.

Substance Abuse and Mental Health Services Administration (SAMHSA). (2007). *Results from the 2006 National Survey on Drug Use and Health: National Findings.* Office of Applied Studies, NSDUH Series H-30, DHHS Publication No. SMA 06-4194. Rockville, MD: SAMHSA.

Sue, D. W., & Sue, D. (1990). *Counseling the culturally different: Theory and practice.* New York, NY: Wiley.

Sullivan, P. (1998). Sexual identity development: The importance of target or dominant group membership. In R. C. Sanlo (Ed.), *Working with lesbian, gay, bisexual, and transgender college students: A handbook for faculty and administrators* (pp. 3–12). Westport, CT: Greenwood Press.

Sun, R., & Walsh, C. A. (2006). Approaches to brain asymmetry and handedness. *Nature Reviews Neuroscience, 7,* 655–662.

Sung, K.-T. (2001). Elder respect: Exploration of ideals and forms in East Asia. *Journal of Aging Studies, 15,* 13–26. doi: 10.1016/S0890 -4065(00)00014-1

Super, C., & Harkness, S. (1986). The developmental niche: A conceptualization at the interface of child and culture. *International Journal of Behavioral Development, 9,* 545–569. doi: 10.1177/016502548600900409

Super, C. M., & Harkness, S. (1994). The developmental niche. In W. J. Lonner & R. Malpass (Eds.), *Psychology and culture* (pp. 95–99). Boston, MA: Allyn & Bacon.

Super, D. E. (1953). A theory of vocational development. *American Psychologist, 8,* 185–190. doi: 10.1037/h0056046

Super, D. E. (1980). A life-span, life-space approach to career development. *Journal of Vocational Behavior, 16,* 282–298. doi: 10.1016/0001-8791(80)90056-1

Surgeon General. (2011). *Children and mental health.* Retrieved from http://www.surgeongeneral.gov/library/mentalhealth/chapter3 /sec1.html

Sussman, R., & Hart, D. (2008). *Man the hunted: Primates, predators and human evolutions.* Boulder, CO: Westview Press.

Sutin, A. R., Costa, P. T., Wethington, E., & Eaton, W. (2010). Turning points and lessons learned: Stressful life events and personality trait development across middle-adulthood. *Psychology of Aging, 25,* 524–533. doi: 10.1037/a0018751

Svanberg, P. O. G. (1998). Attachment, resilience, and prevention. *Journal of Mental Health, 7,* 543–578. doi: 10.1080 /09638239817716

Swidler, A. (2001). *Talk of love: How culture matters.* Chicago, IL: University of Chicago Press.

Tamis-LeMonda, C. S., Bornstein, M. H., & Baumwell, L. (2001). Maternal responsiveness and children's achievement of language milestones. *Child Development, 72,* 748–767. doi: 10.1111/1467 -8624.00313

Tamis-LeMonda, C. S., Cristofaro, T. N., Rodriguez, E. T., & Bornstein, M. H. (2006). Early language development: Social influences in the first years of life. In L. Balter & C. S. Tamis-LeMonda (Eds.), *Child psychology: A handbook of contemporary issues* (2nd ed., pp. 79–108). New York, NY: Psychology Press.

Tapon, D. (2010). Prenatal testing for Down syndrome: Comparison of screening practices in the UK and USA. *Journal of Genetic Counseling, 19,* 112–130. doi: 10.1007/s10897-009-9269-1

Tardif, T., Gelman, S. A., & Xu, F. (1999). Putting the "noun bias" in context: A comparison of English and Mandarin. *Child Development, 70,* 620–635. doi: 10.1111/1467-8624.00045

Tasker, F. (2005). Lesbian mothers, gay fathers, and their children: A review. *Journal of Developmental & Behavioral Pediatrics, 26,* 224–240. doi: 10.1097/00004703-200506000-00012

Tasker, F. (2010). Same-sex parenting and child development: Reviewing the contribution of parental gender. *Journal of Marriage and Family, 72,* 35–40. doi: 10.1111/j.1741.3737 .2009.00681.x

Tauriac, J. J., & Scruggs, N. (2006). Elder abuse among African Americans. *Educational Gerontology, 32*(1), 37–48. doi: 10.1080/03601270500338625

Tavris, C. (1992). *The mismeasure of woman.* New York, NY: Simon & Schuster.

Taylor, D., Purswell, D., Lindo, K., Jayne, N., & Fernando, K. (2011). The impact of child parent relationship therapy on child behavior and parent-child relationships: An examination of parental divorce. *International Journal of Play Therapy, 20*(3), 124–137. doi: 10.1037/a0024469

Taylor, S. E. (2010). Mechanisms linking early stress to adult health outcomes. *Proceedings of the National Academy of Sciences, 107*(19), 8507–8512. doi: 10.1073/pnas.1003890107

Terman, L. M. (1916). *The measurement of intelligence.* Boston, MA: Houghton Mifflin Co.

Tesser, A., & Crelia, R. (1994). Attitude heritability and attitude reinforcement: A test of the niche building hypothesis. *Personality and Individual Differences, 16,* 571–577. doi: 10.1016/0191 -8869(96)00141-9

Thelen, E. (1995). Motor development: A new synthesis. *American Psychologist, 50*(2), 79–95. doi: 10.1037/0003-066X.50.2.79

Thelen, E. (2000). Grounded in the world: Developmental origins of the embodied mind. *Infancy, 1*(1), 3–28. doi: 10.1207 /S15327078IN0101_02

Thelen, E., & Adolph, K. E. (1992). Arnold L. Gesell: The paradox of nature and nurture. *Developmental Psychology, 28,* 368–380. doi: 10.1037/0012-1649.28.3.368

Thomas, A., & Chess, S. (1977). *Temperament and development.* New York, NY: Brunner/Mazel.

Thompson, K., Biddle, K. R., Robinson-Long, M., Poger, J., Wang, J., Yang, Q. X., & Eslinger, P. J. (2009). Cerebral plasticity and recovery of function after childhood prefrontal cortex damage. *Developmental Neurohabilitation, 12,* 298–312. doi: 10.3109/17518420903236262

Thompson, N. S., Dessureau, B., & Olson, C. (1998). Infant cries as evolutionary melodrama: Extortion or deception? *Evolution of Communication, 2*(1), 25–43. doi: 10.1075/eoc.2.1.03tho

Thompson, R. A. (2003). The legacy of early attachments. *Child Development, 71*(1), 145–152. doi: 10.1111/1467-8624.00128

Thompson, R. H., Cotnoir-Bichelman, N. M., McKerchar, P. M., Tate, T. L., & Dancho, K. A. (2007). Enhancing early communication through infant sign training. *Journal of Applied Behavior Analysis, 40*(1), 15–23. doi: 10.1901/jaba.2007.23-06

Thorndike, E. (1932). *The fundamentals of learning.* New York, NY: Teachers College Press.

Thornstam, L. (1997). Gerotranscendence: The contemplative dimension in again. *Journal of Aging Studies, 11,* 143–154. doi: 10.1016/S0890-4065(97)90018-9

Tiefer, L. (2006). The Viagra phenomenon. *Sexualities, 9,* 273–294. doi: 10.1177/1363460706065049

Tikotzky, L., & Sadeh, A. (2009). Maternal sleep-related cognitions and infant sleep: A longitudinal study from pregnancy through the 1st year. *Child Development, 80,* 860–874. doi: 10.1111/j.1467 -8624.2009.01302.x

Timmons, B., Naylor, P., & Pfeiffer, K. (2007). Physical activity for preschoolers: How much and how? *Applied Physiology, Nutrition and Metabolism, 32,* 122–134.

Tourangeau, R., & Yan, T. (2007). Sensitive questions in surveys. *Psychological Bulletin, 133,* 859–883. doi: 10.1037/0033-2909 .133.5.859

Townsend, B. (2001). Dual-earner couples and long work hours: A structural and life course perspective. *Berkeley Journal of Sociology, 45,* 161–179.

Tranter, L. J., & Koutstaal, W. (2008). Age and flexible thinking: An experimental demonstration of the beneficial effects of increased cognitively stimulating activity on fluid intelligence in healthy older adults. *Aging, Neuropsychology, and Cognition, 15,* 184–207. doi: 10.1080/13825580701322163

Triandis, H. C. (1988). Collectivism and individualism: A reconceptualization of a basic concept in cross-cultural social psychology. In B. K. Verma & C. Bagley (Eds.), *Personality, attitudes, and cognitions* (pp. 60–95). London, UK: Macmillan.

Triffletti, P. (2010). Helping mother die. *North American Journal of Medical Sciences. 3*(1), 39–40.

Troiden, R. R. (1989). The formation of homosexual identities. *Journal of Homosexuality, 17,* 43–73. doi: 10.1300/J082v17n01_02

Trommsdorff, G. (2006). Development of emotions as organized by culture. *International Society for the Study of Behavioural Development Newsletter, 49,* 1–4.

Tunnicliffe, P., & Oliver, C. (2011). Phenotype-environment interactions in genetic syndromes associated with severe or profound intellectual disability. *Research in Developmental Disabilities, 32,* 404–418. doi: 10.1016/j.ridd.2010.12.008

Tur-Kaspa, I., Segal, S., Moffa, F., Massobrio, M., & Meltzer, S. (1999). Viagra for temporary erectile dysfunction during treatments with assisted reproductive technologies: Case report. *Human Reproduction, 14,* 1783–1784. doi: 10.1093/humrep/14.7.1783

Umberson, D., Pudrovska, T., & Reczek, C. (2010). Parenthood, childlessness, and well-being: A life course perspective. *Journal of Marriage and Family, 72,* 612–629. doi: 10.1111/j.1741-3737 .2010.00721.x

United Nations International Children's Emergency Fund (UNICEF). (2013). *How does immunization work?* Retrieved from http:// www.unicef.org/immunization/index_how.html

United Nations International Children's Emergency Fund (UNICEF). (2014). *The state of the world's children 2014 in numbers: Every child counts, revealing disparities, advancing children's rights.* New York, NY: Author.

U.S. Bureau of Labor Statistics. (2010). *Summary 10-04/March 2010.* Retrieved from http://www.bls.gov/opub/ils/pdf/opbils81.pdf

U.S. Bureau of Labor Statistics. (2011). *Education pays.* Retrieved from http://www.bls.gov/emp/ep_chart_001.htm

U.S. Census Bureau. (2007). *Educational attainment in the United States: 2006.* Retrieved from www.census.Gov/population /www/socdemo/educ-attn.html

U.S. Census Bureau. (2010a). *Marital status: 2010 American Community Survey.* Retrieved from http://factfinder2.census .gov/faces/tableservices/jsf/pages/productview.xhtml?pid =ACS_10_1YR_S1201&prodType=table\

U.S. Census Bureau. (2010b). *Table C9. Children by presence and type of parent(s), race, and Hispanic origin, 2009. Current Population Survey, 2009. Annual Social and Economic Supplement.* Retrieved from http://www.census.gov/population/www/socdemo/hh-fam /cps2009.html

U.S. Census Bureau. (2011a). *National population projections.* Retrieved from http://www.census.gov/population/www/pop -profile/natproj.html

U.S. Census Bureau. (2011b). *2010 Census shows 65 and older population growing faster than total U.S. population.* Retrieved from http://2010.census.gov/news/releases/operations/cb11-cn192.html

U.S. Census Bureau. (2011c). *Facts for features.* CB11-FF.08 March 23. Retrieved from http://www.census.gov/newsroom/releases/pdf /cb11-ff08_olderamericans.pdf

U.S. Census Bureau. (2011d). *2010 Census brief: The older population—2010.* Retrieved from http://www.census.gov/prod /cen2010/briefs/c2010br-09.pdf

U.S. Census Bureau. (2012a). *Statistical abstract of the United States: 2011 (131st edition). Table 104. Expectations of life at birth, 1970 to 2008, and projections, 2010 to 2020.* Retrieved from http://www.census.gov/compendia/statab/

U.S. Census Bureau. (2012b). *2009 American community survey.* Retrieved from http://www.census.gov/newsroom/releases/archives/facts_for_features_special_editions/cb11-ff17.html

U.S. Department of Agriculture & U.S. Department of Health and Human Services. (2010). *Dietary guidelines for Americans* (7th ed.). Washington, DC: U.S. Government Printing Office.

U.S. Department of Education, National Center for Education Statistics. (2011). *Digest of education statistics, 2010.* NCES 2011-015. Washington, DC: U.S. Government Printing Office.

U.S. Department of Education, Office of Special Education. (2012). *IDEA 2004: Building the legacy. Part C (birth–2 years old).* Retrieved from http://idea.ed.gov/part-c/search/new

U.S. Department of Health and Human Services. (2002). *Physical activity and older Americans: Benefits and strategies.* Retrieved from http://www.ahrq.gov/ppip/activity.htm

U.S. Department of Health and Human Services. (2004). *Bone health and osteoporosis: A report of the Surgeon General.* Rockville, MD: U.S. Department of Health and Human Services.

U.S. Department of Health and Human Services. (2006). *Early Head Start benefits children and families: Early Head Start research and evaluation project.* Retrieved from http://www.acf.hhs.gov/programs/opre/ehs/ehs_resrch/index.html

U.S. Department of Health and Human Services. (2007). *ASPE research brief: Effects of marriage on health.* Washington, DC: Office of the Assistant Secretary of Planning and Evaluation.

U.S. Department of Health and Human Services. (2008). *2008 physical activity guidelines for Americans.* Washington DC: U.S. Government Printing Office.

U.S. Department of Health and Human Services. (2010a). *A report of the Surgeon General: How tobacco smoke causes disease: The biology and behavioral basis for smoking-attributable disease fact sheet.* Retrieved from http://www.surgeongeneral.gov/library/tobaccosmoke/factsheet.html

U.S. Department of Health and Human Services. (2010b). Births, marriages, divorces, and deaths: Provisional data for 2009. *National Vital Statistics Reports.* Series report 58, Number 25.

U.S. Department of Health and Human Services. (2010c). *A report of the Surgeon General: How tobacco smoke causes disease: The biological and behavioral basis for smoking-attributable disease.* Retrieved from http://www.surgeongeneral.gov/library/tobaccosmoke/index.html

U.S. Department of Health and Human Services. (2011). *Summary health statistics for U.S. children: National Health Interview Survey 2010. Vital and health statistics, 10(250).* DHHS Publication No. (PHS)-2012-1578. Hyattsville, MD: National Center for Health Statistics.

U.S. Department of Health and Human Services. (2012). *EHS fact sheet.* Retrieved from http://www.ehsnrc.org/AboutUs/ehs.htm

U.S. Department of Health and Human Services. (2013). *National Prevention, Health Promotion and Public Health Council.* Retrieved from http://www.healthcare.gov/prevention/nphpphc/index.html

U.S. Department of Labor. (2010). *The employment situation.* Retrieved from http://www.bls.gov/news.release/pdf/empsit.pdf

U.S. Department of Labor. (2011). *Women's employment during the recovery.* Retrieved from http://www.dol.gov/_sec/media/reports/femalelaborforce/

U.S. Food and Drug Administration. (2009). *Menopause and hormones.* Retrieved from http://www.fda.gov/forconsumers/byaudience/forwomen/ucm118624.htm

Upadhyay, U. D., Cockrill, K., & Freedman, L. R. (2010). Informing abortion counseling: An examination of evidence-based practices used in emotional care for other stigmatized and sensitive health issues. *Patient Education and Counseling, 81,* 415–421. doi: 10.1016/j.pec.2010.08.026

Vaillant, G. E. (1977). *Adaptation to life.* Boston, MA: Little Brown.

Vaillant, G. E. (2002). *Aging well: Surprising guideposts to a happier life from the landmark Harvard Study of Adult Development.* New York, NY: Little, Brown and Company.

Vaillant, G. E., & Milofsky, E. S. (1980). Natural history of male psychological health, IX: Empirical evidence for Erikson's model of the life cycle. *American Journal of Psychiatry, 137,* 1348–1359.

Vaillant, G., & Mukamal, K. (2001). Successful aging. *The American Journal of Psychiatry, 158,* 839–847. doi: 10.1093/geront/37.4.433

Vaillant, G. E., & Vaillant, C. O. (1990). Natural history of male psychological health, XII: A 45-year study of predictors of successful aging at age 65. *American Journal of Psychiatry, 147,* 31–37.

Vaillant, G. E., Van Bogaert, P., Wikler, D., Damhaut, P., Szliwowski, H. B., & Goldman, S. (1998). Regional changes in glucose metabolism during brain development from the age of 6 years. *Neuroimage, 8,* 62–68. doi: 10.1006/nimg.1998.0346

Vallotton, C. D. (2008). Signs of emotions: What can preverbal children "say" about internal states? *Infant Mental Health Journal, 29,* 234–258. doi: 10..1002/imhj.20175

Vallotton, C., & Ayoub, C. (2010). Use your words: The role of language in the development of toddlers' self-regulation. *Early Childhood Research Quarterly, 26,* 169–181. doi: 10.1016/j.ecresq.2010.09.002

Van Aken, M., Denissen, J. J., Branje, S. J., Dubas, J. S., & Goossens, L. (2006). Midlife concerns and short term personality change in middle-adulthood. *The European Journal of Personality, 20,* 497–513. doi: 10.1002/per.603

Van Balen, F. (2005). Late parenthood among sub-fertile and fertile couples: Motivations and educational goals. *Patient Education and Counseling, 59,* 276–282. doi: 10.1016/j.pec.2004.09.002

Vande Weerd, C., & Paveza, G. (2006). Verbal mistreatment in older adults: A look at persons with Alzheimer's disease and their caregivers in the state of Florida. *Journal of Elder Abuse & Neglect, 17*(4), 11–30. doi: 10.1300/J084v17n04_02

Vanfossen, B., Brown, C. H., Kellam, S., Sokoloff, N., & Doering, S. (2010). Neighborhood context and the development of aggression in boys and girls. *Journal of Community Psychology, 38,* 329–349. doi: 10.1002/jcop.20367

Van IJzendoorn, M. H., Bakermans-Kranenburg, M. J., & Sagi-Schwartz, A. (2006). Attachment across diverse sociocultural contexts: The limits of universality. In K. H. Rubin & O. B. Chung (Eds.), *Parenting beliefs, behaviors, and parent–child relations: A cross-cultural perspective* (pp. 107–142). New York, NY: Psychology Press.

Van Ijzendoorn, M. H., & Kroonenberg, P. M. (1988). Cross-cultural patterns of attachment: A meta-analysis of the Strange Situation. *Child Development, 59,* 147–156. doi: 10.2307/1130396

Van Noorden, T. H. J., Haselager, G. J. T., Cillessen, A. H. N., & Bukowski, W. M. (2014). Empathy and involvement in bullying in children and adolescents: A systematic review. *Journal of Youth and Adolescence.* doi: 10.1007/s10964-014-0135-6

Van Volkom, M. (2006). Sibling relationships in middle and older adulthood: A review of the literature. *Marriage and Family Review, 40,* 151–170. doi: 10.1300/J002v40n02_08

Van Wagenen, A., Driskell, J. D., & Bradford, J. (2013). "I'm still raring to go": Successful aging among lesbian, gay, bisexual and transgender older adults. *Journal of Aging Studies, 27,* 1–14.

Vasile, C. (2010). Developmental metacognition: Aspects in young children. *Petroleum-Gas University of Ploiesti Bulletin, Educational Sciences Series, 62*(2), 120–125.

Vaupel, J. (2010). Biodemography of human ageing. *Nature, 464,* 536–542. doi: 10.1038/nature08984

Vazsonyi, A. T., & Huang, L. (2010). Where self-control comes from: On the development of self-control and its relationship to deviance over time. *Developmental Psychology, 46*(1), 245–257. doi: 10.1037/a0016538

Veenman, M. V. J., Van Hout-Walters, B. H. A. M., & Afflerbach, P. (2006). Metacognition and learning: Conceptual and methodological considerations. *Metacognition and Learning, 1,* 14. doi: 10.1007/s11409-006-6893-0

Venetsanou, F., & Kambas, A. (2010). Environmental factors affecting preschoolers motor development. *Early Childhood Education Journal, 37,* 319–327. doi: 10.1007/s10643-009-0350-z

Verhagen, M, van der Meij, A., Franke, B., Vollebergh, W., Graaf, de Graaf, R., . . . & Janzing, J. G. (2008). Familiality of major depressive disorder and gender differences in comorbidity. *Acta Psychiatrica Scandinavica, 118,* 130–138. doi: 10.1111/j.1600-0447.2008.01186.x

Verheijde, J., Rady, M., McGregor, J., & Murray, C. (2008). Legislation of presumed consent for end-of-life organ donation in the United Kingdom (U.K.): Undermining values in a multicultural society. *Clinics, 63,* 297–300. doi: 10.1590/S1807-59322008000300002

Vermeulen, M. E., & Minor, C. W. (1998). Context of career decisions: Women reared in a rural community. *Career Development Quarterly, 46,* 230–245. doi: 10.1002/j.2161-0045.1998.tb00698.x

Vernon, A. (1998). *The passport program: A journey through emotional, social, cognitive, and self-development (grades 9–12).* Champaign, IL: Research Press.

Vernon, A. (2002). *What works when with children and adolescents: A handbook of individual counseling techniques.* Champaign, IL: Research Press.

Vernon, A. (2006). Depression in children and adolescents: REBT approaches to assessment and treatment. In A. Ellis & M. E. Bernard (Eds.), *Rational emotive behavioral approaches to childhood disorders: Theory, practice, and research* (pp. 212–231). New York, NY: Springer.

Vernon, A. (2009). Working with children, adolescents, and their parents: Practical application of developmental theory. In A. Vernon (Ed.), *Counseling children and adolescents* (4th ed., pp. 1–37). Denver, CO: Love Publishing.

Vernon, A., & Clemente, R. (2005). *Assessment and intervention with children and adolescents: Developmental and multicultural approaches.* Alexandria, VA: American Counseling Association.

Vitaro, F., Boivin, M., & Bukowski, W. M. (2009). The role of friendship in child and adolescent psychosocial development. In K. H. Rubin, W. M. Bukowski, & B. Laursen (Eds.), *Handbook of peer interactions, relations, and groups* (pp. 568–585). New York, NY: Guilford.

Voigt, B., Aberle, I., Schonfeld, J., & Kliegel, M. (2011). Time-based prospective memory in school children: The role of self-initiation and strategic time monitoring. *Journal of Psychology, 219*(2), 92–99. doi: 10.1027/2151-2604/a000053

Von Wachter, T. (2002). *The end of mandatory retirement in the US: Effects on retirement and implicit contracts.* Retrieved from http://www.eea-esem.com/papers/eea-esem/2003/1037/tvw_mr.pdf

Votruba-Drzal, E. (2006). Economic disparities in middle childhood development: Does income matter? *Developmental Psychology, 42,* 1154–1167. doi: 10.1037/0012-1649.42.6.1154

Vygotsky, L. S. (1978). *Mind in society.* Cambridge MA: Harvard University Press.

Waddington, C. H. (1966). *Principles of development and differentiation.* New York, NY: Macmillan.

Wagner, K. D., Ritt-Olson, A., Chou, C.-P., Pokhrel, P., Duan, L., Baezconde-Garbanati, L., & Soto, D. W. (2010). Associations between family structure, family functioning, and substance use among Hispanic/Latino adolescents. *Psychology of Addictive Behaviors, 24,* 98–108. doi: 10.1037/a0018497

Wahba, M. A., & Bridwell, L. G. (1976). Maslow reconsidered: A review of research on the need hierarchy theory. *Organizational Behavior and Human Performance, 15,* 212–240. doi: 10.1016/0030-5073(76)90038-6

Wainright, J. L., Russell, S. T., & Patterson, C. J. (2004). Psychosocial adjustment, school utcomes, and romantic relationships of adolescents with same-sex parents. *Child Development, 75,* 1886–1898. doi: 10.1111/j.1467-8624.2004.00823.x

Waite, L. J., & Joyner, K. (2001). Emotional and physical satisfaction with sex in married, cohabiting and dating sexual unions: Do men and women differ? In E. O. Laumann & R. Michael (Eds.), *Studies on sex* (pp. 239–269). Chicago, IL: University of Chicago Press.

Waite, L. J., Luo, Y., & Lewin, A. C. (2009). Marital happiness and marital stability: Consequences for psychological well-being. *Social Science Research, 38,* 201–212. doi: 10.1016/j.ssresearch.2008.07.001

Waldrop, D. P., & Weber, J. A. (2001). From grandparent to caregiver: The stress and satisfaction of raising grandchildren. *Families in Society: The Journal of Contemporary Human Services, 82,* 461–472. doi: 10.1606/1044-3894.177

Walker, M. P., Brakefield, J., Seidman, A., Morgan, J., Hobson, T., & Stickgold, R. (2003). Sleep and the time course of motor skill learning. *Learning and Memory, 10,* 275–284. doi: 10.1101/lm.58503

Wallerstein, J. S., & Lewis, J. M. (2004). The unexpected legacy of divorce: Report of a 25 year study. *Psychoanalytic Psychology, 21,* 353–370. doi: 10.1037/0736-9735.21.3.353

Walsh, M. E., & Buckley, M. A. (1994). Children's experiences of homelessness: Implications for school counselors. *Elementary School Guidance & Counseling, 29,* 4–15.

Wang, H., & Amato, P. R. (2008). Predictors of divorce adjustment: Stressors, resources, and definition. *Journal of Marriage & Family, 62,* 655–668. doi: 10.1111/j.1741-3737.2000.00655.x

Wang, Q. (2006a). Relations of maternal style and child self-concept to autobiographical memories in Chinese, Chinese immigrant, and European American 3-year-olds. *Child Development, 77,* 1794–1809.

Wang, Q. (2006b). Developing emotion knowledge in cultural context. *International Journal of Behavioral Development, 30*(Suppl. 1), 8–12.

Warner, H. (2011). Biology of aging. In M. R. Katlic (Ed.), *Cardiothoracic surgery in the elderly—Evidence-based practice* (pp. 197–206). New York, NY: Springer.

Warr, P., Butcher, V., Robertson, I., & Callinan, M. (2004). Older people's well-being as a function of employment, retirement, environmental characteristics and role preference. *British Journal of Psychology, 95,* 297–324. doi: 10.1348/0007126041528095

Watson, J. B., & Rayner, R. (1920). Conditioned emotional reactions. *Journal of Experimental Psychology, 3,* 1–14. doi: 10.1037/h0069608

Watt, H. M. G. (2006). The role of motivation in gendered educational and occupational trajectories related to math. *Educational Research and Evaluation, 21,* 305–322. doi: 10.1080 /13803610600765562

Webb, S., Jones, E. H., Merkle, K., Namkung, J., Toth, K., Greenson, J., & Dawson, G. (2010). Toddlers with elevated autism symptoms show slowed habituation to faces. *Child Neuropsychology, 16,* 255–278. doi: 10.1080/09297041003601454

Weber, J. A., & Waldrop, D. P. (2000). Grandparents raising grandchildren: Families in transition. *Journal of Gerontological Social Work, 33,* 27–46. doi: 10.1300/J083v33n02_03

Webster, J., & McCall, M. E. (1999). Reminiscence functions across adulthood: A replication and extension. *Journal of Adult Development, 6*(1), 73–85. doi: 10.1023/A:1021628525902

Wechsler, D. (1958). *The measurement and appraisal of adult intelligence* (4th ed.). Baltimore, MD: Williams & Wilkins Co.

Wechsler, H., Davenport, A., Dowdall, G., Moeykens, B., & Castillo, S. (1994). Health and behavioral consequences of binge drinking in college: A national survey of students at 140 campuses. *The Journal of the American Medical Association, 272*(21), 1672–1677. doi: 10.1001/jama.1994.03520210056032

Wechsler, H., & Nelson, T. F. (2008). What we have learned from the Harvard School of Public Health College Alcohol Study: Focusing attention on college student alcohol consumption and the environmental conditions that promote it. *Journal of Studies on Alcohol and Drugs, 69,* 481–490.

Wehr, T. (2010). The phenomenology of exception times: Qualitative differences between problem-focused and solution-focused interventions. *Applied Cognitive Psychology, 24,* 467–480. doi: 10.1002/acp.1562

Weinstock, H., Berman, S., & Cates, W. (2004). Sexually transmitted diseases among American youth: Incidence and prevalence estimates. *Perspectives on Sexual Reproductive Health, 36,* 6–10. doi: 10.1363/3600604

Weinstock, M. (2008). The long-term behavioural consequences of prenatal stress. *Neuroscience and Biobehavioral Reviews, 32,* 1073–1086. doi: 10.1016/j.neubiorev.2008.03.002

Weisfeldt, M. L., & Zieman, S. J. (2007). Advances in the prevention and treatment of cardiovascular disease. *Health Affairs, 26*(1), 25–37. doi: 10.1377/hlthaff.26.1.25

Weisgram, E. S., Bigler, R. S., & Liben, L. S. (2010). Gender, values, and occupational interests among children, adolescents, and adults. *Child Development, 81,* 757–777. doi: 10.1111/j.1467 -8624.2010.01433.x

Weiss, J. C. (1995). Cognitive therapy and life review therapy: Theoretical and therapeutic implications for mental health counselors. *Journal of Mental Health Counseling, 17*(2), 157–172.

Weiss, L. H., & Schwarz, J. C. (1996). The relationship between parenting types and older adolescents' personality, academic achievement, adjustment, and substance use. *Child Development, 67,* 2101–2114. doi: 10.1111/j.1467-8624.1996.tb01846.x

Wenar, C., & Kerig, P. (2006). *Developmental psychology: From infancy through adolescence.* New York, NY: McGraw-Hill.

Weng, X., Odouli, R., & Li, D. K. (2008). Maternal caffeine consumption during pregnancy and the risk of miscarriage: A prospective cohort study. *American Journal of Obstetrics & Gynecology, 198,* 279.e1–279.e8. doi: 10.1016/j.ajog.2007.10.803

Wentling, R. M. (2002). Work and family issues impact on women. *New Directions for Adult and Continuing Education, 80,* 15–24. doi: 10.1002/ace.8002

Wermter, A., Laucht, M., Schimmelmann, B. G., Banaschweski, T., Sonuga-Barke, E. J. S., Rietschel, M., & Becker, K. (2010). From nature versus nurture, via nature and nurture, to gene x environment interaction in mental disorders. *European Child & Adolescent Psychiatry, 19,* 199–210. doi: 10.1007/s00787-009 -0082-z

West, R., & Hastings, E. (2011). Self-regulation and recall: Growth curve modeling of intervention outcomes for older adults. *Psychology of Aging, 26,* 803–812. doi: 10.1037/a0023784

Westerhof, G. J. (2008). Age identity. In D. Carr (Ed.), *Encyclopedia of the life course and human development* (pp. 10–14). Farmington Hills, MI: Macmillan.

Wethington, E. (2000). Expecting stress: Americans and the "midlife crisis." *Motivation and Emotion, 24,* 85–103. doi: 10.1023/A:1005611230993

Wettig, H. G., Coleman, A. R., & Geider, F. J. (2011). Evaluating the effectiveness of theraplay in treating shy, socially withdrawn children. *International Journal of Play Therapy, 20*(1), 26–37.

Whisman, M. A., & Snyder, D. K. (2007). Sexual infidelity in a national survey of American women: Differences in prevalence and correlates as a function of method of assessment. *Journal of Family Psychology, 21,* 147–154. doi: 10.1037/0893-3200.21.2.147

Whitehead, B. D., & Popenoe, D. (2004). *The state of our unions 2004.* National Marriage Project. Retrieved from http://marriage .rutgers.edu/Publications/SOOU/SOOU2004.

Whitton, S. W., Rhoades, G. K., Stanley, S. M., & Markman, H. J. (2008). Effects of parental divorce on marital commitment and confidence. *Journal of Family Psychology, 22,* 789–793. doi: 10.1037/a0012800

Widaman, K. F. (2009). Phenylketonuria in children and mothers: Genes, environments, behavior. *Current Directions in Psychological Science, 18,* 48–52. doi: 10.1111/j.1467-8721 .2009.01604.x

Widiger, T. A., & Samuel, D. B. (2005). Diagnostic categories or dimensions? A question for the Diagnostic and statistical manual of mental disorders—fifth edition. *Journal of Abnormal Psychology, 114,* 494–504. doi: 10.1037/0021-843X.114.4.494

Widrick, R. M., & Raskin, J. D. (2010). Age-related stigma and the golden section hypothesis. *Aging & Mental Health, 14,* 375–385. doi: 10.1080/13607860903167846

Willford, J. A., Chandler, L. S., Goldschmidt, L., & Day, N. L. (2010). Effects of prenatal tobacco, alcohol and marijuana exposure on processing speed, visual–motor coordination, and interhemispheric transfer. *Neurotoxicology and Teratology, 32,* 580–588. doi: 10.1016/j.ntt.2010.06.004

William T. Grant Foundation Commission on Work, Family, and Citizenship. (1988). The forgotten half: Pathways to success for America's youth and young families. *Phi Delta Kappan, 70*(4), 280.

Williams, H. G., Pfeiffer, K. A., Dowda, M., Jeter, C. Jones, S. & Pate, R. R. (2009). A field based testing protocol for assessment of gross motor skills in preschool children: The children's activity and movement in preschool study motor skills protocol. *Measurement in Physical Education and Exercise Science, 13,* 151–165. doi: 10.1080 /10913670903048036

Williams, J. (1979). Wear and tear injuries in athletes: An overview. *British Journal of Sports Medicine, 12,* 211–214. doi: 10.1136 /bjsm.12.4.211

Willis, P. (1977). *Learning to labour: How working class kids get working class jobs.* Westmead, UK: Saxon House.

Willis, S. L., & Schaie, K. W. (1999). Intellectual functioning in midlife. In S. L. Willis & J. D. Reid (Eds.), *Life in the middle* (pp. 234–247). San Diego, CA: Academic Press.

Wilmoth, J., Skythe, A., Friou, D., & Jeune, B. (1996). The oldest man ever? A case study of exceptional longevity. *The Gerontologist, 36,* 783–788. doi: 10.1093/geront/36.6.783

Wilson, B., & Stuchbury, R. (2010). Do partnerships last? Comparing marriage and cohabitation using longitudinal census data. *Population Trends, 139*(1), 37–63. doi: 10.1057/pt.2010.4

Wilson, D., Mitchell, J., Kemp, B., Adkins, R., & Mann, W. (2009). Effects of assistive technology on functional decline in people aging with a disability. *Assistive Technology, 21,* 208–217. doi: 10.1080/10400430903246068

Wilson, K. L., & Sirois, F. M. (2010). Birth attendant choice and satisfaction with antenatal care: The role of birth philosophy, relational style, and health self-efficacy. *Journal of Reproductive and Infant Psychology, 28,* 69–83. doi: 10.1080/02646830903190946

Wingo, P. A., Smith, R. A., Tevendale, H. D., & Ferre, C. (2011). Recent changes in the trends of teen birth rates, 1981–2006. *Journal of Adolescent Health, 48,* 281–288. doi: 10.1016/j.jadohealth.2010.07.007

Wink, P., & Dillon, M. (2003). Religiousness, spirituality, and psychosocial functioning in late adulthood: Findings from a longitudinal study. *Psychology and Aging, 18,* 916–924. doi: 10.1037/1941-1022.S.1.102

Winkler, S., & Garg, A. K. (1999). Depressed taste and smell in geriatric patients. *Journal of the American Dental Association, 130,* 1759–1765. doi: 10.14219/jada.archive.1999.0133

Winters, K. C., Botzet, A. M., Fahnhorst, T., Baumel, L., & Lee, S. (2009). Impulsivity and its relationship to risky sexual behaviors and drug abuse. *Journal of Child and Adolescent Substance Abuse, 18,* 43–56. doi: 10.1080/15470650802541095

Wolraich, M. L., & Tippins, S. (2003). *American Academy of Pediatrics guide to toilet training.* New York, NY: Bantam.

Wong, P. T. P. (2011). Positive psychology 2.0: Towards a balanced interactive model of the good life. *Canadian Psychology, 52,* 69–81. doi: 10.1037/a0022511

Wood, A. C., Rijsdijk, F., Saudino, K. J., Asherson, P, & Kuntsi, J. (2008). High heritability for a composite index of children's activity level measures. *Behavior Genetics, 38,* 266–276. doi: 10.1007/s10519-008-9196-1

Woodard, J. L., Sugarman, M. A., Nielson, K. A., Smith, J. C., Seidenberg, M., & Durgerian, S. (2012). Lifestyle and genetic contributions to cognitive decline and hippocampal structure and function in healthy aging. *Current Alzheimer Research, 9,* 436–446. doi: 10.2174/156720512800492477

Worden, J. W. (1996). *Children and grief: When a parent dies.* New York, NY: Guilford.

Worden, J. W. (2002). *Grief counseling and grief therapy: A handbook for the mental health practitioner* (3rd ed.). New York, NY: Springer.

Worden, J. W., & Winokuer, H. R. (2011). A task-based approach for counseling the bereaved. In R. A. Neimeyer, D. L. Harris, H. R. Winokuer, & G. F. Thornton (Eds.), *Grief and bereavement in contemporary society: Bridging research and practice* (pp. 57–67). New York, NY: Routledge/Taylor & Francis.

Workman, L., Chilvers, L., Yeomans, H., & Taylor, S. (2006). Development of cerebral lateralization for recognition of emotions in chimeric faces in children aged 5 to 11. *Laterality, 11,* 493–507. doi: 10.1080/13576500600724963

World Health Organization (WHO). (2000). Obesity: Preventing and managing the global epidemic. Report of a WHO consultation. *World Health Organization Technical Report Service, 894,* 1–253.

World Health Organization (2001). *The world health report 2001— Mental health: New understanding, new hope.* Retrieved from http://www.who.int/whr/2001/en/index.html

World Health Organization (WHO). (2007). *Global age-friendly cities: A guide.* Retrieved from http://www.who.int/ageing/publications/Global_age_friendly_cities_Guide_English.pdf

World Health Organization (WHO). (2011). *International Classification of Diseases—10th Edition—clinical modification.* ICD-10-CM. Geneva, Switzerland: Author.

World Health Organization (WHO). (2012a). *Obesity and overweight.* Fact Sheet No. 311. Retrieved from http://www.who.int/mediacentre/factsheets/fs311/en/index.html

World Health Organization (2012b). *Children: reducing mortality.* Fact Sheet No. 178. Retrieved from http://www.who.int/mediacentre/factsheets/fs178/en/

World Health Organization (2013). *Nutrition.* Retrieved from http://www.who.int/topics/nutrition/en/

World Health Organization, UNAIDS Inter-Agency Task Team on Young People. (2006). *Preventing HIV/AIDS in young people: A systematic review of the evidence from developing countries.* Retrieved from http://www.who.int/child_adolescent_health/documents/trs_938/en/index.html

Wozniak, D., & Jopp, D. S. (2012) Positive gerontology: Well-being and psychological strengths in old age. *Journal of Gerontology and Geriatric Research, 1,* e109. doi: 10.4172/2167-7182.1000e109

Yalom, I. D., & Leszcz, M. (2005). *The theory and practice of group psychotherapy* (5th ed.). New York, NY: Basic Books.

Yancu, C. (2011). Gender differences in affective suffering among racially/ethnically diverse community-dwelling elders. *Ethnicity and Health, 16,* 167–184. doi: 10.1080/13557858.2010.547249

Yancu, C., Farmer, D., & Leahman, D. (2010). Barriers to hospice and palliative care services use by African American adults. *American Journal of Hospice and Palliative Medicine, 27,* 248–253. doi: 10.1177/1049909109349942

Yang, S. (2000). Guiding children's verbal plan and evaluation during free play: An application of Vygosky's genetic epistemology to the early childhood classroom. *Early Childhood Journal, 28*(1), 3–10. doi: 10.1023/A:1009587218204

Yates, A. (1991). Childhood sexuality. In M. Lewis (Ed.). *Child and adolescent psychiatry* (pp. 195–215). Baltimore, MD: Williams & Wilkins.

Yeager, D. S., & Dweck, C. S. (2012). Mindsets that promote resilience: When students believe that personal characteristics can be developed. *Educational Psychologist, 47,* 302–314. doi: 10.1080/00461520.2012.722805

Yin, L., Bottnell, C., Clarke, N., Shacks, J., & Poulsen, M. K. (2009). Otoacoustic emissions: A valid efficient first-line hearing screen for preschool children. *Journal of School Health, 79*(4), 147–152. doi: 10.1111/j.1746-1561.2009.00383.x

Young, J. S., Cashwell, C. S., & Shcherbakova, J. (2000). The moderating relationship of spirituality on negative life events and psychological adjustment. *Counseling & Values, 45,* 49–57. doi: 10.1002/j.2161-007X.2000.tb00182.x

Zajacova, A., & Burgard, S. (2010). Body weight and health from early to mid-adulthood: A longitudinal analysis. *Journal of Health and Social Behavior, 51,* 92–107. doi: 10.1177/0022146509361183

Zar, H. J. (2005). Neonatal chlamydial infections: Prevention and treatment. *Pediatric Drugs, 7*(2), 103–110. doi: 10.2165/00148581 -200507020-00003

Zarrett, N., Fay, K., Li, Y., Carrano, J., Phelps, E., & Lerner, R. M. (2009). More than child's play: Variable- and pattern-centered approaches for examining effects of sports participation on youth development. *Developmental Psychology, 45,* 368–382. doi: 10.1037/a0014577

Zaslow, M., Bronte-Tinkew, J., Capps, R., Horowitz, A., Moore, K. A., & Weinstein, D. (2009). Food security during infancy: Implications for attachment and mental proficiency in toddlerhood. *Maternal and Child Health Journal, 13,* 66–80. doi: 10.1007/s10995-008-0329-1

Zehr, M. A. (2011). Studies shed light on teaching immigrant preschoolers. *Education Week, 30*(30), 17.

Zeiders, K. H., Roosa, M. W., & Tein, J.-Y. (2011). Family structure and family processes in Mexican-American families. *Family Process, 50,* 77–91. doi: 10.1111/j.1545-5300.2010.01347.x

Zeifman, D., & Hazan, C. (2008). Pair bonds as attachments: Reevaluating the evidence. In J. Cassidy & P. R. Shaver (Eds.), *The handbook of attachment* (pp. 436–455). New York, NY: Guilford Press.

Zeitlin, M. (1996). My child is my crown: Yoruba parental theories and practices in early childhood. In S. Harkness & C. M. Super (Eds.), *Parents' cultural belief systems* (pp. 407–427). New York, NY: Guilford.

Zelizer, V. A. R. (1994). *Pricing the priceless child: The changing social value of children.* Princeton, NJ: Princeton University Press.

Zimprich, D., Hofer, S. M., & Aartsen, M. J. (2004). Short-term versus long-term longitudinal changes in processing speed. *Gerontology, 50,* 17–21.

Author Index

Subject Index